Current Progress in Renal Replacement Therapy

Current Progress in Renal Replacement Therapy

Edited by Penny Summers

hayle medical

New York

Hayle Medical,
750 Third Avenue, 9th Floor,
New York, NY 10017, USA

Visit us on the World Wide Web at:
www.haylemedical.com

ISBN: 978-1-63241-774-9

Cataloging-in-Publication Data

Current progress in renal replacement therapy / edited by Penny Summers.
     p. cm.
Includes bibliographical references and index.
ISBN 978-1-63241-774-9
1. Acute renal failure--Treatment. 2. Kidneys--Transplantation. 3. Kidneys--Diseases--Treatment.
4. Hemodialysis. I. Summers, Penny.
RC901.7.H45 C87 2019
617.461 059 2--dc23

Table of Contents

Permissions

List of Contributors

Index

Preface

The main aim of this book is to educate learners and enhance their research focus by presenting diverse topics covering this vast field. This is an advanced book which compiles significant studies by distinguished experts in the area of analysis. This book addresses successive solutions to the challenges arising in the area of application, along with it; the book provides scope for future developments.

Renal replacement therapy refers to the therapy concerned with the normal blood-filtering function of the kidneys. It is a treatment method for cases of acute kidney injury, chronic kidney disease, and cases where the kidneys are no longer able to function properly. Renal replacement therapy includes kidney treatment methods like, hemodialysis, peritoneal dialysis, hemofiltration, hemodiafiltration and kidney transplantation. Processes like, hemodialysis, hemofiltration and hemodiafiltration can be both continuous and intermittent. They can use a venovenous route or an arteriovenous route. In hemofiltration, the patient's blood passes through a set of tubing with the help of a machine to a semipermeable membrane, in which the waste products and water get removed by convection. The various advancements in renal replacement therapy are glanced at in this book and their applications as well as ramifications are looked at in detail. Most of the topics introduced in this book cover new techniques and the applications of renal replacement therapy. Students, doctors, experts and all associated with nephrology will benefit alike from this book.

It was a great honour to edit this book, though there were challenges, as it involved a lot of communication and networking between me and the editorial team. However, the end result was this all-inclusive book covering diverse themes in the field.

Finally, it is important to acknowledge the efforts of the contributors for their excellent chapters, through which a wide variety of issues have been addressed. I would also like to thank my colleagues for their valuable feedback during the making of this book.

Editor

Serum albumin level adjusted with C-reactive protein predicts hemodialysis patient survival

Norio Hanafusa[1], Kosaku Nitta[2*], Masayuki Okazaki[3], Mizuki Komatsu[3], Shunji Shiohira[2,3], Hiroshi Kawaguchi[3] and Ken Tsuchiya[1]

Abstract

Background: Malnutrition-related conditions such as protein energy wasting are affecting poor outcome of the dialysis population. The serum albumin level is often used as a marker of wasting and malnutrition. However, the serum albumin level can be affected by the presence of inflammation as well as by nutritional status. We investigated associations between serum albumin values adjusted with C-reactive protein (CRP) and mortality in hemodialysis (HD) patients.

Methods: A total of 397 HD patients were included in this study. The patient characteristics and laboratory data, including serum albumin and CRP levels, were obtained in July 2012. Survival as of the end of August 2014 (maximum follow-up period 25 months) was investigated. First, the regression line was obtained from the entire population between serum albumin and CRP levels. Next, the CRP-adjusted albumin levels were determined as a dichotomized variable with the patients having higher albumin values above the regression line. We investigated associations between three albumin indices (the actual values, the dichotomized index by median, and CRP-adjusted values) and mortality by using Cox proportional hazard models.

Results: The average age of the 397 HD patients was 70.6 years old; 258 were male, and 44.6% were diabetic. Median dialysis vintage was 3.6 years. There were 73 deaths during the observation period. A univariate Cox analysis demonstrated that all three indices were associated with survival, and the hazard ratio (HR) was 0.40 (95% confidence interval (CI) 0.25–0.68) for increase in albumin level, 0.41 (95% CI 0.25–0.68) for higher dichotomized albumin level by median, and 0.46 (95% CI 0.28–0.74) for higher CRP-adjusted albumin level, but only higher CRP-adjusted albumin level was associated with better survival (HR 0.51, 95% CI 0.30–0.85). The degree to which the deviation of albumin was attributable to that of CRP was 12.6%. The analyses on cause-specific mortality revealed that lower albumin levels were associated significantly with infection-related mortality but were not significantly associated with death due to congestive heart failure.

Conclusions: CRP-adjusted albumin was shown to be a better predictor of mortality among the HD patients. When assessing serum albumin values, inflammatory status should be taken into account. Malnutrition or wasting was shown to be associated with a poor outcome independent of inflammation.

Keywords: Albumin, C-reactive protein, Cohort study, Hemodialysis, Mortality, Protein energy wasting

* Correspondence: knitta@kc.twmu.ac.jp
[2]Department of Medicine, Kidney Center, Tokyo Women's Medical University, 8-1 Kawada-cho, Shinjuku-ku, Tokyo 162-8666, Japan
Full list of author information is available at the end of the article

Background

The dialysis population in Japan is becoming older. Malnutrition-related conditions such as protein energy wasting (PEW) [1–4], sarcopenia [5, 6], and frailty [4, 7] draw attentions among such older dialysis populations. Many studies have investigated the relationship between malnutrition and patient outcome, and the results have revealed that malnutrition-related conditions are associated with a poor outcome [5–7].

To investigate the best index that reflects malnutrition is a matter of debate [8–12]. The serum albumin level is one of the most popular indexes of malnutrition [2, 8, 11, 12]. Albumin reportedly relates to the poor survival in original values [13], together with in a form of geriatric nutritional risk index (GNRI) [11]. However, starvation does not necessarily reduce albumin values [14], and the inflammatory state that often coincides with malnutrition in dialysis populations [1] largely affects the lower albumin values [14]. Thus, the serum albumin level might not be a suitable marker of malnutrition in dialysis patients.

We speculated that the values that deducted the effect of inflammation from the actual albumin might become a better marker of malnutrition compared to the original albumin values independent of the effect of inflammation. We therefore performed a study to investigate the relationship between the serum albumin levels and C-reactive protein (CRP) levels, and thereafter, the albumin values adjusted with CRP were investigated from the perspective of all-cause mortality of hemodialysis (HD) patients.

Methods

Design and population

This was a retrospective, observational cohort study conducted at a single center in Japan. The potential population was the chronic dialysis population that was on HD therapy through an arteriovenous fistula at Jyoban Hospital, Iwaki, Japan, in July 2012. HD patients with a malignancy, active inflammation, liver cirrhosis, gastrointestinal bleeding, cardiac valvular disease, or severe illness were excluded from participation and were transferred to another dialysis unit for intensive care. We also excluded the data of patients who did not consent to participate in this study. The Institutional Review Board of the Jyoban Hospital approved the study protocol; the approval number is 25-(3). The protocols were carried out in accordance with the Declaration of Helsinki guidelines regarding ethical principles for medical research involving human subjects. Informed consent was obtained from every subject.

Laboratory measurements

The laboratory data were obtained on the basis of daily clinical practice. The biochemistry data and complete blood counts were obtained on the first day of each week. All measurements were made except the blood urea nitrogen (BUN) level before a dialysis session. BUN level was measured both before and after the dialysis session. Serum creatinine, calcium, phosphorus, albumin, total cholesterol, high-density lipoprotein (HDL) cholesterol, and triglyceride were measured with an autoanalyzer by standard laboratory methods. The serum calcium values were corrected with albumin level. Intact parathyroid hormone (iPTH) was measured by an immunoradiometric assay. Body mass index (BMI) was expressed in kg/m^2. Body weight was calculated as dry weight, defined as post-dialysis weight in which the patient was normotensive and with no signs of overhydration. Urea kinetics were assessed by measuring a blood-based dialysis parameter, Kt/V [15], and the mean value of the three measurements during each of the 3 months before the start of the study was used in the analysis. The normalized protein catabolic rate (nPCR) was used as an indirect indicator of protein intake and was calculated by using the formula previously reported [16].

The history of cardiovascular disease was defined from medical records showing previous heart failure, myocardial infarction, angina pectoris, stroke, coronary artery disease combined with stent implantation, and peripheral artery disease combined with percutaneous transluminal angioplasty.

Clinical outcomes

Endpoints were obtained from the hospital charts and by telephone interview with patients that were conducted by trained interviewers who were blinded to the study protocol. The primary endpoint of this study was all-cause mortality during the follow-up period, from July 1, 2012 to August 31, 2014. The vital status of the subjects was assessed by searching their electronic dialysis records. Patients were censored if the patient was alive on August 31, 2014.

Statistical analyses

For the descriptive analysis, the mean values and standard deviations or median and interquartile ranges (IQRs) were used for normally or non-normally distributed continuous variables. Categorical variables were summarized by numbers and proportion.

The relationship between serum albumin and CRP levels was determined. Linear regression analysis was performed, and the predictive equation of albumin adjusted with CRP was determined. CRP is known to have a log-transformed normal distribution, and log CRP values were used to evaluate the relationship between the CRP and albumin. From the equation, the predicted albumin values that were adjusted with CRP levels were determined.

We performed the survival analysis by using the albumin indices as the main predictors. We used albumin indices in three ways: actual values, albumin dichotomized by the median, and CRP-adjusted albumin that was determined as high or low values, if the actual albumin values were higher or lower than predicted by the CRP levels. We performed Kaplan-Meier analyses followed by log-rank tests for the dichotomized albumin values by the median and CRP-adjusted albumin. Next, a Cox proportional hazard model was employed to evaluate survival effects of albumin. First, we performed univariate analyses, and then the models were adjusted for age, gender, diabetes, dialysis vintage, nPCR, and logCRP. Dialysis vintages were divided into four groups (<2 years, 2–4 years, 4–8 years, ≥8 years). Because the median dialysis vintage was 3.6 years and IQR was 1.6–7.5, such limits yielded almost quartilized groups in terms of the length of dialysis vintage. We used <2-year dialysis vintage group as the reference group. The effects of variables are expressed in the form of hazard ratios (HRs) and 95% confidence intervals (CIs).

We also performed similar survival analyses for the mortalities due to congestive heart failure and infective diseases. The causes of death were collected as the forms of semi-categorized disease entities. The deaths due to congestive heart failure were defined as the death due to itself, while the deaths due to infection included sepsis, pneumonia, and acute cholecystitis. The numbers of the deaths due to either congestive heart failure or infection were limited. Thus, in the multivariate analyses to investigate the associations of each albumin index with the cause-specific mortalities, we only adjusted age, gender, and diabetes as primary diagnoses. Actually, the numbers of deaths due to infection were small, and there remains a concern that we included more variables to adjust in the models. The degree of model fittings was also evaluated by the corrected Akaike's Information Criteria (AICc). Furthermore, in order to investigate more detailed association, we also made a cross table for the numbers of the deceased patients by dichotomized albumin values and CRP-adjusted albumin values. The significance of this association was investigated by Fisher's exact test.

The JMP 11.2.0 software program (SAS Institute Inc., NC, USA) was used to perform the statistical analysis.

Results

Patient characteristics are shown in Table 1. The average age of the patients was 70.6 years old, which was slightly higher than the average age of total HD population of Japan (67.2 ± 12.5 years old at the end of 2013) [15]. Diabetes and nephrosclerosis were the predominant primary diagnoses. One fourth of the patients had a history of cardiovascular disease.

Table 1 Baseline background factors of the subjects

Items	Values
Age (years)	70.6 ± 13.4 (median 72, IQR 62–81)
Gender (female/male)	139/258
Primary diagnosis (person, %)	
Diabetes	177 (44.6%)
Nephrosclerosis	94 (23.7%)
Glomerulonephritis	76 (19.1%)
Others	50 (12.6%)
Dialysis vintage (years)	Median 3.6, IQR 1.6–7.5
History of cardiovascular diseases (person, %)	103 (25.9%)
History of smoking (persons, %)	152 (43.3%, unknown excluded from the population)
Physical indices	
Body height (cm)	159.3 ± 9.9
Dry weight (kg)	56.6 ± 12.2
Body mass index (kg/m²)	22.1 ± 3.8

The laboratory data are summarized in Table 2. The mean serum albumin value was 3.62 ± 0.38 g/dl (median 3.7, IQR 3.4–3.9). The median serum CRP value was 0.14 mg/dl, and the IQR was 0.05–0.38 mg/dl, which can be rephrased as logCRP −0.84 ± 0.62 (log mg/dl).

Figure 1 shows the relationship between the logCRP and albumin values, and a weak but significant correlation was found between the two sets of values. The regression equation was albumin (g/dl) = 3.438 − 0.215 logCRP (log mg/dl). The degree of fitting was expressed as $R^2 = 0.126$, which means that 12.6% of the albumin distribution was determined by the logCRP value.

The numbers of patients who died during the study period and their causes of death are summarized in Table 3. In total, 73 patients had died from all causes. The most common cause of death was heart failure (42.5%), and it was followed by infection (23.3%) and cerebrovascular disease (11.0%).

Kaplan-Meier analyses followed by log-rank tests demonstrated that both the higher dichotomized and CRP-adjusted albumin level groups were significantly associated with better survival (Fig. 2a, b). The univariate analysis was performed to investigate the relationships between each value and the all-cause mortality, and significant associations were found with age, log CRP, and albumin (Table 4). The relationship between serum albumin levels and mortality was investigated in three ways, as described above. The first was the actual value, the second was the dichotomized value, and the last was the albumin values adjusted with CRP. The CRP-adjusted albumin values were the dichotomized value that was determined by the albumin predicted from CRP values with the use of the regression equation, i.e., predicted

Table 2 Baseline laboratory data of the subjects

Items	Measurements
Systolic blood pressure (mmHg)	153.5 ± 17.6
Diastolic blood pressure (mmHg)	80.0 ± 12.1
Pulse rate (per minute)	73.5 ± 13.4
Albumin (g/dl)	3.62 ± 0.38 (median 3.7, IQR 3.4–3.9)
CRP (mg/dl)	Median 0.14, IQR 0.05–0.38 (range 0.01–15.54)
LogCRP (log mg/dl)	−0.84 ± 0.62 (median −0.85, IQR −1.30 to −0.42)
Hemoglobin (g/dl)	10.5 ± 1.3
Ferritin (ng/ml)	Median 60, IQR 23–123
Transferrin saturation (%)	24.7 ± 13.2
Total cholesterol (mg/dl)	152.7 ± 33.0
HDL cholesterol (mg/dl)	46.2 ± 13.8
Triglyceride (mg/dl)	113.1 ± 71.7 (median 94, IQR 64–138)
LDL cholesterol (mg/dl)	83.8 ± 28.0
Albumin-corrected calcium (mg/dl)	9.08 ± 0.65
Phosphate (mg/dl)	4.67 ± 1.75
Intact PTH (pg/ml)	Median 101, IQR 54–179
Kt/V	1.34 ± 0.27
nPCR (g/kg/day)	0.83 ± 0.19

CRP C-reactive protein, *HDL* high-density lipoprotein, *LDL* low-density lipoprotein, *PTH* parathyroid hormone, and *nPCR* normalized protein catabolic rate

albumin (g/dl) = 3.438 − 0.215 logCRP (log mg/dl). If the predicted values were smaller than the actual values, the CRP-adjusted albumin values were determined as low, vice versa. All three indices were significantly negatively correlated with all-cause mortality.

We investigated the predictive power of three albumin indices adjusted by age, gender, diabetes, dialysis vintage, nPCR, and logCRP. The HR for these indices was 0.60 (95% CI 0.29–1.23) for the actual serum albumin values, 0.64 (95% CI 0.37–1.08) for the dichotomized albumin values, and 0.51 (95% CI 0.30–0.85) for the CRP-adjusted albumin values. As a result, only CRP-adjusted albumin value was significantly associated with the poorer outcome (Table 5).

For cause-specific analyses, the lower groups for the albumin indices tended to be associated with lower mortality due to congestive heart failure but did not reach their significances by crude models. The HRs (and 95% CIs) for albumin indices were 0.44 (0.21–1.03), 0.52 (0.24–1.08), and 0.67 (0.32–1.37), for actual albumin values, dichotomized albumin values by the median, and CRP-adjusted albumin values, respectively. This association did not change even after adjustment of age, gender, and diabetes as primary diagnosis (Table 6). AICc is an index of the degree of model fitting, and the lower value demonstrates better model fitting. AICc demonstrated that

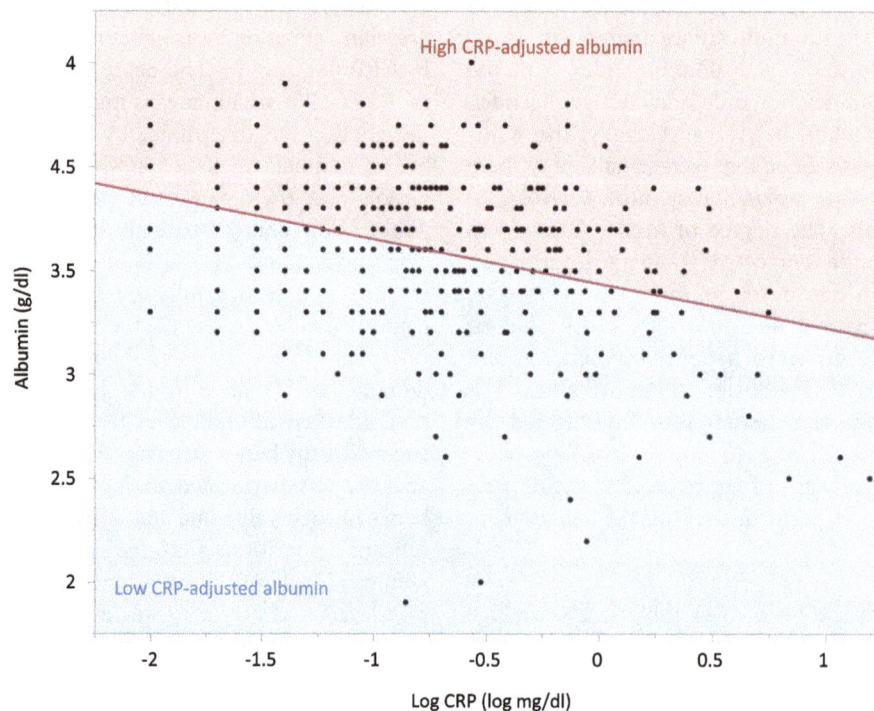

Fig. 1 Relationship between log CRP values and serum albumin values. A scatter plot of log CRP values and serum albumin values is shown. The regression line was obtained by the least squares method. The albumin values above the regression line were considered high CRP-adjusted albumin values, and the values below the regression line low CRP-adjusted serum albumin values

Table 3 Causes of death

Causes for death	Numbers (%)
All causes	73
Cause-specific	
Heart failure	31 (42.5%)
Infection	17 (23.3%)
Cerebrovascular	8 (11.0%)
Malignancy	5 (6.8%)
Myocardial infarction	5 (6.8%)
Gastrointestinal bleeding	4 (5.5%)
Other causes	3 (4.1%)

CRP-adjusted albumin did not improve the degree of model fitting compared to other indices.

On the other hand, the associations between albumin indices and death due to infection were significant for all of the indices investigated by crude models. The HRs (and 95% CIs) for albumin indices were 0.22 (0.09–0.58), 0.12 (0.02–0.42), and 0.12 (0.02–0.41), for actual albumin values, dichotomized albumin values by the median, and CRP-adjusted albumin values, respectively. The associations did not change their significances. However, the CRP-adjusted albumin levels demonstrated the lower HR compared to that of the dichotomized albumin by the median. AICc of the model which included CRP-adjusted albumin was also the lowest among the three models, which indicates the model exhibited the best fitting (Table 7).

Table 8 indicated that the patients in the group with lower dichotomized by the median and lower CRP-adjusted albumin levels demonstrated higher infection-related mortality ($p < 0.001$), while the patients in the group with higher dichotomized by the median and higher CRP-adjusted levels demonstrated better survival ($p = 0.005$).

Discussion

The results of this study showed that 12.6% of the deviation of albumin was determined by CRP. The CRP-adjusted albumin value was the only index associated with a poorer outcome of the chronic HD patients in this study. This result means that malnutrition or wasting itself was associated with survival, independent of the inflammation status, or protein intake of the chronic HD patients in this study. The analyses for cause-specific death demonstrated that such association was evident for death due to infection but not for congestive heart failure.

PEW is a condition in which visceral protein and fat stores decrease as a result of many chronic comorbid conditions, including chronic kidney disease [1, 2]. Since PEW has been shown to be associated with a poor

outcome in many clinical investigations [1, 3, 4], strategies to combat PEW have been anticipated and discussed [1, 3]. The International Society of Renal Nutrition and Metabolism published diagnostic criteria for PEW [2]. The guideline employed four clinical indices: serum chemistry (low serum levels of albumin, prealbumin, and cholesterol), body mass (reduced BMI, weight loss, and reduction of total body fat), muscle mass (muscle wasting, anthropometry, and creatinine appearance), and dietary intake (low dietary protein intake and energy intake) [2]. Thus, reduced serum albumin level is closely related to PEW. Actually, the population with even minimal reduction of albumin as well as low albumin values reportedly experiences poor survival [13]. The results from Kaplan-Meier analyses of this study confirmed such effects of albumin on mortality and demonstrated that lower albumin levels related to worse outcome.

Albumin is synthesized in the liver, and albumin synthesis is influenced by inflammation status [16] and amino acid pools [17, 18]. Moreover, inflammatory status shortens the half-life of serum albumin [19]. Serum albumin level is therefore considered as an index of both inflammation and wasting or malnutrition [1, 14]. However, since dietary restriction does not always lead to a reduction in serum albumin level [14], the significance of inflammation has been postulated and been shown to outweigh the effect of malnutrition in determining the serum albumin levels [14]. Likewise, the reduction of the serum albumin level is not necessarily caused by the malnutrition itself [14]. An experiment in 1944 to 1945 investigated the effect of starvation on the physiological and psychological aspects of healthy volunteers. The results showed that only a limited reduction in serum albumin level (from 4.3 ± 0.5 to 3.9 ± 0.5 g/dl) was observed even after a severe decrease in body mass (BMI: from 21.7 ± 1.7 to 16.4 ± 0.9 kg/m^2) [14]. Moreover, the inflammation-related conditions or wasting are considered to have larger impacts on the reduction of albumin levels [3]. Actually, the results of the present study indicated that 12.6% of deviation in albumin values was derived from those of CRP. Therefore, the degree was not so large, but it was demonstrated that albumin could be influenced by inflammation.

HD patients are prone to have inflammatory status because of the vascular access [20], periodontal diseases [21], bacterial translocation from the altered microbiome in the gut [22], or immunodeficiency [23]. The presence of inflammation can be related to worse survival among HD patients [24, 25]; the HD patients with higher serum CRP level have higher mortality rates [25]. However, the serum CRP levels of our study population were no longer associated with the poor outcome after adjustment for the serum albumin levels. This finding indicated that

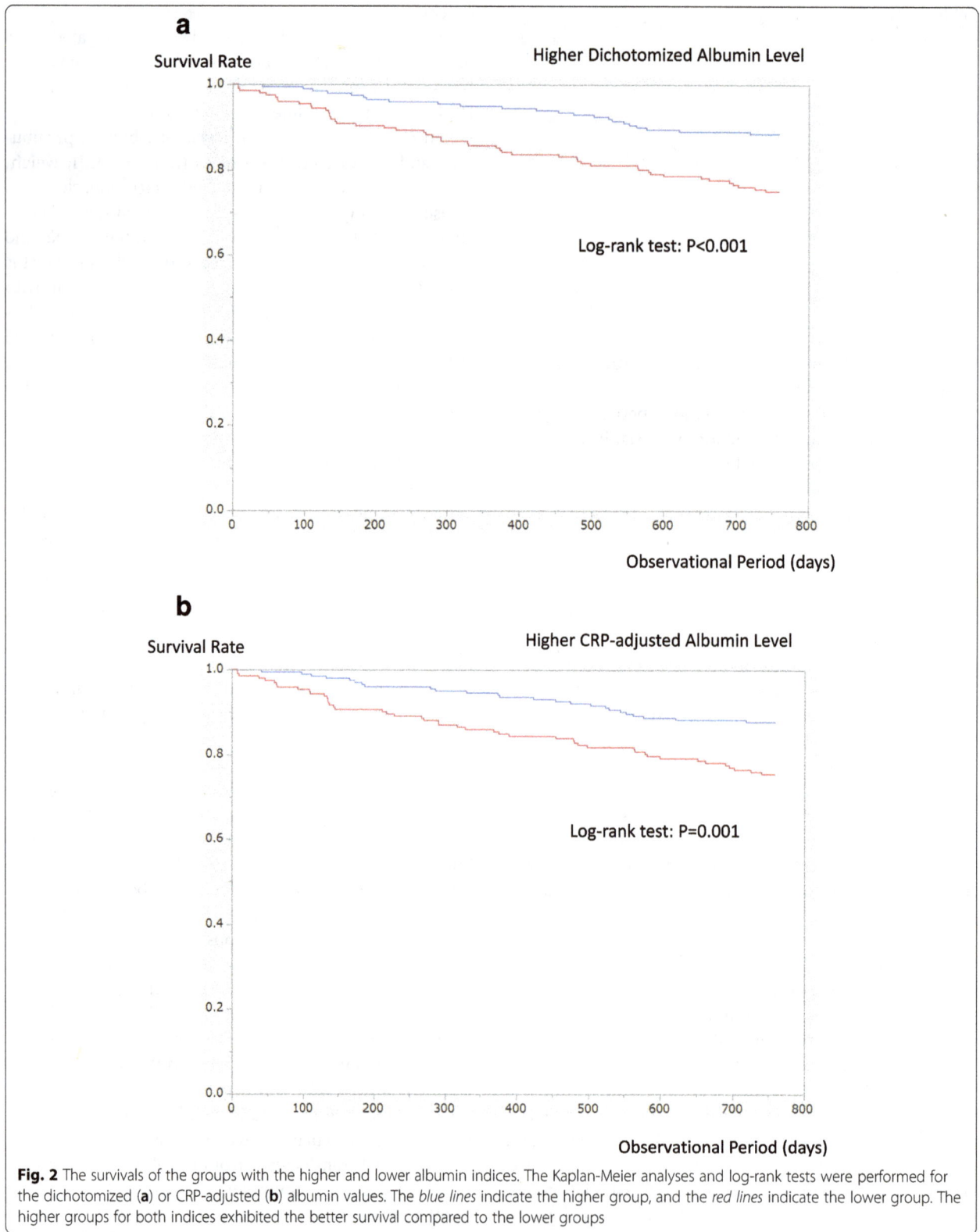

Fig. 2 The survivals of the groups with the higher and lower albumin indices. The Kaplan-Meier analyses and log-rank tests were performed for the dichotomized (**a**) or CRP-adjusted (**b**) albumin values. The blue lines indicate the higher group, and the red lines indicate the lower group. The higher groups for both indices exhibited the better survival compared to the lower groups

the significance of wasting or malnutrition might have larger impact on the better health of HD patients compared to inflammation.

This study demonstrated that such association was most evident for death due to infection. A study investigated the effect of albumin, which was not adjusted for

Table 4 Univariate analysis of the associations between clinical indices and all-cause mortality

Parameters	HR (95% CI)
Age (per 1 year)	1.07 (1.05–1.09)
Gender (female)	0.71 (0.42–1.17)
Diabetes	1.53 (0.96–2.44)
Dialysis vintage (years)	
<2	Reference
≥2 and <4	0.85 (0.45–1.59)
≥4 and <8	0.84 (0.44–1.54)
≥8	0.76 (0.36–1.44)
nPCR (per 1 g/kg/day)	0.61 (0.18–2.02)
LogCRP (per 1 log mg/dl)	1.79 (1.25–2.54)
Actual albumin (per 1 g/dl)	0.40 (0.25–0.68)
Dichotomized albumin by median (the higher group)	0.41 (0.25–0.68)
CRP-adjusted albumin (the higher group)	0.46 (0.28–0.74)

nPCR normalized protein catabolic rate, *CRP* C-reactive protein, *HR* hazard ratio, and *CI* confidence intervals

CRP, on cause-specific mortality across hemodialysis and peritoneal dialysis [26]. The study found that the HRs of low albumin levels for infection-related mortality were higher than those for cardiovascular mortality irrespective of dialysis modalities. Our study confirmed this result even by CRP-adjusted albumin. Moreover, the group with the lower CRP-adjusted albumin values more

Table 5 Predictive power of each of the different albumin indices

Parameters	Model 1	Model 2	Model 3
Age (per 1 year)	1.08 (1.05–1.11)	1.08 (1.05–1.11)	1.08 (1.05–1.10)
Gender (female)	0.50 (0.28–0.87)	0.49 (0.27–0.84)	0.50 (0.28–0.86)
Diabetes	1.82 (1.12–2.96)	1.77 (1.09–2.88)	1.84 (1.14–3.00)
Dialysis vintage (years)			
<2	Reference	Reference	Reference
≥2 and <4	0.84 (0.42–1.66)	0.78 (0.40–1.47)	0.89 (0.45–1.70)
≥4 and <8	0.90 (0.46–1.72)	0.84 (0.44–1.56)	0.92 (0.48–1.73)
≥8	1.35 (0.65–2.71)	1.31 (0.64–2.57)	1.39 (0.68–2.70)
nPCR (per 1 g/kg/day)	2.30 (0.64–7.90)	2.16 (0.62–7.29)	2.28 (0.66–7.55)
Log CRP (per 1 log mg/dl)	1.21 (0.81–1.80)	1.24 (0.84–1.82)	1.43 (0.97–2.10)
Actual albumin (per 1 g/dl)	0.60 (0.29–1.23)	–	–
Dichotomized albumin by median (the higher group)	–	0.64 (0.37–1.08)	–
CRP-adjusted albumin (the higher group)	–	–	0.51 (0.30–0.85)

nPCR normalized protein catabolic rate, *CRP* C-reactive protein, *HR* hazard ratio, and *CI* confidence interval

Table 6 Predictive power of each of the different albumin indices on mortality due to congestive heart failure

Parameters	Model 1	Model 2	Model 3
Age (per 1 year)	1.09 (1.05–1.13)	1.09 (1.05–1.14)	1.09 (1.05–1.13)
Gender (female)	0.57 (0.25–1.23)	0.56 (0.24–1.19)	0.55 (0.24–1.19)
Diabetes	1.65 (0.79–3.46)	1.64 (0.78–3.44)	1.66 (0.80–3.47)
Actual albumin (per 1 g/dl)	0.71 (0.27–1.89)	–	–
Dichotomized albumin by median (the higher group)	–	0.85 (0.38–1.82)	–
CRP-adjusted albumin (the higher group)	–	–	0.87 (0.41–1.80)
Corrected Akaike's Information Criteria	335.1	335.4	335.4

CRP C-reactive protein

significantly associated, which was shown by the lower AICc score, with higher infection-related mortality compared to albumin indices. The fact indicated that lower albumin without the effect of inflammatory status was more likely associated with the death due to infection. Further studies are required to investigate whether hypoalbuminemia itself [13] or malnutrition existing in the background [27] is associated with infection-related mortality.

On the other hand, albumin values were not significantly associated with survival for the death due to congestive heart failure, though the point estimates of HRs favored the higher albumin values for all indices. This fact indicates that low albumin values can relate to the death due to congestive heart failure, but other factors seemed more likely to be associated with such mortality. Moreover, interestingly enough, CRP-adjusted albumin levels were no longer significant compared to other albumin indices. The previous reports demonstrated that

Table 7 Predictive power of each of the different albumin indices on mortality due to infection

Parameters	Model 1	Model 2	Model 3
Age (per 1 year)	1.15 (1.08–1.22)	1.14 (1.07–1.21)	1.14 (1.07–1.21)
Gender (female)	0.60 (0.20–1.66)	0.53 (0.18–1.44)	0.49 (0.16–1.34)
Diabetes	4.21 (1.52–13.5)	3.81 (1.38–12.2)	4.04 (1.46–13.0)
Actual albumin (per 1 g/dl)	0.24 (0.07–0.93)	–	–
Dichotomized albumin by median (the higher group)	–	0.25 (0.04–0.93)	–
CRP-adjusted albumin (the higher group)	–	–	0.17 (0.03–0.62)
Corrected Akaike's Information Criteria	169.4	169.3	165.9

nPCR normalized protein catabolic rate, *CRP* C-reactive protein, *HR* hazard ratio, and *CI* confidence interval

Table 8 Distribution of the numbers of deceased patients. Predictive power of each of the different albumin indices on mortality due to infection

		CRP-adjusted albumin	
		The higher group	The lower group
Dichotomized albumin by median	The higher group	2/180 (1.11%)	0/21 (0%)
	The lower group	0/25 (0%)	15/170 (8.82%)

hypoalbuminemia can relate to cardiovascular diseases [28, 29]. However, it has been demonstrated that there are many other cardiovascular risk factors, and the condition is known as cardiorenal syndrome type 4 [30]. The present study confirmed that the death due to congestive heart failure might be associated with hypoalbuminemia itself, but more substantially with other risk factors as well. These associations require further investigations among larger cohorts.

Several indices, including the malnutrition-inflammation score [8] or GNRI [12], have been proposed to monitor the nutritional status of HD populations, and they have been reported to be good predictors of patient outcome [8, 11]. However, from a clinical standpoint, serum albumin levels can be monitored easily and are widely used to assess global nutritional status. The results of the present study demonstrated that it is important to consider inflammatory status of HD patients when assessing their serum albumin levels. This finding also indicates that malnutrition or wasting can affect the outcome of the patients independent of their inflammation status, thereby confirming the value of nutritional interventions to combat malnutrition in HD populations [1].

Limitations
This study had several limitations. The first limitation was that it was performed on the basis of observational study, and thus, the cause result relationship cannot be drawn whether the outcome can be improved by the increase of serum albumin levels in face of higher CRP or the reduction of CRP in face of lower albumin levels. Second, this study was performed on the database of a single center. Further generalizability of the present investigation will be required by the study using the data of other cohorts. The final limitation was that only the baseline data were analyzed, and no changes in clinical indices, including albumin or CRP values, were considered. Substantial changes in the clinical parameters could take place afterward during the course. However, this study had several advantages. First, the total number of patients was substantial, and we were able to obtain a conclusion from this HD population. Second,

the follow-up period and the numbers of outcomes are also sufficient to be investigated. Third, since the patient background factors almost matched those of the entire Japanese HD population. Therefore, the cohort in our study was the representative of the Japanese HD population.

Conclusions
When assessing the serum albumin levels of HD population, the inflammation status of the patients should be taken into consideration. Wasting or malnutrition itself can predict a worse outcome independent of inflammation.

Abbreviations
BMI: Body mass index; CRP: C-reactive protein; GNRI: Geriatric nutritional risk index; HDL: High-density lipoprotein; HR: Hazard ratio; IQR: Interquartile range; LDL: Low-density lipoprotein; nPCR: Normalized protein catabolic rate; PEW: Protein energy wasting; PTH: Parathyroid hormone

Acknowledgements
Authors acknowledge all the participants and medical staffs who were engaged in the present investigations.

Funding
The authors did not have specific funding source to be disclosed.

Authors' contributions
NH performed the statistical analysis and wrote the draft version of this article. KN and KT planned, organized, and directed the investigation, as well as finalized the manuscript. MO, MK, SS, and HK were in charge of the investigated patients, collected clinical data, and finalizing and reviewing the manuscript. All authors read and approved the final manuscript.

Competing interests
NH was a former member of the division funded by the Terumo Corporation. NH had a research contract concerning oral nutritional support on dialysis patients with Meiji Co., Ltd.

Author details
[1]Department of Blood Purification, Tokyo Women's Medical University, Tokyo, Japan. [2]Department of Medicine, Kidney Center, Tokyo Women's Medical University, 8-1 Kawada-cho, Shinjuku-ku, Tokyo 162-8666, Japan. [3]Department of Nephrology, Jyoban Hospital, Fukushima, Japan.

References

1. Nitta K, Tsuchiya K. Recent advances in the pathophysiology and management of protein-energy wasting in chronic kidney disease. Ren Replace Ther. 2016;2:4.
2. Fouque D, Kalantar-Zadeh K, Kopple J, Cano N, Chauveau P, Cuppari L, Franch H, Guarnieri G, Ikizler TA, Kaysen G, et al. A proposed nomenclature and diagnostic criteria for protein-energy wasting in acute and chronic kidney disease. Kidney Int. 2008;73:391–8.
3. Ikizler TA, Cano NJ, Franch H, Fouque D, Himmelfarb J, Kalantar-Zadeh K, Kuhlmann MK, Stenvinkel P, TerWee P, Teta D, et al. Prevention and treatment of protein energy wasting in chronic kidney disease patients: a consensus statement by the International Society of Renal Nutrition and Metabolism. Kidney Int. 2013;84:1096–107.
4. Kim JC, Kalantar-Zadeh K, Kopple JD. Frailty and protein-energy wasting in elderly patients with end stage kidney disease. J Am Soc Nephrol. 2013;24:337–51.
5. Heimburger O, Qureshi AR, Blaner WS, Berglund L, Stenvinkel P. Hand-grip muscle strength, lean body mass, and plasma proteins as markers of nutritional status in patients with chronic renal failure close to start of dialysis therapy. Am J Kidney Dis. 2000;36:1213–25.
6. Isoyama N, Qureshi AR, Avesani CM, Lindholm B, Barany P, Heimburger O, Cederholm T, Stenvinkel P, Carrero JJ. Comparative associations of muscle mass and muscle strength with mortality in dialysis patients. Clin J Am Soc Nephrol. 2014;9:1720–8.
7. Johansen KL, Chertow GM, Jin C, Kutner NG. Significance of frailty among dialysis patients. J Am Soc Nephrol. 2007;18:2960–7.
8. Kalantar-Zadeh K, Kopple JD, Block G, Humphreys MH. A malnutrition-inflammation score is correlated with morbidity and mortality in maintenance hemodialysis patients. Am J Kidney Dis. 2001;38:1251–63.
9. Steiber AL, Kalantar-Zadeh K, Secker D, McCarthy M, Sehgal A, McCann L. Subjective global assessment in chronic kidney disease: a review. J Ren Nutr. 2004;14:191–200.
10. Kalantar-Zadeh K, Kleiner M, Dunne E, Lee GH, Luft FC. A modified quantitative subjective global assessment of nutrition for dialysis patients. Nephrol Dial Transplant. 1999;14:1732–8.
11. Kobayashi I, Ishimura E, Kato Y, Okuno S, Yamamoto T, Yamakawa T, Mori K, Inaba M, Nishizawa Y. Geriatric Nutritional Risk Index, a simplified nutritional screening index, is a significant predictor of mortality in chronic dialysis patients. Nephrol Dial Transplant. 2010;25:3361–5.
12. Yamada K, Furuya R, Takita T, Maruyama Y, Yamaguchi Y, Ohkawa S, Kumagai H. Simplified nutritional screening tools for patients on maintenance hemodialysis. Am J Clin Nutr. 2008;87:106–13.
13. Kalantar-Zadeh K, Kilpatrick RD, Kuwae N, McAllister CJ, Alcorn Jr H, Kopple JD, Greenland S. Revisiting mortality predictability of serum albumin in the dialysis population: time dependency, longitudinal changes and population-attributable fraction. Nephrol Dial Transplant. 2005;20:1880–8.
14. Friedman AN, Fadem SZ. Reassessment of albumin as a nutritional marker in kidney disease. J Am Soc Nephrol. 2010;21:223–30.
15. Masakane I, Nakai S, Ogata S, Kimata N, Hanafusa N, Hamano T, Wakai K, Wada A, Nitta K. An overview of regular dialysis treatment in Japan (as of 31 December 2013). Ther Apher Dial. 2015;19:540–74.
16. Kaysen GA, Dubin JA, Muller HG, Rosales L, Levin NW, Mitch WE, NIDDK HSG. Inflammation and reduced albumin synthesis associated with stable decline in serum albumin in hemodialysis patients. Kidney Int. 2004;65:1408–15.
17. Eustace JA, Coresh J, Kutchey C, Te PL, Gimenez LF, Scheel PJ, Walser M. Randomized double-blind trial of oral essential amino acids for dialysis-associated hypoalbuminemia. Kidney Int. 2000;57:2527–38.
18. Hiroshige K, Sonta T, Suda T, Kanegae K, Ohtani A. Oral supplementation of branched-chain amino acid improves nutritional status in elderly patients on chronic haemodialysis. Nephrol Dial Transplant. 2001;16:1856–62.
19. Kaysen GA, Greene T, Daugirdas JT, Kimmel PL, Schulman GW, Toto RD, Levin NW, Yan G, Group HS. Longitudinal and cross-sectional effects of C-reactive protein, equilibrated normalized protein catabolic rate, and serum bicarbonate on creatinine and albumin levels in dialysis patients. Am J Kidney Dis. 2003;42:1200–11.
20. Nassar GM, Fishbane S, Ayus JC. Occult infection of old nonfunctioning arteriovenous grafts: a novel cause of erythropoietin resistance and chronic inflammation in hemodialysis patients. Kidney Int. 2002; 61(Suppl 80): S49–54.

21. Chen LP, Chiang CK, Chan CP, Hung KY, Huang CS. Does periodontitis reflect inflammation and malnutrition status in hemodialysis patients? Am J Kidney Dis. 2006;47:815–22.
22. Anders HJ, Andersen K, Stecher B. The intestinal microbiota, a leaky gut, and abnormal immunity in kidney disease. Kidney Int. 2013;83:1010–6.
23. Girndt M, Sester M, Sester U, Kaul H, Kohler H. Molecular aspects of T- and B-cell function in uremia. Kidney Int Suppl. 2001;78:S206–211.
24. Rao M, Guo D, Perianayagam MC, Tighiouart H, Jaber BL, Pereira BJ, Balakrishnan VS. Plasma interleukin-6 predicts cardiovascular mortality in hemodialysis patients. Am J Kidney Dis. 2005;45:324–33.
25. Honda H, Qureshi AR, Heimburger O, Barany P, Wang K, Pecoits-Filho R, Stenvinkel P, Lindholm B. Serum albumin, C-reactive protein, interleukin 6, and fetuin a as predictors of malnutrition, cardiovascular disease, and mortality in patients with ESRD. Am J Kidney Dis. 2006;47:139–48.
26. Mehrotra R, Duong U, Jiwakanon S, Kovesdy CP, Moran J, Kopple JD, Kalantar-Zadeh K. Serum albumin as a predictor of mortality in peritoneal dialysis: comparisons with hemodialysis. Am J Kidney Dis. 2011;58:418–28.
27. Bergstrom J, Lindholm B. Malnutrition, cardiac disease, and mortality: an integrated point of view. Am J Kidney Dis. 1998;32:834–41.
28. Harnett JD, Foley RN, Kent GM, Barre PE, Murray D, Parfrey PS. Congestive heart failure in dialysis patients: prevalence, incidence, prognosis and risk factors. Kidney Int. 1995;47:884–90.
29. Foley RN, Parfrey PS, Harnett JD, Kent GM, Murray DC, Barre PE. Hypoalbuminemia, cardiac morbidity, and mortality in end-stage renal disease. J Am Soc Nephrol. 1996;7:728–36.
30. Ronco C, Haapio M, House AA, Anavekar N, Bellomo R. Cardiorenal syndrome. J Am Coll Cardiol. 2008;52:1527–39.

2

Relationship between mortality and Geriatric Nutritional Risk Index (GNRI) at the time of dialysis initiation: a prospective multicenter cohort study

Akihito Tanaka[1*], Daijo Inaguma[1,2,3], Hibiki Shinjo[1], Minako Murata[1] and Asami Takeda[1]

Abstract

Background: The Geriatric Nutritional Risk Index (GNRI) is a nutritional screening method primarily developed for elderly people; it is also reported to be useful for predicting mortality in patients on maintenance dialysis. However, it is unclear whether it is useful at the time of dialysis initiation, which is accompanied by large weight fluctuations and unstable nutritional status.

Methods: The study included 1524 patients with chronic kidney disease who commenced dialysis therapy at 17 centers. Patients commenced dialysis between October 2011 and September 2013 and were followed up until March 2015.

Results: We analyzed 1489 patients whose GNRI could be calculated and whose prognosis was clear. The mean GNRI was 87.60 (median 87.86). We divided patients based on the median value into a high (H) and low (L) group. The H group included 728 patients (mean GNRI 95.2 ± 4.9, mean age 65.8 ± 13.2 years, 69.3% men), and the L group included 761 patients (mean GNRI 80.3 ± 6.1, mean age 69.1 ± 12.8 years, 66.0% men). Mortality was significantly higher in the L group (L, 22.2% vs. H, 12.6%, $P < 0.001$). The rates of infection-associated death in the L group was significantly higher (L, 5.5% vs. H, 1.9%, $P < 0.001$), although no significant difference was observed regarding cardiovascular disease-associated death (L, 7.6% vs. H, 5.2%, $P = 0.059$) and malignancy-associated death (L, 3.0% vs. H, 3.0%, $P = 1.000$). Multivariate analysis showed an association between GNRI and all-cause mortality (HR 0.9852, 95%CI 0.9707–0.9999, $P = 0.049$) and infection-associated death (HR 0.9484, 95%CI 0.9191–0.9786, $P < 0.001$).

Conclusions: GNRI is useful for predicting mortality even at the time of dialysis initiation. Among the causes of death, GNRI was strongly associated with infection-associated death.

Keywords: GNRI, Dialysis, Infection, Mortality

Background

The number of patients receiving dialysis therapy is increasing yearly, and these patients show high mortality from various causes, the main causes being cardiovascular and infectious diseases [1]. Therefore, to improve the prognosis of patients who commence dialysis therapy, it is important to understand the characteristics of those at a high risk of mortality.

The Geriatric Nutritional Risk Index (GNRI) is a nutritional screening method primarily developed for elderly people and is reported to be useful for ascertaining disease prognosis [2]. Its usefulness in predicting poor outcomes has also been reported for various co-morbidities such as stroke [3], heart failure [4, 5], and for hospitalized patients [6, 7]. Moreover, GNRI is useful in ascertaining disease prognosis in patients on maintenance dialysis [8–10]. However, it remains unclear whether this index is also beneficial at the time of dialysis initiation, where the tendency exists for weight fluctuation due to fluid retention and malnutrition because of uremia.

* Correspondence: zhangren_at_23@yahoo.co.jp
[1]Kidney Disease Center, Japanese Red Cross Nagoya Daini Hospital, 2-9, Myoken-cho, Showa-ku, Nagoya 466-8650, Japan
Full list of author information is available at the end of the article

Therefore, we compared the prognosis of patients with high and low GNRI at the time of dialysis initiation. We also examined various causes of death with respect to GNRI.

Methods

Patients and data collection

Data from the Aichi Cohort Study of Prognosis in Patients Newly Initiated into Dialysis [11, 12] were used in this prospective multicenter study. Patients who commenced dialysis between October 2011 and September 2013 at 17 Japanese institutions were included. This study was approved by the Ethics Committee of the Institutional Review Board of Nagoya Daini Red Cross Hospital (No. IRB20110823-3), and all patients provided written informed consent. Patients who were not discharged and died in the hospital were excluded (Fig. 1). Data regarding patient background, medical history, co-morbidities, medications, and laboratory data during the period of dialysis initiation were collected. Serologic data were obtained at the first dialysis session and just before dialysis initiation. Patients were followed until the end of March 2015.

Method for calculating GNRI

Ideal body weight (IBW) was calculated from height, and GNRI was calculated using IBW, albumin (ALB) level, and body weight (BW).

$$IBW = Height \times Height \times 22$$
$$GNRI = 14.89 \times ALB\ (g/dL) + 41.7 \times (BW/IBW)$$
$$(If\ BW > IBW,\ we\ set\ BW/IBW\ =\ 1)$$

Mortality

Patients were divided into two groups—high and low levels of GNRI—and outcomes and hazard ratios (HRs) were compared between groups. The primary endpoint was mortality. Causes of death were ascertained. The incidence of death was investigated via survey slips sent to the dialysis facilities at the end of March 2015.

Statistics

Baseline characteristics were descriptively presented and were tested using Student's t test or chi squared test. Survival was represented graphically using the Kaplan-Meier method and analyzed using univariate and multivariate Cox regression. HRs were represented graphically using forest plots. Receiver operative characteristic (ROC) curves were used to evaluate the value of GNRI that could detect various causes of death. P values of <0.05 were considered significant.

Results

Baseline characteristics

We analyzed 1489 patients whose GNRI could be calculated and whose prognosis was clear. Table 1 shows baseline characteristics of patients based on GNRI. The

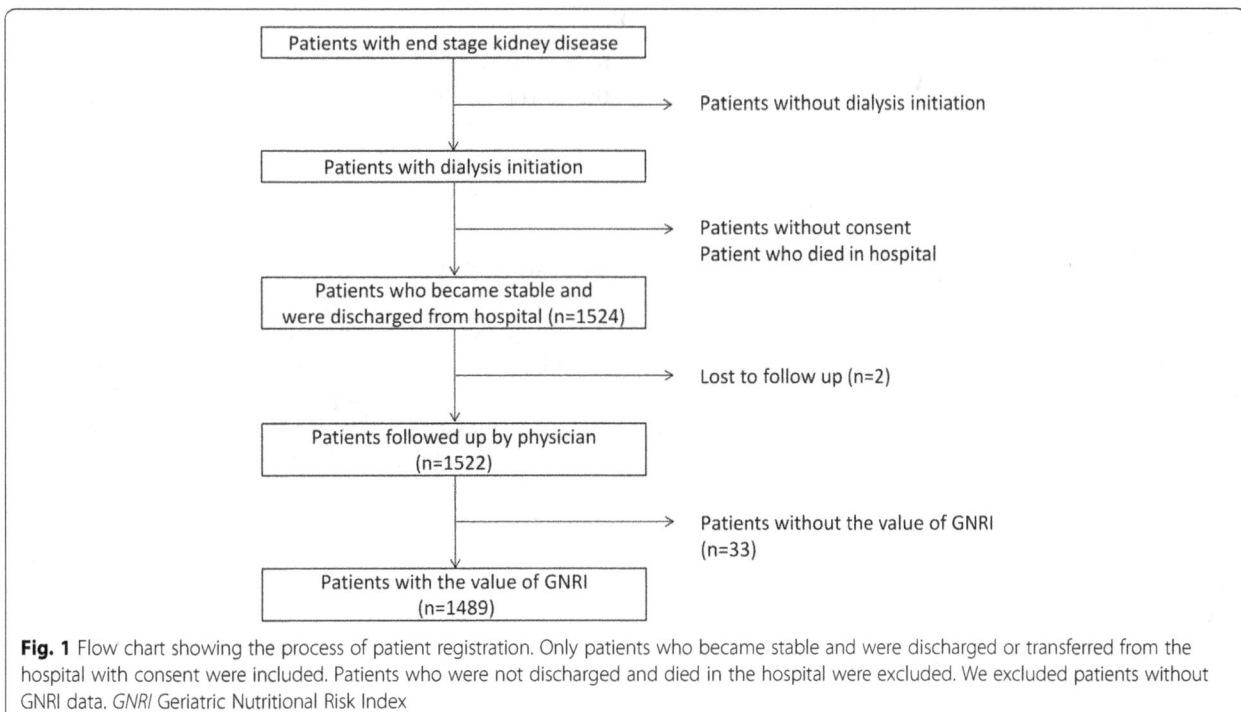

Fig. 1 Flow chart showing the process of patient registration. Only patients who became stable and were discharged or transferred from the hospital with consent were included. Patients who were not discharged and died in the hospital were excluded. We excluded patients without GNRI data. *GNRI* Geriatric Nutritional Risk Index

Table 1 Baseline characteristics of patients in two groups divided by GNRI

Parameter	High group (n = 728)	Low group (n = 761)	P value
Male (%)	69.4	66.0	0.1607
Age (years)	65.8 ± 13.2	69.1 ± 12.8	<0.001
Height (cm)	160.1 ± 9.2	158.8 ± 9.7	0.0059
Body weight (kg)	62.0 ± 13.1	58.2 ± 14.1	<0.001
BMI (kg/cm2)	24.0 ± 4.0	22.9 ± 4.5	<0.001
GNRI	95.2 ± 4.9	80.3 ± 6.1	<0.001
UFV (L)	0.801 ± 0.827	0.967 ± 0.919	<0.001
ACEi or ARB (%)	64.0	57.4	0.0093
β blocker (%)	36.7	33.2	0.1652
Statin (%)	39.7	40.5	0.7603
VDRA (%)	32.6	22.9	<0.001
ESA (%)	88.9	84.1	0.0072
Diabetes (%)	44.5	57.6	<0.001
History of CAD (%)	14.7	18.8	0.0347
History of PCI (%)	9.5	10.9	0.3627
History of CABG (%)	3.7	4.6	0.3899
History of HF Ad (%)	16.6	24.3	0.0002
History of CI (%)	12.6	14.6	0.2733
History of ICH (%)	3.2	2.6	0.5406
History of AD (%)	5.1	6.0	0.4185
History of PAD, F2 (%)	3.6	5.7	0.0564
Amputation (%)	1.0	2.1	0.0743
CVD (%)	40.1	49.5	0.0003
Comorbid MI (%)	4.0	7.2	0.0067
Comorbid HF (%)	18.3	31.5	<0.001
Comorbid PAD (%)	3.7	6.4	0.0167
Comorbid stroke (%)	7.4	10.1	0.0659
SBP (mmHg)	152.5 ± 25.4	150.1 ± 26.4	0.0694
CTR (%)	54.1 ± 7.2	56.2 ± 6.9	<0.001
WBC (1000/μL)	6.3 ± 2.9	7.1 ± 3.3	<0.001
Hb (g/dL)	9.77 ± 1.45	9.00 ± 1.54	<0.001
Plt (10000/μL)	17.3 ± 7.2	19.0 ± 7.9	<0.001
ALB (g/dL)	3.67 ± 0.34	2.75 ± 0.41	<0.001
eGFR (ml/min/1.7m2)	5.21 ± 1.84	5.67 ± 2.52	<0.001
Na (mEq/L)	138.2 ± 4.0	137.6 ± 4.7	0.0045
K (mEq/L)	4.61 ± 0.77	4.48 ± 0.838	0.0020
cCa (mg/dL)	8.44 ± 1.05	8.78 ± 1.03	<0.001
P (mg/dL)	6.23 ± 1.61	6.48 ± 2.10	0.0095
Mg (mg/dL)	2.20 ± 0.50	2.10 ± 0.44	<0.001
UA (mg/dL)	8.71 ± 2.33	8.82 ± 2.45	0.3660
LDL-C (mg/dL)	87.5 ± 31.9	92.0 ± 36.6	0.0168
CRP (mg/dL)	0.88 ± 2.48	2.68 ± 5.10	<0.001

Table 1 Baseline characteristics of patients in two groups divided by GNRI (Continued)

TSAT (%)	28.4 ± 16.3	25.9 ± 16.9	0.0130
Ferritin (ng/mL)	221.6 ± 1328.5	220.5 ± 506.0	0.9846
LVEF (%)	60.8 ± 12.5	60.6 ± 12.0	0.7771
All-cause death (%)	12.6	22.2	<0.001
Infection death (%)	1.9	5.5	0.0003
CVD death (%)	5.2	7.6	0.0593
Malignancy death (%)	3.0	3.0	0.9998

GNRI Geriatric Nutritional Risk Index, *UFV* ultrafiltlation volume, *BMI* body mass index, *ACEi* angiotensin-converting enzyme inhibitor, *ARB* angiotensin receptor blocker, *VDRA* vitamin D receptor agonist, *ESA* erythropoietin stimulating agent, *CAD* coronary artery disease, *PCI* percutaneous coronary intervention, *CABG* coronary artery bypass grafting, *HF* heart failure, *Ad* admission, *CI* cerebral infarction, *ICH* intracerebral hemorrhage, *AD* aortic disease, *PAD, F2* peripheral arterial disease with Fontaine classification 2-4, *CVD* cardiovascular disease, *MI* myocardial infarction, *SBP* systolic blood pressure, *CTR* cardiothoracic ratio, *WBC* white blood cells, *Hb* hemoglobin, *Plt* platelet, *ALB* albumin, *eGFR* estimated glomerular filtration rate, *Na* sodium, *K* potassium, *cCa* corrected calcium, *P* phosphate, *Mg* magnesium, *UA* uric acid, *LDL-C* low-density lipoprotein cholesterol, *CRP* C-reactive protein, *TSAT* transferrin saturation, *LVEF* left ventricular ejection fraction, *CVD* cardiovascular disease

mean value of GNRI was 87.60 (median 87.86). We divided patients based on the median value into a high (H) and low (L) group. The L group was older, and the percentage of ACE inhibitor, angiotensin receptor blocker, and vitamin D receptor agonist administration was lower. The L group had a higher rate of cardiovascular disease (CVD) history. Expectedly, the L group had a lower body mass index (BMI) and ALB values. Overall, the L group had significantly lower levels of electrolytes, which may have been due to a lack of intake. However, it is unknown whether the lower electrolyte levels is clinically meaningful. C-reactive protein levels were higher in the L group. All-cause death and infection-associated death were higher in the L group.

Mortality and causes of death

Figure 2 shows the Kaplan-Meier plot for survival rate in patients according to GNRI levels. Figures 3, 4, and 5 show Kaplan-Meier plots for cumulative incidence rates regarding infection-, CVD-, and malignancy-associated deaths. In the univariate analysis (Kaplan-Meier plot), the incidence of all-cause, infection-associated, and CVD-associated death was significantly higher in the L group. Multivariate analysis was then performed. Figure 6 shows the forest plot, which presents HRs of GNRI for death. In the multivariate analysis, there was no significant difference in CVD-associated death, and only all-cause and infection-associated death showed a significant association. These results indicate the usefulness of GNRI

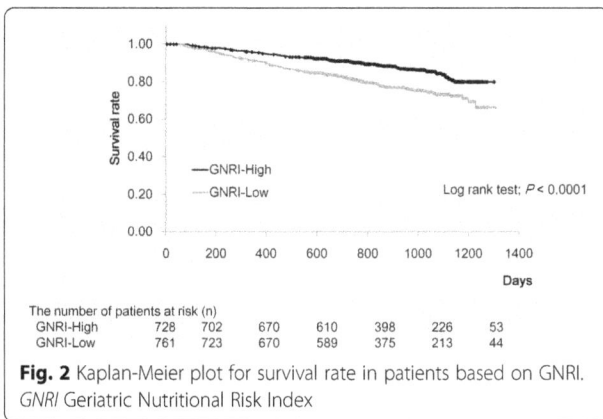

Fig. 2 Kaplan-Meier plot for survival rate in patients based on GNRI. *GNRI* Geriatric Nutritional Risk Index

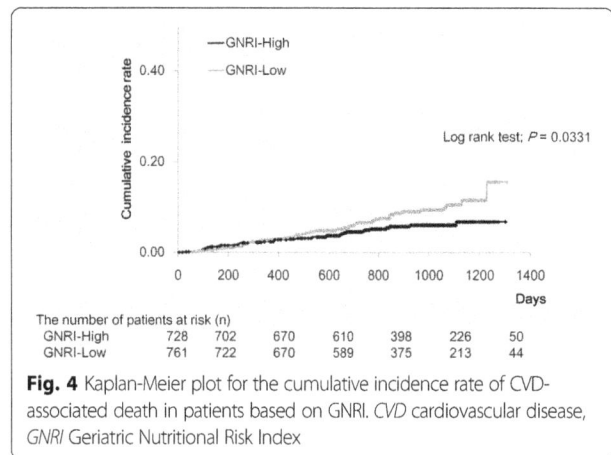

Fig. 4 Kaplan-Meier plot for the cumulative incidence rate of CVD-associated death in patients based on GNRI. *CVD* cardiovascular disease, *GNRI* Geriatric Nutritional Risk Index

for disease prognosis, especially for infection-associated death.

ROC curve of GNRI for predicting death

Because GNRI was originally synthesized from BW and ALB, we assessed whether BMI or ALB alone could sufficiently predict mortality. Figure 7 shows the ROC curve of GNRI predicting all-cause death, and Fig. 8 shows the ROC curve of GNRI predicting infection-associated death. GNRI had a superior ability to predict all-cause and infection-associated death compared to ALB alone. Although there was no significant difference in comparison with BMI, the area under the curve (AUC) of GNRI was higher for both all-cause and infection-associated death in appearance, and the predictive ability tended to be higher. Figure 9 shows stratified analysis by the ultrafiltration volume at first dialysis session for all-cause death. With high amount of ultrafiltration, the accuracy of prediction value of GNRI reduced.

Discussion

We compared the mortality of patients with high and low GNRI at the time of dialysis initiation. GNRI exhibited a good predictive ability not only

during the maintenance dialysis phase but also during dialysis induction when the body weight is unstable or dietary intake may be decreasing. Further, among mortality rates, GNRI was strongly related to infection-associated death.

GNRI is a nutritional evaluation scale that was primarily developed for the elderly but is becoming increasingly used as a simple and objective indicator of prognosis in other conditions. In this study, there is novelty and clinically very meaningful in the point of usefulness of GNRI even when the items for calculating it is modified.

From our findings, patients with low GNRI exhibited a poor prognosis. In this group, there was a prevalence of factors associated with poor prognoses, such as old age, CVD history, and diabetes. Since the patient background is quite different, simple comparison with GNRI alone is difficult. It seems that the L group contains many patients with poor overall medical condition. Despite the mathematical adjustment for these factors above, complete adjustment is difficult. GNRI may comprehensively detect such "poor status." Regarding the

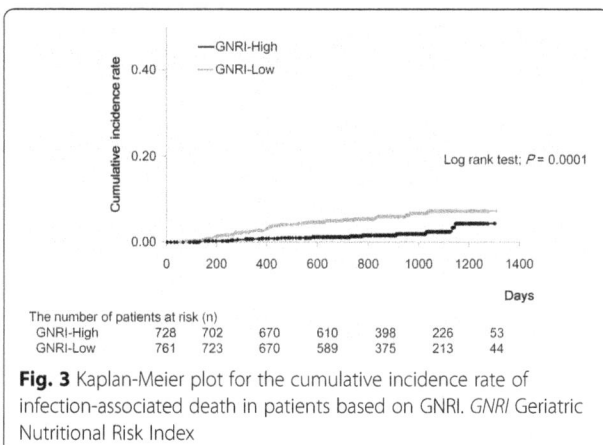

Fig. 3 Kaplan-Meier plot for the cumulative incidence rate of infection-associated death in patients based on GNRI. *GNRI* Geriatric Nutritional Risk Index

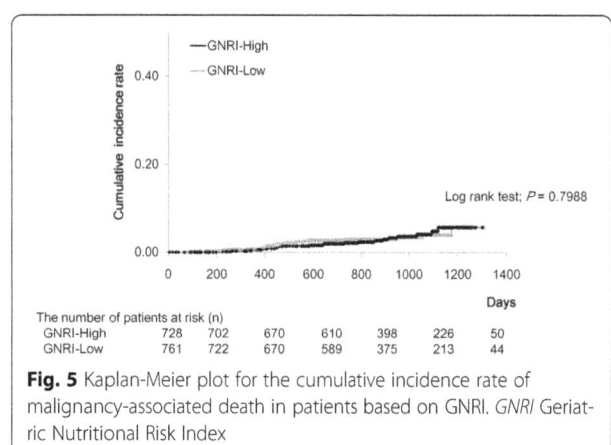

Fig. 5 Kaplan-Meier plot for the cumulative incidence rate of malignancy-associated death in patients based on GNRI. *GNRI* Geriatric Nutritional Risk Index

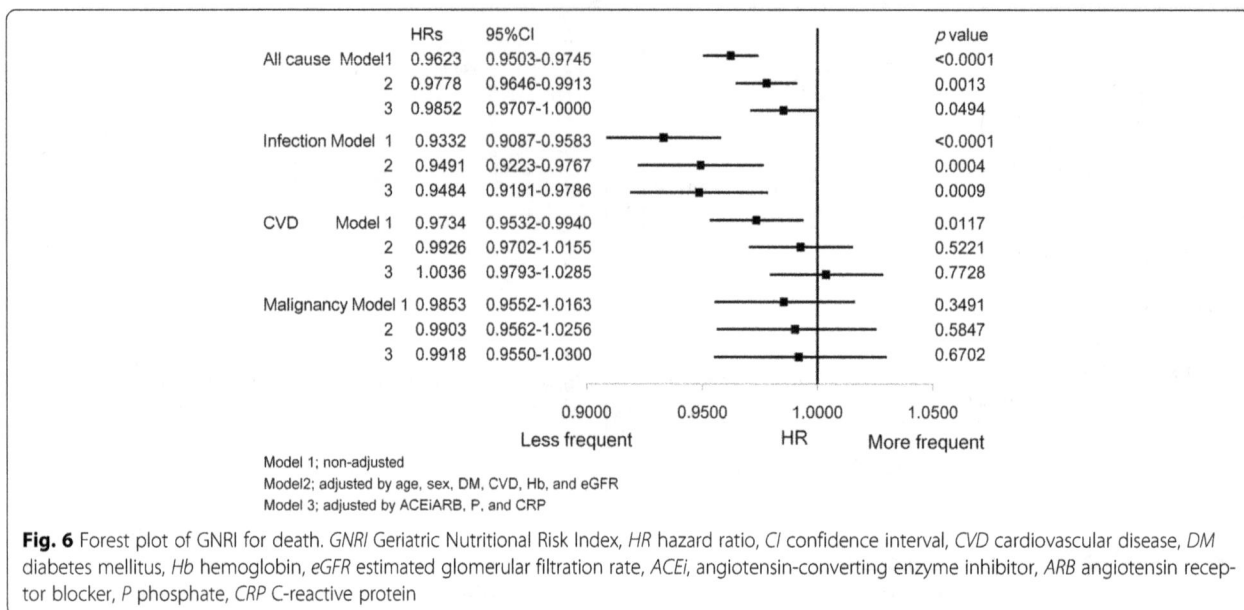

Fig. 6 Forest plot of GNRI for death. *GNRI* Geriatric Nutritional Risk Index, *HR* hazard ratio, *CI* confidence interval, *CVD* cardiovascular disease, *DM* diabetes mellitus, *Hb* hemoglobin, *eGFR* estimated glomerular filtration rate, *ACEi*, angiotensin-converting enzyme inhibitor, *ARB* angiotensin receptor blocker, *P* phosphate, *CRP* C-reactive protein

cause of the strong association with infection-associated death, an immunocompromised status caused by malnutrition [13, 14] may be a reason. However, a definite conclusion cannot be arrived at because leukocyte fraction or immunoglobulin was not measured. We are considering these assessments in the future.

At the time of dialysis initiation, BW and BMI increase because of body fluid retention, and ALB decreases because of dilution. These modifications impair the accuracy of GNRI as shown in Fig. 9. However, our results showed the usability of GNRI

in this condition. Probably the value of GNRI would be more accurate to predict the prognosis if there are no factors to modify. However, this research is meaningful because it shows that prognosis prediction is possible to some extent even if predictive accuracy is lowered by additional modifying factors. It is already known that the stable GNRI value during maintenance dialysis period is useful for prognosis prediction. Hence, this will be a more wonderful research if we can compare the prediction accuracy of GNRI values during the introduction period and stable period. Unfortunately, values of GNRI after

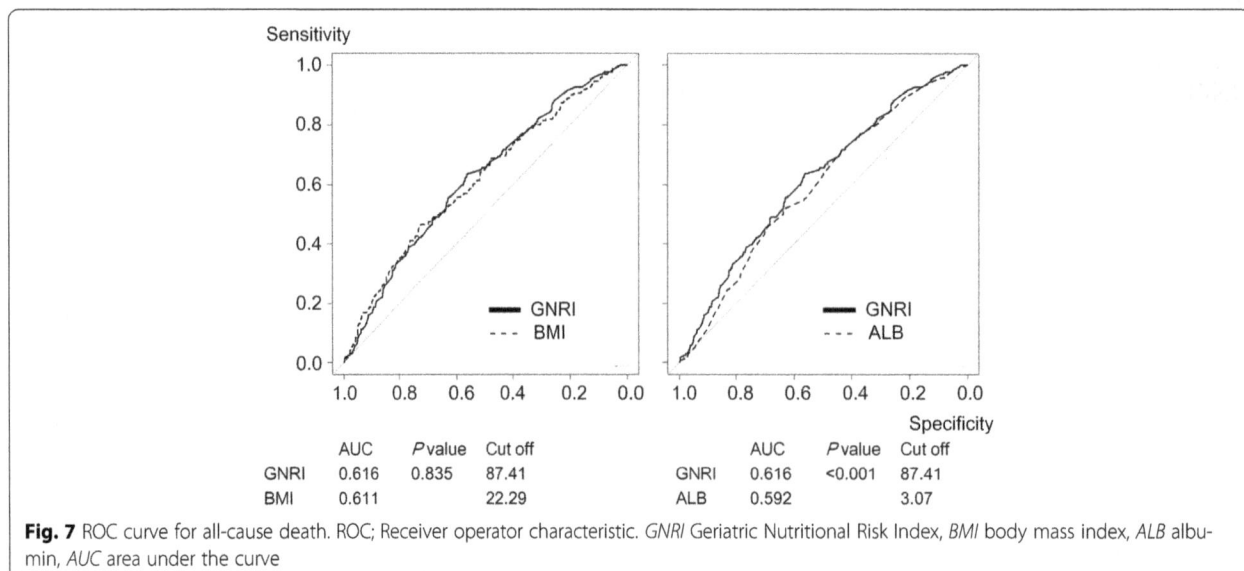

Fig. 7 ROC curve for all-cause death. ROC; Receiver operator characteristic. *GNRI* Geriatric Nutritional Risk Index, *BMI* body mass index, *ALB* albumin, *AUC* area under the curve

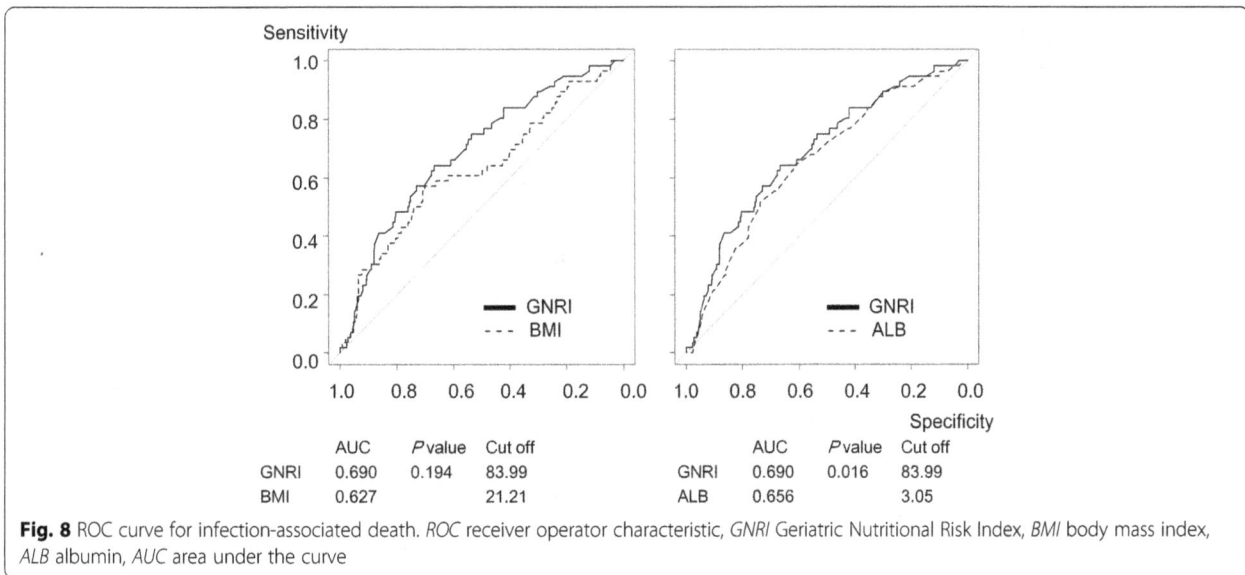

Fig. 8 ROC curve for infection-associated death. *ROC* receiver operator characteristic, *GNRI* Geriatric Nutritional Risk Index, *BMI* body mass index, *ALB* albumin, *AUC* area under the curve

discharge cannot be collected and are unknown because many patients are transferring to other clinics after dialysis initiation. Although it is regrettable that there is no data during stable maintenance period, but in the sense of indicating that GNRI works effectively with the novelty of "dialysis induction period," large number of patients, and with a tremendously high tracking rate, this report seems to be very meaningful.

Our study had some limitations. First, since this was an observational study, a selection bias is expected regarding whether physicians treated patients with end-stage kidney disease and whether poor nutritional status may have resulted in a poor prognosis. Second, regarding the reason for the strong association between GNRI and infection-

associated death, we did not measure values such as fractionation of white blood cells or immunoglobulin levels. Hence, further investigation of this association could not be conducted. Third, when the amount of fluid removal was excessive, the accuracy of predictive value reduced. Therefore, in the cases with too much fluid removal compared to this study, the results of this study may not be applicable.

Conclusions

At the time of dialysis initiation, patients with low GNRI values are associated with a poor prognosis, particularly with regard to infection-associated death. The prediction accuracy of GNRI for all-cause and infection-associated death seems better than that of BMI or ALB alone.

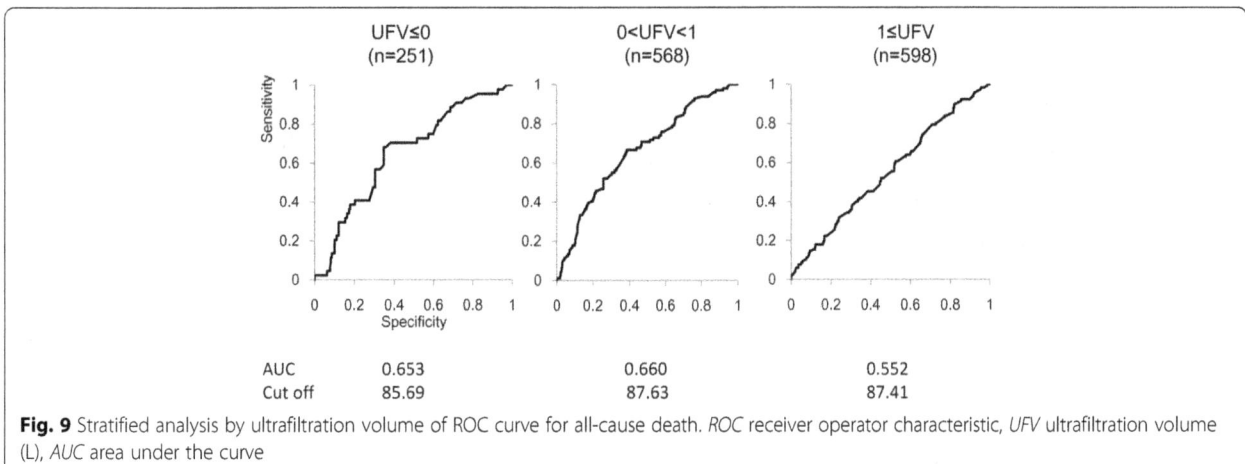

Fig. 9 Stratified analysis by ultrafiltration volume of ROC curve for all-cause death. *ROC* receiver operator characteristic, *UFV* ultrafiltration volume (L), *AUC* area under the curve

Abbreviations

ALB: Albumin; AUC: Area under the curve; BMI: Body mass index; BW: Body weight; CVD: Cardiovascular disease; GNRI: Geriatric nutritional risk index; HR: Hazard ratio; IBW: Ideal body weight; ROC: Receiver operator characteristic; UFV: Ultrafiltration volume

Acknowledgements

We acknowledge the support of the following members of the Aichi Cohort Study of Prognosis in Patients Newly Initiated into Dialysis (AICOPP) who participated in this study: Hirofumi Tamai (Anjo Kosei Hospital), Tomohiko Naruse (Kasugai Municipal Hospital), Kei Kurata (Tosei General Hospital), Hideto Oishi (Komaki City Hospital), Isao Aoyama (Japan Community Healthcare Organization Chukyo Hospital), Hiroshi Ogawa (Shinseikai Daiichi Hospital), Hiroko Kushimoto (Nishichita General Hospital), Hideaki Shimizu (Chubu-Rosai Hospital), Junichiro Yamamoto (Tsushima City Hospital), Hisashi Kurata (Toyota Kosei Hospital), Taishi Yamakawa (Toyohashi Municipal Hospital), Takaaki Yaomura (Nagoya Medical Center), Hirotake Kasuga (Nagoya Kyouritsu Hospital), Shizunori Ichida (Japanese Red Cross Nagoya Daiichi Hospital), Shoichi Maruyama (Nagoya University Graduate School of Medicine), Noritoshi Kato (Nagoya University Graduate School of Medicine), Seiichi Matsuo (Nagoya University Graduate School of Medicine), Shigehisa Koide (Fujita Health University Hospital), and Yukio Yuzawa (Fujita Health University Hospital).
We would like to thank Editage (www.editage.jp) for the English language editing.

Funding

Not applicable.

Authors' contributions

DI designed the study. AT performed the statistical analysis and wrote the manuscript. All authors participated in the care of the patients. All authors read and approved the final manuscript.

Competing interests

The authors declare that they have no competing interests.

Author details

[1]Kidney Disease Center, Japanese Red Cross Nagoya Daini Hospital, 2-9, Myoken-cho, Showa-ku, Nagoya 466-8650, Japan. [2]Department of Nephrology, Fujita Health University School of Medicine, Toyoake, Aichi, Japan. [3]Aichi Cohort Study of Prognosis in Patients Newly Initiated Into Dialysis (AICOPP), Aichi, Japan.

References

1. Masakane I, Nakai S, Ogata S, Kimata N, Hanafusa N, Hamano T, et al. An overview of regular dialysis treatment in Japan (As of 31 December 2013). Ther Apher Dial. 2015;19:540–74.
2. Bouillanne O, Morineau G, Dupont C, Coulombel I, Vincent JP, Nicolis I, et al. Geriatric Nutritional Risk Index: a new index for evaluating at-risk elderly medical patients. Am J Clin Nutr. 2005;82:777–83.
3. Kokura Y, Maeda K, Wakabayashi H, Nishioka S, Higashi S. High nutritional-related risk on admission predicts less improvement of functional independence measure in geriatric stroke patients: a retrospective cohort study. J Stroke Cerebrovasc Dis. 2016;25:1335–41.
4. Kinugasa Y, Kato M, Sugihara S, Hirai M, Yamada K, Yanagihara K, et al. Geriatric nutritional risk index predicts functional dependency and mortality in patients with heart failure with preserved ejection fraction. Circ J. 2013;77:705–11.
5. Kalantar-Zadeh K, Anker SD, Horwich TB, Fonarow GC. Nutritional and anti-inflammatory interventions in chronic heart failure. Am J Cardiol. 2008; 101(11A):89E–103E.
6. Abd-El-Gawad WM, Abou-Hashem RM, El Maraghy MO, Amin GE. The validity of Geriatric Nutrition Risk Index: simple tool for prediction of nutritional-related complication of hospitalized elderly patients. Comparison with mini nutritional assessment. Clin Nutr. 2014;33:1108–16.
7. Gamaletsou MN, Poulia KA, Karageorgou D, Yannakoulia M, Ziakas PD, Zampelas A, et al. Nutritional risk as predictor for healthcare-associated infection among hospitalized elderly patients in the acute care setting. J Hosp Infect. 2012;80:168–72.
8. Edalat-Nejad M, Zameni F, Qlich-Khani M, Salehi F. Geriatric Nutritional Risk Index: a mortality predictor in hemodialysis patients. Saudi J Kidney Dis Transpl. 2015;26:302–8.
9. Chen HY, Chiu YL, Hsu SP, Pai MF, Yang JY, Wu HY, et al. Reappraisal of effects of serum chemerin and adiponectin levels and nutritional status on cardiovascular outcomes in prevalent hemodialysis patients. Sci Rep. 2016;6:34128.
10. Tsai MT, Liu HC, Huang TP. The impact of malnutritional status on survival in elderly hemodialysis patients. J Chin Med Assoc. 2016;79:309–13.
11. Tanaka A, Inaguma D, Shinjo H, Murata M, Takeda A, Aichi Cohort Study of Prognosis in Patients Newly Initiated into Dialysis Study G. Presence of atrial fibrillation at the time of dialysis initiation is associated with mortality and cardiovascular events. Nephron. 2016;132:86–92.
12. Hishida M, Tamai H, Morinaga T, Maekawa M, Aoki T, Tomida H, et al. Aichi cohort study of the prognosis in patients newly initiated into dialysis (AICOPP): baseline characteristics and trends observed in diabetic nephropathy. Clin Exp Nephrol. 2016;20:795–807.
13. Chandra RK. Nutritional regulation of immunity and risk of infection in old age. Immunology. 1989;67:141–7.
14. Pifer TB, McCullough KP, Port FK, Goodkin DA, Maroni BJ, Held PJ, et al. Mortality risk in hemodialysis patients and changes in nutritional indicators: DOPPS. Kidney Int. 2002;62:2238–45.

3

Effect of continuous hemodiafiltration using an AN69ST membrane in patients with sepsis

Akihito Tanaka[1*], Daijo Inaguma[1,2,3], Tomoaki Nakamura[3], Yu Watanabe[1], Eri Ito[1], Naoki Kamegai[1], Hiroya Shimogushi[1], Minako Murata[1], Hibiki Shinjo[1], Kiyomi Koike[1], Yasuhiro Otsuka[1] and Asami Takeda[1]

Abstract

Background: Sepsis is a systemic inflammatory response syndrome caused by infectious disease. Severe sepsis and septic shock are extremely serious conditions with poor prognoses. It is reported that cytokines are deeply involved in the disease mechanism. Continuous hemodiafiltration (CHDF) using a poly(methyl methacrylate) (PMMA) membrane is reported to adsorb various cytokines and improve the status of patients with sepsis. Recently, another cytokine-adsorbing hemofilter, acrylonitrile-co-methallyl sulfonate surface-treated (AN69ST) membrane, has become available for CHDF in patients with sepsis. However, the clinical efficacy of this membrane remains unclear. Therefore, in this study, we compared the efficacy of AN69ST and PMMA membranes.

Methods: This retrospective study included patients with severe sepsis or septic shock who underwent CHDF for at least 24 h in the intensive care unit from January 2013 to August 2016.

Results: This study included 49 patients who underwent CHDF, 32 using an AN69ST membrane and 17 using a PMMA membrane. In the AN69ST and PMMA groups, average age was 71.1 ± 11.4 years and 74.7 ± 9.4 years, respectively, and percentage of men was 71.9 and 88.2%, respectively. Severity of sepsis and vital signs were not significantly different between groups at the start of CHDF. In addition, 28-day mortality was not significantly different between groups (43.8 vs. 35.3%, $P = 0.1625$). However, heart rate in the AN69ST group decreased significantly early in the course of CHDF (6, 12, and 24 h, $P < 0.05$) compared with the PMMA group.

Conclusions: AN69ST and PMMA membranes showed equivalent efficacy. Furthermore, CHDF using an AN69ST membrane may be effective for early stabilization of vital signs.

Keywords: AN69ST, Continuous renal replacement therapy, Continuous hemodiafiltration, Sepsis

Background

Sepsis is a systemic inflammatory response syndrome caused by infectious disease [1]. Severe sepsis and septic shock are extremely serious conditions with poor prognoses [2, 3]. It is reported that cytokines are deeply involved in the disease mechanism. Although various treatments for sepsis have been used, none has been sufficient. Of the available options, blood purification therapy for cytokine removal is reported to be successful [4]. With regard to high-flow and high-volume renal replacement therapy, results have been positive [5, 6] or negative [7, 8], with no clear conclusion. However, continuous renal replacement therapy (CRRT), which removes cytokines by taking advantage of the characteristics of membranes, such as poly(methyl methacrylate) (PMMA), is often used [9, 10]. Although another hemofilter, acrylonitrile-co-methallyl sulfonate surface-treated (AN69ST) membrane, has recently become available in Japan [11], results regarding its clinical efficacy are scarce. In addition, there is no study comparing the AN69ST membrane with another hemofilter with cytokine-adsorption ability, such as PMMA. Therefore, in this study, we investigated the clinical efficacy of the AN69ST membrane in the acute phase.

* Correspondence: zhangren_at_23@yahoo.co.jp
[1]Kidney Disease Center, Japanese Red Cross Nagoya Daini Hospital, 2-9, Myoken-cho, Showa-ku, Nagoya 466-8650, Japan
Full list of author information is available at the end of the article

Table 1 Baseline characteristics of patients treated with CHDF

Parameter	AN69ST ($n = 32$)	PMMA ($n = 17$)	P value
Male (%)	71.9	88.2	0.1914
Age (years)	71.1 ± 11.4	74.7 ± 9.4	0.1123
Height (cm)	159.8 ± 8.9	160.7 ± 9.2	0.7845
BMI	22.4 ± 4.7	21.6 ± 3.8	0.4371
Cause of sepsis			
Peritonitis (%)	46.9	64.7	0.2339
UTI (%)	6.3	11.8	0.5022
Pneumoniae (%)	15.6	11.8	0.7132
Infection bacteria			
Gram-positive coccus (%)	40.6	41.2	0.9702
Gram-negative rod (%)	34.4	47.1	0.3857
Unknown (%)	31.3	23.5	0.5691
Past history			
Diabetes (%)	21.9	23.5	0.8949
Hypertension (%)	53.1	35.3	0.2339
Maintenance dialysis (%)	12.5	29.4	0.1456
Ventilator (%)	84.4	94.1	0.3220
Surgical treatment (%)	50.0	76.5	0.0727
SBP (mmHg)	105.2 ± 26.8	107.9 ± 21.7	0.4945
DBP (mmHg)	54.3 ± 13.2	57.6 ± 15.7	0.5012
MBP (mmHg)	71.3 ± 15.9	74.3 ± 16.6	0.5777
HR (bpm)	99.1 ± 22.0	99.8 ± 17.2	0.9828
BT (°C)	37.3 ± 1.0	36.9 ± 1.1	0.0740
CAI	38.5 ± 27.3	28.4 ± 19.2	0.1689
DOA (µg/kg/min)	0.00 ± 0.00	0.55 ± 2.28	0.1573
DOB (µg/kg/min)	0.89 ± 2.00	0.55 ± 2.28	0.1918
NA (µg/kg/min)	0.38 ± 0.26	0.27 ± 0.19	0.1472
WBC (1000/µL)	15.4 ± 9.5	11.8 ± 11.0	0.1035
Hb (g/dL)	10.6 ± 2.1	10.3 ± 1.4	0.4749
Plt (10,000/µL)	14.5 ± 10.8	13.6 ± 7.4	0.8091
ALB (g/dL)	2.0 ± 0.5	1.9 ± 0.5	0.6591
AST (IU/L)	310.1 ± 754.4	285.7 ± 999.8	0.2610
ALT (IU/L)	172.2 ± 440.3	118.2 ± 388.2	0.1753
UN (mg/dL)	57.2 ± 24.3	48.0 ± 26.1	0.1252
Cr (mg/dL)	3.6 ± 2.2	3.9 ± 3.6	0.4067
eGFR (ml/min/1.7 m^2)	19.0 ± 12.9	25.8 ± 19.0	0.4127
Na (mEq/L)	138.2 ± 4.1	137.8 ± 6.3	0.2291
K (mEq/L)	4.5 ± 1.0	4.3 ± 0.8	0.3714
cCa (mg/dL)	9.4 ± 0.9	9.4 ± 0.9	0.8058
P (mg/dL)	4.6 ± 1.7	4.7 ± 1.9	0.8148
Mg (mg/dL)	2.0 ± 0.5	1.8 ± 0.3	0.3516
CRP (mg/dL)	20.4 ± 12.5	14.8 ± 12.2	0.0991
HCO$_3^-$ (mEq/L)	16.9 ± 5.6	17.0 ± 4.3	0.8500
Lactate (mg/dL)	40.4 ± 32.3	23.9 ± 15.3	0.0928

Table 1 Baseline characteristics of patients treated with CHDF (Continued)

APACHE 2	32.1 ± 7.0	32.5 ± 4.8	0.8086
APACHE2 without kidney	29.3 ± 7.1	30.2 ± 4.9	0.7120
SOFA	13.1 ± 2.7	11.9 ± 2.7	0.0807
SOFA without kidney	10.4 ± 2.3	9.5 ± 2.8	0.4709
PMX (%)	25.0	58.8	0.0194*
CRRT (days)	4.4 ± 2.9	5.3 ± 4.9	0.8970
Death at 28 days (%)	43.8	35.3	0.1625
Cr at 28 days (mg/dL)	1.4 ± 1.3 ($n = 14$)	2.5 ± 1.9 ($n = 9$)	0.0777

CHDF continuous hemodiafiltration, *AN* polyacrylonitrile, *PMMA* polymethyl methacrylate, *BMI* body-mass index, *UTI* urinary tract infection, *SBP* systolic blood pressure, *DBP* diastolic blood pressure, *MBP* mean blood pressure, *HR* heart rate, *BT* body temperature, *CAI* catecholamine index, *DOA* dopamine, *DOB* dobutamine, *NA* noradrenalin, *WBC* white blood cells, *Hb* hemoglobin, *Plt* platelet, *ALB* albumin, *AST* aspartate aminotransferase, *ALT* alanine amino-transferase, *eGFR* estimated glomerular filtration rate, *Na* sodium, *K* potassium, *cCa* corrected calcium, *P* phosphate, *Mg* magnesium, *CRP* C-reactive protein, *HCO$_3^-$* bicarbonate, *APACHE 2* Acute Physiology and Chronic Health Evaluation II score, *SOFA* sequential organ failure assessment score, *PMX* polymyxin B-immobilized fiber column hemoperfusion, *CRRT* continuous renal replacement therapy
*$p < 0.05$

Methods

Patients and data collection

This retrospective study included patients with severe sepsis or septic shock who underwent CRRT for at least 24 h in the intensive care unit from January 2013 to August 2016. Sepsis was diagnosed by meeting at least two systemic inflammatory response syndrome criteria due to a presumed infection [1]. Severe sepsis is that causing organ dysfunction. As CRRT, continuous hemo-diafiltration (CHDF) was performed, starting with a dialysate flow rate of 400 mL/h and a replacement solution flow rate of 400 mL/h, which was adjusted appropriately. A double-lumen catheter was placed in the internal jugular vein as vascular access. Heparin and/or nafamostat mesylate was used with judgment in each case. Judgment of when to start and finish CHDF was determined by consultation with multiple intensive care staff members and nephrologists. The membranes used for CHDF were PMMA and AN69ST.

At the start of CHDF, patients' age, sex, physical findings, cause of sepsis, and laboratory data were collected from their medical records. Acute Physiology and Chronic Health Evaluation II (APACHE II) [12] and sequential organ failure assessment (SOFA) [13] scores also were calculated. Vital signs and catecholamine index (CAI) were evaluated at the start of CHDF and at 6, 12, 24, 48, and 72 h. Twenty-eight-day survival rate was also calculated. Patients' vital signs and CAI at 72 h were included even if CHDF was already finished at that time. CAI was calculated as follows: dopamine level (µg/kg/min) + dobutamine level (µg/kg/min) + noradrenaline level (µg/kg/min) × 100.

Statistical analysis

Baseline characteristics were presented descriptively with average and SD values and were tested using the Mann-Whitney U test for parametrical data and χ^2 test for nonparametrical data. Logistic regression analysis and stratified analysis were performed to evaluate 28-day survival. P values of <0.05 were considered statistically significant.

Results

Baseline characteristics

Table 1 shows the clinical characteristics of the 49 patients included in this study. Of them, 32 underwent CHDF using an AN69ST membrane, while 17 used a PMMA membrane; average age was 71.1 ± 11.4 years and 74.7 ± 9.4 years, respectively, and percentage of men was 71.9 and 88.2%, respectively. As a result, almost all CHDF was performed with AN69ST membrane after becoming available although discussed by multiple intensive care staff members and nephrologists. Severity of sepsis and vital signs at the start of CHDF were not significantly different between groups. The percentage of ventilator user did not show significant difference between both groups. Compared with patients using an AN69ST membrane, those using a PMMA membrane received combination therapy with polymyxin B-immobilized fiber column hemoperfusion (PMX) more frequently (58.8 vs. 25.0%, $P = 0.0194$).

Comparison of 28-day mortality

Figure 1 shows the Kaplan-Meier plot of 28-day survival in patients who underwent CHDF using an AN69ST or PMMA membrane. Twenty-eight-day mortality was not significantly different between groups (43.8 vs. 35.3%, $P = 0.1625$). Figures 2 and 3 show

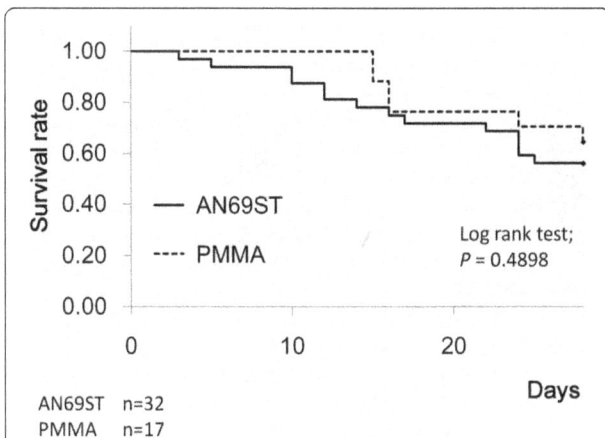

Fig. 2 Survival rates among subgroups stratified according to Acute Physiology and Chronic Health Evaluation II (APACHE II) score without kidney score. *AN69ST* acrylonitrile-co-methallyl sulfonate surface-treated, *NS* not significant, *PMMA* poly(methyl methacrylate)

stratified analysis according to APACHE II and SOFA scores without kidney score. Figure 4 shows the forest plot of odds ratios for 28-day survival. Stratified and multivariate analyses showed no significant difference in mortality between groups. Furthermore, the level of creatinine at 28 days was not different significantly (Table 1).

Time course of vital signs and CAI

Figure 5a shows blood pressure in patients who underwent CHDF using an AN69ST or PMMA membrane.

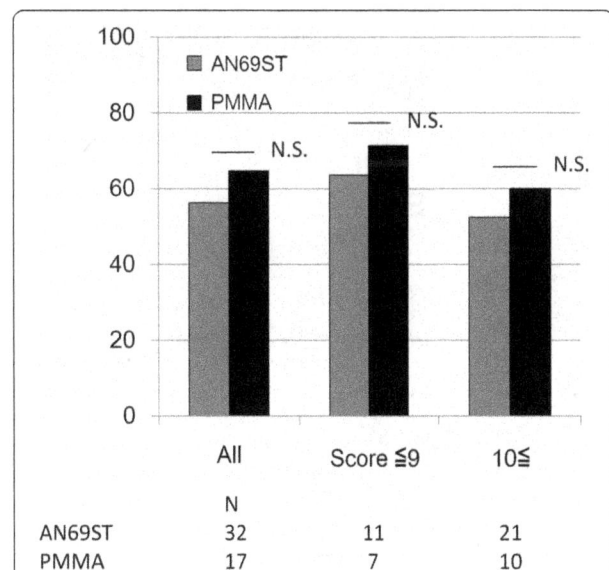

Fig. 1 Kaplan-Meier plot of 28-day survival in patients who underwent continuous hemodiafiltration using a poly(methyl methacrylate) (PMMA) or acrylonitrile-co-methallyl sulfonate surface-treated (AN69ST) membrane

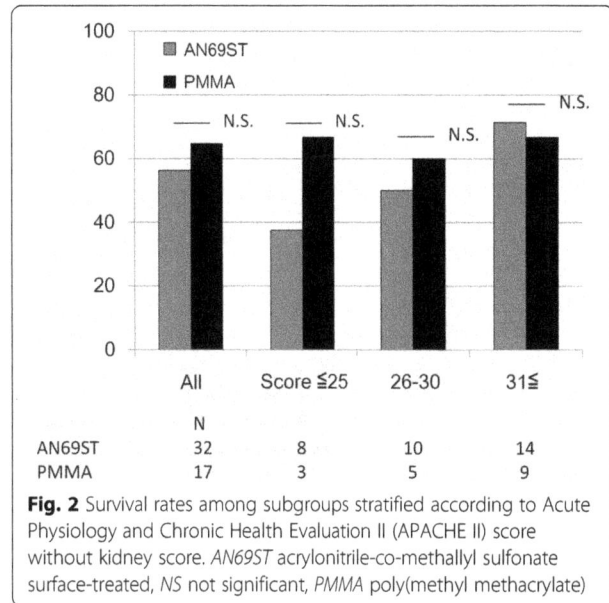

Fig. 3 Survival rates among subgroups stratified according to Sequential Organ Failure Assessment (SOFA) score without kidney score. *AN69ST* acrylonitrile-co-methallyl sulfonate surface-treated, *NS* not significant, *PMMA* poly(methyl methacrylate)

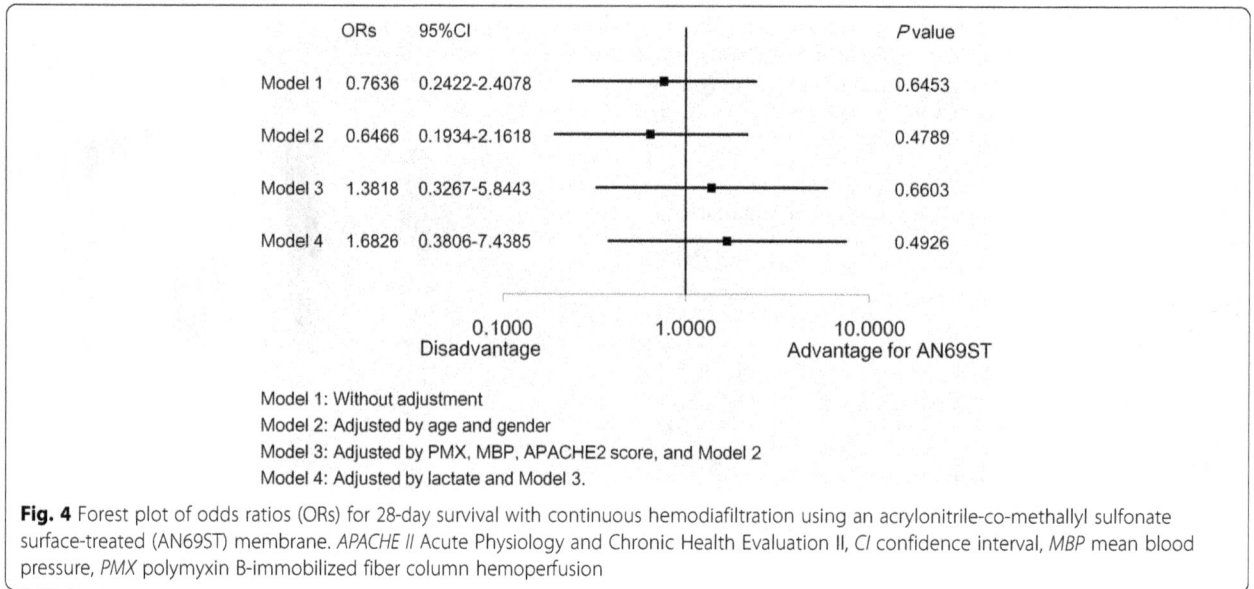

Fig. 4 Forest plot of odds ratios (ORs) for 28-day survival with continuous hemodiafiltration using an acrylonitrile-co-methallyl sulfonate surface-treated (AN69ST) membrane. *APACHE II* Acute Physiology and Chronic Health Evaluation II, *CI* confidence interval, *MBP* mean blood pressure, *PMX* polymyxin B-immobilized fiber column hemoperfusion

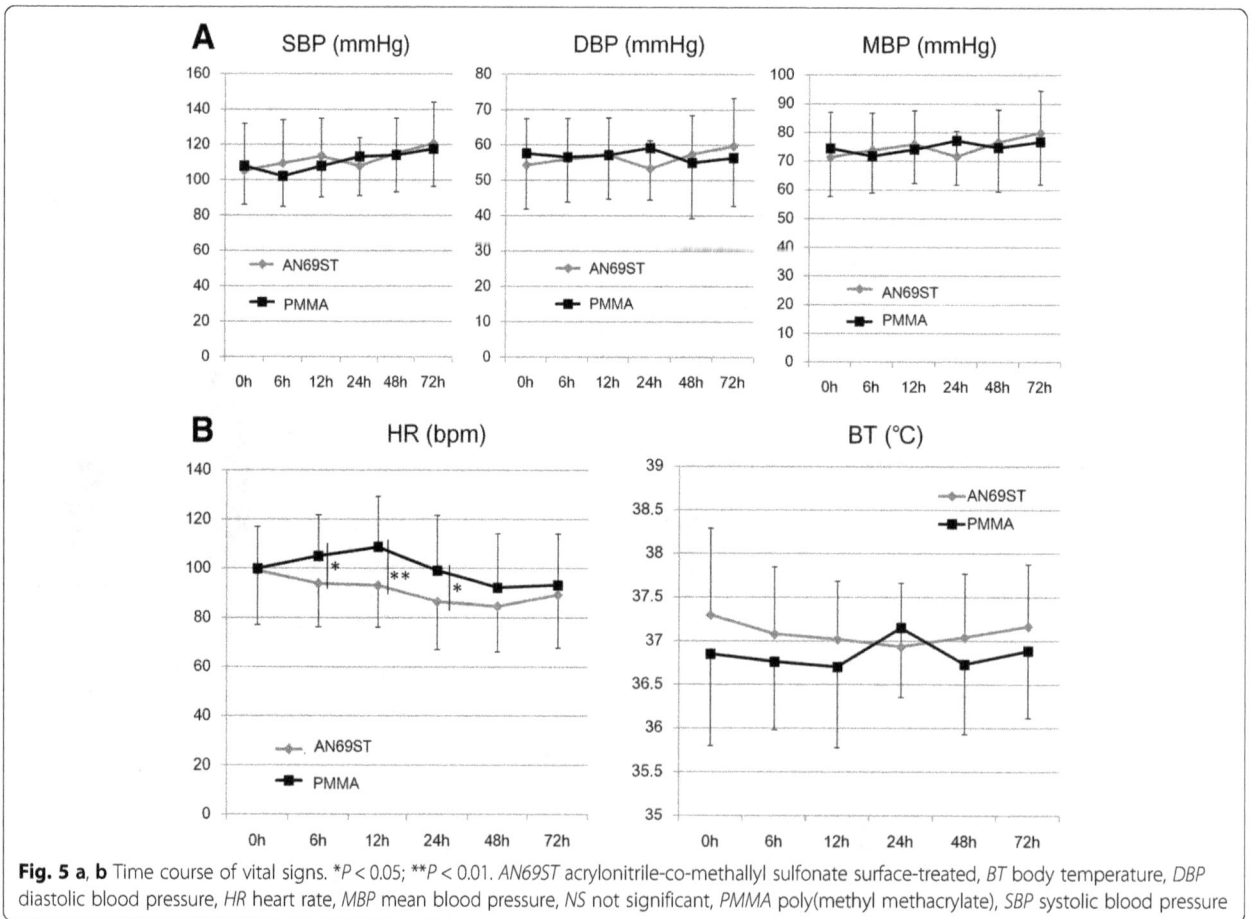

Fig. 5 a, **b** Time course of vital signs. *P < 0.05; **P < 0.01. *AN69ST* acrylonitrile-co-methallyl sulfonate surface-treated, *BT* body temperature, *DBP* diastolic blood pressure, *HR* heart rate, *MBP* mean blood pressure, *NS* not significant, *PMMA* poly(methyl methacrylate), *SBP* systolic blood pressure

There were no significant differences between groups. Figure 5b shows heart rate (HR) and body temperature in such patients. Early in the course of CHDF (6, 12, and 24 h), patients using an AN69ST membrane showed more stable HR than those using a PMMA membrane. Figure 6 shows various parameters which affect vital signs. There was no difference in CAI, fluid removal rate, or the level of albumin.

Discussion

In this study, we compared patients with sepsis who underwent CHDF using an AN69ST or PMMA membrane. AN69ST and PMMA membranes showed equivalent survival. Furthermore, patients using an AN69ST membrane demonstrated rapid stabilization of HR.

There has been no report comparing the clinical efficacy of AN69ST and PMMA membranes. Our study is distinctive in that we focused on patients with sepsis. Some previous studies have reported that CHDF using an AN69ST membrane showed significantly better survival than expected in patients with sepsis [14, 15]. The present report showed nearly equal survival between AN69ST and PMMA membranes, indicating the effectiveness of AN69ST. However, the expected survival rate from APACHE II scores is of a considerably old age, and caution is necessary because survival is considered to be further improved by the current progress in treatment.

When performing CHDF, there are renal and nonrenal indications. In the latter case, cytokine removal is the main purpose. In patients with sepsis, cytokine storm plays a central role in the pathologic condition, and cytokine removal is considered to be effective, as in this study. In the present study, there were no significant differences in urea nitrogen or creatinine levels at the start of CHDF between groups. Furthermore, because multiple intensive care unit physicians and nephrologists at a single institution decided when to start and finish CHDF by discussion, there was little deviation in the criteria for CHDF, even though different membranes with cytokine-adsorption ability were selected. In this study, although we did not measure the levels of cytokines, we presumed that rapid HR stabilization was due to cytokine removal because other parameters which affect HR, such as body temperature, dose of dopamine, fluid removal rate, and the level of albumin, did not show significant difference between both groups.

In our study, although the differences were not significant, the AN69ST group tended to have more severe values for SOFA score, lactate level, and CAI. However, the equivalent survival between groups seems to indicate the effectiveness of the AN69ST membrane. In addition, HR stabilized faster in the AN69ST group than in the PMMA group. We consider that this may be due to the difference in mechanisms: the AN69ST membrane adsorbs cytokines by utilizing an electrical charge, while the PMMA membrane adsorbs cytokines by ensnaring them in the surface pores [16]. However, because we did not measure cytokine level, we are not able to discuss this point further. Nonetheless, it is possible that cytokine easily removed by the AN69ST membrane contributed to earlier improvement of vital signs.

For comparison between membranes, we targeted patients who underwent CHDF for more than 24 h. Patients who died within 24 h after the start of CHDF were too critical to evaluate the differences between membranes. These most severe cases have pathologic conditions with advanced organ dysfunction and may require intensive treatment at an earlier stage.

The prevalence of PMX usage was significantly higher in PMMA group. In this study, after becoming available, almost all CHDF was performed using AN69ST membrane without PMX. It may be a facility trend. Because

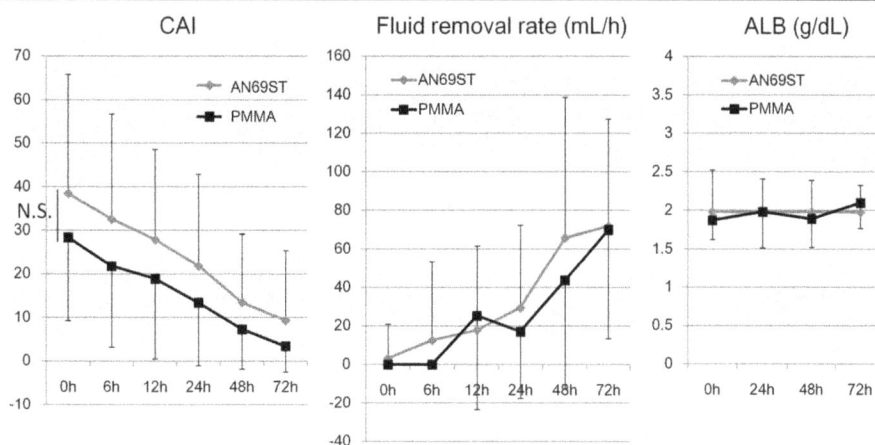

Fig. 6 Time course of various parameters. *ALB* albumin, *AN69ST* acrylonitrile-co-methallyl sulfonate surface-treated, *CAI* catecholamine index, *NS* not significant, *PMMA* poly(methyl methacrylate)

the efficacy of PMX is reported [17], identical prognosis in AN69ST membrane group with low prevalence of PMX usage may be showing advantageous aspect, comparing to PMMA group with higher prevalence of PMX usage.

On the other hand, cost of medical equipments is an important problem. As of 2016 in Japan, AN69ST membrane is about 10% more expensive than PMMA membrane. In this study, we did not examine the life span of membranes because we changed membranes every 24 h before clotting. If life span of AN69ST membrane is longer, the cost problem may be solved.

Our study has some limitations. First, because this was a retrospective study, the backgrounds of both groups were not completely matched. In addition, criteria for the start of CHDF were not clearly defined. However, because multiple physicians determined when to start and finish CHDF by discussion, it is considered that there was no large deviation in judgment. Nonetheless, the start and end criteria for CHDF should be clear. Second, we did not measure the cytokine level. Because HR was stabilized early in the AN69ST group, we should determine whether this was due to the type of cytokines that can be removed.

Conclusions
Patients who underwent CHDF using an AN69ST or PMMA membrane showed similar prognoses. Furthermore, CHDF using an AN69ST membrane may be effective for early stabilization of vital signs.

Abbreviations
AN69ST: Acrylonitrile-co-methallyl sulfonate surface-treated; APACHE II: Acute Physiology and Chronic Health Evaluation II; CAI: Catecholamine index; CHDF: Continuous hemodiafiltration; CRRT: Continuous renal replacement therapy; HR: Heart rate; PMMA: Poly(methyl methacrylate); PMX: Polymyxin B-immobilized fiber column hemoperfusion; SOFA: Sequential organ failure assessment

Acknowledgements
We would like to thank Editage (www.editage.jp) for the English language editing.

Funding
Not applicable.

Authors' contributions
AT and DI designed the study. AT performed the statistical analysis and wrote the manuscript. All authors participated in the care of the patients. All authors read and approved the final manuscript.

Competing interests
The authors declare that they have no competing interests.

Author details
[1]Kidney Disease Center, Japanese Red Cross Nagoya Daini Hospital, 2-9, Myoken-cho, Showa-ku, Nagoya 466-8650, Japan. [2]Department of Nephrology, Fujita Health University School of Medicine, Toyoake, Aichi, Japan. [3]Blood Purification Center, Japanese Red Cross Nagoya Daini Hospital, Nagoya, Japan.

References
1. Levy MM, Fink MP, Marshall JC, Abraham E, Angus D, Cook D, et al. 2001 SCCM/ESICM/ACCP/ATS/SIS International Sepsis Definitions Conference. Crit Care Med. 2003;31:1250–6.
2. Moreno RP, Metnitz B, Adler L, Hoechtl A, Bauer P, Metnitz PG, et al. Sepsis mortality prediction based on predisposition, infection and response. Intensive Care Med. 2008;34:496–504.
3. Silva E, Pedro Mde A, Sogayar AC, Mohovic T, Silva CL, Janiszewski M, et al. Brazilian Sepsis Epidemiological Study (BASES study). Crit Care. 2004;8:R251–60.
4. Bellomo R, Tipping P, Boyce N. Continuous veno-venous hemofiltration with dialysis removes cytokines from the circulation of septic patients. Crit Care Med. 1993;21:522–6.
5. Ronco C, Bellomo R, Homel P, Brendolan A, Dan M, Piccinni P, et al. Effects of different doses in continuous veno-venous haemofiltration on outcomes of acute renal failure: a prospective randomised trial. Lancet. 2000;356:26–30.
6. Saudan P, Niederberger M, De Seigneux S, Romand J, Pugin J, Perneger T, et al. Adding a dialysis dose to continuous hemofiltration increases survival in patients with acute renal failure. Kidney Int. 2006;70:1312–7.
7. RENAL Replacement Therapy Study Investigators, Bellomo R, Cass A, Cole L, Finfer S, Gallagher M, et al. Intensity of continuous renal-replacement therapy in critically ill patients. N Engl J Med. 2009;361:1627–38.
8. VA/NIH Acute Renal Failure Trial Network, Palevsky PM, Zhang JH, O'Connor TZ, Chertow GM, Crowley ST, et al. Intensity of renal support in critically ill patients with acute kidney injury. N Engl J Med. 2008;359:7–20.
9. Nakamura M, Oda S, Sadaishi T, Hirayama Y, Watanabe E, Tateishi Y, et al. Treatment of severe sepsis and septic shock by CHDF using a PMMA membrane hemofilter as a cytokine modulator. Contrib Nephrol. 2010;166:73–82.
10. Matsuda K, Moriguchi T, Harii N, Yanagisawa M, Harada D, Sugawara H. Comparison of efficacy between continuous hemodiafiltration with a PMMA high-performance membrane dialyzer and a PAN membrane hemofilter in the treatment of septic shock patients with acute renal failure. Contrib Nephrol. 2011;173:182–90.
11. Haase M, Bellomo R, Baldwin I, Haase-Fielitz A, Fealy N, Davenport P, et al. Hemodialysis membrane with a high-molecular-weight cutoff and cytokine levels in sepsis complicated by acute renal failure: a phase 1 randomized trial. Am J Kidney Dis. 2007;50:296–304.
12. Knaus WA, Draper EA, Wagner DP, Zimmerman JE. APACHE II: a severity of disease classification system. Crit Care Med. 1985;13:818–29.
13. Vincent JL, Moreno R, Takala J, Willatts S, De Mendonca A, Bruining H, et al. The SOFA (Sepsis-related Organ Failure Assessment) score to describe organ dysfunction/failure. On behalf of the Working Group on Sepsis-Related Problems of the European Society of Intensive Care Medicine. Intensive Care Med. 1996;22:707–10.
14. Shiga H, Hirasawa H, Nishida O, Oda S, Nakamura M, Mashiko K, et al. Continuous hemodiafiltration with a cytokine-adsorbing hemofilter in patients with septic shock: a preliminary report. Blood Purif. 2014;38:211–8.
15. Hirasawa H, Oda S, Nakamura M, Watanabe E, Shiga H, Matsuda K. Continuous hemodiafiltration with a cytokine-adsorbing hemofilter for sepsis. Blood Purif. 2012;34:164–70.
16. Yumoto M, Nishida O, Moriyama K, Shimomura Y, Nakamura T, Kuriyama N, et al. In vitro evaluation of high mobility group box 1 protein removal with various membranes for continuous hemofiltration. Ther Apher Dial. 2011;15:385–93.
17. Cruz DN, Antonelli M, Fumagalli R, Foltran F, Brienza N, Donati A, et al. Early use of polymyxin B hemoperfusion in abdominal septic shock: the EUPHAS randomized controlled trial. JAMA. 2009;301:2445–52.

4

Peritonitis-induced peritoneal injury models for research in peritoneal dialysis review of infectious and non-infectious models

Yasuhiko Ito[1*], Hiroshi Kinashi[1,2], Takayuki Katsuno[1], Yasuhiro Suzuki[1] and Masashi Mizuno[1]

Abstract

Peritonitis is an important complication of peritoneal dialysis. Several animal peritonitis models have been described, including bacterial and fungal models that are useful for studying inflammation in peritonitis. However, these models have limitations for investigating peritoneal fibrosis induced by acute inflammation and present difficulties in handling the infected animals. Animal models of peritonitis which induced peritoneal fibrosis are important for establishing new therapies to improve peritoneal damage induced by peritonitis. Here, we present an overview of representative animal models of peritoneal dialysis-associated infectious and non-infectious peritonitis, including our novel animal models (scraping and zymosan models) that mimic peritoneal injury associated with fibrosis and neoangiogenesis caused by bacterial or fungal peritonitis.

Keywords: Peritonitis, Non-infectious peritonitis model, Scraping model, Zymosan model

Background

There are several reasons why peritonitis is important in peritoneal dialysis (PD) treatment. First, peritonitis remains an important cause of death in PD patients. The mortality rate for peritonitis is approximately 3% [1, 2], and peritonitis is a contributing cause of death in more than 10% of PD patients [3]. Second, peritonitis remains an important factor in withdrawal from PD. In the PD registry of the Nagoya group from both 2005 to 2007 [4] and 2010 to 2012 [5], the most common reasons for withdrawal from PD have been PD-related peritonitis, followed by dialysis failure/ultrafiltration failure and social problems such as lack of family support. PD peritonitis is primarily caused by gram-positive organisms that typically result from touch contamination. The mean incidence of peritonitis as reported twice from a study over a 3-year period was one episode every 42.8 [4] and 47.3 [5] patient-months. Third, peritonitis presents a risk for the development of encapsulating peritoneal sclerosis (EPS) [6]. The duration of peritonitis is independently

associated with EPS [7]. In particular, fungal and *Pseudomonas* infections put patients at a higher risk for the development of EPS [8]. Fourth, peritonitis is one of the risks for a decrease in residual renal function. The number of peritonitis episodes has been reported to be an independent predictor of the development of anuria [9]. Fifth, peritonitis is an important cause of peritoneal membrane injury, which leads to peritoneal fibrosis, neoangiogenesis, and peritoneal dysfunction [10].

The characteristic features of chronic peritoneal damage in PD treatment are the loss of ultrafiltration capacity associated with morphological submesothelial fibrosis with extracellular matrix accumulation, and neoangiogenesis. The pathogenesis of peritoneal fibrosis is attributed to a combination of bioincompatible factors in PD fluid (PDF) and peritonitis, especially repeated episodes of peritonitis [11]. We have reported that uremia is associated with inflammation of the peritoneal membrane [12]. Histologically, acute peritonitis can cause morphological damage to the peritoneum [10, 13]. Detachment and disintegration of mesothelial cells is observed, along with the appearance of fibrin exudation and numerous infiltrating cells, ultimately resulting in internal structures becoming unrecognizable [6]. Therefore, peritonitis plays a crucial role in the

* Correspondence: yasuito@med.nagoya-u.ac.jp
[1]Department of Nephrology and Renal Replacement Therapy, Nagoya University Graduate School of Medicine, 65 Tsurumai-cho, Showa-ku, Nagoya 466-8550, Japan
Full list of author information is available at the end of the article

development of peritoneal damage leading to peritoneal membrane failure.

Animal models of peritonitis-induced peritoneal fibrosis are important for establishing new therapies to improve peritoneal damage induced by peritonitis.

Peritonitis models induced by bacteria or fungus

There are several reports of animal models of peritonitis induced by bacteria or fungi (Table 1). The pathogenic microorganisms used to induce peritonitis include *Staphylococcus aureus* [14–18], *Staphylococcus epidermidis* [19, 20], *Pseudomonas aeruginosa* [21], and *Candida albicans* [22]. These models of infectious peritonitis have been mainly used to elucidate the mechanism of inflammation in the membrane and the mechanism of acute peritoneal membrane failure. However, the acute peritonitis model is not typically used to study peritoneal fibrosis.

A catheter-induced model of gram-positive bacterial peritonitis has been developed, which is an acute bacterial peritonitis model with bacteria originating from skin flora due to lack of aseptic precautions [23–25]. In subsequent studies, these researchers used a model of lipopolysaccharide (LPS)-induced peritonitis instead of the gram-positive bacteria-induced peritonitis model [26, 27]. They investigated the role of nitric oxide (NO) released by endothelial NO synthase (eNOS) in the gram-positive bacterial peritonitis model [23] and the LPS-induced peritonitis model [27] and suggested that the selective inhibition of eNOS might ameliorate the poor peritoneal function caused by acute peritonitis. They reported that mice injected with LPS developed a cloudy dialysate with increased white blood cell counts and NO metabolite levels and inflammatory cell infiltration in the peritoneum. These observations are similar to those of the gram-positive peritonitis model.

The mechanisms of inflammation were studied in the bacterial and fungal peritonitis models; however, these models were not used to investigate the long-term complications such as fibrosis and neoangiogenesis.

Table 1 Summary of representative rodent models used to study peritoneal dialysis and its associated complications

Representative animal models		Methods	Species	Experimental period	Peritoneal dysfunction	Neoangiogenesis	Fibrosis	EPS	References
Peritonitis model									
Infectious model	Bacteria	*Staphylococcus aureus*	Mouse	2 days	No report	No report	No report	–	[14]
			Rat	2 weeks	No report	No report	±	–	[15–18]
		Staphylococcus epidermidis	Mouse	2 weeks	No report	No report	No report	–	[20]
		Pseudomonas aeruginosa	Rat	1 week	No report	No report	No report	–	[21]
	Fungus	*Candida albicans*	Mouse	1 day	No report	No report	No report	–	[22]
	Performance without aseptic precautions		Mouse	1 week	+	+	No report	–	[23]
			Rat	1 week	+	+	No report	–	[23–25]
Non-infectious model		LPS	Mouse	1 day	+	No report	No report	–	[26, 27]
			Rat	1 day	+	No report	No report	–	[28, 29]
		PDF with LPS	Rat	3–6 weeks	+	+	+	–	[29–36]
		SES	Mouse	2 days	No report	No report	No report	–	[11, 37]
		Scraping	Rat	2 weeks	+	+	+	–	[38, 39]
		Zymosan with scraping	Rat	5 weeks	No report	+	+	±	[64, 67]
		PDF	Mouse	4–5 weeks	+	+	+	–	[78–83]
			Rat	1–20 weeks	+	+	+	–	[69–77]
		Chlorhexidine	Mouse	1–8 weeks	+	+	+	+	[97–108]
			Rat	1–8 weeks	+	+	+	+	[84–96]
		Methylglyoxal	Mouse	3–7 weeks	+	+	+	+	[113, 114]
			Rat	3 weeks	+	+	+	+	[109–112]
		TGF-β1	Mouse	1–10 weeks	No report	+	+	+	[115–118]
			Rat	1–4 weeks	+	+	+	–	[119, 120]

LPS lipopolysaccharide, *PDF* peritoneal dialysis fluid, *SES* a lyophilized cell-free supernatant, *TGF-β1* transforming growth factor-β1, *EPS* encapsulating peritoneal sclerosis

Non-infectious peritonitis models

Currently, the number of reports in which investigators use the non-infectious peritonitis model is increasing. The non-infectious model is convenient and useful for handling animals and performing experiments. We suggest that a model of peritoneal fibrosis induced in a peritonitis model will help identify new strategies for preventing peritoneal fibrosis. Many studies have used the LPS-induced peritoneal injury model [26–36]. LPS derived from *Escherichia coli* (Sigma, St. Louis, MO) is frequently used [26–30, 33, 35]. A method involving a single LPS dose was used to study peritoneal inflammation and dysfunction [26–29]. Rat peritoneal inflammation and significant changes in neoangiogenesis were caused by daily administration of PDF over 3 weeks following an initial exposure to LPS [29–35].

Another non-infectious peritonitis model induced by administration of lyophilized cell-free supernatants from *Staphylococcus epidermidis* has been used to study the regulation of inflammation and leukocyte trafficking [11, 37].

Hurst et al. showed that interleukin-6 (IL-6)/soluble IL-6 receptor trans-signaling, which involves signal transducer and activator of transcription 3 (STAT3) activation, regulates chemokine secretion and polymorphonuclear neutrophil apoptosis in the peritoneal cavity. These mechanisms of inflammation and leukocyte trafficking have been clearly shown in the non-infectious model.

Here, we introduce a model of peritoneal fibrosis that we generated in rats and mice that is induced by acute inflammation with mechanical scraping, the so-called "scraping model."

Scraping model

We first reported the scraping model as a non-infectious, peritonitis-induced peritoneal fibrosis model [38]. After opening the rat abdomen under anesthesia, the right parietal peritoneum received hand-driven scratching for 1 min using the edge of a 15-ml centrifuge tube (Fig. 1). Rats freely consumed food with or without NaCl loading after surgery [38–40]. Similarly, in mice, the right parietal

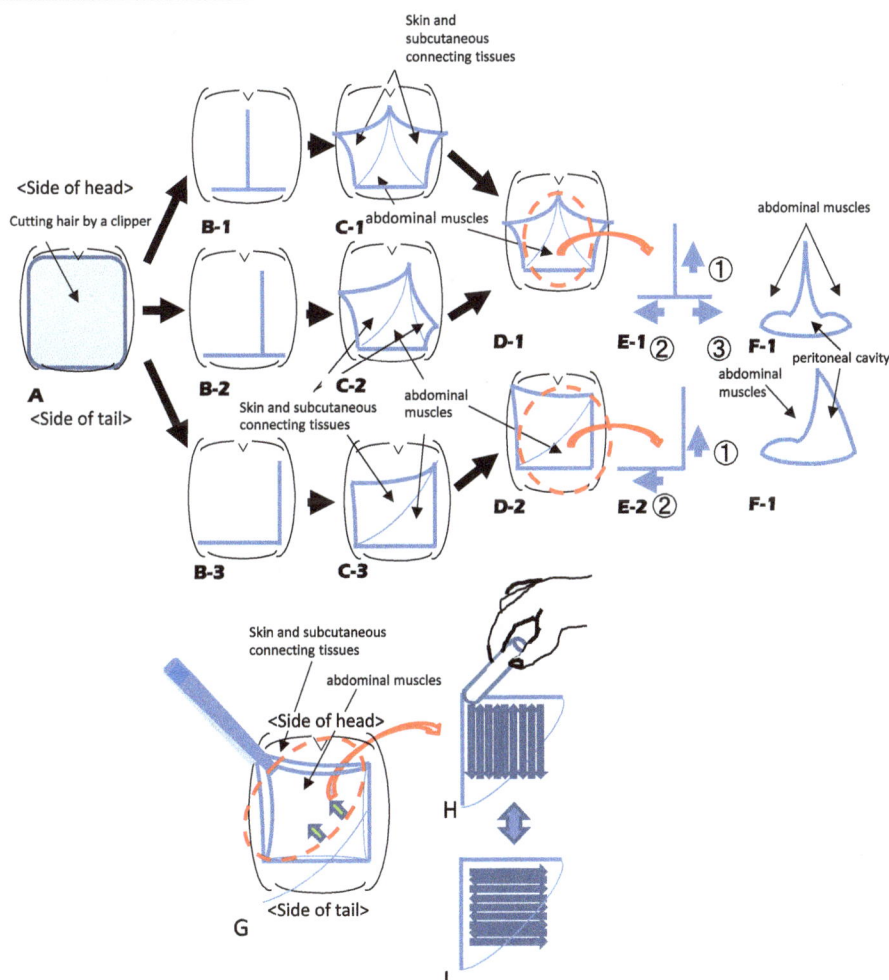

Fig. 1 Procedures to generate scraping model. Used by permission from *Methods Mol Biol* [40]

peritoneum was scraped for 90 s with the cap of an injection needle.

In this model (Fig. 2), neutrophil infiltration with fibrin exudation from the scraped peritoneum was demonstrated in 6 to 24 h after surgery. The predominant infiltrating cells switched to a mononuclear population on day 3, and inflammation gradually decreased thereafter. From days 7 to 14, the peritoneum became markedly thickened with the accumulation of alpha-smooth muscle actin (α-SMA)-positive fibroblasts and type III collagen. Mesothelial cells were not detected in 6 to 24 h after scraping, while approximately 30 and 70% of the total peritoneal length was covered with mesothelial cells on days 3 and 14, respectively. Increased CD31-positive blood vessel density was observed, which peaked at day 14. Transforming growth factor-β (TGF-β) and plasminogen activator inhibitor-1 (PAI-1), mainly expressed in the submesothelial compact zone, increased rapidly starting on day 3 and peaked at day 14. TGF-β and PAI-1 messenger RNA (mRNA) expression was upregulated from day 3 and peaked at day 7. In contrast, monocyte chemotactic protein-1 (MCP-1) mRNA rapidly increased and peaked at day 3. The pathology of this model in the early stage is characterized by strong infiltration of neutrophils and macrophages. The latter stage of this model is characterized by fibrosis and neoangiogenesis. In addition, peritoneal membrane permeability increased in rats that underwent bilateral scraping [38]. The pathological features and time course of this model are summarized in Figs. 2 and 3a.

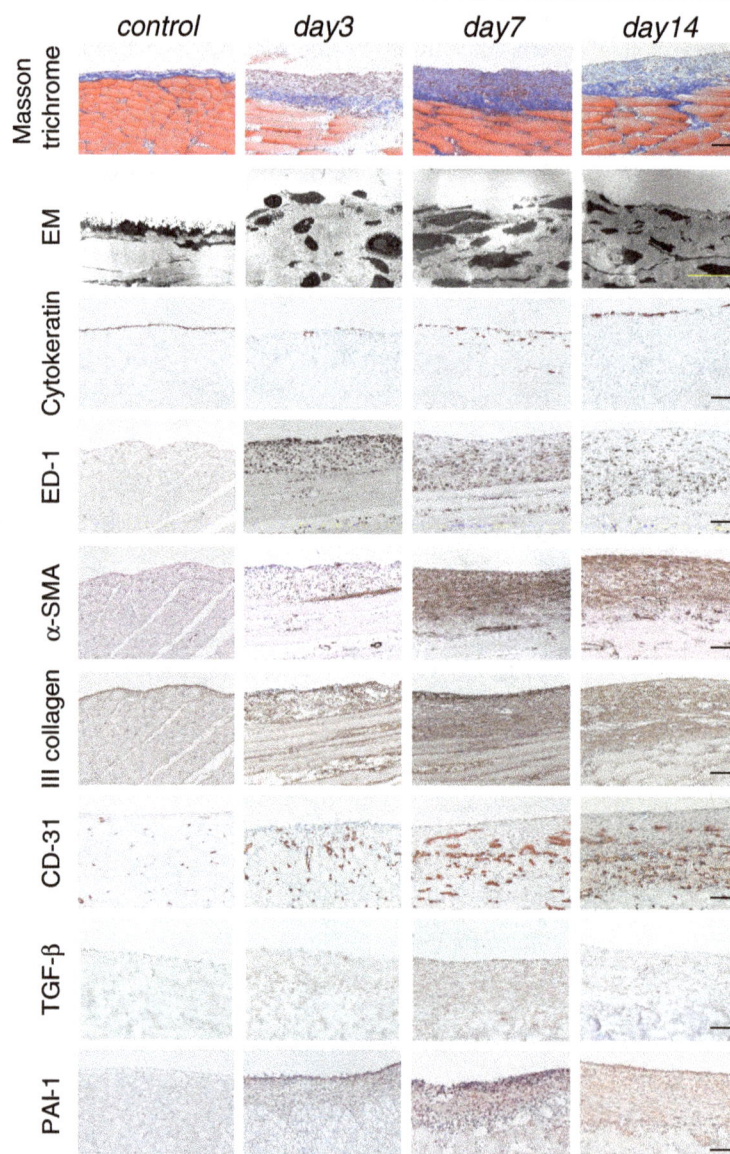

Fig. 2 Pathological findings of rat scraping model. Used by permission from *Am J Physiology* [38]

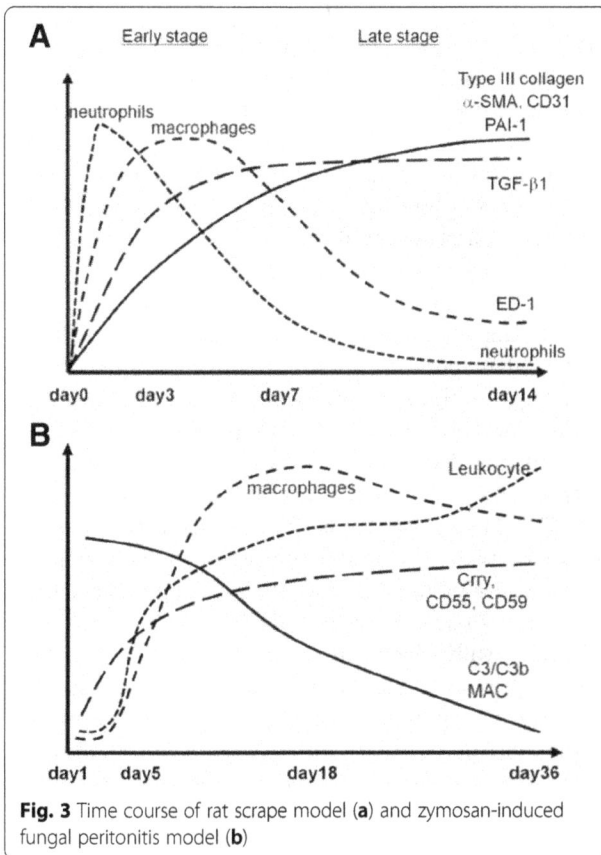

Fig. 3 Time course of rat scrape model (**a**) and zymosan-induced fungal peritonitis model (**b**)

Using this model, we investigated the effects of mineralocorticoid receptor (MR) blockade with salt loading [38]. The local renin-angiotensin-aldosterone system (RAAS) is thought to play a role in peritoneal injury in PD patients [41]. Peritoneal mesothelial cells have been observed to express angiotensinogen, angiotensin-converting enzyme (ACE), and angiotensin II type 1 receptors (AT1R) [42, 43]. We found that MRs were expressed by rat fibroblasts and scraped peritoneum. Treatment with spironolactone suppressed macrophage infiltration, neoangiogenesis, and fibrosis, which is associated with the suppression of TGF-β and PAI-1 expression, thereby resulting in improvement of peritoneal dysfunction, including ultrafiltration, glucose transport, and albumin leakage [38]. The effects of spironolactone have also been shown in the LPS-induced peritoneal injury model [36].

In addition, we demonstrated the effects of atrial natriuretic peptide (ANP) in this model [39]. ANP has been used as a diuretic and vasodilator in clinical settings. ANP has been shown to play an important function in the inhibition of RAAS [44, 45]. ANP and brain natriuretic peptide (BNP) have been reported to prevent cardiac fibrosis [44, 46] and renal fibrosis [47–49], and to reduce infarct size in acute myocardial infarction [50]. We demonstrated that AT1R, ACE, and atrial natriuretic peptide receptor (NPR-A) mRNA expression were increased and

peaked at days 14, 7, and 7, respectively. ANP administration resulted in a significant reduction in macrophage infiltration, fibrosis, and neoangiogenesis [39]. In this model, the salt loading progression of peritoneal fibrosis is likely to be involved in local RAAS activation. Administration of an MR blocker or ANP with antibiotics may prevent peritoneal membrane dysfunction associated with fibrosis and neoangiogenesis in human bacterial peritonitis. In a small study, 25 mg/day of spironolactone for 6 months was shown to reduce CD20 and collagen IV levels in the human peritoneal membrane [51]. Recently, the scraping model was used to study the effectiveness of cell therapy using the mesothelial cells to prevent peritoneal damage in PD patients [52].

Zymosan-induced fungal peritonitis model

By modifying the scraping model, we established the zymosan-induced fungal peritonitis model. Although fungal peritonitis is not common, yeast infection with the most common *Candida* species results in a poor outcome with high mortality [53–55]. The 2016 International Society for Peritoneal Dialysis guidelines recommends removal of the PD catheter in fungal peritonitis [56]. Several clinical observations have suggested that EPS could be induced by a single occurrence of fungal peritonitis [56–60]. The cell walls of many types of yeast activate various signaling reactions, including the complement system [61]. Complement maintains host homeostasis by eliminating microorganisms and irregular cells and also regulates cellular immunity. The complement system in the peritoneum is continuously active at low levels, and complement regulators (CRegs) regulate complement activation. Irregular activation of complement leads to tissue damage in many diseases [62, 63].

We demonstrated the expression of CRegs, Crry, CD55, and CD59 in rat peritoneum, especially along the mesothelial cell layer [64]. In rat peritoneum, combined blockade of Crry and CD59 induced severe focal inflammation with edema [65]. We examined the state of complement activation in the aforementioned rat scraping model, and C3 and C3b were transiently present in the inflammatory stage at day 3 [64]. Zymosan is abundant in the cell walls of fungi and activates the complement system through the alternative pathway [66].

We demonstrated that administration of zymosan after scraping promoted severe peritoneal injury that is pathologically similar to human fungal peritonitis. Zymosan (5 mg/rat/day, 2 mg/mouse/day) mixed with PDF was intraperitoneally injected into the rat or mouse abdominal cavity for up to 5 days after scraping the rat or mouse peritoneum [40, 64, 67]. Macroscopic findings in the zymosan rats showed the presence of a few white plaques at day 3, and yellow-white plaques at day 5, while no plaques were found in the control scraping model.

Plaque fusion resulted in the formation of a yellow-white sheet covering the peritoneum with numerous small vessels running into the plaques, which suggests the occurrence of peritoneal neovascularization in the zymosan model at day 5. Peritoneal thickening associated with severe infiltration of inflammatory cells continued and remained present in the zymosan model at day 36, while the peritoneum was of normal appearance in the control scraping rats.

In recent experiments, we found that disease severity was affected by the lots of the zymosan (Sigma-Aldrich, St. Louis, MO). Expression of CRegs, Crry, CD55, and CD59 transiently decreased in the control scraping model at day 5. In contrast, CRegs expression was further decreased in the zymosan model at day 5 and continued decreasing up to day 18. Complement activation products, C3b and membrane attack complex (MAC), were clearly found in the zymosan model from days 1 to 5, and small amounts of these products remained at days 18 and 36. The time course of this model is summarized in Fig. 3b.

Systemic complement depletion by cobra venom factor or local suppression of complement activation by Crry-immunoglobulin or soluble complement receptor 1 dramatically reduced complement activation, peritoneal thickening, and inflammation. These findings clearly indicated that the zymosan model is a complement-dependent model of severe proliferative peritonitis [64]. Fungal peritonitis is known to be one of the causes of EPS. Subsequently, we successfully demonstrated that further enhancement of complement activation by inhibiting CRegs and enhancing systemic activation with cobra venom factor in the zymosan model induced fibrin exudation, which is the initial event of EPS [68].

Other models of non-infectious peritoneal injury associated with inflammation and fibrosis

Administration of PDF into the abdominal cavity of rats and mice by repeated intraperitoneal injection or implanting a catheter is a method used to study the pathophysiological changes of the peritoneum associated with PD [69–83], but a non-peritonitis model. Daily intraperitoneal injection of 4.25% glucose dialysate into the rat abdominal cavity for 1 week induced an increased peritoneal membrane transport rate and the absence of the peritoneal surface layer, as observed by electron microscopy [69, 70]. Daily injection of PDF (100 ml/kg, once or twice daily) was performed for up to 8 or 12 weeks to obtain morphological changes in the rat peritoneum [71–73]. Implantation of a silicon catheter into the rat abdomen was reported to amplify peritoneal inflammation from PDF through a foreign body reaction [74]. However, the peritoneum of rats that received only a puncture without infusion of any solution showed no functional or pathological changes [73, 75].

A model of renal insufficiency, such as 5/6 nephrectomy, was used in combination with PDF infusion to closely model the clinical situation of peritoneal dialysis patients and to understand the influence of PD on residual renal function [76, 77]. Daily intraperitoneal exposure of 1.5–3.0 ml of 4.25% glucose PDF for 4 or 5 weeks, with or without implanting a catheter, produced peritoneal dysfunction and morphological changes, such as fibrosis and neoangiogenesis, in mice [78–83].

Chronic intraperitoneal exposure to chemical irritation (chlorhexidine gluconate (CG)) is used as an experimental model of peritoneal fibrosis with inflammation and EPS. Suga et al. developed a CG-induced peritoneal fibrosis model in rats [84]. Daily injection of 0.1% CG in 15% ethanol, dissolved in 2–3 ml saline per 200 g body weight, was administered in the rat peritoneal cavity [85–87]. At day 7, the peritoneal tissue was partially thickened with edema and showed initial accumulation of connective tissues and modest cell migration. At day 14, significant alterations were found, including peritoneal thickening with edema, cell infiltration, and neoangiogenesis. At days 21 to 28, the peritoneal tissue was markedly thickened and showed remarkable proliferation of collagen fibers. The number of macrophages gradually increased in the thickened areas and reached a maximum at day 21. At day 28, neoangiogenesis had decreased, whereas collagen fibrils had accumulated. At day 35, fibrillary elements with cell infiltration occupied the submesothelial zone. Peritoneal resting for 3 weeks after 3 weeks of CG exposure ameliorated some functional parameters in the peritoneum; however, elevated peritoneal thickness and fibrosis continued during the resting period [88–91]. Placing an infusion pump in the rat abdominal cavity was reported as an alternative administration route for CG [92–94].

A lower dosage of CG is an option for producing mild peritoneal injury [95, 96]. Mice were given daily intraperitoneal administration of 0.3 ml or 10 ml saline/kg body weight containing 0.1% CG in 15% ethanol [97, 98]. Peritoneal fibrosis and increased infiltration of mononuclear cells were observed over time. Peritoneal fibrosis reached the chronic inflammatory stage, and macroscopic evidence of EPS was observed by 8 weeks. Lower doses of CG or shorter time courses produced milder and more infrequent development of peritoneal fibrosis [99, 100]. Recent studies showed that a standard peritoneal fibrosis model could be produced in mice following treatment with 0.1% CG every other day or three times a week for 1–3 weeks [101–108].

Glucose degradation products contained in PDF contribute to the biocompatibility of conventional PDF and are risk factors for EPS. Methylglyoxal (MGO) is an extremely toxic glucose degradation product, and administration of PDF containing MGO can be used as an animal peritoneal fibrosis model. Rats were given intraperitoneal injections of 100 ml/kg of 2.5% glucose PDF (pH 5.0) containing 20 mM MGO every day for 3 weeks [109–111]. Peritoneal function decreased significantly, and fibrous peritoneal thickening with proliferation of mesenchymal-like mesothelial cells and abdominal cocoon was induced. The combination of low doses of MGO and adenine-induced renal failure accelerated the progression of fibrous peritoneal thickening, whereas both MGO and renal failure alone did not [112]. Intraperitoneal injection of PDF (100 ml/kg) containing 20 or 40 mM MGO for five consecutive days per week for 3 weeks induced peritoneal injury in mice [113, 114]. We clearly showed the presence of severe lymphangiogenesis in the diaphragm of both CG and MGO models [96, 114]. TGF-β is a central mediator of peritoneal fibrosis. Overexpression of TGF-β1 driven by intraperitoneal adenovirus administration induced peritoneal fibrosis through epithelial mesenchymal transition, neoangiogenesis, and poor peritoneal function in mice [115–118] and rats [119, 120]. Other chemical irritants, such as deoxycholate [121], household bleach [122] and acidic solutions [123], were also reported to produce peritoneal inflammation, fibrosis, and abdominal cocoon in rats.

Conclusions

Non-infectious peritonitis models are convenient and useful for animal handling and performing experiments. The peritoneum in the scraping model showed signs of peritonitis initially and fibrosis at a later stage. These pathological changes, along with alterations in solute transport, mimic those observed in bacterial peritonitis. This model is useful for exploring strategies for the treatment and prevention of peritoneal fibrosis and membrane failure. The zymosan model is useful for studying the mechanisms of fungal peritonitis and the drugs used to reduce peritoneal damage induced by fungal peritonitis. Anti-complement therapy might be useful as a therapeutic in human fungal peritonitis and related peritoneal damage. Other non-infectious models, such as CG and MGO models, are also useful for investigating the pathophysiology of fibrosis with inflammation, angiogenesis, and lymphangiogenesis.

Abbreviations
ACE: Angiotensin-converting enzyme; ANP: Atrial natriuretic peptide; AT1R: Angiotensin II type 1 receptors; BNP: Brain natriuretic peptide; CG: Chlorhexidine gluconate; CRegs: Complement regulators; eNOS: Endothelial NO synthase; IL-6: Interleukin-6; LPS: Lipopolysaccharide; MAC: Membrane attack complex; MCP-1: Monocyte chemotactic protein-1; MGO: Methylglyoxal; MR: Mineralocorticoid receptor; NO: Nitric oxide; NPR-A: Natriuretic peptide receptor; PD: Peritoneal dialysis; PDF: PD fluid; RAAS: Renin-angiotensin-aldosterone system; STAT3: Signal transducer and activator of transcription 3; TGF-β: Transforming growth factor-β; α-SMA: Alpha-smooth muscle actin

Acknowledgements
This work was supported in part by a Grant-in-Aid for Scientific Research from the Ministry of Education, Science and Culture of Japan (YI, # 20590972).

Funding
There is no funding. The authors declare that no financial conflict of interest exists.

Authors' contributions
YI and HK planned the study, searched and collected the literatures, and wrote the manuscript. All the authors wrote the manuscript partly. TK, YS, and MM discussed the contents of the manuscript with YI and HK. All authors read and approved the final manuscript.

Competing interests
The authors declare that they have no competing interests.

Author details
[1]Department of Nephrology and Renal Replacement Therapy, Nagoya University Graduate School of Medicine, 65 Tsurumai-cho, Showa-ku, Nagoya 466-8550, Japan. [2]Department of Pathology, University Medical Center Utrecht, Utrecht, The Netherlands.

References
1. Brown MC, Simpson K, Kerssens JJ, Mactier RA, Scottish Renal Registry. Peritoneal dialysis-associated peritonitis rates and outcomes in a national cohort are not improving in the post-millennium (2000–2007). Perit Dial Int. 2011;31:639–50.
2. Davenport A. Peritonitis remains the major clinical complication of peritoneal dialysis: the London, UK, peritonitis audit 2002–2003. Perit Dial Int. 2009;29:297–302.
3. Pajek J, Hutchison AJ, Bhutani S, Brenchley PE, Hurst H, Perme MP, et al. Outcomes of peritoneal dialysis patients and switching to hemodialysis: a competing risks analysis. Perit Dial Int. 2014;34:289–98.
4. Mizuno M, Ito Y, Tanaka A, Suzuki Y, Hiramatsu H, Watanabe M, et al. Peritonitis is still an important factor for withdrawal from peritoneal dialysis therapy in the Tokai area of Japan. Clin Exp Nephrol. 2011;15:727–37.
5. Mizuno M, Ito Y, Suzuki Y, Sakata F, Saka Y, Hiramatsu T, et al. Recent analysis of status and outcomes of peritoneal dialysis in the Tokai area of Japan: the second report of the Tokai peritoneal dialysis registry. Clin Exp Nephrol. 2016;20:960–97.
6. Tawada M, Ito Y, Hamada C, Honda K, Mizuno M, Suzuki Y, et al. Vascular endothelial cell injury is an important factor in the development of encapsulating peritoneal sclerosis in long-term peritoneal dialysis patients. PLoS One. 2016;11:e0154644.
7. Nakao M, Yokoyama K, Yamamoto I, Matsuo N, Tanno Y, Ohkido I, et al. Risk factors for encapsulating peritoneal sclerosis in long-term peritoneal dialysis: a retrospective observational study. Ther Apher Dial. 2014;18:68–73.
8. Kawanishi H, Moriishi M. Epidemiology of encapsulating peritoneal sclerosis in Japan. Perit Dial Int. 2005;25(Suppl 4):S14–8.
9. Szeto CC, Kwan BC, Chow KM, Chung S, Yu V, Cheng PM, et al. Predictors of residual renal function decline in patients undergoing continuous ambulatory peritoneal dialysis. Perit Dial Int. 2015;35:180–8.
10. Williams JD, Craig KJ, Topley N, Von Ruhland C, Fallon M, Newman GR, et al. Morphologic changes in the peritoneal membrane of patients with renal disease. J Am Soc Nephrol. 2002;13:470–9.
11. Devuyst O, Margetts PJ, Topley N. The pathophysiology of the peritoneal membrane. J Am Soc Nephrol. 2010;21:1077–85.
12. Sawai A, Ito Y, Mizuno M, Suzuki Y, Toda S, Ito I, et al. Peritoneal macrophage infiltration is correlated with baseline peritoneal solute transport rate in peritoneal dialysis patients. Nephrol Dial Transplant. 2011;26:2322–32.

13. Verger C, Luger A, Moore HL, Nolph KD. Acute changes in peritoneal morphology and transport properties with infectious peritonitis and mechanical injury. Kidney Int. 1983;23:823–31.

14. Catalan MP, Esteban J, Subirá D, Egido J, Ortiz A, Grupo de Estudios Peritoneales de Madrid-FRIAT/IRSIN. Inhibition of caspases improves bacterial clearance in experimental peritonitis. Perit Dial Int. 2003;23:123–6.

15. Calame W, Afram C, Blijleven N, Hendrickx RJ, Namavar F, Beelen RH. Establishing an experimental infection model for peritoneal dialysis: effect of inoculum and volume. Perit Dial Int. 1993;13(Suppl 2):S79–80.

16. Welten AG, Zareie M, van den Born J, ter Wee PM, Schalkwijk CG, Driesprong BA, et al. In vitro and in vivo models for peritonitis demonstrate unchanged neutrophil migration after exposure to dialysis fluids. Nephrol Dial Transplant. 2004;19:831–9.

17. van Westrhenen R, Westra WM, van den Born J, Krediet RT, Keuning ED, Hiralall J, et al. Alpha-2-macroglobulin and albumin are useful serum proteins to detect subclinical peritonitis in the rat. Perit Dial Int. 2006;26:101–7.

18. Akman S, Koyun M, Gelen T, Coskun M. Comparison of intraperitoneal antithrombin III and heparin in experimental peritonitis. Pediatr Nephrol. 2008;23:1327–30.

19. Mactier RA, Moore H, Khanna R, Shah J. Effect of peritonitis on insulin and glucose absorption during peritoneal dialysis in diabetic rats. Nephron. 1990;54:240–4.

20. Gallimore B, Gagnon RF, Richards GK. Response of chronic renal failure mice to peritoneal Staphylococcus epidermidis challenge: impact of repeated peritoneal instillation of dialysis solution. Am J Kidney Dis. 1989;14:184–95.

21. Finelli A, Burrows LL, DiCosmo FA, DiTizio V, Sinnadurai S, Oreopoulos DG, et al. Colonization-resistant antimicrobial-coated peritoneal dialysis catheters: evaluation in a newly developed rat model of persistent Pseudomonas aeruginosa peritonitis. Perit Dial Int. 2002;22:27–31.

22. Kretschmar M, Hube B, Bertsch T, Sanglard D, Merker R, Schröder M, et al. Germ tubes and proteinase activity contribute to virulence of Candida albicans in murine peritonitis. Infect Immun. 1999;67:6637–42.

23. Ni J, Moulin P, Gianello P, Feron O, Balligand JL, Devuyst O. Mice that lack endothelial nitric oxide synthase are protected against functional and structural modifications induced by acute peritonitis. J Am Soc Nephrol. 2003;14:3205–16.

24. Combet S, Van Landschoot M, Moulin P, Piech A, Verbavatz JM, Goffin E, et al. Regulation of aquaporin-1 and nitric oxide synthase isoforms in a rat model of acute peritonitis. J Am Soc Nephrol. 1999;10:2185–96.

25. Ferrier ML, Combet S, van Landschoot M, Stoenoiu MS, Cnops Y, Lameire N, et al. Inhibition of nitric oxide synthase reverses changes in peritoneal permeability in a rat model of acute peritonitis. Kidney Int. 2001;60:2343–50.

26. Ni J, Cnops Y, McLoughlin RM, Topley N, Devuyst O. Inhibition of nitric oxide synthase reverses permeability changes in a mouse model of acute peritonitis. Perit Dial Int. 2005;25(Suppl 3):S11–4.

27. Ni J, McLoughlin RM, Brodovitch A, Moulin P, Brouckaert P, Casadei B, et al. Nitric oxide synthase isoforms play distinct roles during acute peritonitis. Nephrol Dial Transplant. 2010;25:86–96.

28. Breborowicz A, Połubinska A, Wu G, Tam P, Oreopoulos DG. N-acetylglucosamine reduces inflammatory response during acute peritonitis in uremic rats. Blood Purif. 2006;24:274–81.

29. Korybalska K, Wieczorowska-Tobis K, Polubinska A, Wisniewska J, Moberly J, Martis L, et al. L-2-oxothiazolidine-4-carboxylate: an agent that modulates lipopolysaccharide-induced peritonitis in rats. Perit Dial Int. 2002;22:293–300.

30. Kim YL, Kim SH, Kim JH, Kim SJ, Kim CD, Cho DK, et al. Effects of peritoneal rest on peritoneal transport and peritoneal membrane thickening in continuous ambulatory peritoneal dialysis rats. Perit Dial Int. 1999;19(Suppl 2):S384–7.

31. Margetts PJ, Kolb M, Yu L, Hoff CM, Gauldie J. A chronic inflammatory infusion model of peritoneal dialysis in rats. Perit Dial Int. 2001;21(Suppl 3):S368–72.

32. Margetts PJ, Gyorffy S, Kolb M, Yu L, Hoff CM, Holmes CJ, et al. Antiangiogenic and antifibrotic gene therapy in a chronic infusion model of peritoneal dialysis in rats. J Am Soc Nephrol. 2002;13:721–8.

33. Park SH, Lee EG, Kim IS, Kim YJ, Cho DK, Kim YL. Effect of glucose degradation products on the peritoneal membrane in a chronic inflammatory infusion model of peritoneal dialysis in the rat. Perit Dial Int. 2004;24:115–22.

34. Nie J, Hao W, Dou X, Wang X, Luo N, Lan HY, et al. Effects of Smad7 overexpression on peritoneal inflammation in a rat peritoneal dialysis model. Perit Dial Int. 2007;27:580–8.

35. Song SH, Kwak IS, Yang BY, Lee DW, Lee SB, Lee MY. Role of rosiglitazone in lipopolysaccharide-induced peritonitis: a rat peritoneal dialysis model. Nephrology (Carlton). 2009;14:155–63.

36. Zhang L, Hao JB, Ren LS, Ding JL, Hao LR. The aldosterone receptor antagonist spironolactone prevents peritoneal inflammation and fibrosis. Lab Invest. 2014;94:839–50.

37. Hurst SM, Wilkinson TS, McLoughlin RM, Jones S, Horiuchi S, Yamamoto N, et al. Il-6 and its soluble receptor orchestrate a temporal switch in the pattern of leukocyte recruitment seen during acute inflammation. Immunity. 2001;14:705–14.

38. Nishimura H, Ito Y, Mizuno M, Tanaka A, Morita Y, Maruyama S, et al. Mineralocorticoid receptor blockade ameliorates peritoneal fibrosis in new rat peritonitis model. Am J Physiol Renal Physiol. 2008;294:F1084–93.

39. Kato H, Mizuno T, Mizuno M, Sawai A, Suzuki Y, Kinashi H, et al. Atrial natriuretic peptide ameliorates peritoneal fibrosis in rat peritonitis model. Nephrol Dial Transplant. 2012;27:526–36.

40. Mizuno M, Ito Y. Rat models of acute and/or chronic peritoneal injuries including peritoneal fibrosis and peritoneal dialysis complications. Methods Mol Biol. 2016;1397:35–43.

41. Nessim SJ, Perl J, Bargman JM. The renin-angiotensin-aldosterone system in peritoneal dialysis: is what is good for the kidney also good for the peritoneum? Kidney Int. 2010;78:23–8.

42. Noh H, Ha H, Yu MR, Kim YO, Kim JH, Lee HB. Angiotensin II mediates high glucose-induced TGF-beta1 and fibronectin upregulation in HPMC through reactive oxygen species. Perit Dial Int. 2005;25:38–47.

43. Kiribayashi K, Masaki T, Naito T, Ogawa T, Ito T, Yorioka N, et al. Angiotensin II induces fibronectin expression in human peritoneal mesothelial cells via ERK1/2 and p38 MAPK. Kidney Int. 2005;67:1126–35.

44. Tsuneyoshi H, Nishina T, Nomoto T, Kanemitsu H, Kawakami R, Unimonh O, et al. Atrial natriuretic peptide helps prevent late remodeling after left ventricular aneurysm repair. Circulation. 2004;110(11 Suppl 1):II174–9.

45. Kasama S, Furuya M, Toyama T, Ichikawa S, Kurabayashi M. Effect of atrial natriuretic peptide on left ventricular remodelling in patients with acute myocardial infarction. Eur Heart J. 2008;29:1485–94.

46. Ito T, Yoshimura M, Nakamura S, Nakayama M, Shimasaki Y, Harada E, et al. Inhibitory effect of natriuretic peptides on aldosterone synthase gene expression in cultured neonatal rat cardiocytes. Circulation. 2003;107:807–10.

47. Kasahara M, Mukoyama M, Sugawara A, Makino H, Suganami T, Ogawa Y, et al. Ameliorated glomerular injury in mice overexpressing brain natriuretic peptide with renal ablation. J Am Soc Nephrol. 2000;11:1691–701.

48. Suganami T, Mukoyama M, Sugawara A, Mori K, Nagae T, Kasahara M, et al. Overexpression of brain natriuretic peptide in mice ameliorates immune-mediated renal injury. J Am Soc Nephrol. 2001;12:2652–63.

49. Makino H, Mukoyama M, Mori K, Suganami T, Kasahara M, Yahata K, et al. Transgenic overexpression of brain natriuretic peptide prevents the progression of diabetic nephropathy in mice. Diabetologia. 2006;49:2514–24.

50. Kitakaze M, Asakura M, Kim J, Shintani Y, Asanuma H, Hamasaki I, et al. Human atrial natriuretic peptide and nicorandil as adjuncts to reperfusion treatment for acute myocardial infarction (J-WIND): two randomised trials. Lancet. 2007;370:1483–92.

51. Vazquez-Rangel A, Soto V, Escalona M, Toledo RG, Castillo EA, Polanco Flores NA, et al. Spironolactone to prevent peritoneal fibrosis in peritoneal dialysis patients: a randomized controlled trial. Am J Kidney Dis. 2014;63:1072–4.

52. Kitamura S, Horimoto N, Tsuji K, Inoue A, Takiue K, Sugiyama H, et al. The selection of peritoneal mesothelial cells is important for cell therapy to prevent peritoneal fibrosis. Tissue Eng Part A. 2014;20:529–39.

53. Nagappan R, Collins JF, Lee WT. Fungal peritonitis in continuous ambulatory peritoneal dialysis—the Auckland experience. Am J Kidney Dis. 1992;20:492–6.

54. Wang AY, Yu AW, Li PK, Lam PK, Leung CB, Lai KN, et al. Factors predicting outcome of fungal peritonitis in peritoneal dialysis: analysis of a 9-year experience of fungal peritonitis in a single center. Am J Kidney Dis. 2000;36:1183–92.

55. Felgueiras J, del Peso G, Bajo A, Hevia C, Romero S, Celadilla O, et al. Risk of technique failure and death in fungal peritonitis is determined mainly by duration on peritoneal dialysis: single-center experience of 24 years. Adv Perit Dial. 2006;22:77–81.

56. Li PK, Szeto CC, Piraino B, de Arteaga J, Fan S, Figueiredo AE, et al. ISPD peritonitis recommendations: 2016 update on prevention and treatment. Perit Dial Int. 2016;36:481–508.

57. Rigby RJ, Hawley CM. Sclerosing peritonitis: the experience in Australia. Nephrol Dial Transplant. 1998;13:154–9.

58. Lee HY, Kim BS, Choi HY, Park HC, Kang SW, Choi KH, et al. Sclerosing encapsulating peritonitis as a complication of long-term continuous ambulatory peritoneal dialysis in Korea. Nephrology (Carlton). 2003;8(Suppl 1):S33–9.

59. Gupta S, Woodrow G. Successful treatment of fulminant encapsulating peritoneal sclerosis following fungal peritonitis with tamoxifen. Clin Nephrol. 2007;68:125–9.

60. Trigka K, Dousdampanis P, Chu M, Khan S, Ahmad M, Bargman JM, et al. Encapsulating peritoneal sclerosis: a single-center experience and review of the literature. Int Urol Nephrol. 2011;43:519–26.

61. Sorenson WG, Shahan TA, Simpson J. Cell wall preparations from environmental yeasts: effect on alveolar macrophage function in vitro. Ann Agric Environ Med. 1998;5:65–71.

62. Mizuno M, Morgan BP. The possibilities and pitfalls for anti-complement therapies in inflammatory diseases. Curr Drug Targets Inflamm Allergy. 2004;3;87–96.

63. Mizuno M. A review of current knowledge of the complement system and the therapeutic opportunities in inflammatory arthritis. Curr Med Chem. 2006;13:1707–17.

64. Mizuno M, Ito Y, Hepburn N, Mizuno T, Noda Y, Yuzawa Y, et al. Zymosan, but not lipopolysaccharide, triggers severe and progressive peritoneal injury accompanied by complement activation in a rat peritonitis model. J Immunol. 2009;183:1403–12.

65. Mizuno T, Mizuno M, Morgan BP, Noda Y, Yamada K, Okada N, et al. Specific collaboration between rat membrane complement regulators Crry and CD59 protects peritoneum from damage by autologous complement activation. Nephrol Dial Transplant. 2011;26:1821–30.

66. Rawal N, Pangburn MK. C5 convertase of the alternative pathway of complement. Kinetic analysis of the free and surface-bound forms of the enzyme. J Biol Chem. 1998;273:16828–35.

67. Kim H, Mizuno M, Furuhashi K, Katsuno T, Ozaki T, Yasuda K, et al. Rat adipose tissue-derived stem cells attenuate peritoneal injuries in rat zymosan-induced peritonitis accompanied by complement activation. Cytotherapy. 2014;16:357–68.

68. Mizuno M, Ito Y, Mizuno T, Harris CL, Suzuki Y, Okada N, et al. Membrane complement regulators protect against fibrin exudation increases in a severe peritoneal inflammation model in rats. Am J Physiol Renal Physiol. 2012;302:F1245–51.

69. Guo QY, Peng WX, Cheng HH, Ye RG, Lindholm B, Wang T. Hyaluronan preserves peritoneal membrane transport properties. Perit Dial Int. 2001;21:136–42.

70. Wang T, Cheng HH, Liu SM, Wang Y, Wu JL, Peng WX, et al. Increased peritoneal membrane permeability is associated with abnormal peritoneal surface layer. Perit Dial Int. 2001;21(Suppl 3):S345–8.

71. Chunming J, Miao Z, Cheng S, Nana T, Wei Z, Dongwei C, et al. Tanshinone IIA attenuates peritoneal fibrosis through inhibition of fibrogenic growth factors expression in peritoneum in a peritoneal dialysis rat model. Ren Fail. 2011;33:355–62.

72. Lee EA, Oh JH, Lee HA, Kim SI, Park EW, Park KB, et al. Structural and functional alterations of the peritoneum after prolonged exposure to dialysis solutions: role of aminoguanidine. Perit Dial Int. 2001;21:245–53.

73. Musi B, Braide M, Carlsson O, Wieslander A, Albrektsson A, Ketteler M, et al. Biocompatibility of peritoneal dialysis fluids: long-term exposure of nonuremic rats. Perit Dial Int. 2004;24:37–47.

74. Flessner MF, Credit K, Richardson K, Potter R, Li X, He Z, et al. Peritoneal inflammation after twenty-week exposure to dialysis solution: effect of solution versus catheter-foreign body reaction. Perit Dial Int. 2010;30:284–93.

75. Zeltzer E, Klein O, Rashid G, Katz D, Korzets Z, Bernheim J. Intraperitoneal infusion of glucose-based dialysate in the rat—an animal model for the study of peritoneal advanced glycation end-products formation and effect on peritoneal transport. Perit Dial Int. 2000;20:656–61.

76. Nakao A, Nakao K, Takatori Y, Kojo S, Inoue J, Akagi S, et al. Effects of icodextrin peritoneal dialysis solution on the peritoneal membrane in the STZ-induced diabetic rat model with partial nephrectomy. Nephrol Dial Transplant. 2010;25:1479–88.

77. Kihm LP, Müller-Krebs S, Klein J, Ehrlich G, Mertes L, Gross ML, et al. Benfotiamine protects against peritoneal and kidney damage in peritoneal dialysis. J Am Soc Nephrol. 2011;22:914–26.

78. Wang J, Jiang ZP, Su N, Fan JJ, Ruan YP, Peng WX, et al. The role of peritoneal alternatively activated macrophages in the process of peritoneal fibrosis related to peritoneal dialysis. Int J Mol Sci. 2013;14:10369–82.

79. Duan WJ, Yu X, Huang XR, Yu JW, Lan HY. Opposing roles for Smad2 and Smad3 in peritoneal fibrosis in vivo and in vitro. Am J Pathol. 2014;184:2275–84.

80. Yu JW, Duan WJ, Huang XR, Meng XM, Yu XQ, Lan HY. MicroRNA-29b inhibits peritoneal fibrosis in a mouse model of peritoneal dialysis. Lab Invest. 2014;94:978–90.

81. Aroeira LS, Lara-Pezzi E, Loureiro J, Aguilera A, Ramírez-Huesca M, González-Mateo G, et al. Cyclooxygenase-2 mediates dialysate-induced alterations of the peritoneal membrane. J Am Soc Nephrol. 2009;20:582–92.

82. Loureiro J, Aguilera A, Selgas R, Sandoval P, Albar-Vizcaíno P, Pérez-Lozano ML, et al. Blocking TGF-β1 protects the peritoneal membrane from dialysate-induced damage. J Am Soc Nephrol. 2011;22:1682–95.

83. Loureiro J, Sandoval P, del Peso G, Gónzalez-Mateo G, Fernández-Millara V, Santamaria B, et al. Tamoxifen ameliorates peritoneal membrane damage by blocking mesothelial to mesenchymal transition in peritoneal dialysis. PLoS One. 2013;8:e61165.

84. Suga H, Teraoka S, Ota K, Komemushi S, Furutani S, Yamauchi S, et al. Preventive effect of pirfenidone against experimental sclerosing peritonitis in rats. Exp Toxicol Pathol. 1995;47:287–91.

85. Mishima Y, Miyazaki M, Abe K, Ozono Y, Shioshita K, Xia Z, et al. Enhanced expression of heat shock protein 47 in rat model of peritoneal fibrosis. Perit Dial Int. 2003;23:14–22.

86. Nishino T, Miyazaki M, Abe K, Furusu A, Mishima Y, Harada T, et al. Antisense oligonucleotides against collagen-binding stress protein HSP47 suppress peritoneal fibrosis in rats. Kidney Int. 2003;64:887–96.

87. Io H, Hamada C, Ro Y, Ito Y, Hirahara I, Tomino Y. Morphologic changes of peritoneum and expression of VEGF in encapsulated peritoneal sclerosis rat models. Kidney Int. 2004;65:1927–36.

88. Bozkurt D, Hur E, Ulkuden B, Sezak M, Nar H, Purclutepe O, et al. Can N-acetylcysteine preserve peritoneal function and morphology in encapsulating peritoneal sclerosis? Perit Dial Int. 2009;29(Suppl 2):S202–5.

89. Bozkurt D, Sipahi S, Cetin P, Hur E, Ozdemir O, Ertilav M, et al. Does immunosuppressive treatment ameliorate morphology changes in encapsulating peritoneal sclerosis? Perit Dial Int. 2009;29(Suppl 2):S206–10.

90. Ertilav M, Hur E, Bozkurt D, Sipahi S, Timur O, Sarsik B, et al. Octreotide lessens peritoneal injury in experimental encapsulated peritoneal sclerosis model. Nephrology (Carlton). 2011;16:552–7.

91. Huddam B, Başaran M, Koçak G, Azak A, Yalçın F, Reyhan NH, et al. The use of mycophenolate mofetil in experimental encapsulating peritoneal sclerosis. Int Urol Nephrol. 2015;47:1423–8.

92. Komatsu H, Uchiyama K, Tsuchida M, Isoyama N, Matsumura M, Hara T, et al. Development of a peritoneal sclerosis rat model using a continuous-infusion pump. Perit Dial Int. 2008;28:641–7.

93. Kanda R, Hamada C, Kaneko K, Nakano T, Wakabayashi K, Hara K, et al. Paracrine effects of transplanted mesothelial cells isolated from temperature-sensitive SV40 large T-antigen gene transgenic rats during peritoneal repair. Nephrol Dial Transplant. 2014;29:289–300.

94. Wakabayashi K, Hamada C, Kanda R, Nakano T, Io H, Horikoshi S, et al. Adipose-derived mesenchymal stem cells transplantation facilitate experimental peritoneal fibrosis repair by suppressing epithelial-mesenchymal transition. J Nephrol. 2014;27:507–14.

95. Saito H, Kitamoto M, Kato K, Liu N, Kitamura H, Uemura K, et al. Tissue factor and factor v involvement in rat peritoneal fibrosis. Perit Dial Int. 2009;29:340–51.

96. Kinashi H, Ito Y, Mizuno M, Suzuki Y, Terabayashi T, Nagura F, et al. TGF-β1 promotes lymphangiogenesis during peritoneal fibrosis. J Am Soc Nephrol. 2013;24:1627–42.

97. Ishii Y, Sawada T, Shimizu A, Tojimbara T, Nakajima I, Fuchinoue S, et al. An experimental sclerosing encapsulating peritonitis model in mice. Nephrol Dial Transplant. 2001;16:1262–6.

98. Sawada T, Ishii Y, Tojimbara T, Nakajima I, Fuchinoue S, Teraoka S. The ACE inhibitor, quinapril, ameliorates peritoneal fibrosis in an encapsulating peritoneal sclerosis model in mice. Pharmacol Res. 2002;46:505–10.

99. Tanabe K, Maeshima Y, Ichinose K, Kitayama H, Takazawa Y, Hirokoshi K, et al. Endostatin peptide, an inhibitor of angiogenesis, prevents the progression of peritoneal sclerosis in a mouse experimental model. Kidney Int. 2007;71:227–38.

100. Fukuoka N, Sugiyama H, Inoue K, Kikumoto Y, Takiue K, Morinaga H, et al. Increased susceptibility to oxidant-mediated tissue injury and peritoneal fibrosis in acatalasemic mice. Am J Nephrol. 2008;28:661–8.

101. Yoshio Y, Miyazaki M, Abe K, Nishino T, Furusu A, Mizuta Y, et al. TNP-470, an angiogenesis inhibitor, suppresses the progression of peritoneal fibrosis in mouse experimental model. Kidney Int. 2004;66:1677–85.

102. Nakav S, Kachko L, Vorobiov M, Rogachev B, Chaimovitz C, Zlotnik M, et al. Blocking adenosine A2A receptor reduces peritoneal fibrosis in two independent experimental models. Nephrol Dial Transplant. 2009;24:2392–9.

103. Kokubo S, Sakai N, Furuichi K, Toyama T, Kitajima S, Okumura T, et al. Activation of p38 mitogen-activated protein kinase promotes peritoneal fibrosis by regulating fibrocytes. Perit Dial Int. 2012;32:10–9.

104. Yokoi H, Kasahara M, Mori K, Ogawa Y, Kuwabara T, Imamaki H, et al. Pleiotrophin triggers inflammation and increased peritoneal permeability leading to peritoneal fibrosis. Kidney Int. 2012;81:160–9.

105. Nishino T, Ashida R, Obata Y, Furusu A, Abe K, Miyazaki M, et al. Involvement of lymphocyte infiltration in the progression of mouse peritoneal fibrosis model. Ren Fail. 2012;34:760–6.

106. Sekiguchi Y, Hamada C, Ro Y, Nakamoto H, Inaba M, Shimaoka T, et al. Differentiation of bone marrow-derived cells into regenerated mesothelial cells in peritoneal remodeling using a peritoneal fibrosis mouse model. J Artif Organs. 2012;15:272–82.

107. Hirose M, Nishino T, Obata Y, Nakazawa M, Nakazawa Y, Furusu A, et al. 22-Oxacalcitriol prevents progression of peritoneal fibrosis in a mouse model. Perit Dial Int. 2013;33:132–42.

108. Yokoi H, Kasahara M, Mori K, Kuwabara T, Toda N, Yamada R, et al. Peritoneal fibrosis and high transport are induced in mildly pre-injured peritoneum by 3,4-dideoxyglucosone-3-ene in mice. Perit Dial Int. 2013;33:143–54.

109. Hirahara I, Kusano E, Yanagiba S, Miyata Y, Ando Y, Muto S, et al. Peritoneal injury by methylglyoxal in peritoneal dialysis. Perit Dial Int. 2006;26:380–92.

110. Hirahara I, Ishibashi Y, Kaname S, Kusano E, Fujita T. Methylglyoxal induces peritoneal thickening by mesenchymal-like mesothelial cells in rats. Nephrol Dial Transplant. 2009;24:437–47.

111. Hirahara I, Sato H, Imai T, Onishi A, Morishita Y, Muto S, et al. Methylglyoxal induced basophilic spindle cells with podoplanin at the surface of peritoneum in rat peritoneal dialysis model. Biomed Res Int. 2015;2015: 289751.

112. Onishi A, Akimoto T, Morishita Y, Hirahara I, Inoue M, Kusano E, et al. Peritoneal fibrosis induced by intraperitoneal methylglyoxal injection: the role of concurrent renal dysfunction. Am J Nephrol. 2014;40:381–90.

113. Kitamura M, Nishino T, Obata Y, Furusu A, Hishikawa Y, Koji T, et al. Epigallocatechin gallate suppresses peritoneal fibrosis in mice. Chem Biol Interact. 2012;195:95–104.

114. Terabayashi T, Ito Y, Mizuno M, Suzuki Y, Kinashi H, Sakata F, et al. Vascular endothelial growth factor receptor-3 is a novel target to improve net ultrafiltration in methylglyoxal-induced peritoneal injury. Lab Invest. 2015;95:1029–43.

115. Liu L, Shi CX, Ghayur A, Zhang C, Su JY, Hoff CM, et al. Prolonged peritoneal gene expression using a helper-dependent adenovirus. Perit Dial Int. 2009;29:508–16.

116. Patel P, Sekiguchi Y, Oh KH, Patterson SE, Kolb MR, Margetts PJ. Smad3-dependent and -independent pathways are involved in peritoneal membrane injury. Kidney Int. 2010;77:319–28.

117. Margetts PJ, Hoff C, Liu L, Korstanje R, Walkin L, Summers A, et al. Transforming growth factor β-induced peritoneal fibrosis is mouse strain dependent. Nephrol Dial Transplant. 2013;28:2015–27.

118. Padwal M, Siddique I, Wu L, Tang K, Boivin F, Liu L, et al. Matrix metalloproteinase 9 is associated with peritoneal membrane solute transport and induces angiogenesis through β-catenin signaling. Nephrol Dial Transplant. 2016. doi:10.1093/ndt/gfw076.

119. Margetts PJ, Kolb M, Galt T, Hoff CM, Shockley TR, Gauldie J. Gene transfer of transforming growth factor-beta1 to the rat peritoneum: effects on membrane function. J Am Soc Nephrol. 2001;12:2029–39.

120. Margetts PJ, Bonniaud P, Liu L, Hoff CM, Holmes CJ, West-Mays JA, et al. Transient overexpression of TGF-β1 induces epithelial mesenchymal transition in the rodent peritoneum. J Am Soc Nephrol. 2005;16:425–36.

121. Gotloib L, Wajsbrot V, Cuperman Y, Shostak A. Acute oxidative stress induces peritoneal hyperpermeability, mesothelial loss, and fibrosis. J Lab Clin Med. 2004;143:31–40.

122. Levine S, Saltzman A. Abdominal cocoon: an animal model for a complication of peritoneal dialysis. Perit Dial Int. 1996;16:613–6.

123. Nakamoto H, Imai H, Ishida Y, Yamanouchi Y, Inoue T, Okada H, et al. New animal models for encapsulating peritoneal sclerosis—role of acidic solution. Perit Dial Int. 2001;21(Suppl 3):S349–53.

5

Psychonephrology in Japan

Yoichi Ohtake

Abstract

Psychonephrology is the field of study encompassing nephrology, psychiatry, and psychosomatic medicine, which is based on the concept of consultation-liaison within the biopsychosocial model of mind–body unity. The Japanese Society for Psychonephrology was founded in Japan in 1990 to resolve psychological problems in dialysis patients and renal transplant patients, for whom survival time has increased. Patients with chronic kidney disease (CKD) face various psychological burdens during the time leading up to the initiation of renal replacement therapy (RRT) or through to the continuation of RRT. Patients with CKD may experience high levels of stress, poor physical conditions, medication side effects, as well as adjustment disorders and anxiety/depression. Additionally, close relationships between these patients and their family and medical staff can cause psychological stress in these other individuals. The three main domains in psychonephrology concern psychological care for patients, which includes drug therapy, psychotherapy, and environmental adjustments; interventions for psychosomatic disorders; and mental health care for staff involved in RRT. Interdisciplinary collaboration among psychiatrists, psychotherapists, nephrologists, transplant surgeons, and paramedics to resolve patients' problems has been promoted. Future developments in psychonephrology include adhering to patients' desires regarding discontinuation/withholding of dialysis and palliative care and shared decision-making during the time leading up to RRT. Further development of psychonephrology in Japan will help to maintain higher levels of quality of life in CKD patients and provide relief for their psychological issues.

Keywords: Psychonephrology, Psychosomatic medicine, Japan, Chronic kidney disease, Renal replacement therapy, Psychotherapy, Quality of life

Background

Psychonephrology is the field of study that focuses on nephrology and mental health fields such as psychiatry and psychosomatic medicine [1]. During the time leading up to the initiation of renal replacement therapy (RRT) or through to the continuation of RRT, patients with kidney disease face various psychological burdens. As a result, the area of psychonephrology has been expanding over time. Patients with kidney disease are now in need of a broad range of medical services beyond management of their psychological pain. Also required are support for decision-making during the time from conservative management of renal failure to the initiation of RRT, judgments on the discontinuation/withholding of RRT, and non-cancer palliative care for patients with chronic kidney disease (CKD). There are several reasons why the new field of psychonephrology focusing on CKD was established rather than other serious physical diseases. First, CKD patients (especially with dialysis) usually experience high levels of stress and have characteristics not found in patients with other diseases. Second, CKD patients often suffer from poor physical conditions aside from their primary disease and medication side effects, which commonly manifest as psychological reactions. Third, close relationships between these patients and their family and medical staff can cause psychological stress in these other individuals.

Brief overview of psychonephrology
History of psychonephrology

The origin of psychonephrology is considered to date back to 1978, when three liaison psychiatrists coined the term to highlight an aspect of American consultation-liaison psychiatry and initiated a conference on this topic [1]. Since then, the conference has evolved into an international event held once every 2 years. Levy [2] later compiled the conference papers into a book entitled *Psychonephrology*.

Correspondence: yohtake.jp@gmail.com
1-1-1 Ebaraji-cho Nishi-ku Sakai, Osaka 593-8304, Japan

Psychonephrology in Japan

The Japanese Society for Psychonephrology (JSPN) [3] was founded in Japan in 1990 under the leadership of Dr. Kazuo Ohta and Dr. Shigekazu Haruki, mainly to resolve various psychological problems in dialysis patients and renal transplant patients. Around the same time, treatment outcomes of RRT in CKD patients dramatically improved in Japan, notably extending their survival. However, the intervention environments for CKD patients were far from ideal, and medical care for their psychological problems was particularly lacking. Since its inception, JSPN has held a convention every year, with the 26th installment having taken place in 2016. Aside from its national conventions, JSPN also organizes many regional study groups and workshops. In addition, the Japanese Society for Dialysis Therapy (JSDT) and other nephrology-related medical conferences have also seen an increase in symposiums or presentations on psychonephrology, with focus on providing support for patients' decision-making about RRT and the discontinuation/withholding of dialysis.

With the recent specialization and advancement in medical technologies, the need for team medical care has been re-recognized. As such, attempts have been made in the field of psychonephrology to promote interdisciplinary collaboration among psychiatrists, psychotherapists, nephrologists, transplant surgeons, and paramedics to resolve patients' problems, rather than each profession providing specialized care.

Psychosomatic medicine in psychonephrology

Along with psychiatric medicine, psychosomatic medicine has long been studied in Japan. Psychosomatic medicine is based on an academic framework that developed mainly in Japan and Germany and is characterized by a biopsychosocial model approach based on the notion of mind–body unity, rather than mind–body split. The history of psychosomatic medicine in Japan dates back to 1960, when Yujiro Ikemi and others established the Japanese Society of Psychosomatic Medicine [4]. Since then, departments of psychosomatic medicine have been established in some institutions across Japan (currently eight).

Similar to consultation-liaison psychiatry, the concept of consultation-liaison exists in psychosomatic medicine and is known as psychonephrology. Psychosomatic medicine is also involved in various other fields, such as psychosomatic respiratory disease, psychosomatic cardiovascular disease, and psycho-oncology. The field of primary care has a high affinity for the biopsychosocial model approach, which is also characterized by a particular focus on collaboration with paramedical staff in team medical care.

Three domains of psychonephrology

Three main domains in psychonephrology exist: (1) care for CKD patients, particularly psychological care associated with RRT; (2) interventions for psychosomatic disorders in CKD patients; and (3) mental health care for staff involved in RRT.

Psychological care associated with CKD

During the time leading up to the initiation of RRT, CKD patients experience a range of different kinds of psychological pain and use various defense mechanisms to cope with these pain types. Specifically, many experience anxiety, anger, resentment, tension, despair, and depression before finally coming to accept the necessity of undergoing RRT. However, some CKD patients continue to remain in denial even after the initiation of RRT, which often manifests as physical symptoms or nonadherence to treatment.

Similar to patients receiving a cancer diagnosis in general, it typically takes approximately 2 weeks for CKD patients to regain their psychological equilibrium after being notified of the need for RRT, which is a normal psychological reaction. However, some CKD patients may have a reaction known as an adjustment disorder, which delays their psychological recovery. Depending on the patients, anxiety/depression may last much longer than 2 weeks after notification, or in some cases, anxiety/depression may worsen beyond the severity of an adjustment disorder and remain as a mood disorder (depressive state) (Fig. 1). Psychonephrology is also involved in the psychological care of these types of patients.

Interventions for psychosomatic disorder in CKD patients

The Japanese Society of Psychosomatic Medicine defines a psychosomatic disorder as "a physical condition with a structural or functional disorder in which psychological or social factors are closely involved in its onset or progress, with the exclusion of physical symptoms caused by other mental disorders such as neurosis and depression." The most common psychosomatic disorders include irritable bowel syndrome, migraine, and atopic dermatitis.

Patients with CKD may present with psychosomatically pathologic conditions or unidentified complaints. In the case of psychosomatically pathologic conditions, it is important to listen to the patient to elicit their explanatory model and to share hypotheses about the condition with the patient. Unidentified complaints can be regarded as physical manifestations of psychological suffering; therefore, it is necessary to explore and consider the patient's mental state underlying the condition.

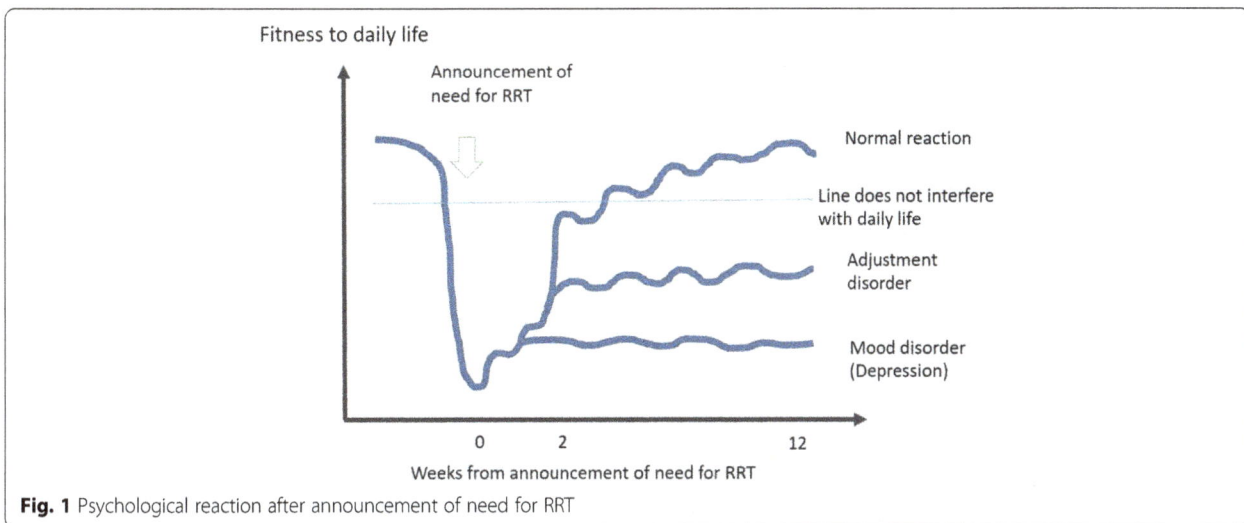

Fig. 1 Psychological reaction after announcement of need for RRT

Mental health care for dialysis staff

The majority of RRT performed in Japan is hemodialysis, which is most commonly administered in-center three times a week. Unlike with regular outpatient treatment, a much closer relationship can develop between hemodialysis patients and attending medical staff. It is ideal when this relationship produces positive effects on the patient's quality of life (QOL); however, unfortunately, this is not always the case. Because patients with kidney disease must cope with chronic conditions, they are sensitive to changes in their health and test results. A certain proportion is considered "difficult patients," who may persistently complain of their physical problems until they feel understood or think that their conditions are not being understood by their physicians. Therefore, a very close patient–doctor relationship must be maintained, which is also likely to cause psychological problems among dialysis staff.

In Japan, the "Amendment to the Industrial Safety and Health Act Industrial Safety and Health Act" was passed in June 2014, which requires employers of ≥50 workers to offer Stress Checks in their workplaces at least once a year to assess levels of mental stress experienced by workers. Such mental health care for dialysis staff is also one of the domains of psychonephrology.

The mental state of patients prior to receiving RRT

The mental process leading to the initiation of RRT

After years of undergoing outpatient treatment, many CKD patients come to somewhat accept their declining kidney function. However, RRT is sometimes required earlier than originally expected because of rapid deterioration or unexpected acute exacerbation of kidney function. In such cases, various psychological reactions may be seen in patients when notified that they need to undergo RRT; they usually experience disappointment/

hopelessness in the beginning, followed by denial, anxiety, anger, and depression before finally accepting RRT. This is very similar to the process of accepting death described in "On Death and Dying" by Elisabeth Kübler-Ross [5]. However, unlike terminal cancer patients, CKD patients experience kidney death but continue to live. For this reason, the mental process leading to the initiation of RRT varies from case to case. It is also important to keep in mind that not all patients undergoing RRT have come to terms with the disease.

Total pain

Total pain is a concept of suffering mainly used in the area of palliative care, which was introduced by Cicely Saunders, a pioneer of modern hospice care [6]. Total pain is considered to be suffering that encompasses a person's physical, psychological, social, and spiritual pain. Figure 2 illustrates total pain experienced by CKD patients. It is essential that these problems be examined in a comprehensive and holistic manner. Particularly, psychological, social, and spiritual pain can easily be overlooked and thus require careful attention. While physical pain can be controlled to some degree by changing dialysis conditions, switching RRT modalities, or adjusting oral medications, the management of psychological pain is, as mentioned, a key part of psychonephrology.

Defense mechanisms

Reactions of the mind triggered by psychological crises during the time leading up to the initiation of RRT or during RRT are called defense mechanisms. Common defense mechanisms are presented in Table 1. These defense mechanisms come in all manners and forms; they are essential to everyday life and include social adjustment behaviors such as sublimation and humor. The various defense mechanisms underlying the behavior of

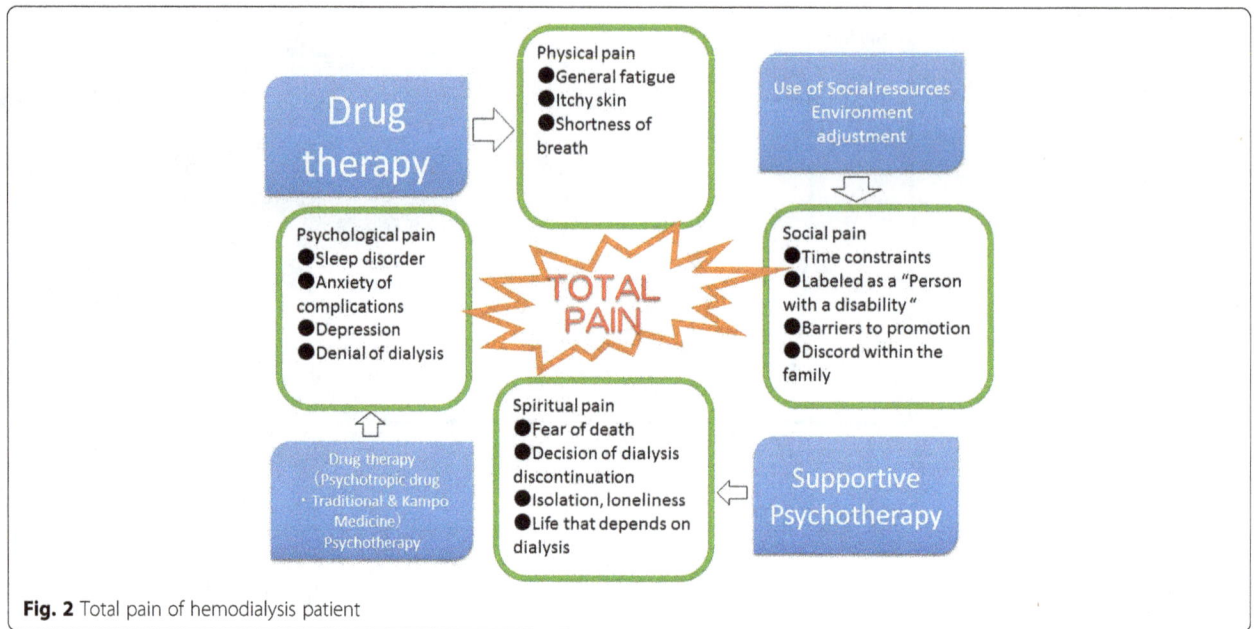

Fig. 2 Total pain of hemodialysis patient

patients with kidney disease should be considered and given close attention. In some patients, these defense mechanisms do not fully function, which may lead to the development of psychiatric diseases, such as depression and schizophrenia. Such cases should be referred to a psychiatrist immediately.

Anxiety and depression

According to studies published overseas, psychological tests conducted among dialysis patients have shown approximately 15–60% have "severe depressive symptoms" and 12–52% have "anxiety." With respect to disorders, approximately 10–20% of dialysis patients have been shown to meet DSM-IV criteria for major depressive disorder and 46% met criteria for some type of anxiety disorder. Among the variants in anxiety disorders, "panic disorder" is considered to be the most common in dialysis patients [7–9].

To treat such psychiatric conditions/diseases in patients with CKD, regular dialysis physicians are likely to use benzodiazepines. Benzodiazepines are easy to use in CKD patients because no renal function-based dose adjustment is necessary, which are primarily metabolized by the liver. In terms of their action mechanism, however,

benzodiazepines are considered to be merely symptomatic treatment and have a high potential for dependence/tolerance. Conversely, patients with impaired kidney function and referred to a psychiatric or psychosomatic medicine department are often turned away or given no medication because of their kidney problems. Because many antidepressants and antipsychotics can be used in patients with impaired kidney function, it is optimal to work closely with a psychiatrist to support CKD patients with psychological problems.

Effective psychotherapeutic approaches in psychonephrology

Treatments for various psychological conditions can roughly be divided into (1) drug therapy, (2) psychotherapy, and (3) environmental adjustments. Particularly, rapid progress has been made in the field of psychotherapy, with a variety of approaches having been proposed in quick succession worldwide.

The psychotherapeutic approaches that are considered effective in psychonephrology are shown in Table 2. Although these approaches may employ various techniques and skills, all should focus on how patients can improve their self-control abilities using the resources

Table 1 Various defense mechanisms

Repression	Conversion
Projection	Somatization
Rationalization	Acting out
Sublimation	Denial
Displacement	Humor

Table 2 Psychotherapy used in psychonephrology

Supportive psychotherapy	Transactional analysis
Behavioral therapy	Autogenic training
Cognitive behavioral therapy	Family therapy
Solution-focused brief therapy	Interpersonal therapy
Motivational interviewing	Autonomy training

currently available to them. Furthermore, it is desirable to choose a psychotherapeutic approach that can help to manage decreased self-efficacy and self-control commonly seen in CKD patients.

Future developments in psychonephrology

As mentioned, psychonephrology was originally developed to resolve psychological problems in CKD patients. However, the area of psychonephrology is gradually expanding to assist with various problems occurring at clinical sites. Two future development paths for psychonephrology are described in the following sections.

Discontinuation/withholding of dialysis and non-cancer palliative care

In Japan, the primary reason for the introduction of dialysis treatment is diabetic nephropathy, and the age of patients at the start of dialysis is growing older each year, reaching 69 years old at present time. Under such circumstances, ethical issues such as whether to introduce dialysis to CKD patients with complications and when to stop dialysis in patients currently receiving it need to be dealt with urgently. At the 53rd annual meeting of the JSDT, Seiji Ohira gave a presentation entitled "Consideration for not Starting Dialysis (Withholding) and Discontinuing Dialysis (Withdrawal)." In 2014, the study subgroup on withholding and withdrawal of dialysis established as a subsidiary organization of the hemodialysis guidelines commission of the JSDT published "Proposal for the Shared Decision-Making Process Regarding Initiation and Continuation of Maintenance Hemodialysis." [10] This proposal described the importance of respecting patients' autonomous decisions and providing support for patients' decision-making process as a medical team. It is evident that patients' desires should be regarded as the highest priority. However, in reality, patients are often unable to make decisions on their own due to dementia or old age and require family members to make decisions for them. This can place psychological burdens on family members, often hindering smooth decision-making. In such situations, medical staff in psychonephrology units need to assess the psychological status of the people concerned and take on a catalytic role in communication among different professionals, patients/family members, and medical staff.

Such advance care planning, which includes advance directives (AD), is being increasingly advocated in the field of palliative care (Fig. 3). In Japan, the Kidney Disease Therapy Society has created an AD form based on survival with dignity, rather than death with dignity [11].

Additionally, the Japan Association for Clinical Ethics recommends the Physical Orders for Life Sustaining Treatment (POLST) developed in the USA [12]. The POLST is a document that includes specific instructions

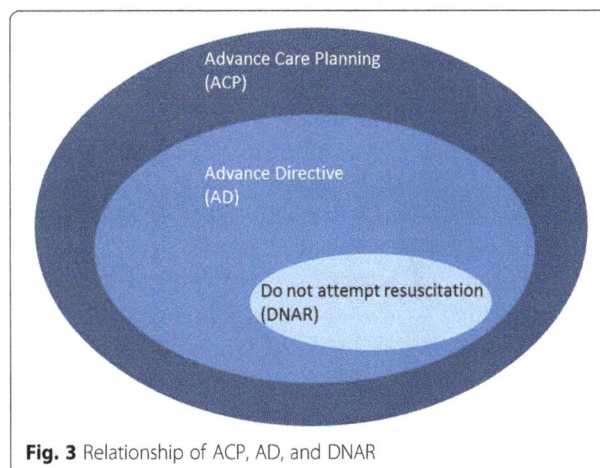

Fig. 3 Relationship of ACP, AD, and DNAR

regarding end-of-life care created based on the will of patients with severe progressive disease or chronic disease and contains more detailed instructions on medical interventions than Do Not Attempt Resuscitation instructions. The POLST form is created after consent has been obtained through in-depth discussion with patients or those who represent the patients. The POLST also contains an item about dialysis in Section C: other medical interventions.

At any rate, with the further aging of Japanese dialysis patients, the involvement of psychonephrology will be unavoidable to support decision making regarding discontinuation/withholding of dialysis and other matters, as well as the creation of AD forms.

In addition, in Japan, more than 90% of patients receiving palliative care are said to be cancer patients. However, palliative care is defined as an approach for addressing "life-threatening diseases," which include CKD. The Ministry of Health, Labour and Welfare (MHLW) formulated the Basic Plan to Promote Cancer Control based on the Cancer Control Act. As part of the plan, the PEACE Project (Palliative care Emphasis program on symptom management and Assessment for Continuous medical Education) was launched and has been implemented to help health care professionals engaged in cancer care to acquire basic knowledge and skills required in palliative care [13]. This 2-day program aims to enable participants to learn how to provide basic care to alleviate physical and psychological symptoms in typical cancer patients. The MHLW plans to disseminate palliative care into non-cancer fields; as its first step, the promotion of palliative care in cardiovascular diseases is already underway. Therefore, CKD will also be included in MHLW's plans, and psychonephrology approaches are expected to play an active role in palliative care for CKD patients, particularly in alleviating their psychological symptoms.

Shared decision-making during the time leading up to RRT

Previously, treatment methods prior to the initiation of RRT were often selected through paternalism, in which doctors make decisions on optimal treatment for their patients. However, this method began to face growing criticism with the spread of informed consent. In contrast to paternalism, an alternative approach was introduced where patients give informed consent after understanding and agreeing to the treatment explained. However, as with RRT, cases exist in which informed consent is impractical. For example, the patient may be unable to choose a treatment from multiple proposed options, the treatment chosen by the patient may not necessarily be the best option, or the patient may later change their mind based on information provided by medical staff. To resolve these concerns, the concept of shared decision-making was developed, through which "doctors provide patients with medical information, and the patients actively convey their values and preferences to the doctors so that the doctors and patients share the same information, thereby making it possible to choose the best treatment approach for the patients." [14] In shared decision-making, communication between patients and doctors is considered of utmost importance [10, 15].

For the implementation of shared decision-making, a three-step model was developed to facilitate the process [14]. The presence of psychiatrists/psychosomatic medicine physicians is also important because of their ability to create an atmosphere of trust and comfort as well as their third-person point of view.

Conclusions

Psychonephrology can be practiced by all health care professionals involved in RRT and is a growing area that is expected to see increased growth in future. Further development of psychonephrology in Japan will help to maintain higher levels of QOL in CKD patients and provide relief for their psychological issues.

Abbreviations
AD: Advance directives; CKD: Chronic kidney disease; JSDT: Japanese Society for Dialysis Therapy; JSPN: Japanese Society for Psychonephrology; MHLW: Ministry of Health, Labour and Welfare; PEACE Project: Palliative care Emphasis program on symptom management and Assessment for Continuous medical Education Project; POLST: Physical Orders for Life Sustaining Treatment; RRT: Renal replacement therapy; QOL: Quality of life

Acknowledgements
The authors would like to thank Dr. Atsuko Koyama who introduced me the world of psychonephrology.

Competing interests
The authors declare that they have no competing interests.

Funding
None.

References
1. Levy NB. What is psychonephrology? J Nephrol. 2008;21:S51–3.
2. Levy NB, editor. Psychonephrology 1. Boston: Springer US; 1981.
3. The Japanese Society for Psychonephrology. http://www.jspn-ndt.com. Accessed 15 Sept 2016.
4. Japanese Society of Psychosomatic Medicine (JSPM). http://www.shinshin-igaku.com/index.html. Accessed 15 Sept 2016.
5. Kübler-Ross E. On death and dying. New York: Routledge; 1969.
6. Richmond C. Dame Cicely Saunders. BMJ Br Med J. 2005;331:238.
7. Murtagh FE, Addington-Hall J, Higginson IJ. The prevalence of symptoms in end-stage renal disease: a systematic review. Adv Chronic Kidney Dis. 2007;14:82–99.
8. Cukor D, Coplan J, Brown C, Friedman S, Newville H, Safier M, et al. Anxiety disorders in adults treated by hemodialysis: a single-center study. Am J Kidney Dis. 2008;52:128–36.
9. Hedayati SS, Finkelstein FO. Epidemiology, diagnosis, and management of depression in patients with CKD. Am J Kidney Dis. 2009;54:741–52.
10. Watanabe Y, Hirakata H, Okada K, Yamamoto H, Tsuruya K, Sakai K, et al. Proposal for the shared decision-making process regarding initiation and continuation of maintenance hemodialysis. Ther Apher Dial. 2015;19:108–17.
11. Kidney Disease Therapy Society. http://www.geocities.jp/chronickidneydisease/paper.html. Accessed 15 Sept 2016.
12. Japan Association for Clinical Ethics. http://www.j-ethics.jp/workinggroup.htm. Accessed 15 Sept 2016.
13. PEACE PROJECT. http://www.jspm-peace.jp. Accessed 15 Sept 2016.
14. Elwyn G, Frosch D, Thomson R, Joseph-Williams N, Lloyd A, Kinnersley P, et al. Shared decision making: a model for clinical practice. J Gen Intern Med. 2012;27:1361–7.
15. Schell JO, Green JA, Tulsky JA, Arnold RM. Communication skills training for dialysis decision-making and end-of-life care in nephrology. Clin J Am Soc Nephrol. 2013;8:675–80.

6

Atypical hemolytic uremic syndrome

Yoko Yoshida, Hideki Kato* and Masaomi Nangaku

Abstract

Atypical hemolytic uremic syndrome (aHUS) is a thrombotic microangiopathy (TMA) characterized by microangiopathic hemolytic anemia, thrombocytopenia, and acute renal failure. Most cases of aHUS are caused by uncontrolled complement activation due to genetic mutations in the alternative pathway of complement. More recently, mutations in the gene of coagulation system have also been identified in patients with aHUS. In Japan, the recent studies of aHUS have identified the unique genetic characteristics in our country and enabled us to revise the diagnostic criteria. In this article, we review the classification of TMAs and describe the pathophysiology, diagnosis, and management of aHUS. We also highlight current progress in clinical and basic research of the patients with aHUS in Japan.

Keywords: Atypical hemolytic uremic syndrome, Complement, Alternative pathway, Complement factor H, Complement component C3, Eculizumab

Background

Thrombotic microangiopathy (TMA) is defined by a histological region characterized by microvascular changes including thrombosis, which results in microangiopathic hemolytic anemia, thrombocytopenia, and organ failure. TMAs are caused by a variety of hereditary or acquired etiologies, and now broadly classified into four categories; hemolytic uremic syndrome caused by Shiga toxin-producing *Escherichia coli* (STEC) infection (STEC-HUS), atypical hemolytic uremic syndrome (aHUS), thrombotic thrombocytopenic purpura (TTP), and secondary TMA.

Historically, HUS was classified into two forms by the presence of diarrhea. Ninety percent of HUS arises from the infection of STEC with severe diarrhea; thus, this form of HUS was previously named "D (diarrhea) (+) HUS", presumably STEC-HUS. On the other hand, the remaining 10% of HUS was named "D (diarrhea) (−) HUS", because it was caused without the infection of STEC. In 1975, several research groups reported that this form of HUS could be familial, implicating the presence of hereditary D(−) HUS [1]. Thus, the term "atypical HUS (aHUS)" was used to describe the patients with D(−) HUS and hereditary D(−) HUS. However, since 1980s, various clinical and experimental studies

have convincingly shown that most cases of aHUS result from uncontrolled complement activation due to genetic mutations or acquired autoantibodies in the alternative pathway of complement. These new findings of aHUS led to differentiate complement-mediated aHUS from other types of TMA. According to these observations, currently, the term of aHUS is generally used to describe complement-mediated aHUS [2–4]. Other TMAs associated with a variety of causes including infection, drug, transplant, and pregnancy are now named "secondary TMA" or etiology-based denomination (e.g., pregnancy TMA).

Recent advances in understanding pathogenesis of aHUS have clearly led to differentiate aHUS from other TMAs and changed the therapeutic approach for aHUS [5, 6]. However, making a solid diagnosis of this disease is still not easy due to poor penetrance and lack of method for identifying excess complement activations. Moreover, recent studies have also found that the mutations in the gene of coagulation system predispose to aHUS leading investigators to reconsider the definition of aHUS. Our aim in this review is not only to describe the pathogenesis, diagnosis, and management of aHUS but also to improve the evidence-based practice of this disease.

* Correspondence: hkatou-tky@umin.ac.jp
Division of Nephrology and Endocrinology, The University of Tokyo Hospital,
7-3-1 Hongo, Bunkyo-ku 113-8655, Tokyo, Japan

Classification of thrombotic microangiopathies

HUS due to Shiga toxin-producing bacteria is most frequently formed and is generally called STEC-HUS (or HUS or typical HUS). Although STEC-HUS occurs at any age, children can be predominantly affected. Severe abdominal pain, diarrhea, and bloody stools are common findings, which appeared several days after taking contaminated foods. The progression to HUS is related to the binding of Shiga toxin to the target cell surface via globotriaosylceramide, which leads to cytotoxic effect via inhibition of protein synthesis and apoptosis. Moreover, the presence of Shiga toxin also induces the secretion of unusually large von Willebrand factor (VWF) from endothelial cells [7]. Prognosis of STEC-HUS is favorable with 90% of child cases being recovered, but 1–2% of patients die during acute phase, and 12% of patients, who recovered from STEC-HUS once, die or progress to end-stage renal disease (ESRD) in long-term follow-up [3, 8].

TTP results from severe deficiency of a disintegrin-like and metalloprotease with thrombospondin type 1 motif, 13 (ADAMTS13), which is a specific cleaving protease of VWF. ADAMTS13 deficiency leads to the secretion of unusually large VWF from vascular endothelial cells, thus leading to the VWF-dependent platelet adhesion in small vessels. Homozygous or compound heterozygous mutations of *ADAMTS13* are the cause of hereditary TTP [9, 10]. Moreover, acquired TTP arises from autoantibodies against ADAMTS13 [11].

A link between complement system and aHUS has been highlighted since the 1970s [12], and subsequent study identified that genetic mutation of *complement factor H* (*CFH*), a major complement regulatory factor, is associated with pathophysiology of aHUS [13]. Since then, various genetic mutations in multiple complement factors belonging to alternative pathway have been found in 60% of patients with aHUS. Two types of variants are associated with this disease; one is loss-of-function mutation of the complement regulatory factors, and the other is gain-of-function mutation of complement itself or complement activation factors. Of note, autoantibodies against CFH also predispose to aHUS. These genetic or acquired defects result in excess complement activation on the cell surface, leading to endothelial damage, inflammation, and thrombosis formation. More recently, a link between coagulation system and aHUS has also been highlighted.

Secondary TMA arises from diverse factors and diseases (metabolic disorder, infection, drug, pregnancy, autoimmune disease, systemic disease, hematopoietic stem cell transplantation/solid organ transplantation, malignant hypertension, and malignancy). In pediatric cases, both *Streptococcus pneumoniae* infection and Cobalamin C deficiency are highly related to the cause of secondary TMA. In contrast to STEC-HUS, aHUS, and

TTP, the pathogenesis of secondary TMA is still unclear. Especially, the distinction between aHUS and secondary TMA is sometimes not clear. In fact, complement genetic mutations or anti-CFH autoantibodies have been found in a part of patients with post-transplant-mediated TMA [14] and patients with hemolysis, elevated liver enzyme, low platelet count (HELLP) syndrome [15, 16]. It is unclear whether aHUS is underlying the disease or not in these cases; thus, more studies are needed to confirm these findings.

In Japan, the classification of TMAs was originally described in a diagnostic criteria for aHUS proposed by the Joint Committee of the Japanese Society of Nephrology and the Japan Pediatric Society in 2013 [17, 18]. In this criterion, aHUS was defined as TMA excluding STEC-HUS and TTP; therefore, TMA caused by a variety of etiology, now named secondary TMA, was also included in the category of aHUS. This classification has led to the early diagnosis of aHUS and timely initiation of treatment. However, the term of aHUS is now generally accepted to describe only complement-mediated aHUS as described above. To address this situation, the Joint Committee developed a novel guideline for aHUS including recommendation for treating this disease in 2016 [19, 20]. This guideline redefined aHUS as TMA caused by complement dysregulation, and the exclusion of secondary TMA is needed for diagnosing aHUS in addition to the exclusion of STEC-HUS and TTP (ADAMTS13 <10%). Current problem of this field is that there are some cases of aHUS among secondary TMA [14, 21]; however, there are no crucial clinical characteristics and laboratory parameters to distinguish them. To overcome this problem, further research regarding both clinical characteristics and laboratory biomarkers and the establishment of rapid genetic diagnostic system for aHUS are required.

We hope that this novel guideline will improve the understanding of physiopathology and diagnosis of individual TMA, leading to a rapid and correct diagnosis, and more judicious treatment for individual cases in Japan.

Epidemiology

aHUS is considered a rare disease, but its incidence is not known precisely. The annual incidence of aHUS is estimated to be two cases per million in the USA [22], and the prevalence are reported to be 3.3 per million among patients below the age of 18 [5]. More recently, the research group from France reported an incidence of 0.23 cases per million [23]. aHUS affects at any age, and approximately half of this disease usually occurs before the age of 18, without sex difference [24]. Although, the epidemiology of patients with aHUS in Japan has not been well clarified, based on our cohort study, 100 to 200 patients seem to have been diagnosed.

Pathophysiology

The complement system is an essential component of innate immunity for protecting host from invading pathogens. Complement system, which consists of over 30 proteins, can be mostly present as inactivated forms, and the activation of it is caused through three main pathways; classical pathway, alternative pathway, and lectin pathway. These three pathways promote the formation of C3 convertase, which degrades C3 into C3a and C3b. The C3b molecule functions as a major opsonin, and binds covalently to pathogens or to any surface. The binding of C3b to Gram-positive bacteria leads to the phagocytosis by neutrophils, macrophages, and monocytes. In the case of Gram-negative bacteria, bound C3b induces the progression of complement cascade and the generation of the lytic membrane attack complex. The activation of the classical and the lectin pathways is initiated by the recognition of invading microorganisms via the Fc moieties of antigen-bound antibody or mannose-binding lectin, respectively. On the other hand, the activation of alternative pathway needs no specific initiator.

The activation process of alternative pathway is illustrated in Fig. 1. In the alternative pathway, C3 is easily converted to $C3(H_2O)$ and rapidly reacted with complement factor B (CFB) and complement factor D (CFD). This reaction leads to the formation of $C3(H_2O)Bb$, which works as an initial fluid phase C3 convertase and prompt to generate more C3b. This spontaneous activation system called "tick over" is potentially dangerous; thus, it is strictly controlled by complement regulatory factors including CFH, complement factor I (CFI), and membrane cofactor protein (MCP). Generally, $C3(H_2O)Bb$ or C3b is rapidly and proteolytically inactivated by CFI collaborated with CFH in the fluid phase. On the self-cell surface like endothelial cells, CFH also acts as a complement regulator by binding to sialic acids or sulfated glycosaminoglycans on self-surface via its C-terminal basic domains. A transmembrane protein MCP helps to inactivate C3b by CFI. Thrombomodulin (THBD), a transmembrane protein, which generates anticoagulant active protein C to reduce blood coagulation, is also associated with the downregulation of alternative pathway by accelerating CFI-mediated inactivation of C3b. On the other hand, once C3b binds to pathogens lacking complement regulatory proteins, bound C3b preferentially reacts with CFB and CFD, which results in formation of a C3 convertase and generating more C3b. The C3 convertase can recruit another C3b to form C3bBbC3b (C5 convertase), which generates a potent anaphylatoxin C5a through cleavage of C5. The binding of C5b to C6, C7, C8, and C9 causes the formation of membrane attack complex (C5b–9) for eliminating pathogens.

Several research groups have shown that approximately 60% of patients with aHUS have mutations in

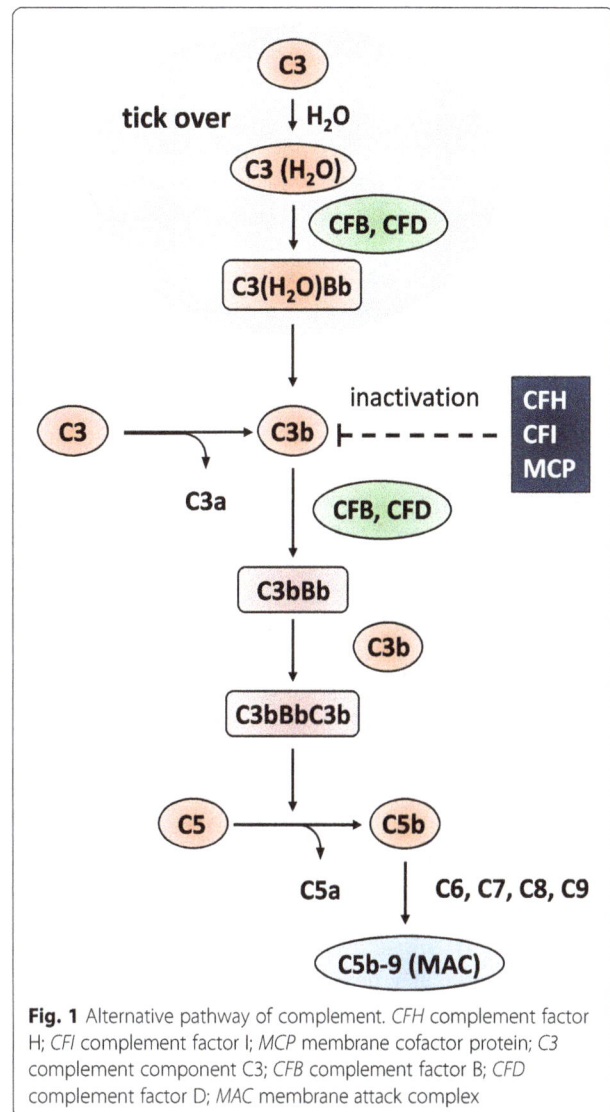

Fig. 1 Alternative pathway of complement. *CFH* complement factor H; *CFI* complement factor I; *MCP* membrane cofactor protein; *C3* complement component C3; *CFB* complement factor B; *CFD* complement factor D; *MAC* membrane attack complex

complement regulatory or complement factors in the alternative pathway (CFH, CFI, MCP, THBD, C3, and CFB). Loss of function mutations in complement regulatory factors (CFH [13, 25–27], CFI [28, 29], MCP [30, 31], and THBD [32]) cause the impairment of inactivating C3b both on the cell surface and fluid phase. On the other hand, gain of function mutations in complement activation factors, C3 and CFB reduce the binding affinity for CFH and/or MCP leading to impaired CFI-mediated inactivation [33–36]. These aHUS-associated mutations cause excess complement activation on host-cell surface leading endothelial damage. Moreover, combined mutations in the foregoing six genes seem to increase susceptibility to aHUS [37]. Acquired autoantibodies against CFH have been identified in 5–10% of patients with aHUS [38–40]. These antibodies are highly associated with the alteration in *CFH-related* (*CFHR*) genes. The genes encoding the five CFHR (CFHR1-5) proteins are characterized by several large genomic repeat regions having a high sequence identity. Thus, these regions occur nonallelic homologous recombination leading to the deletion or duplication within *CFH* and *CFHR* genes. Notably, homozygous gene deletion of *CFHR1* is specifically linked with the production of autoantibodies against CFH [39–41]. A majority of these antibodies recognize the C-terminal region of CFH and inhibit the complement regulatory function of CFH on the cell surface [42]. Moreover, nonallelic homologous recombination of *CFHR* gene region predisposes to the formation of hybrid gene of *CFH-CFHR*, which causes aHUS [6].

Currently, several research groups have shown the correlation between coagulation system and aHUS. In 2013, Lemaire et al. have identified that the homozygous or compound heterozygous mutations in the *diacylglycerol kinase epsilon* (*DGKE*) gene in 13 aHUS patients who belong to nine unrelated families by whole-exome sequencing [43]. DGKE is a lipid kinase family protein, and is expressed in endothelium, platelets, and podocytes. The underlying pathology of DGKE-associated aHUS is still unclear, but one possibility is that the loss of function of DGKE results in upregulation of prothrombotic factors and platelet activations. It is still debatable whether DGKE-associated aHUS is linked with complement activation or not.

More recently, one published paper has identified four genetic variants in the gene of plasminogen in the patients with aHUS, and three of these variants were known plasminogen deficiency mutations [44]. Miyata et al. have shown that one genetic variant p.Ala620Thr in plasminogen, which is commonly observed in the northeast Asian populations including Japanese and causes dysplasminogenemia, is not predisposing variant for aHUS [45]. Further studies are required to confirm whether the coagulation system is additional pathogenesis for aHUS or not.

In addition to disease-associated mutations mentioned above, some environmental factors are related to increase the risk of developing aHUS. The onset of aHUS seems to be facilitated by various triggers such as infection and pregnancy [14, 24]. One retrospective study has shown that 21 of 100 adult female patients with aHUS developed pregnancy-associated TMA mainly in postpartum period [46].

Diagnosis of aHUS
Clinical diagnosis of aHUS
Rapid diagnosis of aHUS is critical for early initiation of treatment that prevents the patient's kidney from ESRD. Clinically, initial diagnosis of aHUS is made by microangiopathic hemolytic anemia (Hb <10 g/dL, negative direct Coombs test, elevated LDH, decreased haptoglobin, and

the presence of schistocytes), thrombocytopenia (platelet count $<150 \times 10^9/L$), and renal failure (elevated serum creatinine, low glomerular filtration rate, proteinuria, and hematuria). Other diseases which show similar clinical presentation to TMA such as disseminated intravascular coagulation or heparin-induced thrombocytopenia should be carefully excluded. In patients with aHUS, the major target organ is the kidney, but the heart, lungs, gastrointestinal tract, pancreas, and brain can also be affected. Although the presence of diarrhea is a representative manifestation of STEC-HUS, it has also been identified in 10–30% of aHUS patients [14, 24].

To differentiate aHUS from TTP, the activity of ADAMTS13 should be measured before the initiation of plasma therapy. Severe deficiency of ADAMTS13 activity (<10%) is common findings in patients with TTP. One study of 214 patients with TMA has shown that severe low platelet count ($<30 \times 10^9/L$) and serum creatinine (<2.26 mg/dL) were commonly detected in 157 of 160 patients with patients having severe ADAMTS13 deficiency [47] implicating that kidney damage is not generally severe in TTP. Of note, these laboratory data do not always differentiate aHUS from TTP. The confirmation of STEC-HUS needs the direct detection of Shiga toxins in feces and anti-lipopolysaccharide immunoglobulin M antibody measurements. Moreover, the screening of various diseases or specific laboratory data associated with TMA is critical for diagnosing secondary TMA.

Complement assessment in aHUS
To confirm the clinical diagnosis of aHUS, a variety of specific diagnostic tests are recommended as follows: quantification of complement components (C3 and C4), regulators (CFH, CFI, MCP, and CFB), and complement activity (CH50 for classical pathway, AP50 for alternative pathway), screening of anti-CFH autoantibodies, and genetic test of candidate gene (*CFH, CFI, MCP, C3, CFB, THBD*, and *DGKE*) [5]. The low level of C3, but not C4, may reflect the excess activation of the alternative pathway, but only 30–40% of patients with aHUS show a low level of C3 [14, 23]. Thus, a normal C3 level does not exclude the diagnosis of aHUS. Similarly, normal levels of abovementioned complement factors do not rule out the diagnosis of aHUS, because a majority of mutations cause functional impairment instead of quantitative defects. The hemolytic assay can be used to assess the CFH function [48–50]. In this assay, patient specimens are incubated with sheep red blood cells (RBCs) that have been known as "non-activating cells" leading no amplification of C3b on its cell surface. CFH is a major complement regulatory factor in the alternative pathway, and consists of 20 short consensus repeats (SCRs) with each about 60 amino residues. CFH is capable of protecting sheep RBCs from complement-mediated lysis via

binding of CFH SCRs19-20 to sialic acids richly expressed on surface of sheep RBCs. Thus, *CFH* mutations or anti-CFH autoantibodies having a defect in the protection of cell surfaces lyse the sheep RBCs [50]. The anti-CFH autoantibodies are generally measured by ELISA. Although several ELISA methods have been reported, Watson et al. have recommended the use of the Paris method, which is the most robust, cost-effective, and easy to establish [51].

Various biomarkers have been studied to reveal the underlying complement perturbations of aHUS to differentiate it from other TMAs. The significantly increased levels of C5a and soluble C5b-9 (sC5b-9), markers of terminal complement activation, have been identified in the acute phase of aHUS compared with TTP or healthy controls [52, 53]. Moreover, urine C5a, sC5b-9, and alternative pathway activation marker Ba are elevated in acute phase of aHUS, and these markers are decreased by eculizumab administration, with the exception of Ba [54]. However, Noris et al. has reported that plasma C5a and sC5b-9 were not suitable markers for diagnosing aHUS, because these values were normal in 9 out of 19 cases even during the acute phase [55]. Recent study has described a new technique for detecting excess complement activation by using modified HAM test, which is classically used to diagnose the patients with paroxysmal nocturnal hemoglobinuria (PNH). Gavriilaki and their colleagues have established the GPI-anchored protein-deficient cells, that is, PNH-like reagent cells [56]. When this cells are treated with the serum from TMA patients, significantly reduced cell viability are found in aHUS, compared to TTP. This novel method might be used for rapid diagnosis for aHUS to differentiate it from other TMAs.

Degradation of C3 spontaneously occurs after blood collection, which leads to altered complement state in patient specimens. To avoid pre-analytical errors, blood samples should be immediately centrifuged, and serum or plasma should be stored at −80 °C. EDTA plasma is generally used for measuring C5a, sC5b-9, and Ba but cannot be used for measuring ADAMTS13 activity, which can be only determined by using citrated plasma. Storage of EDTA plasma, citrated plasma, and serum before therapy is critical for accurate hemolytic assessment of underlying complement profile in patients suspected with aHUS.

Genetic test

Genetic screening is needed to confirm the clinical diagnosis of aHUS. Direct sequencing of six candidate genes (*CFH, CFI, MCP, C3, CFB,* and *THBD*) should be performed to reveal the predisposing mutations associated with aHUS. The screening of *DGKE* mutations is also recommended for the patients with onset of aHUS before the age of 1–2 years. Multiple ligation-dependent

probe amplification is generally used to identify the copy number variations of the genes encoding CFHR proteins. As shown in the recent finding of *DGKE* mutations, next-generation sequencing analysis is helpful to revealing the undiscovered disease-associated genes in aHUS.

Causality between genetic variants and the development of aHUS should be carefully assessed. A recent important study has shown that 122 of 406 (27%) mutations, which were published as disease-associated mutations in 104 individuals were either common polymorphisms or lacked direct evidence for pathogenicity [57]. Guidelines for genetic analysis have stated the importance of the terms to describe the genetic variants, and recommended the careful assessment to differentiate disease-causing genetic variants from many variants of human genome. To avoid the false-positive reports of causality, various mutations detected in aHUS should be carefully studied, and correctly named by using appropriate nomenclature (e.g., pathogenic, likely pathogenic, uncertain significance, likely benign and benign) instead of simple term like "causative" or "no causative" [58].

Genetic background of aHUS is complicated because of its various hereditary forms (autosomal dominant or autosomal recessive manner) and poor penetrance (about 50%). Therefore, individual and families should be provided an opportunity for genetic consultation by physicians, genetic professionals, and genetic counselors. Patient and patients' family members should be provided the following information: (1) the hereditary forms of aHUS and the importance of genetic test in the patients' parents, siblings, and offspring, (2) the risk of aHUS in the patient's parents, siblings, and offspring, and (3) the risk of aHUS during pregnancy or after delivery.

Treatment for aHUS
Plasma treatment

Since 1980s, plasma infusion (PI) or plasma exchange (PE) had empirically been considered as the first choice for the treatment of aHUS. PI with fresh frozen plasma serves functional complement regulatory factors. In addition to this effect, PE is presumed to remove the abnormal complement related factors like mutant proteins or anti-CFH antibodies. There are no prospective clinical trial data, but the introduction of plasma therapy has decreased the mortality of patients with aHUS and achieved hematological remission in 70% of patients with aHUS. On the contrary, plasma therapy resulted in ESRD or death in 48% of pediatric and 67% of adult cases died or reached ESRD within 3-year follow-up [14]. Especially in aHUS patients with *CFH* or *CFI* mutations, complete hematological remission or renal recovery rates was low.

Although some patients do not achieve complete remission by plasma therapy, it is still an important therapeutic approach for the patients suspected with aHUS. Early initiation of plasma therapy followed by maintenance PI/PE could be effective for attaining hematological remission and preserving renal function. However, evaluation of other TMAs and the diagnosis of aHUS take some times in practical situations. Of note, the efficacy of plasma therapy is uncertain in the treatment for STEC-HUS. In the case of secondary TMA, the necessity and efficacy of plasma therapy depends on the coexisting disease, and PE should be avoided in the cases with *S. pneumoniae*-mediated TMA. Concomitant immunosuppression and plasma therapy may allow better outcomes by reducing antibody titers in the case of anti-CFH antibody positive patients. So far, combined therapy of PE and immunosuppression (steroids with or without immunosuppressants such as cyclophosphamide or rituximab) for the induction and maintenance therapy with steroids and immunosuppresants (mycophenolate mofetil or azathioprine) have been reported to be favorable [5, 59, 60]. Eculizumab also seems to be effective in anti-CFH antibody aHUS patients [5]. However, the optimal treatment combination for anti-CFH antibody positive patients remains to be elucidated in the future. Catheter-related complications should be concerned in pediatric cases, and PI may be recommended when PE is technically difficult to perform. Plasma therapy should be tapered based on increased platelet count, improvement of hemolysis, and lactate dehydrogenase level.

Eculizumab

Eculizumab, a monoclonal humanized antibody against C5, was originally approved for treating the patients with PNH. This antibody specifically binds to C5 and blocks the terminal complement activation by inhibiting the cleavage of C5 into C5a and C5b. The efficacy and safety of eculizumab for the treatment of aHUS have been reported since 2009 [61–63], and both the USA Food and Drug Administration and the European Medicines Agency approved the indication of aHUS in the treatment of aHUS in 2011. Subsequent reports also showed that the use of eculizumab was effective for the patients with aHUS who underwent the renal transplantation [64].

In pediatric cases, eculizumab administration is recommended as a first-line therapy when the diagnosis of aHUS is made, because these patients have a high risk of catheter-related complications and a lower incidence of secondary TMA than adults. Contrary, in adult patients, the initial choice of PE or eculizumab is often difficult because adults have higher incidence of secondary TMA, some secondary TMA have the indication of PE, and currently eculizumab is not approved for secondary TMA in our country. The authors recommend evaluating STEC-HUS, TTP, and secondary TMA before the initial use of eculizumab. In adult cases, eculizumab

administration may be recommended as a first choice in the following situations: (1) the patients have repeated episode of aHUS or family history (especially, one or more family members have renal failure caused by TMA), (2) the patients are already diagnosed with aHUS, and (3) the probability of the diagnosis of aHUS is high. Although the reports are limited, eculizumab treatment for aHUS during pregnancy stabilizes clinical and laboratory markers and shows no overt safety issues [65]. However, further investigations are needed to ascertain the efficacy and safety of eculizumab in the treatment of the patients with aHUS during pregnancy.

The appearance of eculizumab opened a new era for treatment of aHUS; however, it is still unclear how long eculizumab therapy should be continued. Eculizumab treatment requires the patients to visit the hospital once every 2 weeks, which may lead to the impaired quality of life. Moreover, lifelong treatment may cause the compromised vascular access. The extremely high cost of eculizumab is also important limitation of this drug. The current report concerning the eculizumab withdrawal has shown that 24 patients discontinued the treatment, and 6 out of 24 patients (25%) had recurrence at the time of publication [66]. Four of these six patients had *CFH* mutation or anti-CFH antibodies, suggesting that the patients having CFH-related abnormalities were frequently associated with the recurrence of aHUS [5, 66]. On the other hand, patients with MCP mutation, CFI mutation, or no mutation showed no recurrence. Although more studies are needed to confirm these observations, lifelong treatment may not be needed for all patients with aHUS, and clarifying the genetic background may help to discontinue the anti-complement drug [67].

Prognosis

Before the use of eculizumab for treating aHUS, a poor prognosis of this disease has historically been described, with higher than 50% mortality and ESRD. The clinical outcomes vary depending on the genetic alterations [14, 24]. The worst prognosis is the patients with *CFH* mutations, with over 50% mortality or ESRD rates within 1 year from the first episode of aHUS [14, 24]. On the contrary, the cases of the patients with MCP mutations have a good prognosis; none of the children and only 25% of adults reached to ESRD at first episode although they have a high risk of relapse [2]. Of note, these data come from the historical studies treated with plasma therapy [14, 23, 24]. Recent advances of therapy including early initiation of plasma therapy or eculizumab administration significantly improved the mortality and prognosis of aHUS [62, 68]. In the near future, the data showing prognosis of aHUS patients depending on the genetic background treated with eculizumab will be clarified. Systemic management including blood pressure control is also important as short- and long-term treatment; however, the effects of different antihypertensive drug classes remain to be elucidated.

Current studies for the patients with aHUS in Japan

Since the early 2000s, some patients with clinically suspected aHUS have been identified in Japan. In 2008, Mukai et al. reported the predisposing mutation of CFH in a 1-year-old female aHUS patient by using both hemolytic assay and genetic analysis [69]. Further study was performed by Fujimura et al., who have studied Japanese patients with TMA by measuring ADAMTS13 activity since 1998. In 2009, they reported the characteristics of 919 TMA patients and noted that 24 of 919 were suspected to be "congenital aHUS" because of having repeated and familial TMA episodes with ADAMTS13 levels of more than 10% [70]. To reveal the underlying pathogenic mechanisms of these patients, they established the diagnostic system for aHUS (the quantitative hemolytic assay, the screening of anti-CFH antibody, and the genetic tests of *CFH, CFI, MCP, C3, CFB, and THBD*) [45, 50, 71, 72]. In the hemolytic assay, Yoshida et al. [50] produced inhibitory monoclonal antibodies against CFH and used one of these antibodies as a positive control, which enabled to quantitatively calculate the degree of hemolysis in patient plasma. They revealed that patient plasma with CFH mutation or anti-CFH autoantibodies had >50% hemolysis. In addition, patient plasma with the C3 p.K1105Q mutation positioned at the CFH binding interface also showed >50% hemolysis.

The genetic analysis of 45 patients with aHUS has shown that the frequency of *C3* mutation (43%) was greater than that in Western countries (2–10%). In contrast, only 7% of patients with aHUS carried the *CFH* mutations in Japan, which is much less than the frequency reported by Western countries [50]. Interestingly, about 80% patients with *C3* mutations have the same variants of I1157T, and the patients carrying this variants were only found in an extremely restricted area (Kansai district including Mie, Nara, Kyoto and Osaka prefectures) of West Japan [50, 73]. These observations suggested that the genetic background of aHUS in Japan differs from that of Western countries. However, because study population was small and 60% of the patients with aHUS were from West Japan, further assessments are required to reveal the genetic characteristics in Japan. Complement-related genes have also been investigated in the patients with congenital TTP having renal damage by Fan et al [74]. Six complement and complement regulatory genes of aHUS were sequenced, and they have suggested that rare predisposing complement genetic mutations of aHUS do not contribute to renal insufficiency in congenital TTP patients.

In 2013, the use of eculizumab was approved for treating complement-mediated aHUS patients by Ministry of Health, Labour and Welfare in Japan. Several case reports have described the efficacy and safety of this drug for aHUS in Japan. Ito et al. have retrospectively analyzed the clinical course of 10 pediatric aHUS cases treated with eculizumab, and shown that all patients achieved the rapid hematological remission with withdrawal from plasma therapy [75]. Ohta et al. have reported that one infant patient with compound heterozygous *DGKE* mutation, who significantly recovered from severe hypertensions and peritoneal dialysis by eculizumab administration [72, 76]. Of note, this patient showed the severely decreased level of C3 suggesting unregulated complement activation; however, it is unclear whether the mutation in *DGKE* is associated with exhausted C3 or not in this particular patient. In contrast to pediatric cases with aHUS, little has been reported on adult cases in Japan. The study published by Okumi et al. has shown one male patient with *CFH* mutation, who received living-related kidney transplant after first episode of aHUS [77]. This patient developed aHUS again after transplantation, but his hematological parameters and renal function was fully recovered by initiation of eculizumab treatment.

Currently, the diagnostic system of aHUS was moved from Nara Medical University to the Division of Nephrology and Endocrinology, the University of Tokyo Hospital. Protein-based analyses (the hemolytic assay and the screening of anti-CFH autoantibodies) are performed in the University of Tokyo Hospital, and the DNA analyses of six candidate genes (*CFH, CFI, MCP, C3, CFB, and THBD*) are in National Cerebral and Cardiovascular Center. Moreover, epidemiologic study of aHUS is ongoing in the University of Tokyo Hospital. Consultation for diagnostic test of aHUS is available by e-mail (ahus-office@umin.ac.jp).

Conclusions

The recent progresses in the field of aHUS during the last two decade have significantly clarified the underlying pathology of aHUS, which led to new era for complement blockade; eculizumab therapy. Early administration of eculizumab has dramatically prevented the progression to ESRD in the patients with aHUS. In Japan, an established structured diagnostic system of aHUS has gradually revealed both clinical characteristic and genetic background of this disease. On the other hand, the data on the prognosis (risk of ESRD, death, relapse, and recurrence after renal transplantation) or outcome of eculizumab therapy still have not been well documented. Now, our groups are addressing these issues, and we hope that this ongoing study will lead to early diagnosis and appropriate treatment for patients with aHUS in Japan.

Abbreviations

ADAMTS13: A disintegrin-like and metalloprotease with thrombospondin type 1 motif, 13; aHUS: Atypical hemolytic uremic syndrome; CFB: Complement factor B; CFD: complement factor D; CFH: Complement factor H; CFHR: Complement factor H related; CFI: Complement factor I; DGKE: Diacylglycerol kinase epsilon; EDTA: Ethylenediaminetetraacetic acid; ESRD: End-stage renal disease; HELLP: Hemolysis, elevated liver enzyme, low platelet count; MCP: Membrane cofactor protein; RBC: Red blood cell; STEC: Shiga toxin-producing *Escherichia coli*; TMA: Thrombotic microangiopathy; TTP: Thrombotic thrombocytopenic purpura; VWF: von Willebrand factor

Acknowledgements

The authors would like to express their gratitude to emeritus professor Yoshiro Fujimura, professor Masanori Matsumoto of Nara Medical University and Toshiyuki Miyata of National Cerebral and Cardiovascular Center who originally established epidemiology and diagnostic system of TMA in Japan.

Funding

This study was supported by research grants from the Ministry of Health, Labour and Welfare of Japan and from Japan Society for the Promotion of Science, Grant-in-Aid for Scientific Research (C) (15K09246), and the Japanese Association for Complement Research.

Authors' contributions

YY and HK made the original form of this manuscript. MN organized the comprehensive study project and edited of this manuscript. All authors read and approved the final manuscript.

Competing interests

MN received lecture fees and research funding from Alexion Pharmaceuticals, Inc. HK received lecture fees from Alexion Pharmaceuticals, Inc.

References

1. Kaplan BS, Chesney RW, Drummond KN. Hemolytic uremic syndrome in families. N Engl J Med. 1975;292:1090–3.
2. Loirat C, Fremeaux-Bacchi V. Atypical hemolytic uremic syndrome. Orphanet J Rare Dis. 2011;6:60.
3. Mele C, Remuzzi G, Noris M. Hemolytic uremic syndrome. Semin Immunopathol. 2014;36:399–420.
4. Campistol JM, Arias M, Ariceta G, Blasco M, Espinosa L, Espinosa M, et al. An update for atypical haemolytic uraemic syndrome: diagnosis and treatment. A consensus document. Nefrologia. 2015;35:421–47.
5. Loirat C, Fakhouri F, Ariceta G, Besbas N, Bitzan M, Bjerre A, et al. An international consensus approach to the management of atypical hemolytic uremic syndrome in children. Pediatr Nephrol. 2016;31:15–39.
6. Nester CM, Barbour T, de Cordoba SR, Dragon-Durey MA, Fremeaux-Bacchi V, Goodship TH, et al. Atypical aHUS: state of the art. Mol Immunol. 2015;67:31–42.
7. Huang J, Motto DG, Bundle DR, Sadler JE. Shiga toxin B subunits induce VWF secretion by human endothelial cells and thrombotic microangiopathy in ADAMTS13-deficient mice. Blood. 2010;116:3653–9.
8. Garg AX, Suri RS, Barrowman N, Rehman F, Matsell D, Rosas-Arellano MP, et al. Long-term renal prognosis of diarrhea-associated hemolytic uremic syndrome: a systematic review, meta-analysis, and meta-regression. JAMA. 2003;290:1360–70.
9. Levy GG, Nichols WC, Lian EC, Foroud T, McClintick JN, McGee BM, et al. Mutations in a member of the ADAMTS gene family cause thrombotic thrombocytopenic purpura. Nature. 2001;413:488–94.
10. Kokame K, Matsumoto M, Soejima K, Yagi H, Ishizashi H, Funato M, et al. Mutations and common polymorphisms in ADAMTS13 gene responsible for von Willebrand factor-cleaving protease activity. Proc Natl Acad Sci U S A. 2002;99:11902–7.
11. Tsai HM, Lian EC. Antibodies to von Willebrand factor-cleaving protease in acute thrombotic thrombocytopenic purpura. N Engl J Med. 1998;339:1585–94.
12. Thompson RA, Winterborn MH. Hypocomplementaemia due to a genetic deficiency of beta 1H globulin. Clin Exp Immunol. 1981;46:110–9.
13. Warwicker P, Goodship TH, Donne RL, Pirson Y, Nicholls A, Ward RM, et al. Genetic studies into inherited and sporadic hemolytic uremic syndrome. Kidney Int. 1998;53:836–44.
14. Noris M, Caprioli J, Bresin E, Mossali C, Pianetti G, Gamba S, et al. Relative role of genetic complement abnormalities in sporadic and familial aHUS and their impact on clinical phenotype. Clin J Am Soc Nephrol. 2010;5: 1844–59.
15. Fakhouri F, Jablonski M, Lepercq J, Blouin J, Benachi A, Hourmant M, et al. Factor H, membrane cofactor protein, and factor I mutations in patients with hemolysis, elevated liver enzymes, and low platelet count syndrome. Blood. 2008;112:4542–5.
16. Crovetto F, Borsa N, Acaia B, Nishimura C, Frees K, Smith RJ, et al. The genetics of the alternative pathway of complement in the pathogenesis of HELLP syndrome. J Matern Fetal Neonatal Med. 2012;25:2322–5.
17. Sawai T, Nangaku M, Ashida A, Fujimaru R, Hataya H, Hidaka Y, et al. Diagnostic criteria for atypical hemolytic uremic syndrome proposed by the Joint Committee of the Japanese Society of Nephrology and the Japan Pediatric Society. Clin Exp Nephrol. 2014;18:4–9.
18. Sawai T, Nangaku M, Ashida A, Fujimaru R, Hataya H, Hidaka Y, et al. Diagnostic criteria for atypical hemolytic uremic syndrome proposed by the Joint Committee of the Japanese Society of Nephrology and the Japan Pediatric Society. Pediatr Int. 2014;56:1–5.
19. Kato H, Nangaku M, Hataya H, Sawai T, Ashida A, Fujimaru R, et al. Clinical guides for atypical hemolytic uremic syndrome in Japan. Pediatr Int. 2016; 58:549–55.
20. Kato H, Nangaku M, Hataya H, Sawai T, Ashida A, Fujimaru R, et al. Clinical guides for atypical hemolytic uremic syndrome in Japan. Clin Exp Nephrol. 2016;20:536–43.
21. Le Quintrec M, Lionet A, Kamar N, Karras A, Barbier S, Buchler M, et al. Complement mutation-associated de novo thrombotic microangiopathy following kidney transplantation. Am J Transplant. 2008;8:1694–701.
22. Constantinescu AR, Bitzan M, Weiss LS, Christen E, Kaplan BS, Cnaan A, et al. Non-enteropathic hemolytic uremic syndrome: causes and short-term course. Am J Kidney Dis. 2004;43:976–82.
23. Fremeaux-Bacchi V, Fakhouri F, Garnier A, Bienaime F, Dragon-Durey MA, Ngo S, et al. Genetics and outcome of atypical hemolytic uremic syndrome: a nationwide French series comparing children and adults. Clin J Am Soc Nephrol. 2013;8:554–62.
24. Sellier-Leclerc AL, Fremeaux-Bacchi V, Dragon-Durey MA, Macher MA, Niaudet P, Guest G, et al. Differential impact of complement mutations on clinical characteristics in atypical hemolytic uremic syndrome. J Am Soc Nephrol. 2007;18:2392–400.
25. Richards A, Buddles MR, Donne RL, Kaplan BS, Kirk E, Venning MC, et al. Factor H mutations in hemolytic uremic syndrome cluster in exons 18-20, a domain important for host cell recognition. Am J Hum Genet. 2001;68:485–90.
26. Caprioli J, Bettinaglio P, Zipfel PF, Amadei B, Daina E, Gamba S, et al. The molecular basis of familial hemolytic uremic syndrome: mutation analysis of factor H gene reveals a hot spot in short consensus repeat 20. J Am Soc Nephrol. 2001;12:297–307.
27. Perez-Caballero D, Gonzalez-Rubio C, Gallardo ME, Vera M, Lopez-Trascasa M, RodriguezdeCordoba S, et al. Clustering of missense mutations in the C-terminal region of factor H in atypical hemolytic uremic syndrome. Am J Hum Genet. 2001;68:478–84.
28. Fremeaux-Bacchi V, Dragon-Durey MA, Blouin J, Vigneau C, Kuypers D, Boudailliez B, et al. Complement factor I: a susceptibility gene for atypical haemolytic uraemic syndrome. J Med Genet. 2004;41:e84.

29. Kavanagh D, Kemp EJ, Mayland E, Winney RJ, Duffield JS, Warwick G, et al. Mutations in complement factor I predispose to development of atypical hemolytic uremic syndrome. J Am Soc Nephrol. 2005;16:2150–5.

30. Richards A, Kemp EJ, Liszewski MK, Goodship JA, Lampe AK, Decorte R, et al. Mutations in human complement regulator, membrane cofactor protein (CD46), predispose to development of familial hemolytic uremic syndrome. Proc Natl Acad Sci U S A. 2003;100:12966–71.

31. Noris M, Brioschi S, Caprioli J, Todeschini M, Bresin E, Porrati F, et al. Familial haemolytic uraemic syndrome and an MCP mutation. Lancet. 2003;362:1542–7.

32. Delvaeye M, Noris M, De Vriese A, Esmon CT, Esmon NL, Ferrell G, et al. Thrombomodulin mutations in atypical hemolytic-uremic syndrome. N Engl J Med. 2009;361:345–57.

33. Fremeaux-Bacchi V, Miller EC, Liszewski MK, Strain L, Blouin J, Brown AL, et al. Mutations in complement C3 predispose to development of atypical hemolytic uremic syndrome. Blood. 2008;112:4948–52.

34. Schramm EC, Roumenina LT, Rybkine T, Chauvet S, Vieira-Martins P, Hue C, et al. Mapping interactions between complement C3 and regulators using mutations in atypical hemolytic uremic syndrome. Blood. 2015;125:2359–69.

35. Goicoechea de Jorge E, Harris CL, Esparza-Gordillo J, Carreras L, Arranz EA, Garrido CA, et al. Gain-of-function mutations in complement factor B are associated with atypical hemolytic uremic syndrome. Proc Natl Acad Sci U S A. 2007;104:240–5.

36. Roumenina LT, Jablonski M, Hue C, Blouin J, Dimitrov JD, Dragon-Durey MA, et al. Hyperfunctional C3 convertase leads to complement deposition on endothelial cells and contributes to atypical hemolytic uremic syndrome. Blood. 2009;114:2837–45.

37. Bresin E, Rurali E, Caprioli J, Sanchez-Corral P, Fremeaux-Bacchi V, Rodriguez de Cordoba S, et al. Combined complement gene mutations in atypical hemolytic uremic syndrome influence clinical phenotype. J Am Soc Nephrol. 2013;24:475–86.

38. Dragon-Durey MA, Loirat C, Cloarec S, Macher MA, Blouin J, Nivet H, et al. Anti-factor H autoantibodies associated with atypical hemolytic uremic syndrome. J Am Soc Nephrol. 2005;16:555–63.

39. Jozsi M, Licht C, Strobel S, Zipfel SL, Richter H, Heinen S, et al. Factor H autoantibodies in atypical hemolytic uremic syndrome correlate with CFHR1/CFHR3 deficiency. Blood. 2008;111:1512–4.

40. Moore I, Strain L, Pappworth I, Kavanagh D, Barlow PN, Herbert AP, et al. Association of factor H autoantibodies with deletions of CFHR1, CFHR3, CFHR4, and with mutations in CFH, CFI, CD46, and C3 in patients with atypical hemolytic uremic syndrome. Blood. 2010;115:379–87.

41. Bhattacharjee A, Reuter S, Trojnar E, Kolodziejczyk R, Seeberger H, Hyvarinen S, et al. The major autoantibody epitope on factor H in atypical hemolytic uremic syndrome is structurally different from its homologous site in factor H-related protein 1, supporting a novel model for induction of autoimmunity in this disease. J Biol Chem. 2015;290:9500–10.

42. Jozsi M, Strobel S, Dahse HM, Liu WS, Hoyer PF, Oppermann M, et al. Anti factor H autoantibodies block C-terminal recognition function of factor H in hemolytic uremic syndrome. Blood. 2007;110:1516–8.

43. Lemaire M, Fremeaux-Bacchi V, Schaefer F, Choi M, Tang WH, Le Quintrec M, et al. Recessive mutations in DGKE cause atypical hemolytic-uremic syndrome. Nat Genet. 2013;45:531–6.

44. Bu F, Maga T, Meyer NC, Wang K, Thomas CP, Nester CM, et al. Comprehensive genetic analysis of complement and coagulation genes in atypical hemolytic uremic syndrome. J Am Soc Nephrol. 2014;25:55–64.

45. Miyata T, Uchida Y, Yoshida Y, Kato H, Matsumoto M, Kokame K, et al. No association between dysplasminogenemia with p.Ala620Thr mutation and atypical hemolytic uremic syndrome. Int J Hematol. 2016;104:223–7.

46. Fakhouri F, Roumenina L, Provot F, Sallee M, Caillard S, Couzi L, et al. Pregnancy-associated hemolytic uremic syndrome revisited in the era of complement gene mutations. J Am Soc Nephrol. 2010;21:859–67.

47. Coppo P, Schwarzinger M, Buffet M, Wynckel A, Clabault K, Presne C, et al. Predictive features of severe acquired ADAMTS13 deficiency in idiopathic thrombotic microangiopathies: the French TMA reference center experience. PLoS One. 2010;5:e10208.

48. Sanchez-Corral P, Gonzalez-Rubio C, Rodriguez de Cordoba S, Lopez-Trascasa M. Functional analysis in serum from atypical hemolytic uremic syndrome patients reveals impaired protection of host cells associated with mutations in factor H. Mol Immunol. 2004;41:81–4.

49. Roumenina LT, Roquigny R, Blanc C, Poulain N, Ngo S, Dragon-Durey MA, et al. Functional evaluation of factor H genetic and acquired abnormalities: application for atypical hemolytic uremic syndrome (aHUS). Methods Mol Biol. 2014;1100:237–47.

50. Yoshida Y, Miyata T, Matsumoto M, Shirotani-Ikejima H, Uchida Y, Ohyama Y, et al. A novel quantitative hemolytic assay coupled with restriction fragment length polymorphisms analysis enabled early diagnosis of atypical hemolytic uremic syndrome and identified unique predisposing mutations in Japan. PLoS One. 2015;10:e0124655.

51. Watson R, Lindner S, Bordereau P, Hunze EM, Tak F, Ngo S, et al. Standardisation of the factor H autoantibody assay. Immunobiology. 2014;219:9–16.

52. Volokhina EB, Westra D, van der Velden TJ, van de Kar NC, Mollnes TE, van den Heuvel LP. Complement activation patterns in atypical haemolytic uraemic syndrome during acute phase and in remission. Clin Exp Immunol. 2015;181:306–13.

53. Cataland SR, Holers VM, Geyer S, Yang S, Wu HM. Biomarkers of terminal complement activation confirm the diagnosis of aHUS and differentiate aHUS from TTP. Blood. 2014;123:3733–8.

54. Cofiell R, Kukreja A, Bedard K, Yan Y, Mickle AP, Ogawa M, et al. Eculizumab reduces complement activation, inflammation, endothelial damage, thrombosis, and renal injury markers in aHUS. Blood. 2015;125:3253–62.

55. Noris M, Galbusera M, Gastoldi S, Macor P, Banterla F, Bresin E, et al. Dynamics of complement activation in aHUS and how to monitor eculizumab therapy. Blood. 2014;124:1715–26.

56. Gavriilaki E, Yuan X, Ye Z, Ambinder AJ, Shanbhag SP, Streiff MB, et al. Modified Ham test for atypical hemolytic uremic syndrome. Blood. 2015;125:3637–46.

57. Bell CJ, Dinwiddie DL, Miller NA, Hateley SL, Ganusova EE, Mudge J, et al. Carrier testing for severe childhood recessive diseases by next-generation sequencing. Sci Transl Med. 2011;3:65ra4.

58. Richards S, Aziz N, Bale S, Bick D, Das S, Gastier-Foster J, et al. Standards and guidelines for the interpretation of sequence variants: a joint consensus recommendation of the American College of Medical Genetics and Genomics and the Association for Molecular Pathology. Genet Med. 2015;17:405–24.

59. Dragon-Durey MA, Sethi SK, Bagga A, Blanc C, Blouin J, Ranchin B, et al. Clinical features of anti-factor H autoantibody-associated hemolytic uremic syndrome. J Am Soc Nephrol. 2010;21:2180–7.

60. Sinha A, Gulati A, Saini S, Blanc C, Gupta A, Gurjar BS, et al. Prompt plasma exchanges and immunosuppressive treatment improves the outcomes of anti-factor H autoantibody-associated hemolytic uremic syndrome in children. Kidney Int. 2014;85:1151–60.

61. Nürnberger J, Philipp T, Witzke O, Opazo Saez A, Vester U, Baba HA, et al. Eculizumab for atypical hemolytic-uremic syndrome. N Engl J Med. 2009;360:542–4.

62. Legendre CM, Licht C, Muus P, Greenbaum LA, Babu S, Bedrosian C, et al. Terminal complement inhibitor eculizumab in atypical hemolytic-uremic syndrome. N Engl J Med. 2013;368:2169–81.

63. Licht C, Ardissino G, Ariceta G, Cohen D, Cole JA, Gasteyger C, et al. The global aHUS registry: methodology and initial patient characteristics. BMC Nephrol. 2015;16:207.

64. Zuber J, Le Quintrec M, Krid S, Bertoye C, Gueutin V, Lahoche A, et al. Eculizumab for atypical hemolytic uremic syndrome recurrence in renal transplantation. Am J Transplant. 2012;12:3337–54.

65. Servais A, Devillard N, Fremeaux-Bacchi V, Hummel A, Salomon L, Contin-Bordes C, et al. Atypical haemolytic uraemic syndrome and pregnancy: outcome with ongoing eculizumab. Nephrol Dial Transplant. 2016; doi:10.1093/ndt/gfw314.

66. Nester CM. Managing atypical hemolytic uremic syndrome: chapter 2. Kidney Int. 2015;87:882–4.

67. Fakhouri F, Fila M, Provot F, Delmas Y, Barbet C, Chatelet V, et al. Pathogenic variants in complement genes and risk of atypical hemolytic uremic syndrome relapse after eculizumab discontinuation. Clin J Am Soc Nephrol. 2016; doi:10.2215/CJN.06440616.

68. Licht C, Greenbaum LA, Muus P, Babu S, Bedrosian CL, Cohen DJ, et al. Efficacy and safety of eculizumab in atypical hemolytic uremic syndrome from 2-year extensions of phase 2 studies. Kidney Int. 2015;87:1061–73.

69. Mukai S, Hidaka Y, Hirota-Kawadobora M, Matsuda K, Fujihara N, Takezawa Y, et al. Factor H gene variants in Japanese: its relation to atypical hemolytic uremic syndrome. Mol Immunol. 2011;49:48–55.

70. Fujimura Y, Matsumoto M. Registry of 919 patients with thrombotic microangiopathies across Japan: database of Nara Medical University during 1998-2008. Intern Med. 2010;49:7–15.

71. Fan X, Yoshida Y, Honda S, Matsumoto M, Sawada Y, Hattori M, et al. Analysis of genetic and predisposing factors in Japanese patients with atypical hemolytic uremic syndrome. Mol Immunol. 2013;54:238–46.

72. Miyata T, Uchida Y, Ohta T, Urayama K, Yoshida Y, Fujimura Y. Atypical haemolytic uraemic syndrome in a Japanese patient with DGKE genetic mutations. Thromb Haemost. 2015;114:862–3.

73. Matsumoto T, Fan X, Ishikawa E, Ito M, Amano K, Toyoda H, et al. Analysis of patients with atypical hemolytic uremic syndrome treated at the Mie University Hospital: concentration of C3 p.I1157T mutation. Int J Hematol. 2014;100:437–42.

74. Fan X, Kremer Hovinga JA, Shirotani-Ikejima H, Eura Y, Hirai H, Honda S, et al. Genetic variations in complement factors in patients with congenital thrombotic thrombocytopenic purpura with renal insufficiency. Int J Hematol. 2016;103:283–91.

75. Ito N, Hataya H, Saida K, Amano Y, Hidaka Y, Motoyoshi Y, et al. Efficacy and safety of eculizumab in childhood atypical hemolytic uremic syndrome in Japan. Clin Exp Nephrol. 2016;20:265–72.

76. Ohta T, Urayama K, Tada Y, Furue T, Imai S, Matsubara K, et al. Eculizumab in the treatment of atypical hemolytic uremic syndrome in an infant leads to cessation of peritoneal dialysis and improvement of severe hypertension. Pediatr Nephrol. 2015;30:603–8.

77. Okumi M, Omoto K, Unagami K, Ishida H, Tanabe K. Eculizumab for the treatment of atypical hemolytic uremic syndrome recurrence after kidney transplantation associated with complement factor H mutations: a case report with a 5-year follow-up. Int Urol Nephrol. 2016;48:817–8.

7

Association between chronic kidney disease and physical activity level in patients with ischemic heart disease

Ryota Matsuzawa[1], Takashi Masuda[2,3*], Kentaro Kamiya[1], Nobuaki Hamazaki[1,3], Kohei Nozaki[1], Shinya Tanaka[3], Emi Maekawa[4] and Junya Ako[3,4]

Abstract

Background: Although it is believed that chronic kidney disease (CKD) in patients with ischemic heart disease (IHD) negatively affects physical activity after discharge, its actual influence on the physical activity of patients with IHD remains unclear. This study aimed to investigate the association between CKD and the acquirement of appropriate physical activity after hospital discharge in patients with IHD.

Methods: Subjects were 245 patients with IHD (65 ± 11 years, 203 males) admitted to Kitasato University Hospital from July 2007 to January 2014 due to unstable angina pectoris or acute myocardial infarction. Appropriate physical activity was defined according to the American Heart Association/the American College of Cardiology guidelines, which recommend ≥150 min/week of moderate-to-vigorous activity. We assessed intervention for IHD, comorbidities, smoking habits, serum high-sensitivity C-reactive protein, estimated glomerular filtration rate (eGFR), left ventricular ejection fraction, duration of hospital stay, 6-min walk distance during hospitalization, and physical activity 3 months after discharge. Patients with eGFR ≥60 mL/min/1.73 m^2 and 15 ≤ eGFR < 60 mL/min/1.73 m^2 were diagnosed with stage G1-G2 CKD and stage G3-G4 CKD, respectively.

Results: Only 87 patients (35.5%) achieved appropriate levels of physical activity. Stepwise multivariate logistic regression analysis identified stage G3-G4 CKD (odds ratio, 1.91; 95%CI, 1.02–3.55; $P = 0.04$) and a 6-min walk distance <400 m (odds ratio, 17.8; 95%CI, 4.16–76.6; $P < 0.001$) as significant independent factors that hinder acquiring appropriate physical activity.

Conclusions: Stage G3-G4 CKD was associated with poor acquirement of appropriate physical activity after hospital discharge in patients with IHD.

Keywords: CKD, Ischemic heart disease, Coronary artery disease, Physical activity

Background

Increased physical activity reduces cardiovascular mortality risk in general populations [1]. Furthermore, recent meta-analyses revealed that the physically active had a 20–50% less risk of coronary heart disease than the physically inactive [2, 3]. The American Heart Association (AHA) presented seven impact goals for maintaining healthy cardiovascular conditions in all adults that included a physically active lifestyle and management of cholesterol, blood pressure, blood sugar, smoking status, weight, and diet [4]. The lifestyle management guidelines published by the AHA and the American College of Cardiology (ACC) in 2013 stated that physical activity of moderate-to-vigorous intensity for at least 150 min a week is appropriate for obtaining a variety of health benefits [5]. In addition, maintaining a physically active lifestyle is important for both primary and secondary prevention of ischemic heart disease (IHD). Many patients with IHD, however, tend to have poor physical activity after hospital discharge [6]. Increased physical activity also provides a large variety of health benefits to

* Correspondence: tak9999@med.kitasato-u.ac.jp
[2]Department of Rehabilitation, School of Allied Health Sciences, Kitasato University, 1-15-1 Kitasato, Sagamihara, Kanagawa 252-0373, Japan
[3]Department of Cardio-Angiology, Graduate School of Medical Sciences, Kitasato University, Sagamihara, Japan
Full list of author information is available at the end of the article

chronic kidney disease (CKD) patients [7, 8]. However, previous studies reported that the majority of CKD patients were physically inactive in their daily living [7, 9, 10]. Although it is believed that CKD in patients with IHD negatively affects physical activity after discharge, its actual influence on the physical activity of patients with IHD remains unclear.

The purpose of this study was to investigate the association between CKD and the acquirement of appropriate physical activity after hospital discharge in patients with IHD.

Methods

Study population

This study was approved by the Kitasato University Hospital Research Ethic Committee. After receiving an explanation of the study purpose and protocol, all patients gave their informed consent.

Subjects were 245 patients with IHD admitted to Kitasato University Hospital from July 2007 to January 2014 due to unstable angina pectoris or acute myocardial infarction and underwent cardiac rehabilitation during hospitalization. The patients included 203 men and 42 women (mean age, 65 years; range, 31 to 86 years). Of the 245 patients, 54 (22.0%) received coronary artery bypass graft surgery and 191 (78.0%) received percutaneous coronary intervention. All patients were successfully treated for coronary artery reperfusion and experienced no myocardial ischemia, as determined by electrocardiograph changes or chest pain after hospital discharge. Patients were excluded from the study if they received maintenance hemodialysis therapy (stage 5D) or needed any assistance with walking, occurred with heart failure, and refused to be measured the physical activity at 3 months after hospital discharge. Because the health benefits of increased physical activity are unclear in patients with stage G5 CKD who are not on hemodialysis and medical staffs did not educate and enhance them to participate in exercise aggressively in contrast to patients with stages G1-G4 CKD and 5D, the patients with stage G5 CKD were also excluded.

Clinical characteristics

Patient information on age, gender, height, employment, intervention for IHD, smoking habits, and comorbid conditions such as cerebrovascular disease, peripheral arterial disease, orthopedic disorder, or diabetes mellitus were collected from medical records or by interview at study entry. Body weight, body mass index, left ventricular ejection fraction on an echocardiogram, ankle-brachial index, and duration of hospital stay, were determined at hospital discharge. We measured blood hemoglobin and serum levels of albumin, creatine kinase, and high-sensitivity C-reactive protein and assessed

the estimated glomerular filtration rate (eGFR) after admission. The parameter of eGFR was re-assessed at 3 months after hospital discharge, and the difference in eGFR between at baseline and 3 months was calculated. Peak creatine kinase levels in patients with acute myocardial infarction were also confirmed during hospitalization. In patients with diabetes, HbA1c levels were investigated at hospital discharge. Peripheral arterial disease was assessed using an ankle-brachial index (Form PWV/ABI, Omron Colin, Tokyo, Japan). Patients with an eGFR ≥ 60 mL/min/1.73 m^2, 15–60 mL/min/ 1.73 m^2, and <15 mL/min/1.73 m^2 were diagnosed with stage G1-G2 CKD, stage G3-G4 CKD, and stage G5 CKD, respectively.

Exercise capacity

Six-minute walk distance was measured at hospital discharge and 3 months as an indicator of exercise capacity, in accordance with guidelines established by the American Thoracic Society [11]. The difference in 6-min walk distance between at baseline and 3 months was calculated. After patients received a detailed explanation of the procedure from a physical therapist, they were instructed to walk as fast and long as possible along a 30-m walkway marked at 1-m intervals. Patients were allowed to stop and rest or reduce their walking speed if they felt shortness of breath or fatigue. The physical therapist encouraged patients during the test (e.g., "you are doing well", "keep up the good work"). Measurement was suspended if patients experienced chest pain, dyspnea, leg cramps, hyperhidrosis, cyanosis, or facial pallor during the test. The Society of Sarcopenia, Cachexia and Wasting Disorders defined individuals with 6-min walk distance <400 m as having reduced physical activity [12]. In the present study, 6-min walk distance ≥ 400 m was adopted as an appropriate level of exercise capacity for patients with IHD.

Physical activity

Physical activity was assessed using an accelerometer (Lifecorder; Suzuken, Nagoya, Japan) 3 months after hospital discharge. The accelerometer was worn at the waist for 7 days, except during bathing and sleeping, to record vertical acceleration of the body and number of steps. Instrument accuracy and reliability was confirmed in previous study [13]. Vertical vector magnitude was analyzed every 2 min and then digitally divided into 11 grades of 0, 0.5, and 1.0 to 9.0, with a lower grade indicating lower intensity of physical activity. Briefly, grades <3.0, 4.0–6.0, and >7.0 corresponded to physical activity at light (1.8–2.9 Mets), moderate (3.6–5.2 Mets), and vigorous (>6.1 Mets) intensity, respectively [14]. According to the AHA/ACC guidelines, adults should engage in physical activity at moderate-to-vigorous intensity, such as brisk walking, for at least 150 min a week [5]. To evaluate this activity, the time patients spent moving at moderate-to-vigorous intensity per week was aggregated. An aggregated time ≥150 min/week was defined as appropriate physical activity. In addition to time spent moving per week, the number of steps per day was also counted for physical activity.

Statistical analysis

The chi-square test or unpaired t test was used to compare differences in patient characteristics, 6-min walk distance, and physical activity between patients with stage G1-G2 CKD and patients with stage G3-G4 CKD. In comparison of physical activity levels between the two groups, the patients were stratified by age (<65 years or ≥65 years. Additionally, after we selected the active patients with higher frequency of attendance to ambulant cardiac rehabilitation (≥1.1 time per week) [15] from our study participants, we evaluated the differences in patient characteristics, renal function, and exercise capacity of the active participants. To evaluate whether CKD disrupted acquirement of appropriate physical activity after hospital discharge, a stepwise multivariate logistic regression analysis was performed using CKD stage, age, sex, body mass index, employment, intervention for IHD, comorbid conditions, smoking habits, blood hemoglobin, serum albumin and high-sensitivity C-reactive protein, left ventricular ejection fraction, duration of hospital stay and 6-min walk distance as exploratory variables, with physical activity as a dependent variable. Data are presented as mean ± standard deviation or a percentage, with a P value less than 0.05 considered statistically significant. Analyses were performed using SPSS software, version 22.0 (IBM Corporation, Armonk, NY, USA).

Results

Clinical characteristics and exercise capacity

Clinical characteristics and exercise capacity are summarized in Table 1. Patients with stage G3-G4 CKD were significantly older compared to those with stage G1-G2 CKD ($P < 0.001$), while the ratio of patients who were unemployed or had a smoking history were significantly higher ($P = 0.002$ and $P = 0.007$, respectively). Blood hemoglobin, eGFR, and left ventricular ejection fraction were significantly lower in patients with stage G3-G4 CKD ($P = 0.008$, $P < 0.001$, and $P = 0.001$, respectively), and their duration at the hospital was significantly longer ($P = 0.04$). The 6-min walk distance was 465 ± 101 m for all patients, 470 ± 104 m for patients with stage G1-G2 CKD, and 459 ± 98 m for patients with stage G3-G4 CKD. There was no significant difference in 6-min walk distance between patients with stage G1-G2 CKD and those with stage G3-G4 CKD.

Physical activity

Physical activity after hospital discharge is shown in Fig. 1. The number of steps and moderate-to-vigorous physical activity were significantly lower in patients with stage G3-G4 CKD than in those with stage G1-G2 CKD ($P = 0.01$ and $P < 0.001$, respectively). Of the 245 patients, 87 patients (35.5%) acquired appropriate physical activity, that is, 29 (25.4%) among patients with stage G3-G4 CKD and 58 (44.3%) among those with stage G1-G2 CKD. The ratio was significantly lower in stage G3-G4 CKD than in stage G1-G2 CKD ($P = 0.002$). Although the significant associations of CKD stage with acquirement rate of appropriate physical activity and moderate-to-vigorous physical activity were seen in patients aged 65 years and older, there was no association between CKD stage and physical activity levels in patients aged 64 years or younger.

Logistic regression analyses

The results of univariate and multivariate logistic regression analyses are presented in Table 2. In the univariate logistic regression analysis, stage G3-G4 CKD, an older age, female gender, unemployment, lower blood hemoglobin and albumin levels, longer duration of hospital stay, and a 6-min walk distance <400 m significantly contributed to reduced physical activity. Stepwise multivariate analysis identified stage G3-G4 CKD (odds ratio, 1.91; 95% confidence interval, 1.02–3.55; $P = 0.04$) and a 6-min walk distance <400 m (odds ratio, 17.8; 95% confidence interval, 4.16–76.6; $P < 0.001$) as significant independent factors that hinder acquiring appropriate physical activity.

Changes in renal function and exercise capacity

Table 3 shows change in renal function and exercise capacity between patients with stage G1-G2 CKD and G3-G4 CKD. In patients with stages G3-G4, eGFR was significantly increased after 3 months ($P = 0.03$). On the other hand, Δ6-min walk distance was significantly higher in patients with stage G1-G2 CKD than stage G3-G4 CKD, although clinical significant improvement of 6-min walk distance was seen in patients with stage G3-G4 CKD.

Table 4 summarizes baseline characteristics and change in renal function and exercise capacity from hospital discharge to 3 months in active and non-active participants. In active participants, eGFR and 6-min walk distance improved, (eGFR 58.8 ± 20.6 to 61.8 ± 17.2 mL/min/1.73 m^2, Δ +4.77 mL/min/1.73 m^2, 6-min walk distance 451.8 ± 85.3 to 511.9 ± 88.1 m, Δ +60.1 m).

Table 1 Clinical characteristics and exercise capacity

	All patients (n = 245)	Stage G1-G2 CKD (n = 131)	Stage G3-G4 CKD (n = 114)	P
Age (years)	64.6 ± 10.5	61.6 ± 11.0	68.0 ± 8.9	<0.001
Gender (% male)	82.9	81.7	84.2	0.60
Height (m)	1.6 ± 0.1	1.64 ± 0.08	1.62 ± 0.08	0.13
Weight (kg)	63.3 ± 11.5	63.7 ± 12.2	63.0 ± 10.6	0.64
Body mass index (kg/m^2)	23.8 ± 3.3	23.7 ± 3.4	23.9 ± 3.1	0.54
Unemployed (%)	50.2	40.5	60.5	0.002
Intervention for IHD				0.79
CABG (%)	22.0	21.4	22.8	
PCI (%)	78.0	78.6	77.2	
Comorbidities (%)				
Cerebrovascular disease	8.6	6.9	10.5	0.31
Orthopedic disorder	17.6	19.1	15.8	0.50
Diabetes mellitus	39.6	34.4	45.6	0.07
Smoking (%)				0.007
Current	36.1	43.8	27.2	
Former	36.9	28.5	46.5	
Never	27.0	27.7	26.3	
Laboratory data				
Hemoglobin (g/dL)	12.9 ± 1.72	13.1 ± 1.62	12.6 ± 1.80	0.008
Peak creatine kinase (IU/L)	2841 ± 2583	2871 ± 2460	2778 ± 2743	0.83
Albumin (g/dL)	3.9 ± 0.4	4.0 ± 0.4	3.9 ± 0.4	0.15
High-sensitive CRP (mg/dL)	0.76 ± 0.33	0.80 ± 1.19	0.73 ± 1.24	0.67
eGFR (mL/min/1.73 m^2)	61.5 ± 18.4	74.5 ± 11.5	46.5 ± 12.5	0.001
HbA1c (%)	6.03 ± 1.17	6.02 ± 1.29	6.06 ± 1.07	0.87
Left ventricular ejection fraction (%)	50.7 ± 13.3	53.4 ± 11.4	47.5 ± 14.7	0.001
Ankle-brachial index	1.08 ± 0.12	1.09 ± 0.12	1.08 ± 0.13	0.68
Duration of hospital stay (days)	26.8 ± 17.2	24.8 ± 14.4	29.2 ± 19.7	0.04
6-min walk distance (m)	464.6 ± 101.1	470.3 ± 104.2	459.0 ± 97.8	0.43

Values are expressed as mean ± standard deviation or percentage
CABG coronary artery bypass graft, *CKD* chronic kidney disease, *CRP* C-reactive protein, *eGFR* estimated glomerular filtration rate, *IHD* ischemic heart disease, *PCI* percutaneous coronary intervention

Discussion

The present study demonstrated that CKD in patients with IHD prevented the achievement of appropriate physical activity after hospital discharge. In particular, having stage G3-G4 CKD was a significant independent limiting factor. To our knowledge, this is the first study showing the association between CKD and objectively measured physical activity level in patients with IHD.

Many studies have reported that increased physical activity reduces cardiovascular risk and all-cause mortality risk in general populations [1–3] or in patients with end-stage renal disease [16]. Wannamethee et al. also reported that maintaining a physically active lifestyle could decrease the risk of all-cause mortality in patients with IHD [17]. Although it was formerly believed that increasing physical activity worsened renal function in patients with CKD via reduced renal blood flow, recent studies have shown beneficial effects on not only exercise capacity [18, 19] but also renal function [8, 15]. In our data, the patients with higher frequency of attendance to our cardiac rehabilitation program experienced an improvement of renal function as previously reported [15]. A prospective cohort study demonstrated that increasing physical activity delayed the deterioration of renal function in patients with stage G3-G4 CKD [8]. Furthermore, recent study reported that an aerobic exercise program was safely performed by patients with IHD who have CKD and improved their eGFR [15].

Association between chronic kidney disease and physical activity level in patients with ischemic...

53

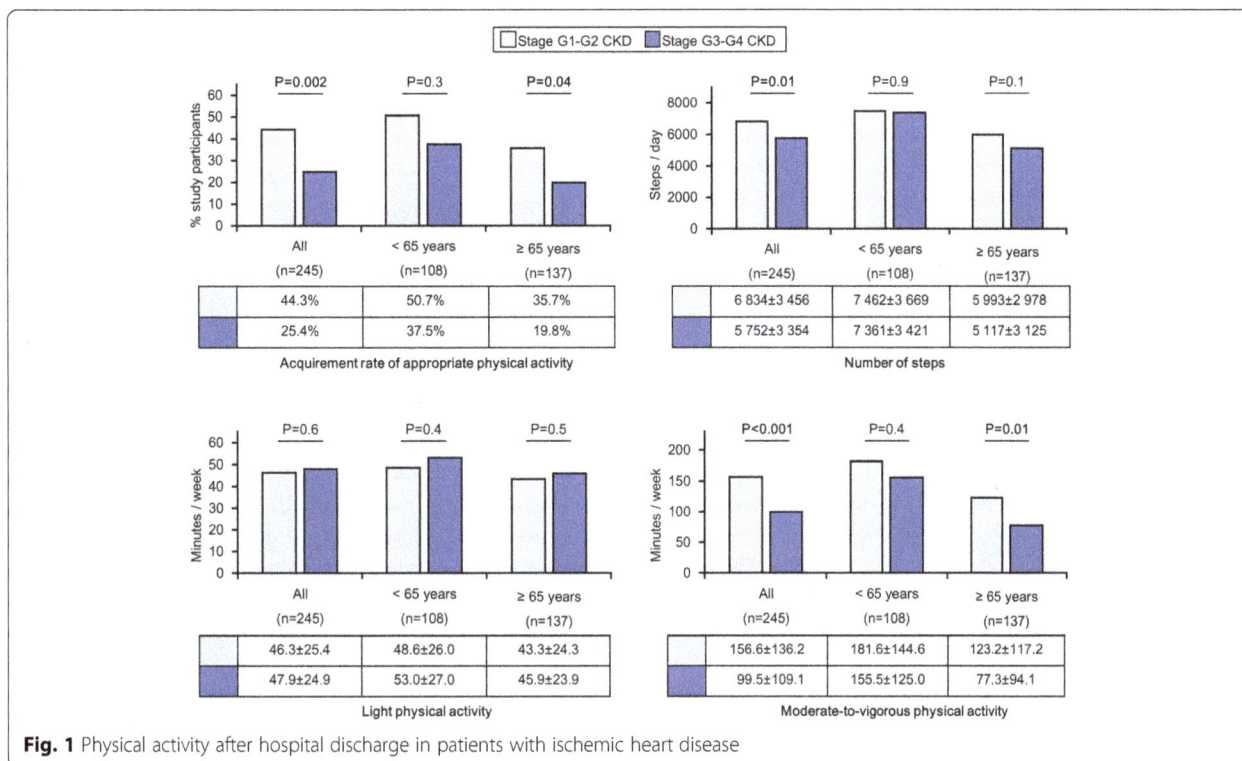

Fig. 1 Physical activity after hospital discharge in patients with ischemic heart disease

Table 2 The univariate and multivariate logistic regression analyses

Factors	Units of increase	Univariate analysis		Multivariate analysis	
		ORs (95% CI)	P	ORs (95% CI)	P
CKD stage G3-G4 to stage G1-G2	–	2.33 (1.35–4.01)	0.002	1.91 (1.02–3.55)	0.04
Age	10 years	1.47 (1.14–1.89)	0.003	–	–
Women to men	–	4.97 (1.88–13.2)	0.001	–	–
Body mass index	1 kg/m^2	0.99 (0.91–1.07)	0.8	–	–
Unemployed to employed	–	2.13 (1.25–3.64)	0.005	–	–
CABG to PCI	–	1.81 (0.92–3.55)	0.08	–	–
CVD to non-CVD	–	2.65 (0.87–8.09)	0.09	–	–
Orthopedic disorder to non-orthopedic disorder	–	1.21 (0.60–2.43)	0.6	–	–
DM to non-DM	–	1.53 (0.89–2.64)	0.1	–	–
Ex-smoker to non-smoker	–	0.56 (0.28–1.11)	0.1	–	–
Current smoker to non-smoker	–	0.53 (0.26–1.06)	0.07	–	–
Hemoglobin	1.0 g/dL	0.78 (0.66–0.92)	0.003	–	–
Albumin	0.1 mg/dL	0.94 (0.88–0.99)	0.04	–	–
High-sensitivity CRP	0.1 mg/dL	1.02 (0.99–1.04)	0.2	–	–
LVEF	10%	1.06 (0.87–1.29)	0.6	–	–
Duration of hospital stay	1 day	1.03 (1.01–1.06)	0.005	–	–
6MWD of <400 m to 6MWD of ≥400 m	–	18.9 (4.43–80.5)	<0.001	17.8 (4.16–76.6)	<0.001

Analyses were performed using univariate and multivariate logistic regression analyses

ORs odds ratios, *CI* confidence interval, *CKD* chronic kidney disease, *CABG* coronary artery bypass grafting, *CVD* cerebrovascular disease, *DM* diabetes mellitus, *CRP* C-reactive protein, *LVEF* left ventricular ejection fraction, *6MWD* 6-min walk distance, *PCI* percutaneous coronary intervention

Table 3 Changes in renal function and exercise capacity

	Stage G1-G2 CKD (n = 95)	Stage G3-G4 CKD (n = 87)	P^a
eGFR (mL/min/1.73 m²)			
At baseline (hospital discharge)	75.8 ± 13.1	45.1 ± 13.7	<0.001
At 3 months	73.3 ± 13.1	47.1 ± 15.6	<0.001
Δ eGFR (mL/min/1.73 m²)	−2.47 ± 11.2	2.02 ± 13.5	0.03
6-min walk distance (m)			
At baseline (hospital discharge)	477.9 ± 99.8	460.4 ± 99.8	0.2
At 3 months	535.9 ± 100.6	495.2 ± 116.6	0.01
Δ 6-min walk distance (m)	58.1 ± 59.6	34.8 ± 63.5	0.01

Values are expressed as mean ± standard deviation
CKD chronic kidney disease, eGFR estimated glomerular filtration rate
[a]Comparison between stage G1-G2 and stage G3-G4

Maintaining a physically active lifestyle is therefore considered necessary for the secondary prevention of IHD after discharge in patients who also have CKD.

We found that stage G3-G4 CKD decreased moderate-to-vigorous physical activity after hospital discharge in patients with IHD. Many studies have reported that both patients on hemodialysis [20] and those with stage G3-G4 CKD have poor physical activity [7, 9, 10], supporting our findings. Three possible reasons may explain the relationship between CKD and physical inactivity. First, anemia is a frequent and inevitable complication of CKD that is detected even in early stages of CKD. Because anemia decreases oxygen delivery to skeletal muscles, patients with anemia might fatigue easily during moderate-to-vigorous physical activity, leading to their inactivity. Second, peripheral arterial disease is a major complication in patients with CKD. Some epidemiological studies have shown that the prevalence of peripheral arterial disease is significantly higher in non-hemodialytic patients with stage G3-G5 CKD than in patients with stage G1-G2 CKD [21, 22]. Ischemic symptoms such as muscle pain or lower extremity discomfort, which are induced by walking and remitted by rest, could hinder increasing physical activity in patients with stage G3-G4 CKD. Finally, depressive symptoms are known to attenuate the urge to leave the home, resulting in physical inactivity for CKD patients [23]. In a previous study surveying approximately 6000 community-dwelling elderly, patients with stage G3-G5 CKD had double the risk of depression compared to those with stage G1-G2 CKD [24]. On the basis of these reasons, stage G3-G4 CKD may hinder acquiring appropriate physical activity after discharge.

Goal-setting of physical activity is well known as one of the most popular techniques to promote in people with chronic illnesses [25, 26]. A meta-analysis, which

investigated the effectiveness of pedometer-used intervention on physical activity in community-dwelling people, concluded that setting a physical activity goal is a key motivational factor for increasing physical activity and is absolutely essential for successful intervention [27], and the same intervention successfully increased physical activity levels in CKD patients [28]. Chase JA et al. systematically reviewed what interventions were helpful in maintaining physical activity in cardiac patients, and suggested the self-monitoring with a pedometer, promoting during clinic visits, and objective feedback [29]. In addition to these approaches, we should promote for cardiac patients to participate in cardiac rehabilitation program more to rebuild self-confidence to exercise.

There are some limitations to the present study. First, the study showed significant differences in age, the ratio of patients who were unemployed or had a smoking history, blood hemoglobin, left ventricular ejection fraction, and duration of hospital stay between patients with stage G1-G2 CKD and those with stage G3-G4 CKD. Therefore, we performed multivariate logistic regression analysis to assess the significant independent effects of stage G3-G4 CKD on physical activity. Consequently, stage G3-G4 CKD was identified as the significant independent factor in the present study. Second, although we considered the effect of clinical characteristics to the extent possible, an effect of albuminuria on physical activity in our patients was not elucidated. Albuminuria is a well-known symptom for CKD patients, and a recent study showed a positive correlation between with albuminuria and frailty or sarcopenia in community-dwelling people [30, 31]. Therefore, albuminuria could disrupt the acquirement of appropriate physical activity after hospital discharge among the patients with IHD. In addition, we will consider the prevalence of sarcopenia in patients with CKD. Sarcopenia would be associated with low physical activity and exercise tolerance and deterioration of renal function. Third, although an aggregated time ≥150 min/week at moderate-to-vigorous intensity was defined as appropriate physical activity in our study according to AHA/ACC guideline, it would be still controversial whether engaging in the physical activity level for Japanese patients with IHD or CKD to have a role in secondary prevention. Fourth, because we studied patients who could be followed up for more than 3 months after hospital discharge, they likely also had better compliance with treatment than patients who dropped out of the study during the follow-up period. If the study included the dropout patients, physical activity after discharge may have been much lower. Although we showed that stage G3-G4 CKD prevented achievement of appropriate physical activity after discharge in patients with

Table 4 Baseline characteristics and changes in renal function and exercise capacity between active and non-active participants

	All patients (n = 182)	Active participants (n = 18)	Non-active participants (n = 164)	P
Age (years)	64.0 ± 10.7	66.2 ± 9.8	63.7 ± 10.8	0.35
Gender (% male)	85.2	83.3	85.4	0.73
Height (m)	1.63 ± 0.08	1.64 ± 0.09	1.63 ± 0.08	0.58
Weight (kg)	64.1 ± 11.8	65.9 ± 14.4	63.9 ± 11.5	0.51
Body mass index (kg/m^2)	23.9 ± 3.4	24.3 ± 4.4	23.9 ± 3.2	0.61
Unemployed (%)	47.8	61.1	46.3	0.32
Intervention for IHD				0.54
CABG (%)	20.3	11.1	21.3	
PCI (%)	79.7	88.9	78.7	
Comorbidities (%)				
Cerebrovascular disease	8.8	11.1	8.5	0.66
Orthopedic disorder	19.9	23.5	19.5	0.75
Diabetes mellitus	40.1	38.9	40.2	1.00
Smoking (%)				0.17
Current	35.9	17.6	37.8	
Former	35.4	53.0	33.5	
Never	28.7	29.4	28.7	
Laboratory data				
Hemoglobin (g/dL)	12.9 ± 1.64	12.7 ± 1.36	13.0 ± 1.70	0.49
Peak creatine kinase (IU/L)	2367 ± 2536	2719 ± 3102	2330 ± 2479	0.55
Albumin (g/dL)	3.94 ± 0.42	3.91 ± 0.45	3.94 ± 0.41	0.74
High-sensitive CRP (mg/dL)	0.76 ± 1.24	0.43 ± 0.44	0.79 ± 1.29	0.25
Left ventricular ejection fraction (%)	51.2 ± 13.7	50.0 ± 13.9	51.3 ± 13.7	0.70
Ankle-brachial index	1.08 ± 0.12	1.09 ± 0.14	1.08 ± 0.12	0.65
Duration of hospital stay (days)	25.9 ± 16.4	22.9 ± 6.73	26.3 ± 17.1	0.41
eGFR (mL/min/1.73 m^2)				
At baseline (hospital discharge)	61.6 ± 19.2	58.8 ± 20.6	61.9 ± 19.1	0.52
At 3 months	59.6 ± 20.5	61.8 ± 17.2	59.4 ± 20.9	0.68
Δ eGFR (mL/min/1.73 m^2)	−0.97 ± 13.9	4.77 ± 19.7	−1.53 ± 13.2	0.12
6-min walk distance (m)				
At baseline (hospital discharge)	469.5 ± 99.8	451.8 ± 85.3	471.5 ± 101.3	0.43
At 3 months	516.5 ± 110.2	511.9 ± 88.1	517.0 ± 112.6	0.86
Δ 6-min walk distance (m)	46.9 ± 62.4	60.1 ± 37.8	45.5 ± 64.5	0.35

Values are expressed as mean ± standard deviation or percentage
CABG coronary artery bypass graft, *CKD* chronic kidney disease, *CRP* C-reactive protein, *eGFR* estimated glomerular filtration rate, *IHD* ischemic heart disease, *PCI* percutaneous coronary intervention

IHD, the underlying mechanisms remain undetermined. We have previously reported that the frailty was detected in approximately half of patients with stage G5 CKD [32], in which the muscle weakness is observed in patients with not only stage G5 CKD but also stage G3-G4 CKD [33]. It is well known that muscle weakness is associated with lower physical activity in older adults. Therefore, further studies are needed to clarify the potential mechanisms underlying the association between CKD and decreased physical activity.

Conclusions

Stage G3-G4 CKD in patients with IHD was associated with poor acquirement of appropriate physical activity after hospital discharge.

Abbreviations

ACC: American College of Cardiology; AHA: American Heart Association; CKD: Chronic kidney disease; eGFR: Estimated glomerular filtration rate; IHD: Ischemic heart disease

Acknowledgements

We are grateful for the help of Chiharu Noda, Takami Iwamura, Mari Kawano, Akiko Igarashi, and other staffs in the cardiac rehabilitation room.

Funding

This research was supported by JSPS KAKENHI (Grant Number 26350585).

Authors' contributions

This article has eight authors. Our study needed a planner of the study (JA, TM, RM), three persons for the measurement (NH, KN, ST), two persons as the study explainer (RM, KK), two persons for the data entry (RM, KK), two persons as analyst (TM, RM), and the head of research (TM). All authors read and approved the final version of the manuscript.

Competing interests

The authors declare that they have no competing interests.

Author details

[1]Department of Rehabilitation, Kitasato University Hospital, Sagamihara, Japan. [2]Department of Rehabilitation, School of Allied Health Sciences, Kitasato University, 1-15-1 Kitasato, Sagamihara, Kanagawa 252-0373, Japan. [3]Department of Cardio-Angiology, Graduate School of Medical Sciences, Kitasato University, Sagamihara, Japan. [4]Department of Cardiovascular Medicine, Kitasato University School of Medicine, Sagamihara, Japan.

References

1. Barengo NC, Hu G, Lakka TA, Pekkarinen H, Nissinen A, Tuomilehto J. Low physical activity as a predictor for total and cardiovascular disease mortality in middle-aged men and women in Finland. Eur Heart J. 2004;25(24):2204–11.
2. Li J, Siegrist J. Physical activity and risk of cardiovascular disease—a meta-analysis of prospective cohort studies. Int J Environ Res Public Health. 2012; 9(2):391–407.
3. Nocon M, Hiemann T, Muller-Riemenschneider F, Thalau F, Roll S, Willich SN. Association of physical activity with all-cause and cardiovascular mortality: a systematic review and meta-analysis. Eur J Cardiovasc Prev Rehabil. 2008; 15(3):239–46.
4. Arnett DK. Wicked problems and worthy pursuits: resolving to meet American Heart Association 2020 Impact Goals. Circulation. 2012;125(21): 2554–6.
5. Eckel RH, Jakicic JM, Ard JD, de Jesus JM, Houston Miller N, Hubbard VS, et al. 2013 AHA/ACC guideline on lifestyle management to reduce cardiovascular risk: a report of the American College of Cardiology/ American Heart Association Task Force on Practice Guidelines. Circulation. 2014;129(25 Suppl 2):S76–99.
6. Stevenson TG, Riggin K, Nagelkirk PR, Hargens TA, Strath SJ, Kaminsky LA. Physical activity habits of cardiac patients participating in an early outpatient rehabilitation program. J Cardiopulm Rehabil Prev. 2009;29(5): 299–303.
7. Beddhu S, Baird BC, Zitterkoph J, Neilson J, Greene T. Physical activity and mortality in chronic kidney disease (NHANES III). Clin J Am Soc Nephrol. 2009;4(12):1901–6.
8. Robinson-Cohen C, Littman AJ, Duncan GE, Weiss NS, Sachs MC, Ruzinski J, et al. Physical activity and change in estimated GFR among persons with CKD. J Am Soc Nephrol. 2014;25(2):399–406.
9. Finkelstein J, Joshi A, Hise MK. Association of physical activity and renal function in subjects with and without metabolic syndrome: a review of the Third National Health and Nutrition Examination Survey (NHANES III). Am J Kidney Dis. 2006;48(3):372–82.
10. Navaneethan SD, Kirwan JP, Arrigain S, Schold JD. Adiposity measures, lean body mass, physical activity and mortality: NHANES 1999–2004. BMC Nephrol. 2014;15:108.
11. Laboratories ATSCoPSfCPF. ATS statement: guidelines for the six-minute walk test. Am J Respir Crit Care Med. 2002;166(1):111–7.
12. Morley JE, Abbatecola AM, Argiles JM, Baracos V, Bauer J, Bhasin S, et al. Sarcopenia with limited mobility: an international consensus. J Am Med Dir Assoc. 2011;12(6):403–9.
13. Schneider PL, Crouter SE, Lukajic O, Bassett Jr DR. Accuracy and reliability of 10 pedometers for measuring steps over a 400-m walk. Med Sci Sports Exerc. 2003;35(10):1779–84.
14. Kumahara H, Schutz Y, Ayabe M, Yoshioka M, Yoshitake Y, Shindo M, et al. The use of uniaxial accelerometry for the assessment of physical-activity-related energy expenditure: a validation study against whole-body indirect calorimetry. Br J Nutr. 2004;91(2):235–43.
15. Takaya Y, Kumasaka R, Arakawa T, Ohara T, Nakanishi M, Noguchi T, et al. Impact of cardiac rehabilitation on renal function in patients with and without chronic kidney disease after acute myocardial infarction. Circ J. 2014;78(2):377–84.
16. Matsuzawa R, Matsunaga A, Wang G, Kutsuna T, Ishii A, Abe Y, et al. Habitual physical activity measured by accelerometer and survival in maintenance hemodialysis patients. Clin J Am Soc Nephrol. 2012;7(12): 2010–6.
17. Wannamethee SG, Shaper AG, Walker M. Physical activity and mortality in older men with diagnosed coronary heart disease. Circulation. 2000;102(12): 1358–63.
18. Castaneda C, Gordon PL, Uhlin KL, Levey AS, Kehayias JJ, Dwyer JT, et al. Resistance training to counteract the catabolism of a low-protein diet in patients with chronic renal insufficiency. A randomized, controlled trial. Ann Intern Med. 2001;135(11):965–76.
19. Eidemak I, Haaber AB, Feldt-Rasmussen B, Kanstrup IL, Strandgaard S. Exercise training and the progression of chronic renal failure. Nephron. 1997;75(1):36–40.
20. Matsuzawa R, Matsunaga A, Kutsuna T, Ishii A, Abe Y, Yoneki K, et al. Association of habitual physical activity measured by an accelerometer with high-density lipoprotein cholesterol levels in maintenance hemodialysis patients. Sci World J. 2013;2013:780783.
21. Lash JP, Go AS, Appel LJ, He J, Ojo A, Rahman M, et al. Chronic Renal Insufficiency Cohort (CRIC) Study: baseline characteristics and associations with kidney function. Clin J Am Soc Nephrol. 2009;4(8): 1302–11.
22. Selvin E, Erlinger TP. Prevalence of and risk factors for peripheral arterial disease in the United States: results from the National Health and Nutrition Examination Survey, 1999–2000. Circulation. 2004;110(6): 738–43.
23. Zhang M, Kim JC, Li Y, Shapiro BB, Porszasz J, Bross R, et al. Relation between anxiety, depression, and physical activity and performance in maintenance hemodialysis patients. J Ren Nutr. 2014; 24(4):252–60.
24. Campbell KH, Huang ES, Dale W, Parker MM, John PM, Young BA, et al. Association between estimated GFR, health-related quality of life, and depression among older adults with diabetes: the Diabetes and Aging Study. Am J Kidney Dis. 2013;62(3):541–8.
25. McEwan D, Harden SM, Zumbo BD, Sylvester BD, Kaulius M, Ruissen GR, et al. The effectiveness of multi-component goal setting interventions for changing physical activity behaviour: a systematic review and meta-analysis. Health Psychol Rev. 2016;10(1):67–88.

26. O'Brien N, McDonald S, Araujo-Soares V, Lara J, Errington L, Godfrey A, et al. The features of interventions associated with long-term effectiveness of physical activity interventions in adults aged 55–70 years: a systematic review and meta-analysis. Health Psychol Rev. 2015;9(4):417–33.

27. Bravata DM, Smith-Spangler C, Sundaram V, Gienger AL, Lin N, Lewis R, et al. Using pedometers to increase physical activity and improve health: a systematic review. JAMA. 2007;298(19):2296–304.

28. Nowicki M, Murlikiewicz K, Jagodzinska M. Pedometers as a means to increase spontaneous physical activity in chronic hemodialysis patients. J Nephrol. 2010;23(3):297–305.

29. Chase JA. Systematic review of physical activity intervention studies after cardiac rehabilitation. J Cardiovasc Nurs. 2011;26(5):351–8.

30. Chang CC, Hsu CY, Chang TY, Huang PH, Liu LK, Chen LK, et al. Association between low-grade albuminuria and frailty among community-dwelling middle-aged and older people: a cross-sectional analysis from I-Lan Longitudinal Aging Study. Sci Rep. 2016;6:39434.

31. Kim TN, Lee EJ, Hong JW, Kim JM, Won JC, Kim MK, et al. Relationship between sarcopenia and albuminuria: the 2011 Korea National Health and Nutrition Examination Survey. Medicine (Baltimore). 2016;95(3), e2500.

32. Matsuzawa R, Matsunaga A, Wang G, Yamamoto S, Kutsuna T, Ishii A, et al. Relationship between lower extremity muscle strength and all-cause mortality in Japanese patients undergoing dialysis. Phys Ther. 2014;94(7): 947–56.

33. Pereira RA, Cordeiro AC, Avesani CM, Carrero JJ, Lindholm B, Amparo FC, et al. Sarcopenia in chronic kidney disease on conservative therapy: prevalence and association with mortality. Nephrol Dial Transplant. 2015.

8

Factors associated with employment in patients undergoing hemodialysis: a mixed methods study

Hideyo Tsutsui[1,2,3*], Kyoko Nomura[2], Aya Ishiguro[2,4], Yoshinari Tsuruta[5], Sawako Kato[6], Yoshinari Yasuda[7], Shunya Uchida[8] and Yoshiharu Oshida[1]

Abstract

Background: For patients undergoing hemodialysis, continuing in labor is very challenging and many patients have difficulty in current and/or previous workplaces. The objective of the present study is to clarify the determinants of being employed in hemodialysis patients by use of the mixed methods approach.

Methods: One hundred and forty-nine patients undergoing hemodialysis were interviewed between 2010 and 2011 using the "100-category checklists" based on the International Classification of Functioning, Disability and Health developed for hemodialysis patients. The categories with which the participants experienced difficulty at workplace were analyzed using the mixed methods approach. In quantitative data, the patients undergoing hemodialysis were divided into two groups if they experienced any difficulty in current and/or previous workplaces (i.e., "experienced" group vs. "not experienced" group). In qualitative data, responses to the open-ended questions were analyzed using a grounded theory approach.

Results: In total of 149 patients (male, 66%; mean age 62 years; mean hemodialysis vintage, 8.6 years), 62% had diabetes and 86% were in labor at the time of investigation. In a quantitative analysis, compared to the unexperienced group, the experienced group was more likely to show the physical problems such as fatigability and decline of physical strength and declined energy level. In a qualitative analysis, three determinants of being unemployed were emerged including hospital visits (i.e., three times a week), vascular access, and physical symptoms. In contrast, a favorable determinant for the work continuation and job opportunities was found to be a flexible dialysis shift.

Conclusions: Our mixed methods study suggests that patients undergoing hemodialysis frequently suffer from physical problems such as frequent hospital visits for hemodialysis, vascular access troubles, and physical distress, resulting in frequent unemployment. One solution for unemployment of the patients undergoing hemodialysis is a dialysis shift flexible for individual lifestyles.

Keywords: Dialysis shift, Employment, Hospital visits, Patients undergoing hemodialysis, Physical symptoms, Vascular access

Background

Changes in socioeconomic status related to work including position, income, contract, and employment status frequently occur in patients undergoing hemodialysis [1–3]. A prospective study investigating 659 patients undergoing dialysis in The Netherlands reported that at

the start of hemodialysis treatment, 31% of the patients were employed, but that the proportion decreased to 25% within 1 year after dialysis initiation [1]. Another study of 4026 patients undergoing dialysis in the US Renal Data System reported that 41.9% of the patients were employed before starting hemodialysis treatment, but the proportion decreased to 21.1% after hemodialysis treatment and decreased even further to 6.6% a year later [2].

In Japan, among very few studies conducted on this issue, Nakayama et al. [3] reported that 63% of their study patients were employed prior to dialysis, 22% of

* Correspondence: htsutsui@med.teikyo-u.ac.jp
[1]Research Center of Health, Physical Fitness, and Sports, Nagoya University, Furo-cho, Chikusa-ku, Nagoya 464-8601, Japan
[2]Department of Hygiene and Public Health, Teikyo University School of Medicine, 2-11-1 Kaga, Itabashi-ku, Tokyo 173-8605, Japan
Full list of author information is available at the end of the article

which became unemployed after the start of hemodialysis treatment. According to the nationwide report of 10,522 dialysis patients conducted by the National Kidney Disease Council in Japan in 2011 [4], 41% of the men and 43% of the women undergoing hemodialysis became unemployed in the last 5 years. These values show an increasing trend compared with the former report published in 2006 [5]. Although receiving hemodialysis treatment at night, patients on hemodialysis must leave the workplace earlier than the regular office hours thrice a week. This disruption of the work shift sometimes makes it difficult to stay in full-time labor; however, the time constraint, though obvious, may not be the only reason.

Therefore, the purpose of this study was to investigate how patients undergoing hemodialysis experience difficulties in the workplace and to clarify the determinants associated with employment in patients undergoing hemodialysis in Japan. The mixed methods approach was employed to incorporate the quantitative and qualitative analyses of our invented questionnaire system, increasing the validity of the results.

Methods

Patients

A total of 149 outpatients undergoing maintenance hemodialysis consisted of 49 patients at Masuko Memorial Hospital in Nagoya and 100 patients at the Meiyo Clinic in Toyohashi, Japan. Exclusion criteria were (i) hemodialysis duration shorter than 5 years, (ii) dementia, and (iii) hearing difficulty. We confirmed these exclusion criteria by medical record review. Interviews were conducted from December 2009 to January 2011 by a single investigator (HT).

Of the 149 patients, 84 were employed and 65 were unemployed (including retirees) at the time of the investigation.

Written informed consents were obtained from all participants. The study protocol was approved by the Internal Review Board of the Research Center of Health, Physical Fitness, and Sports, Nagoya University (approval number #22-9, #23-09).

Procedure

Study design

We used the mixed methods approach to clarify key factors of the difficulties in patients undergoing hemodialysis maintaining employment [6] and collected both quantitative and qualitative data through interviews. We interviewed all 149 patients. One interviewer (HT) conducted a semi-structured interview with each patient for 40 to 60 min.

100-category checklist

The "100-category checklist" included the following categories from the International Classification of Functioning, Disability and Health (ICF): 40 categories from the "Body functions" component; 14 categories from the "Body structures" component; 25 categories from the "Activities and participation" component; and 21 categories from the "Environmental factors" component [7]. The Cronbach's alpha of this checklist was 0.86 [8]. Of the 100-category checklist, three categories regarding employment were as follows:

1. *d845 Acquiring, keeping and terminating a job*: Have you ever been dismissed, demoted, or changed your employment status from full-time to part-time after starting hemodialysis treatment? For example, in a job interview, have you ever been rejected because of undergoing hemodialysis treatment?
2. *d850 Remunerative employment*: Have you often been absent from the workplace since you began hemodialysis treatment? Because of this, have you ever found any difficulty in working itself?
3. *e590 Labour and employment services, systems and policies*: Have you ever felt that you were not supported in finding a job or in being trained for a job due to hemodialysis treatment?

Using the 100-category checklist for hemodialysis patients based on the ICF [7, 8], participants were interviewed and asked whether they had experienced any difficulties in each category of the checklist since the initiation of hemodialysis treatment. Participants answered each question with either "yes" or "no". If a participant answered "yes", the person concerned was further asked to report how and why the patient perceived difficulties; this portion of the study was used for qualitative analysis.

We set up a research question, "What are the factors impeding the work of patients undergoing hemodialysis?" Among the 149 study patients, we conducted qualitative analysis of 87 patients who experienced any difficulty in current or previous workplaces. As the interview progressed, the concept of "existence of vascular access trouble" was generated and the hypothesis that vascular access trouble affects work was formulated, so a question asking about the influence on work during the time of vascular access trouble was added.

Analyses

In quantitative data, the patients undergoing hemodialysis were divided into two groups according to whether they experienced any difficulty in current or previous workplaces (i.e., experienced group vs. not experienced group). The chi-square test or Fisher's exact test was used for categorical variables, and the t test was used for continuous variables showing normal distribution. The baseline clinical characteristics included age and hemodialysis vintage; these are continuous variables that are expressed as mean

± standard deviation. In addition, sex, underlying diseases, complications, hemodialysis shift, and employed status are categorical variables and are expressed as numbers and percentages.

Crude and adjusted odds ratios were computed along with the 95% confidence interval for each 100-category checklist category. Multivariate logistic regression analysis for the effect of each category on experiencing work-related difficulty as outcome was performed by adjusting for age, hemodialysis vintage, presence of diabetic nephropathy, retinopathy or neuropathy, cerebral vascular disorder, anemia, and employment status. All statistical analyses were carried out using SPSS, version 19.0 (IBM Corp, Armonk, NY, USA). Statistical significance was set at $p < 0.05$.

In qualitative data, responses to the open-ended questions were analyzed using the grounded theory approach [9]. Transcript analyses were conducted to interpret data and saturate findings according to the grounded theory. The data were scrutinized line by line with open coding to reach a consensus on a core category that accounted

for the data. During analysis, emerging themes and theories were discussed with our research team. Emerging categories were explored and identified by comparing and contrasting the data. The first author (HT) developed the initial codes, and the third author (AI) reviewed the coding scheme. All codes were reviewed to discover codes that had similarities between them or shared similar properties in order to form categories. These operations were repeated, and categories that best represented the data were created. A diagram was developed with feedback from nephrologists and internists on the properties of emerging categories. Interviews were conducted in the Japanese language, and Japanese words were used to analyze the data. The final diagram was developed with which all collaborators in our research team agreed.

Results
Quantitative results
The characteristics of the study patients undergoing hemodialysis are shown in Table 1. The patients in the

Table 1 Clinical characteristic in patients undergoing hemodialysis

Characteristics	Total ($n = 149$)	Difficulty in current and/or previous workplaces		P
		Experienced ($n = 87$)	Not experienced ($n = 62$)	
Sex (men/women) [n]	98/51	57/30	41/21	0.938
Age (years)	62 ± 11	59 ± 10	66 ± 10	<0.001
Hemodialysis vintage (years)	8.6 ± 5.6	10.7 ± 5.7	5.5 ± 3.7	<0.001
Underlying diseases				
Chronic glomerulonephritis [n (%)]	26 (17.4)	26 (100.0)	0	–
Diabetic nephropathy [n (%)]	93 (62.4)	31 (33.3)	62 (66.7)	0.001
Nephrosclerosis [n (%)]	14 (9.4)	14 (100.0)	0	–
IgA nephropathy [n (%)]	4 (2.7)	4 (100.0)	0	–
Polycystic kidney [n (%)]	3 (2.0)	2 (100.0)	0	–
Others [n (%)]	5 (3.4)	5 (100.0)	0	–
Unidentified [n (%)]	4 (2.7)	4 (100.0)	0	–
Complications				
Diabetic retinopathy [n (%)]	78 (52.3)	26 (29.9)	52 (83.9)	<0.001
Diabetic neuropathy [n (%)]	25 (16.8)	10 (11.5)	15 (24.2)	0.041
Cerebral vascular disorder [n (%)]	50 (33.6)	20 (23.0)	30 (48.4)	0.001
Cardiovascular disorder [n (%)]	78 (52.3)	47 (54.0)	31 (50.0)	0.628
Anemia [n (%)]	43 (28.9)	33 (37.9)	10 (16.1)	0.004
Secondary hyperparathyroidism [n (%)]	29 (19.5)	21 (24.1)	8 (12.9)	0.088
Reshape of vascular access [n (%)]	77 (51.7)	44 (56.6)	33 (53.2)	0.750
Hemodialysis shift				
Daytime [n (%)]	112 (75.2)	70 (80.5)	42 (67.7)	0.011
Night [n (%)]	37 (24.8)	17 (19.5)	20 (32.3)	0.742
Employed at the time of investigation [n (%)]	84 (56.4)	71 (81.6)	13 (21.0)	<0.001

Data on age and hemodialysis vintage are shown as mean ± standard deviation. The chi-square tests were used for comparisons of sex, underlying diseases, complications, and employed at the time of investigation. The t test was used for comparisons of age and hemodialysis vintage

group who experienced employment difficulty (experienced group) were significantly younger, had shorter hemodialysis vintage, were less likely to have diabetic nephropathy, were more likely to have anemia, and were more likely to be employed compared with the patients in the group who had not experienced in an employment difficulty (not experienced group). Because the patients in the experienced group seemed to be in better physical condition than the patients in the not experienced group, the experienced group seemed to more easily remain employed than the not experienced group. However, although the experienced group looked healthy in appearance, they were not able to carry out such activities as going on business trips, working overtime, or carrying heavy baggage, like healthy people. For that reason, they experienced involuntary changes in their work assignments and decreases in salaries because they talked about the fact that they could not accomplish these activities due to hemodialysis therapy. Although they experienced these difficulties, they were not quitting their jobs, thinking that "it is better than unemployment".

The response patterns of the experienced group and not experienced group and the results of the logistic regression models for the 100-category checklist are shown in Tables 2, 3, 4, and 5.

Compared to patients in the not experienced group, participants in the experienced group reported difficulties in the following categories: *attention functions (b140)*; *sensory functions related to temperature and other stimuli (b270)*; *hematological system functions (b430)*; *general physical endurance (b4550)*; *aerobic capacity (b4551)*; *fatigability (b4552)*; *weight maintenance functions (b530)*; *urinary excretory functions (b610)*; *sexual functions (b640)*; *functions of hair (b850)*; *heart (s4100)*; *structure of urinary system (b610)*; *looking after one's health (d570)*; *sports (d9201)*; *socializing (d9205)*; *products or substances for personal consumption (e110)*; *individual attitudes of health professionals (e450)*; *media services, systems and policies (e560)* and *health services, systems and policies (e580)*.

After adjusting for age, hemodialysis vintage, presence of diabetic nephropathy, retinopathy and neuropathy, cerebral vascular disorder, anemia, and employment status, participants in the experienced group were found to report difficulties in the following categories compared with participants in the not experienced group: *energy level (b1300)*; *attention functions (b140)*; and *sensory functions related to temperature and other stimuli (b270)*. They were also more likely to have difficulty in the categories of *fine hand use (d440)*; *looking after one's health (d570)*; *socializing (d9205)*; and *individual attitudes of health professions (e450)*.

Qualitative results

Ten categories were generated including *hospital visit*; *vascular access*; *physical symptoms*; *difficulty in commuting*; *restriction of work* including workload, job contents,

and working hours; *attitude of coworkers in the workplace*; *changes of work conditions* including position, salary, and status; *acceptance of reality by patients*; *balance between work and treatment*; and *decrease in time to spend with family*. These categories were further grouped into two themes including (i) *factors associated with being employed* and (ii) *adjusted hemodialysis shift* (Fig. 1).

Factors associated with being employed

The three properties of hospital visit, vascular access, and physical symptoms emerged as factors associated with being employed in patients undergoing hemodialysis. For example,

> "(For hemodialysis) I was recommended to quit working (because I was not able to contribute to the workplace) due to the 3-times-a-week hospital visits." (Age 59, female)

> "I experienced vascular access occlusions twice and I feel finger-tip numbness and drop things frequently... Under such a physical condition, I had experienced difficulty at work." (Age 62, male)

> "I quit working because I had to leave the workplace early 3 times a week because of hemodialysis. In addition, I had to be absent from the workplace due to unexpected events like a hypoglycemic attack during duty hours and hospitalization to treat vascular access problems." (Age 63, female)

Difficulty in commuting Participants perceived difficulty in commuting due to physical symptoms. For example,

> "If a commuter bus is full, I have to take care that my vascular access is not compressed." (Age 48, male)

> "I feel numbness of my feet frequently; especially in the right toes (as though they were pressed) and...so it is hard to go up and down the stairs of the subway, I am always worn out when I arrive at the company every morning...Thus, I was not able to work very much after I initiated hemodialysis." (Age 60, male)

Restriction of work The three properties of hospital visit, vascular access, and physical symptoms formed restriction of work such as *limitation of workload and job contents* and *reduction of working hours*. For example,

> "It greatly impacted my work because I was not able to go on a business trip on a day of hemodialysis treatment. In addition, I was not able to carry heavy baggage because of my vascular access; this prevents me from going on a business trip." (Age 55, male)

> "I am an interior decorator mechanic. My working hours are shortened because of visiting the hospital

Table 2 Comparison of the categories which reported difficulty in the components of "Body functions" according to employment status (n = 149)

ICF category		Difficulty in current and/or previous workplaces			Logistic regression analysis					
		Experienced (%)	Not experienced (%)		Univariate			Multivariate[a]		
		n = 87	n = 62	P*	OR	95% CI	P	OR	95% CI	P
b110	Consciousness functions	31.0	29.0	0.793	0.74	0.35–1.55	0.416	1.13	0.38–3.39	0.824
b1300	Energy level	50.6	45.2	0.515	1.71	0.85–3.48	0.135	3.78	1.30–11.04	0.015
b1302	Appetite	31.0	27.4	0.633	0.81	0.38–1.72	0.582	0.59	0.18–1.93	0.382
b134	Sleep functions	59.8	56.5	0.685	0.86	0.42–1.75	0.682	1.27	0.45–3.62	0.652
b140	Attention functions	37.9	25.8	0.120	2.61	1.14–5.98	0.023	5.35	1.61–17.73	0.006
b152	Emotional functions	32.2	16.1	0.027	1.95	0.82–4.67	0.133	0.51	0.12–2.14	0.353
b210	Seeing functions	63.2	83.9	0.006	0.35	0.14–0.86	0.022	–	–	–
b240	Sensations associated with hearing and vestibular function	46.0	40.3	0.493	0.89	0.44–1.79	0.739	1.04	0.36–3.00	0.937
b250	Taste function	26.4	22.6	0.591	1.28	0.56–2.92	0.560	0.83	0.26–2.66	0.750
b260	Proprioceptive function	23.0	66.1	<0.001	0.30	0.15–0.62	0.001	0.70	0.25–1.99	0.507
b265	Touch function	13.8	24.2	0.104	0.48	0.21–1.14	0.096	–	–	–
b270	Sensory functions related to temperature and other stimuli	19.5	4.8	0.013	10.18	1.32–78.53	0.026	38.62	2.30–648.65	0.011
b280	Sensory of pain	51.7	38.7	0.116	1.34	0.66–2.71	0.414	0.75	0.26–2.14	0.584
b410	Heart functions	54.0	50.0	0.629	1.48	0.73–2.97	0.275	2.56	0.87–7.52	0.087
b415	Blood vessel functions	23.0	48.4	0.001	0.36	0.17–0.73	0.005	–	–	–
b420	Blood pressure functions	82.8	87.1	0.470	1.24	0.48–3.16	0659	3.00	0.48–18.67	0.238
b430	Hematological system functions	37.9	16.1	0.004	2.45	1.03–5.80	0.043	–	–	–
b440	Respiration functions	34.5	29.0	0.483	0.97	0.46–2.05	0.945	1.35	0.45–4.05	0.597
b4550	General physical endurance	69.0	22.6	<0.001	5.01	2.29–10.99	<0.001	1.97	0.62–6.25	0.251
b4551	Aerobic capacity	62.1	22.6	<0.001	3.94	1.81–8.61	0.001	2.26	0.68–7.10	0.188
b4552	Fatigability	74.7	43.5	<0.001	3.46	1.68–7.14	0.001	2.75	0.95–7.93	0.062
b515	Digestive functions	14.9	21.0	0.399	0.81	0.33–1.99	0.650	0.83	0.22–3.16	0.786
b525	Defecation functions	66.9	72.6	0.139	0.42	0.19–0.94	0.034	0.77	0.25–2.40	0.656
b530	Weight maintenance functions	25.3	14.5	0.110	3.73	1.22–11.38	0.021	1.33	0.30–5.92	0.712
b535	Sensations associated with the digestive system	37.9	35.5	0.760	0.87	0.43–1.78	0.708	0.82	0.29–2.30	0.701
b545	Water, mineral and electrolyte balance functions	17.2	17.7	0.937	2.85	0.92–8.82	0.069	1.13	0.25–5.08	0.869
b555	Endocrine gland functions	32.2	0	<0.001	–	–	–	–	–	–
b610	Urinary excretory functions	86.2	38.7	<0.001	4.94	4.34–10.44	<0.001	1.06	0.34–3.34	0.922
b620	Urination functions	60.9	38.7	0.007	1.83	0.91–3.70	0.092	1.12	0.39–3.25	0.832
b640	Sexual functions	31.0	6.5	<0.001	18.49	2.44–140.34	0.005	0.16	0.02–1.49	0.107
b670	Sensations associated with genital and reproductive functions	0	0	NA	–	–	–	–	–	–
b710	Mobility of joint functions	55.2	61.3	0.456	0.83	0.41–1.68	0.603	1.06	0.37–3.03	0.908
b730	Muscle power functions	8.0	0	0.042	–	–	–	–	–	–
b735	Muscle tone functions	0	0	NA	–	–	–	–	–	–
b780	Sensations related to muscles and movement functions	75.9	69.4	0.377	1.76	0.82–3.75	0.146	1.82	0.57–5.82	0.316
b810	Protective functions of the skin	72.4	54.8	0.027	1.49	0.73–3.06	0.274	1.11	0.40–3.09	0.839

Table 2 Comparison of the categories which reported difficulty in the components of "Body functions" according to employment status (n = 149) (Continued)

b820	Repair functions of the skin	43.7	43.5	0997	1.31	0.64–2.65	0.460	1.24	0.44–3.50	0.685
b840	Sensation related to the skin	70.1	77.4	0.321	0.57	0.24–1.31	0.183	0.81	0.26–2.53	0.711
b850	Functions of hair	46.0	19.4	0.001	2.95	1.29–6.74	0.010	1.76	0.58–5.37	0.319

OR odds ratio, ICF International Classification of Functioning, Disability and Health, CI confidence interval
*Chi-square test
[a]Adjusting for age, hemodialysis vintage, presence of diabetic nephropathy, retinopathy and neuropathy, cerebral vascular disorder, anemia, and employment status

for hemodialysis treatment. Therefore, my salary went down." (Age 51, male)

Attitude of coworkers in the workplace The restriction of work such as the limitation of workload and job contents and reduction of working hours further affects Attitude of coworkers in the workplace such as *reaction of colleagues and superior* and *the response of the employer and coworkers in management positions*. For example,

"I felt guilty that I had to leave my workplace early three times a week due to hemodialysis treatment, especially at the end of a one-year term work schedule (when the workload is maximized). I left work under their cold stares." (Age 60, female)

"It was very difficult to have my employer understand that my working hours were shortened because of hospital visits for hemodialysis." (Age 58, male)

Moreover, Attitude of coworkers in the workplace was affected by *misunderstanding* of coworkers in the workplace and *prejudice* against hospital visits, vascular access, and physical symptoms.

Changes in work conditions Attitudes of coworkers in the workplace driven by misunderstanding and prejudice against patients undergoing hemodialysis determined *changes in work conditions* such as *reshuffling, switch from full-time to part-time labor, decrease in wages,* and *dropping from promotion ladder*. For example,

"Because of leaving the workplace early due to hospital visits or hemodialysis treatment), I was transferred from sales promotion to an office job." (Age 41, male)

"Though I worked full-time, I was switched to part-time because I was not able to go to a business trip." (Age 65, male)

Table 3 Comparison of the categories which reported difficulty in the components of "Body structures" according to employment status (n = 149)

ICF category		Difficulty in current and/or previous workplaces			Logistic regression analysis					
		Experienced (%)	Not experienced (%)		Univariate			Multivariate[a]		
		n = 87	n = 62	P*	OR	95% CI	P	OR	95% CI	P
s220	Structure of eyeball	54.0	80.6	0.001	0.34	0.15–0.78	0.010	1.28	0.15–11.04	0.820
s410	Structure of cardiovascular system	33.3	56.5	0.005	0.45	0.22–0.91	0.027	2.04	0.54–7.72	0.292
s4100	Heart	25.3	1.6	<0.001	12.22	1.59–93.70	0.016	5.33	0.39–72.44	0.209
s550	Structure of pancreas	3.4	1.6	0.641	1.35	0.14–13.34	0.797	–	–	–
s5801	Thyroid gland	8.0	6.5	0763	0.77	0.21–2.76	0.683	0.23	0.02–2.66	0.241
s5802	Parathyroid gland	8.0	6.5	0.763	1.22	0.49–2.99	0.670	6.45	0.11–1.87	0.273
s610	Structure of urinary system	88.5	35.5	<0.001	4.94	2.34–10.44	<0.001	1.00	0.32–3.16	0.998
s6100	Kidneys	100.0	100.0	NA	–	–	–	–	–	–
s630	Structure of reproductive system	9.2	8.1	0.809	0.69	0.21–2.24	0.537	–	–	–
s730	Structure of upper extremity	50.6	53.2	0.750	0.66	0.33–1.34	0.253	0.55	0.20–1.56	0.261
s750	Structure of lower extremity	24.1	25.8	0.816	1.07	0.48–2.42	0.862	1.43	0.43–4.84	0.562
s770	Additional musculoskeletal structures related to movement	4.6	3.2	1.000	2.30	0.26–20.23	0.454	6.28	0.40–98.48	0.191
s830	Structure of nails	62.1	79.0	0.027	0.72	0.33–1.56	0.399	1.79	0.52–6.20	0.359

OR odds ratio, ICF International Classification of Functioning, Disability and Health, CI confidence interval
*Chi-square test
[a]Adjusting for age, hemodialysis vintage, presence of diabetic nephropathy, retinopathy and neuropathy, cerebral vascular disorder, anemia, and employment status
NA refers to "not applicable"

Table 4 Comparison of the categories which reported difficulty in the components of "Activities and participation" according to employment status (n = 149)

ICF category		Difficulty in current and/or previous workplaces			Logistic regression analysis					
		Experienced (%)	Not experienced (%)		Univariate			Multivariate^a		
		n = 87	n = 62	P*	OR	95% CI	P	OR	95% CI	P
d220	Undertaking multiple tasks	26.4	0	<0.001	–	–	–	–	–	–
d240	Handling stress and other psychological demands	10.3	1.6	0.046	–	–	–	–	–	–
d430	Lifting and carrying objects	54.0	33.9	0.015	1.91	0.93–3.93	0.077	2.35	0.82–6.78	0.114
d440	Fine hand use	29.9	33.9	0.606	1.08	0.51–2.09	0.846	5.42	1.61–18.30	0.006
d450	Walking	9.2	27.4	0.003	0.27	0.11–0.66	0.004	0.64	0.18–2.19	0.473
d465	Moving around using equipment	10.3	16.1	0.297	0.57	0.21–1.52	0.261	1.60	0.37–6.87	0.530
d470	Using transportation	20.7	30.6	0.166	0.41	0.19–0.89	0.024	0.74	0.23–2.43	0.619
d475	Driving	31.0	30.6	0.960	0.77	0.37–1.62	0.490	1.21	0.41–3.62	0.728
d510	Washing oneself	10.3	21.0	0.072	0.48	0.19–1.20	0.114	1.06	0.36–3.78	0.931
d520	Caring for body parts	10.3	14.5	0.441	0.67	0.24–1.85	0.435	1.08	0.26–4.42	0.918
d550	Eating	5.7	9.7	0.366	0.77	0.21–2.76	0.683	1.18	0.22–6.53	0.847
d570	Looking after one's health	32.2	24.2	0.289	2.99	1.22–7.37	0.017	4.05	1.24–6.26	0.021
d630	Preparing meals	8.0	14.5	0.209	0.30	0.10–0.86	0.026	1.00	0.18–5.65	0.996
d640	Doing housework	17.2	21.0	0.566	0.43	0.19–1.01	0.052	0.31	0.06–1.50	0.144
d660	Assisting others	4.6	3.2	1.000	0.89	0.16–5/04	0.894	–	–	–
d845	Acquiring, keeping and terminating a job	100.0	0	<0.001	–	–	–	–	–	–
d850	Remunerative employment	89.7	8.1	<0.001	–	–	–	–	–	–
d9201	Sports	33.3	16.1	0.019	5.40	1.79–16.30	0.003	3.71	0.54–14.66	0.062
d9204	Hobbies	43.7	38.7	0.144	1.02	0.50–2.06	0.960	2.53	0.88–7.28	0.085
d9205	Socializing	40.2	19.4	0.007	2.90	1.23–6.84	0.015	5.86	1.63–21.06	0.007

OR odds ratio, ICF International Classification of Functioning, Disability, and Health, CI confidence interval
*Chi-square test
^aAdjusting for age, hemodialysis vintage, presence of diabetic nephropathy, retinopathy and neuropathy, cerebral vascular disorder, anemia, and employment status

"My salary stopped increasing because I had to leave the workplace early due to hospital visits for hemodialysis." (Age 47, male)
"Because I do not have time to visit the hospital and undergo hemodialysis during business trips, I cannot go on business trips. I had no choice regarding this, but I was not able to be promoted because of that. As a result, my subordinate has become my boss." (Age 59, male)

With these aforementioned examples, changes of work conditions led to a change of work conditions or to resignation from the job among patients undergoing hemodialysis. Simultaneously, these patients who experienced changes or resignation from a job have also been exposed to continuous anxiety about work continuation or reemployment.

Acceptance of reality by patients Changes in work conditions make some patients accept what they face (i.e., *so what attitude*) including *hard work for job*

hunting, revocation of unofficial decision due to hemodialysis, and *loss of job*. For example,

"Whenever I confessed, "I am a hemodialysis patient", I was failed in an employment test…I have not obtained a job yet so far." (Age 49, male)
"After I informed my new workplace after my retirement that I have initiated hemodialysis, I was told 'Please abandon the contract'." (Age 60, male)
"When I told my workplace that I was going to start hemodialysis, I was dismissed immediately." (Age 61, female)

Adjusted hemodialysis shift
Balance between work and treatment might go well if hemodialysis shifts were well adjusted for individual needs such as *flexibility of dialysis shift* and *cooperation between dialysis clinics*. Simultaneously, balance between work and treatment may *decrease time to spend with family*. For example,

Table 5 Comparison of the categories which reported difficulty in the components of "Environmental factors" according to employment status (n = 149)

ICF category	Difficulty in current and/or previous workplaces			Logistic regression analysis					
	Experienced (%)	Not experienced (%)		Univariate			Multivariate[a]		
	n = 87	n = 62	P*	OR	95% CI	P	OR	95% CI	P
e110 Products or substances for personal consumption	43.7	30.6	0.107	2.20	1.02–4.72	0.043	2.06	0.73–5.83	0.173
e310 Immediate family	6.9	3.2	0.470	1.36	0.26–7.01	0.713	0.62	0.03–13.20	0.758
e320 Friends	11.5	1.6	0.026	4.84	0.60–38.97	0.139	0.87	0.03–25.77	0.936
e325 Acquaintances, peers, colleagues, neighbors and community members	6.9	1.6	0.240	2.78	0.33–23.81	0.350	0.72	0.02–22.88	0.853
e330 People in positions of authority	2.3	0	0.511	–	–	–	–	–	–
e350 Domesticated animals	0	0	NA	–	–	–	–	–	–
e355 Health professionals	6.9	0	0.041	–	–	–	–	–	–
e410 Individual attitudes of immediate family members	3.4	11.3	0.094	0.27	0.07–1.01	0.051	1.73	0.21–14.39	0.612
e420 Individual attitudes of friends	6.9	1.6	0.240	2.78	0.33–23.81	0.350	5.52	0.34–89.43	0.230
e425 Individual attitudes of acquaintances, peers, colleagues, neighbors and community members	6.9	3.2	0.470	1.36	0.26–7.01	0.713	3.17	0.37–27.51	0.296
e430 Individual attitudes of people in positions of authority	8.0	1.6	0.042	–	–	–	–	–	–
e440 Individual attitudes of personal care providers and personal assistants	1.1	3.2	0.571	0.22	0.02–2.44	0.215	0.46	0.02–13.65	0.655
e450 Individual attitudes of health professionals	23.0	16.1	0.303	3.55	1.16–10.84	0.026	5.77	1.40–23.85	0.015
e465 Social norms, practices, and ideologies	20.7	12.9	0.217	1.61	0.60–4.31	0.347	0.70	0.16–3.13	0.644
e540 Transportation services, systems and policies	10.3	4.8	0.360	5.38	0.67–42.98	0.112	7.35	0.54–100.82	0.136
e555 Associations and organizational services, systems, and policies	12.6	9.7	0.175	1.52	0.47–4.93	0.489	2.36	0.45–12.38	0.309
e560 Media services, systems and policies	18.4	12.9	0.369	3.67	1.04–13.00	0.044	2.59	0.55–12.24	0.230
e570 Social security services, systems and policies	26.4	11.3	0.023	3.55	1.16–10.84	0.026	1.74	0.40–7.55	0.461
e580 Health services, systems and policies	25.3	8.1	0.007	4.35	1.24–0.30	0.022	2.18	0.42–11.34	0.354
e590 Labour and employment services, systems and policies	74.7	25.8	<0.001	–	–	–	–	–	–

OR odds ratio, ICF International Classification of Functioning, Disability and Health, CI confidence interval
*Chi-square test
[a]Adjusting for age, hemodialysis vintage, presence of diabetic nephropathy, retinopathy and neuropathy, cerebral vascular disorder, anemia, and employment status
NA refers to "not applicable"

"Because I was not able to find a job if I underwent hemodialysis in a daytime shift, I switched to a night shift and then I got a new job." (Age 34, male)

"On the day of hemodialysis, I come back home late, and on the day without hemodialysis I come home back late because of compensating for the loss I made for hemodialysis treatment. I do not have enough time to play with my child so I feel pity." (Age 33, male)

The respondents also reported that because adjusted hemodialysis shift is not usually offered at their clinics, the patients always perceived *anxiety about work continuation or reemployment*.

Discussion

Using a mixed methods approach, we demonstrated that the three factors of three times a week hospital visits, vascular access, and physical symptoms rank the main reasons for employment difficulties for patients undergoing hemodialysis. The present results are consistent with the previous study indicated that employment of patients aged 18 to 54 was greater in facilities offering a 5 p.m. or later hemodialysis shift [10]. Muehrer et al. [11] reported that treatment of anemia with erythropoietin before the development of renal insufficiency and education for patients on job friendly home dialysis options may improve work retention. Kutner et al. [10] reported that a facility employment rate was positively associated independently with availability of a 5 p.m. or later dialysis shift,

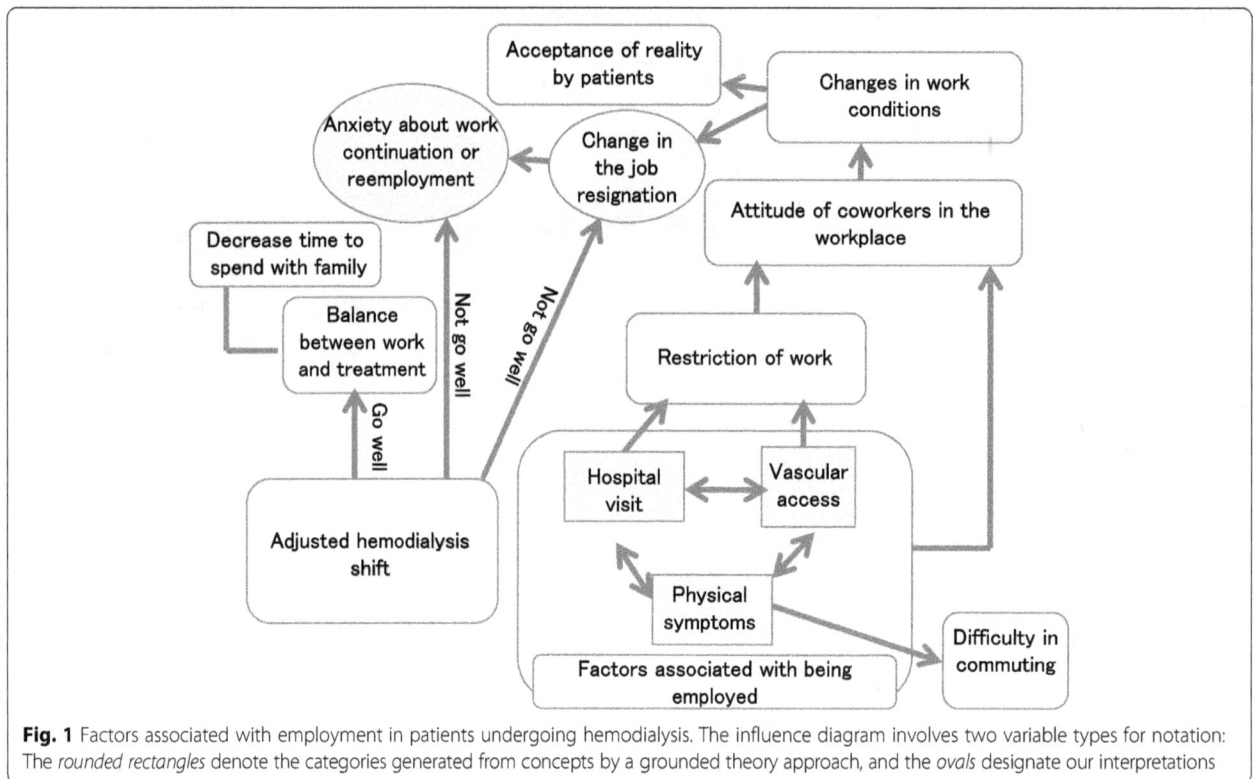

Fig. 1 Factors associated with employment in patients undergoing hemodialysis. The influence diagram involves two variable types for notation: The *rounded rectangles* denote the categories generated from concepts by a grounded theory approach, and the *ovals* designate our interpretations

after adjusting for patient/social-worker ratio, rurality of unit location, and unit size. Although we have not investigated issues regarding anemia treatment or home dialysis, the fact that a 5 p.m. or later dialysis shift improves the working situation has been made clear not only through the results of the quantitative study but also as the actual experience of patients undergoing hemodialysis, as shown by the qualitative study. The strength of our approach was the use of the mixed methods approach.

Although not a mixed methods study, Nakayama et al. reported that working patients who initiated hemodialysis experienced a decline in the average number of working hours and a decrease in their average annual individual income in a Japanese cohort study [3]. Furthermore, depending on the work style (e.g., frequent official trips in trade business), job opportunities were limited in order to protect the vascular access. Indeed, in our quantitative analysis, more than half of the patients in the experienced group agreed on the inconvenience of carrying baggage due to the vascular access.

Moreover, patients who experienced an occlusion of the vascular access had to urgently take days off to be hospitalized for treating the vascular occlusion. For these reasons, patients undergoing hemodialysis are always exposed to such types of discrimination at the workplace as pay cuts, relocation, and so on. These issues frequently occurred in our study sample; approximately 80% of our participants experienced occlusions of the vascular access.

Such a high incidence of vascular access occlusions may be explained by vascular atherosclerosis because the majority of the participants suffered diabetic nephropathy as the underlying kidney disease [12].

Patients in our study manifested various physical symptoms. In particular, patients in the experienced group were more likely to report fatigability and decline in physical strength. According to previous studies, these two physical symptoms are known as two major complaints among patients undergoing hemodialysis [13–15]. Jhamb et al. reported that the incidence of fatigue in patients undergoing hemodialysis ranges from 60 to 97% [13]. Many previous studies have shown that physical activity levels are extremely low in patients undergoing hemodialysis probably because of reduced aerobic capacity [14, 15]. Impairments in physical functions increase the likelihood of loss of unemployment in patients undergoing hemodialysis [1, 4]. In addition to the previous findings, we could show that the participants in the experienced group were more likely to report problems with energy level, attention functions, sensory functions related to temperature and other stimuli, and fine hand use according to the result of the multivariate logistic regression model. A relationship between decline of energy level and maintenance of employment after dialysis initiation has been observed [16]. Indeed, Kutner et al. [17] reported that patients who remained employed had a lower score on the Patient Health Questionnaire 2 (PHQ-2) depression measure; on the basis of the PHQ-2 cutoff score ≥3, 12.1% of the 191 patients who remained employed had possible or probable depression, compared with 32.8% of the 394 patients who were no longer employed.

Misunderstanding and prejudice of superiors and colleagues at the workplace mainly affected employment of the patients undergoing hemodialysis due to the three factors such as frequent hospital visits, vascular access, and physical symptoms. In our quantitative analysis, patients in the experienced group were more likely to report that they had ever been bothered by the attitudes of their superiors and colleagues; some of these patients had actually quit working or changed jobs.

Our study suggested a counteraction to leaving the workplace: if hemodialysis shifts were adapted to the lifestyle of an individual patient, the likelihood of job continuation and job acquisition increased. Indeed, Kutner et al. [10] reported that the strongest predictor of the employment rate among patients on hemodialysis is a night dialysis shift and that the employment rates increased three-fold among facilities which adopted a night shift [10]. According to a Japanese nationwide report [4], 65.4% of patients undergoing hemodialysis in the evening were employed. Among these, 59.6% of civil service workers and 50.4% of general office workers in particular received evening hemodialysis starting after 5:00 p.m. This indicates that patients who use night shift dialysis may not be able to work at night or overtime, but they do not need to leave the workplace early during the day time. To maintain work continuation in patients undergoing hemodialysis, flexible adjustment of dialysis shifts may be a key factor. Mutual use of dialysis shifts among working satellite clinics and flexible shifts to adapt to individual lifestyles may ameliorate the employment rate among patients undergoing hemodialysis.

The present study had several limitations that need to be mentioned. First, our study sample was retrieved from medical charts from two facilities in Aichi prefecture, Japan; thus, the generalizability of our results may be limited to some extent. Second, we only investigated patients who reported difficulties regarding the checklist and who were employed at the time of investigation. We did not evaluate patients who did not report any difficulties even if they were employed. Thus, some information bias might exist. Third, the number of patients does not suffice for a detailed statistical analysis with multiple parameters. Therefore, we performed analysis using the mixed methods approach. Fourth, we did not investigate into the educational status, family income, and marital status which have an impact on the employment. Accordingly, as for our result, influence of these socioeconomic statuses may not be considered. Fifth, laboratory parameters were not evaluated in conjunction with the questionnaire. Despite these limitations, we could clearly show the close relationship between the employment status and the physical status of the patients undergoing hemodialysis by a mixed methods approach.

Conclusions

The present study clearly showed that the negative determinants of employment in patients undergoing hemodialysis were frequent hospital visits, vascular access, and unfavorable physical symptoms. The present result also demonstrated the usefulness of hemodialysis shifts. Specifically, night dialysis starting evening may play a key role in enabling patients to maintain their employment. The mutual use of a night hemodialysis shift among working satellite clinics and flexible shifts to adapt to individual lifestyles may decrease the difficulty in working among patients undergoing hemodialysis.

Abbreviations
ICF: International Classification of Functioning, Disability and Health; PHQ-2: The Patient Health Questionnaire 2

Acknowledgements
This study was supported by a grant from the Kidney Foundation, Aichi. The authors would like to thank M. Ogi, Y. Nagata, K. Kita, M. Natsume, F. Ito, and S. Ozaki—head nurses at Meiyo Clinic; Drs. A. Ito and F. Kato—nephrologists; and H. Sato—director of nursing service department, at Masuko Memorial Hospital, for their support with respect to the interviews.

Funding
This study was in part supported by a grant from the Aichi Kidney Foundation.

Authors' contributions
HT organized the design of the study, implementation of interview survey, and acquisition of the data; performed the statistical analysis; and wrote a draft of the manuscript. KN and SU edited the draft. AI assisted with data analysis. YT, SK, and YY recruited patients and assisted with the interview survey. YO was the person in charge of this research project and made substantial contributions to the conception and design of the study. All authors read and approved the final manuscript.

Authors' information
HT is the associate professor of the General Medical Education and Research Center, Teikyo University. KN is the associate professor of the Department of Hygiene and Public Health, Teikyo University School of Medicine. AI is the researcher of the Jean Hailes Research Unit, School of Public Health and Preventive Medicine, Monash University. YT is the director of the Meiyo Clinic. SK is the associate professor of the Department of Nephrology, Nagoya University Graduate School of Medicine. YY is the associate professor of the Department of Chronic Kidney Disease Initiatives, Nagoya University Graduate School of Medicine. SU is the professor of the Department of Internal Medicine, Teikyo University School of Medicine. YO is the professor of the Research Center of Health, Physical Fitness, and Sports, Nagoya University.

Competing interests
The authors declare that they have no competing interests.

Author details
[1]Research Center of Health, Physical Fitness, and Sports, Nagoya University, Furo-cho, Chikusa-ku, Nagoya 464-8601, Japan. [2]Department of Hygiene and Public Health, Teikyo University School of Medicine, 2-11-1 Kaga, Itabashi-ku, Tokyo 173-8605, Japan. [3]General Medical Education and Research Center, Teikyo University, 2-11-1 Kaga, Itabashi-ku, Tokyo 173-8605, Japan. [4]Jean Hailes Research Unit, School of Public Health and Preventive Medicine, Monash University, Level 1, 549 St Kilda Rd, Melbourne, VIC 3004, Australia. [5]Meiyo Clinic, 64-3 Yatori-cho, Toyohashi 441-8023, Japan. [6]Department of Nephrology, Nagoya University Graduate School of Medicine, 65 Tsurumai, Showa-ku, Nagoya 466-0064, Japan. [7]Department of Chronic Kidney Disease Initiatives, Nagoya University Graduate School of Medicine, 65 Tsurumai, Showa-ku, Nagoya 466-0064, Japan. [8]Department of Internal Medicine, Teikyo University School of Medicine, 2-11-1 Kaga, Itabashi-ku, Tokyo 173-8605, Japan.

References
1. van Manen JG, Korevaar JC, Dekker FW, Reuselaars MC, Boeschoten EW, Krediet RT, et al. Changes in employment status in end-stage renal disease patients during their first year of dialysis. Perit Dial Int. 2001;21:595–601.
2. Tappe K, Turkelson C, Doggett D, Coates V. Disability under Social Security for patients with ESRD: an evidence-based review. Disabil Rehabil. 2001;23:177–85.
3. Nakayama M, Ishida M, Ogihara M, Hanaoka K, Tamura M, Kanai H, et al. Social functioning and socioeconomic changes after introduction of regular dialysis treatment and impact of dialysis modality: a multi-centre survey of Japanese patients. Nephrology. 2015;20:523–30.
4. Japan Association of Kidney Disease Patients, Japanese Association of Dialysis Physicians. Report of research on patients with dialysis treatment in 2011. 2012 (in Japanese).
5. Japan Association of Kidney Disease Patients, Japanese Association of Dialysis Physicians. Report of research on patients with dialysis treatment in 2006. 2007 (in Japanese).
6. John WC. In: John WC, editor. Basic features of mixed methods research. USA: SAGE Publications; 2014.
7. Tsutsui H, Koike T, Yamazaki C, Ito A, Kato F, Sato H, et al. Identification of hemodialysis patients' common problems using the International Classification of Functioning, Disability and Health. Ther Apher Dial. 2009;13:186–92.
8. Tsutsui H, Ojima T, Tsuruta Y, Kato S, Yasuda Y, Oshida Y. Validity of a checklist for hemodialysis patients based on the International Classification of Functioning, Disability and Health. Ther Apher Dial. 2014;18:473–80.
9. Corbin JM, Strauss A. Basics of qualitative research. Techniques and procedures for developing grounded theory. 3rd ed. London: SAGE Publications; 2008.
10. Kutner N, Bowles T, Zhang R, Huang Y, Pastan S. Dialysis facility characteristics and variation in employment rate: a national study. Clin J Am Soc Nephrol. 2008;3:111–6.
11. Muehrer RJ, Schatell D, Witten B, Gangnon R, Becker BN, Hofmann RM. Factors affecting employment at initiation of dialysis. Clin J Am Soc Nephrol. 2011;6:489–96.
12. Alsmady M, Shahait AD, Alawwa IA, Riziq MG, Abusba AM, Al-Quach A. Outcome of upper limb vascular access for hemodialysis. Saudi J Kidney Dis Transpl. 2015;26:1210–42.
13. Jhamb M, Argyropoulos C, Steel JL, Plantinga L, Wu AW, Fink NE, et al. Correlates and outcomes of fatigue among incident dialysis patients. Clin J Am Soc Nephrol. 2009;4:1779–86.
14. Johansen KL, Shubert T, Doyle J, Soher B, Sakkas GK, Kent-Braun JA. Muscle atrophy in patients receiving hemodialysis: effects on muscle strength, muscle quality, and physical function. Kidney Int. 2003;63:291–7.
15. Koufaki P, Mercer TH, Naish PF. Effects of exercise training on aerobic and functional capacity of end-stage renal disease patients. Clin Physiol Funct Imaging. 2002;22:115–24.
16. Murray PD, Dobbels F, Lonsdale DC, Harden PN. Impact of end-stage kidney disease on academic achievement and employment in young adults: a mixed methods study. J Adolesc Health. 2014;55:505–12.
17. Kutner NG, Zhang R, Huang Y, Johansen KL. Depressed mood, usual activity level, and continued employment after starting dialysis. Clin J Am Soc Nephrol. 2010;5:2040–5.

9

The characteristics of the older dialysis population—heterogeneity and another type of altered risk factor patterns

Norio Hanafusa[1]* (iD), Kosaku Nitta[2] and Ken Tsuchiya[1]

Abstract

The number of older dialysis patients is increasing in many countries. For example, the trend is linked to the increase in the dialysis patients 70 years of age and over in Japan. Older dialysis patients often experience deteriorating physical and psychological functions, and special consideration for older patients has been focused on improving or preventing such deteriorations. On the other hand, from the standpoint of clinical studies, the distribution of clinical parameters, clinical outcomes, and their associations of older dialysis patients differ from those of younger patients. Moreover, they exhibit heterogeneous phenotypes. Health age may be more important than the chronological age in considering older patients. Since the age is the most powerful predictor of survival, clinical interventions might have little benefit on the very old dialysis patients. Therefore, maintaining the quality of life or activity of daily living might surpass survival regarding the goal of management of very old dialysis patients. Above all, individualized management according to the heterogeneity or health age are necessary for the older dialysis patients. Future clinical studies of older dialysis patients are needed for the better understanding of this population.

Keywords: Altered risk factor pattern, Clinical parameter, Clinical outcome, Distribution, Health age, Heterogeneity, Individualized management, Older dialysis population

Background

The older dialysis populations are expanding throughout the world. The increase in the older dialysis population can be attributed to increasing in the population 70 years of age and over in Japan (Fig. 1) [1]. Data from the United States Renal Data System (USRDS) show a similar trend in the dialysis population in the USA [2]. The proportion of older dialysis patients is even larger in other countries. The Dialysis Outcome and Practice Patterns Study (DOPPS) showed that nearly half of the dialysis patients in Belgium are 75 years old or more [3].

The older people have many problems and issues. They experience deteriorating physical function, for example, sarcopenia, protein-energy wasting, frailty, and visual or hearing loss. They experience deterioration of psychological or psychiatric conditions. These conditions relate closely to each other. Frailty can be associated with the impaired

cognitive function among end-stage renal disease patients [4] as well as among the general population [5]. They can become a vicious cycle to be broken. They may also suffer from socio-economic difficulties. This malnutrition-cachexia-relating syndrome, or geriatric syndrome, has been reported to associate with worse clinical outcomes [6–9]. The syndrome can include sarcopenia, wasting, and frailty. Sarcopenia focuses on the muscles of the patients, which encompasses muscle mass, strength, and gait speed [10, 11]. Wasting indicates the reduction of visceral proteins, body mass, muscle mass, and dietary intake [12]. Hereinafter, we refer to the reduction of physical component as wasting. On the other hand, frailty is wider meaning and the scope covers psychological, psychiatric, and socio-economic conditions as well as physical conditions [13, 14]. We will refer to the deterioration of the various functions of the patients not limited to physical components as frail or frailty. Withdrawal or withholding of dialysis treatment is a major concern among older dialysis patients.

Older dialysis patients have specific issues from the standpoint of clinical studies or trials. Clinical studies

* Correspondence: hanafusa@twmu.ac.jp
[1]Department of Blood Purification, Tokyo Women's Medical University, 8-1 Kawada-cho, Shinjuku-ku, Tokyo 162-8666, Japan
Full list of author information is available at the end of the article

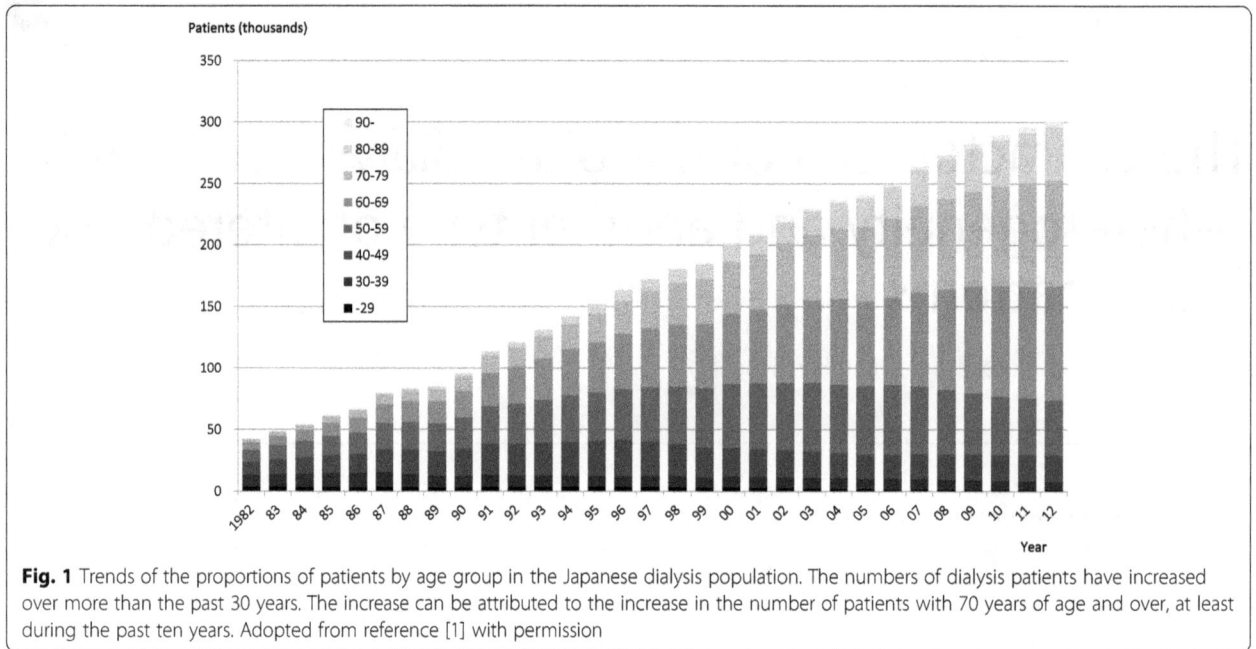

Fig. 1 Trends of the proportions of patients by age group in the Japanese dialysis population. The numbers of dialysis patients have increased over more than the past 30 years. The increase can be attributed to the increase in the number of patients with 70 years of age and over, at least during the past ten years. Adopted from reference [1] with permission

usually attempt to identify associations between certain clinical parameters and outcomes. In this sense, the older population can differ from the younger counterparts in all these parameters which are essential for clinical studies, namely the distribution of clinical parameters, outcomes in both quality and quantity, and the association between clinical parameters and outcomes (Fig. 2). Moreover, there is no consensus definition of the term "older population." Older phenotype might be more important for older patients, and the phenotype can relate to the heterogeneity of the population. In this review, we discuss these issues concerning older dialysis population.

Differences between older and younger dialysis patients

The distribution of clinical parameters

The distributions of clinical parameters sometimes differ across age groups. Figure 3 shows the distributions of several clinical parameters obtained from the Japanese Society for Dialysis Therapy Renal Data Registry (JRDR) by age groups [15]. The patients with the low values were

prevalent among the older age groups for all parameters presented in this figure.

Extracellular volume status is also known to differ between the older and younger dialysis populations. A study based on the Korean registry investigated the bio-impedance parameters of 90 chronic hemodialysis patients and found that their extracellular water to total body water ratios, which are proxies for overhydration, correlated positively with the ages of the patients. Thus, older patients may be more likely to experience overhydration [16].

On the other hand, these changes in the distribution of clinical parameters have been confirmed by the studies that adjusted for the patient characteristics. Lertdumrongluk et al. investigated chronic kidney disease-mineral bone disorder (CKD-MBD) management across age groups in a cohort of 107,817 patients who were receiving their dialysis treatment at DaVita. They found that the odds of developing hyperphosphatemia were lower in the older population, but the odds of developing hypophosphatemia were higher in the same population. Thus, the distribution of serum phosphate levels can differ across age groups even after adjustments for covariates [17].

Differences in clinical outcomes

Many studies have demonstrated that older dialysis patients are more likely to experience worse outcomes than younger patients. This can be partially based on the shorter life expectancy of the older general population. Figure 4 demonstrates the comparison of the life expectancy between the dialysis population and the general population that was investigated in JRDR database. The result indicates that the older persons in the dialysis and

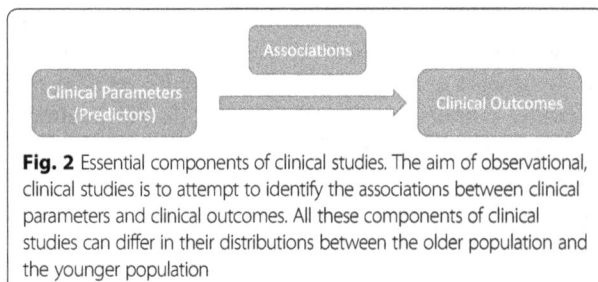

Fig. 2 Essential components of clinical studies. The aim of observational, clinical studies is to attempt to identify the associations between clinical parameters and clinical outcomes. All these components of clinical studies can differ in their distributions between the older population and the younger population

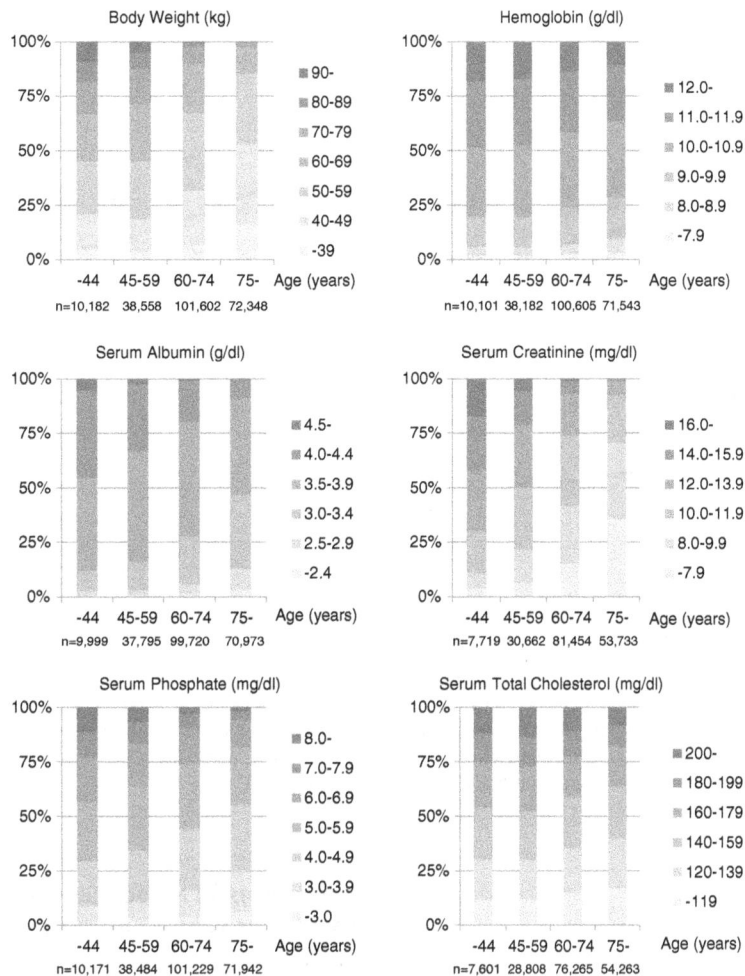

Fig. 3 Distributions of the clinical parameters by age group. The distributions of clinical parameters are shown according to age group. The patients with lower values were more prevalent than younger patients regarding all the clinical parameters shown in this figure. This figure was reproduced from reference [15]

general population experience shorter life expectancy compared to the younger population. Interestingly, the ratios of the life expectancy of the dialysis population to that of the general population were almost 50% irrespective of the age groups of the patients [18]. The fact indicates that the shorter life span of the older dialysis patients is due to the shorter life expectancy of the older general population.

The results of a study that investigated the effects of the older age in the DOPPS cohort showed that the group of patients 75 years of age and over had higher mortality rates than the group under 45 years of age in most of the regions investigated [3]. Moreover, the distribution of the causes of death might also differ across age groups. The proportions of the patients died of cardiovascular disease were smaller in the elderly group except in Japan [3]. JRDR database demonstrated that the proportion of the patients died of cardiovascular disease were almost similar in the elderly patients to the younger patients except for

the group of 45–59 years old, while the proportion that died of infection was larger in the older groups (Fig. 5). A similar result was obtained regarding the quality of life (QOL). The older patients might experience poorer QOL than the younger patients, especially based on the physical component summary scores; although, the mental component summary did not differ across the age groups [3]. Regarding QOL, such association can be controversial; several studies demonstrated that the decline in QOL scores among the older dialysis population was slower than the younger patients [19, 20]. Although the associations between the age groups and QOL scores are not uniform and affected by the criteria investigated, many studies demonstrated that age is one of the major determinants of QOL and that the physical functioning in QOL tended to be worse in the older population [21].

These results indicate that the distribution of clinical outcomes or vulnerability to a worse outcome can differ across age groups.

a

Life Expectancy (years)

Age (years)

b

Life Expectancy (years)

Age (years)

c

Ratios of Life Expectancy (%)

Age (years)

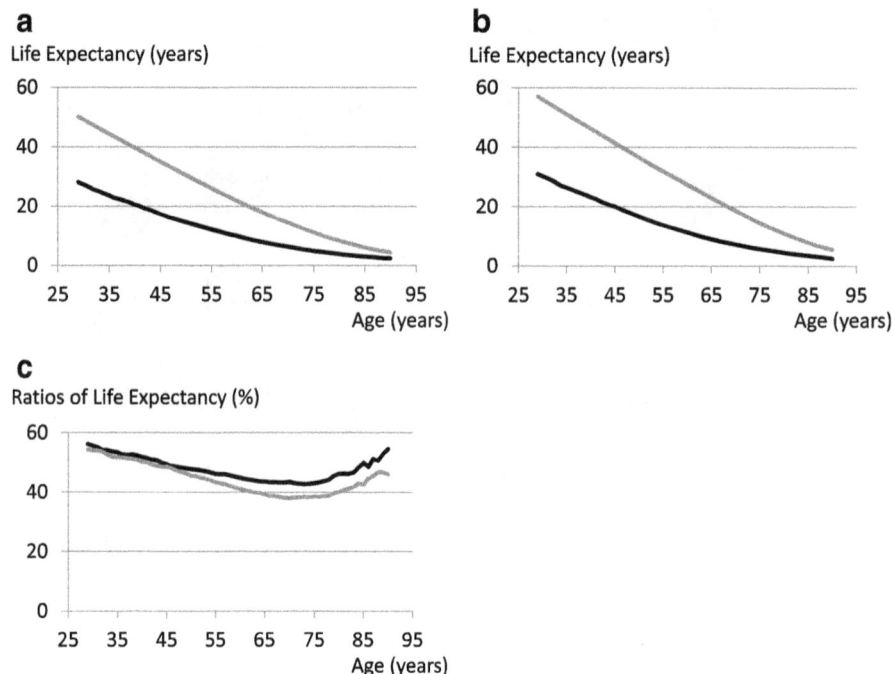

Fig. 4 Life expectancy of the Japanese general population and dialysis population by age. The life expectancy by year were demonstrated among the Japanese general (*gray lines*) and dialysis (*black lines*) population for male (**a**) and female (**b**). The ratios of life expectancy of dialysis patients to the general population by sex (the *black line*, male; the *gray line*, female) were also demonstrated by age (**c**). The ratios were almost uniform and about 50% irrespective of patients' age. This figure was reproduced from reference [18]

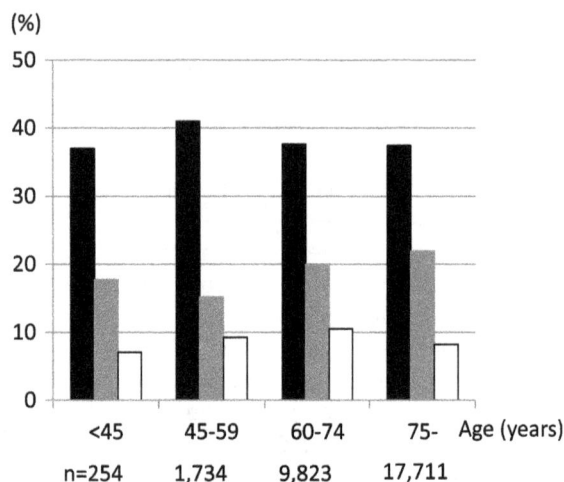

Fig. 5 The breakdown of the causes of death by age groups. The breakdown and proportion of the patients who died of CVD, infection, and malignancy were demonstrated in *black*, *gray*, and *open bars*, respectively. The proportions of CVD as a cause of death were almost equal across age groups except for the group with 45–59 years old. On the other hand, the patients who died of infection were more prevalent in the older patients. Because the patients who died of other causes of death were omitted, the proportions do not sum up to 100%. The figure was produced from the data in reference [15]. CVD, cardiovascular disease

Differences in associations between clinical parameter values and outcomes

The aim of clinical studies is to attempt to identify the association between clinical parameter values and clinical outcomes that can serve as the basis for randomized control trials. Such changes in associations should be considered even in daily clinical practice.

The association between gender and survival may differ across age groups, although somewhat controversial [22]. A study based on the Canadian Organ Replacement Registry investigated associations between gender and all-cause mortality across age groups in a cohort of 28,971 incident chronic hemodialysis patients. This study found that women had survival benefits over men among young patients under 45 years of age, whereas among the older patients 75 years of age and over, women had a lower survival probability than men, even after adjustment for covariates [23]. These results showed that association between gender and survival might differ across age groups.

Hemoglobin (Hb) levels are another example. We investigated the association between Hb levels and survival across age groups in the Japan DOPPS cohort [24] and found differences between the younger group and older group. In the group with Hb levels in the 9–10 g/dl range, only the younger group under 75 years of age had a higher mortality risk than the group with Hb levels in the 10–11 g/dl range (HR 1.46, 95% CI 1.07–2.00), but the older population in the same Hb levels did not experience worse survival (HR 0.83, 95% CI 0.57–1.21). Moreover, a significant interaction between Hb levels and age groups was found in the group with Hb levels in the 9–10 g/dl range ($p = 0.044$).

This result was confirmed by another study based on the Korean cohort. This study found that only the younger group with Hb levels in the 9–10 g/dl range who were under 65 years of age had a significantly higher mortality risk than the group with Hb levels in the 10–11 g/dl range (HR 4.78, 95% CI 1.81–12.62). On the other hand, the older group did not have a significantly worse outcome (HR 1.80, 95% CI 0.95–3.39); although, the interaction between Hb levels and age groups was marginally non-significant ($p = 0.0526$) [25].

The study mentioned above from DaVita investigated the associations between serum phosphate levels and mortality by age groups [17] and found a J-shaped or U-shaped association between serum phosphate levels and all-cause mortality in the crude models. On the other hand, hypophosphatemia (serum phosphate below 3.5 mg/dl) was associated with higher mortality only in the 65 years of age over group after adjustment for covariates, including for malnutrition-inflammation complex syndrome, while hyperphosphatemia (serum phosphate above 5.5 mg/dl) was uniformly associated with higher mortality risks across all age groups [17].

Another type of altered risk factor patterns

Risk-factor patterns have been reported to change as chronic kidney disease (CKD) stages progress. More specifically, the associations between clinical parameters and outcomes found in the end-stage renal disease (ESRD) population may differ from the patterns observed in early stages of CKD or even in the general population. Such alterations encompass body mass index [26], body height [27, 28], blood pressure [29], and serum cholesterol level [30]. These findings are called "altered risk factor patterns" [31, 32] or "reverse epidemiology" [33]. These altered risk factor patterns can be found in other disease conditions, including congestive heart failure [34], cancer [35], acquired immune deficiency syndrome [36], and even in the older general population [37]. On the other hand, as discussed above, associations between risk factors or clinical parameters and clinical outcomes might change again with advancing age even if the population is confined to ESRD. Such change may be another type of risk factor pattern alterations among patients with kidney disease.

Older populations are heterogeneous

Another problem is that older population is heterogeneous. This fact also relates to the definition of older patients, because the cut-off age for older patients can be ambiguous due to the heterogeneities in the health status among them.

The scheme shown in Fig. 6 illustrates the heterogeneity of older dialysis patients. During the normal aging process, actual or chronological age and age based on health status, i.e., health age, are almost identical. Here, the health age is a conceptual age by which we can consider a patient robust or frail, and the health age can closely relate to the clinical outcomes more than the actual or chronological age. However, the relationship between chronological age and health age can vary among the patients. Patients who are considered frail have a higher health age than their chronological age, while patients who are considered robust have a lower health age than their chronological age. Importantly, the disparities between chronological age and health age become wider in older populations. Moreover, health age may be more closely associated with outcomes than biological age. Thus, patients can be classified as old or young by their health age. Although Fig. 6 is only conceptual, the older dialysis patients are more heterogenic than the younger patients in terms of the phenotypes of wasting or the geriatric syndrome as discussed later. This concept can also be supported by clinical experiences in daily practice. The concept should be confirmed, and the definition of the health age itself should be determined by future investigations.

We performed a preliminary study on heterogeneities in the older dialysis population in the JRDR, the Japanese Registry [38], by comparing the coefficients of variances of clinical parameters with those of the 45–59 years of age groups. The heterogeneities of the clinical parameters indicating "wasting," including creatinine generation rate, serum levels of creatinine, and albumin exhibited large heterogeneities. Therefore, these parameters might relate to the frailty or robustness of the patients.

This study confirmed that the older population is heterogeneous, especially regarding clinical parameters related to wasting. This finding was reinforced by the evidence that protein-energy wasting is closely associated with worse outcomes independent of the patient's age [39–41]. The significance of wasting in considering the well-being or outcomes of the older patients requires further investigation. Activities of daily living (ADL) or comorbidities can be the key issues for an understanding of such heterogeneities among the older patients or the health age. The older incident dialysis patients tend to experience worse ADL assessed by Barthel index [42, 43], and the lower ADL can be associated with the worse outcome [43]. The comorbidities of the patients also relate to the worse outcome even among the elderly patients who undergo dialysis treatments [44–46]. The patients with wasting are vulnerable to complications leading to comorbidities, while the patients with multiple comorbidities

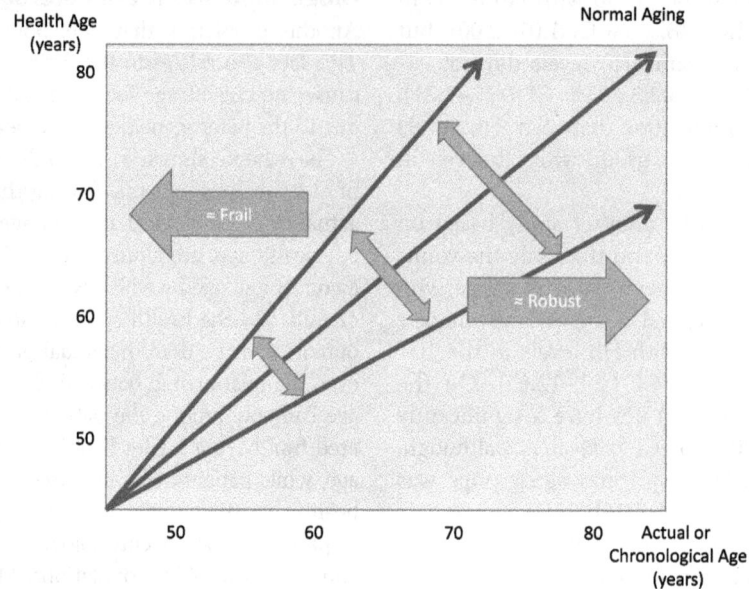

Fig. 6 Scheme of older dialysis patients and heterogeneities. Conceptually, two types of age expression can be considered in a single patient, actual and chronological ages. The chronological age is usually used to determine the age of patients, while health age is a conceptual age and it determines the phenotype of the patients. During the normal aging process, the two ages are identical. Patients are considered frail when their health ages are higher than their actual ages. Importantly, the disparities or the heterogeneities across patients are wider in the older population

often experience wasting conditions. The cause-result relationship between wasting and comorbidities remains unclear because these relationships have been obtained through observational studies. It is possible that interventions against wasting can break the vicious cycle of wasting and comorbidities.

Appropriate goals for the management of older dialysis patients

Age itself is still the most powerful predictor of survival; although, wasting also has a substantial effect on survival. Figure 7 indicates the survival rates by primary diagnoses of the patients [47]. The survival rates were almost identical

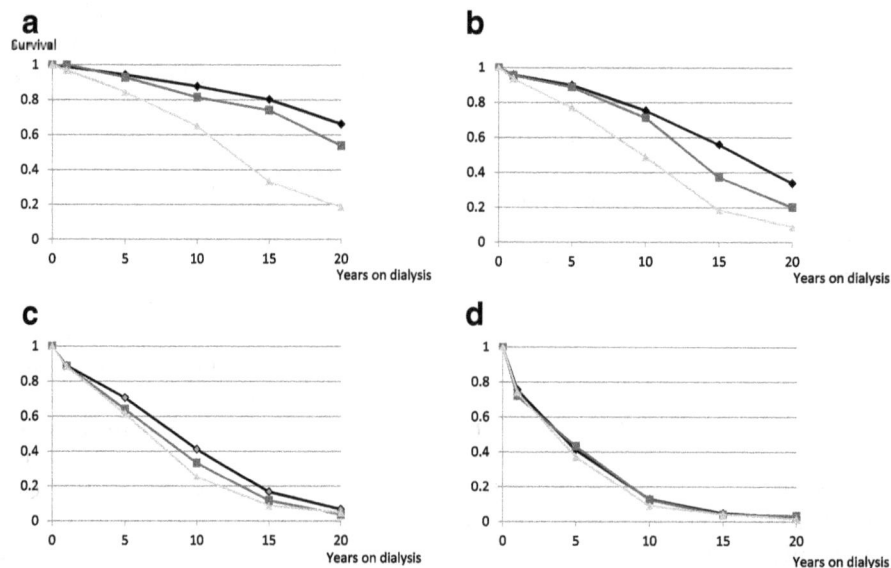

Fig. 7 Crude mortality rates according to primary diagnosis and the age at the start of dialysis. Crude mortality rates are shown according to the primary diagnosis of end-stage renal disease and age at the start of dialysis therapy. The age groups at the start of dialysis therapy were 30–44, 45–59, 60–74, and 75–89 years old in panels **a**, **b**, **c**, and **d**, respectively. Primary diagnoses of glomerulonephritis, nephrosclerosis, and diabetes are shown in *black*, *dark gray*, and *pale gray*, respectively. The differences in survival decreased as the age at the start of dialysis increased. This figure was reproduced from reference [47]

irrespective of the diagnoses, especially among the very old population. This fact suggests that therapeutic interventions on the very old dialysis patients might be of little benefit. Therefore, the goals of the management of such patients could be improving the well-being, QOL, or ADL rather than their survival. Of course, we should prioritize the preferences of patients and their families or caregivers and discuss the goals carefully and comprehensively in decision making.

Conclusions

Older dialysis populations differ from younger dialysis populations in the distributions of their clinical parameters, clinical outcomes, and associations between them. Moreover, there are great heterogeneities within older populations, especially regarding wasting phenotypes, and these heterogeneities require individualized managements. Finally, individualized goals of dialysis management are also necessary, especially for the very old population. However, many points remain to be elucidated regarding the management of older dialysis patients.

Abbreviations

ADL: Activity of daily living; CI: Confidence interval; CVD: Cardiovascular disease; ESRD: End-stage renal disease; CKD-MBD: Chronic kidney disease-mineral bone disorder; DOPPS: The Dialysis Outcome and Practice Patterns Study; Hb: Hemoglobin; HR: Hazard ratio; JRDR: The Japanese Society for Dialysis Therapy Renal Data Registry; JSDT: The Japanese Society for Dialysis Therapy; QOL: Quality of life; USRDS: The United States Renal Data System

Acknowledgements

The data reported here were provided by the JSDT. The interpretation and reporting of these data are the responsibility of the authors and do not reflect the official interpretation or views of the JSDT.

Funding

The authors did not have a specific funding source to be disclosed regarding this article.

Authors' contributions

NH planned the review, searched the literature, and prepared the article. KN and KT searched the literature and assisted in writing the article. All authors read and approved the final manuscript.

Competing interests

NH was a former member of a division that is funded by Terumo Corporation. Other authors have no competing interests to declare regarding the contents of this article.

Author details

[1]Department of Blood Purification, Tokyo Women's Medical University, 8-1 Kawada-cho, Shinjuku-ku, Tokyo 162-8666, Japan. [2]Department of Medicine, Kidney Center, Tokyo Women's Medical University, 8-1 Kawada-cho, Shinjuku-ku, Tokyo 162-8666, Japan.

References

1. Hanafusa N, Nakai S, Iseki K, Tsubakihara Y. Japanese society for dialysis therapy renal data registry—a window through which we can view the details of Japanese dialysis population. Kidney Int Suppl (2011). 2015;5(1):15–22.
2. Saran R, Li Y, Robinson B, Abbott KC, Agodoa LY, Ayanian J, Bragg-Gresham J, Balkrishnan R, Chen JL, Cope E, et al. US Renal Data System 2015 Annual Data Report: epidemiology of kidney disease in the United States. Am J Kidney Dis. 2016;Svii(3 Suppl 1):S1–S305.
3. Canaud B, Tong L, Tentori F, Akiba T, Karaboyas A, Gillespie B, Akizawa T, Pisoni RL, Bommer J, Port FK. Clinical practices and outcomes in elderly hemodialysis patients: results from the Dialysis Outcomes and Practice Patterns Study (DOPPS). Clin J Am Soc Nephrol. 2011;6(7):1651–62.
4. McAdams-DeMarco MA, Tan J, Salter ML, Gross A, Meoni LA, Jaar BG, Kao WH, Parekh RS, Segev DL, Sozio SM. Frailty and cognitive function in incident hemodialysis patients. Clin J Am Soc Nephrol. 2015;10(12):2181–9.
5. Robertson DA, Savva GM, Kenny RA. Frailty and cognitive impairment—a review of the evidence and causal mechanisms. Ageing Res Rev. 2013;12(4): 840–51.
6. Johansen KL, Chertow GM, Jin C, Kutner NG. Significance of frailty among dialysis patients. J Am Soc Nephrol. 2007;18(11):2960–7.
7. Isoyama N, Qureshi AR, Avesani CM, Lindholm B, Barany P, Heimburger O, Cederholm T, Stenvinkel P, Carrero JJ. Comparative associations of muscle mass and muscle strength with mortality in dialysis patients. Clin J Am Soc Nephrol. 2014;9(10):1720–8.
8. Drew DA, Weiner DE, Tighiouart H, Scott T, Lou K, Kantor A, Fan L, Strom JA, Singh AK, Sarnak MJ. Cognitive function and all-cause mortality in maintenance hemodialysis patients. Am J Kidney Dis. 2015;65(2):303–11.
9. Griva K, Stygall J, Hankins M, Davenport A, Harrison M, Newman SP. Cognitive impairment and 7-year mortality in dialysis patients. Am J Kidney Dis. 2010;56(4):693–703.
10. Chen LK, Liu LK, Woo J, Assantachai P, Auyeung TW, Bahyah KS, Chou MY, Chen LY, Hsu PS, Krairit O, et al. Sarcopenia in Asia: consensus report of the Asian Working Group for Sarcopenia. J Am Med Dir Assoc. 2014;15(2):95–101.
11. Cruz-Jentoft AJ, Baeyens JP, Bauer JM, Boirie Y, Cederholm T, Landi F, Martin FC, Michel JP, Rolland Y, Schneider SM, et al. Sarcopenia: European consensus on definition and diagnosis: report of the European working group on sarcopenia in older people. Age Ageing. 2010;39(4):412–23.
12. Fouque D, Kalantar-Zadeh K, Kopple J, Cano N, Chauveau P, Cuppari L, Franch H, Guarnieri G, Ikizler TA, Kaysen G, et al. A proposed nomenclature and diagnostic criteria for protein-energy wasting in acute and chronic kidney disease. Kidney Int. 2008;73(4):391–8.
13. Fried LP, Tangen CM, Walston J, Newman AB, Hirsch C, Gottdiener J, Seeman T, Tracy R, Kop WJ, Burke G, et al. Frailty in older adults: evidence for a phenotype. J Gerontol A Biol Sci Med Sci. 2001;56(3):M146–56.
14. Statement on the frailty from the Japan Geriatrics Society (in Japanese). http://www.jpn-geriat-soc.or.jp/info/topics/pdf/20140513_01_01. Accessed 12 Dec 2016.
15. An Overview of Regular Dialysis Treatment in Japan (As of December 31, 2014) (in Japanese). http://member.jsdt.or.jp/member/contents/cdrom/2014/main.html. Accessed 12 Dec 2016.
16. Lee JE, Jo IY, Lee SM, Kim WJ, Choi HY, Ha SK, Kim HJ, Park HC. Comparison of hydration and nutritional status between young and elderly hemodialysis patients through bioimpedance analysis. Clin Interv Aging. 2015;10:1327–34.
17. Lertdumrongluk P, Rhee CM, Park J, Lau WL, Moradi H, Jing J, Molnar MZ, Brunelli SM, Nissenson AR, Kovesdy CP, et al. Association of serum phosphorus concentration with mortality in elderly and nonelderly hemodialysis patients. J Ren Nutr. 2013;23(6):411–21.
18. The Illustrated Version of An Overview of Regular Dialysis Treatment in Japan (As of December 31, 2005) (in Japanese). http://docs.jsdt.or.jp/overview/pdf2006/p43.pdf. Accessed 12 Dec 2016.
19. Rebollo P, Ortega F, Baltar JM, Alvarez-Ude F, Alvarez Navascues R, Alvarez-Grande J. Is the loss of health-related quality of life during renal

replacement therapy lower in elderly patients than in younger patients? Nephrol Dial Transplant. 2001;16(8):1675–80.

20. Unruh ML, Newman AB, Larive B, Dew MA, Miskulin DC, Greene T, Beddhu S, Rocco MV, Kusek JW, Meyer KB, et al. The influence of age on changes in health-related quality of life over three years in a cohort undergoing hemodialysis. J Am Geriatr Soc. 2008;56(9):1608–17.

21. Apostolou T. Quality of life in the elderly patients on dialysis. Int Urol Nephrol. 2007;39(2):679–83.

22. Hecking M, Bieber BA, Ethier J, Kautzky-Willer A, Sunder-Plassmann G, Saemann MD, Ramirez SP, Gillespie BW, Pisoni RL, Robinson BM, et al. Sex-specific differences in hemodialysis prevalence and practices and the male-to-female mortality rate: the Dialysis Outcomes and Practice Patterns Study (DOPPS). PLoS Med. 2014;11(10):e1001750.

23. Sood MM, Rigatto C, Komenda P, Mojica J, Tangri N. Mortality risk for women on chronic hemodialysis differs by age. Can J Kidney Health Dis. 2014;1:10.

24. Hanafusa N, Nomura T, Hasegawa T, Nangaku M. Age and anemia management: relationship of hemoglobin levels with mortality might differ between elderly and nonelderly hemodialysis patients. Nephrol Dial Transplant. 2014;29(12):2316–26.

25. Kwon O, Jang HM, Jung HY, Kim YS, Kang SW, Yang CW, Kim NH, Choi JY, Cho JH, Kim CD, et al. The Korean Clinical Research Center for End-Stage Renal Disease Study validates the association of hemoglobin and erythropoiesis-stimulating agent dose with mortality in hemodialysis patients. PLoS One. 2015;10(10):e0140241.

26. Kalantar-Zadeh K, Kopple JD, Kilpatrick RD, McAllister CJ, Shinaberger CS, Gjertson DW, Greenland S. Association of morbid obesity and weight change over time with cardiovascular survival in hemodialysis population. Am J Kidney Dis. 2005;46(3):489–500.

27. Elsayed ME, Ferguson JP, Stack AG. Association of height with elevated mortality risk in ESRD: variation by race and gender. J Am Soc Nephrol. 2016;27(2):580–93.

28. Shapiro BB, Streja E, Ravel VA, Kalantar-Zadeh K, Kopple JD. Association of height with mortality in patients undergoing maintenance hemodialysis. Clin J Am Soc Nephrol. 2015;10(6):965–74.

29. Zager PG, Nikolic J, Brown RH, Campbell MA, Hunt WC, Peterson D, Van Stone J, Levey A, Meyer KB, Klag MJ, et al. "U" curve association of blood pressure and mortality in hemodialysis patients. Medical Directors of Dialysis Clinic, Inc. Kidney Int. 1998;54(2):561–9.

30. Iseki K, Yamazato M, Tozawa M, Takishita S. Hypocholesterolemia is a significant predictor of death in a cohort of chronic hemodialysis patients. Kidney Int. 2002;61(5):1887–93.

31. Kopple JD. The phenomenon of altered risk factor patterns or reverse epidemiology in persons with advanced chronic kidney failure. Am J Clin Nutr. 2005;81(6):1257–66.

32. Kopple JD. How to reconcile conventional and altered risk factor patterns in dialysis patients. Semin Dial. 2007;20(6):602–5.

33. Kalantar-Zadeh K, Block G, Humphreys MH, Kopple JD. Reverse epidemiology of cardiovascular risk factors in maintenance dialysis patients. Kidney Int. 2003;63(3):793–808.

34. Kalantar-Zadeh K, Block G, Horwich T, Fonarow GC. Reverse epidemiology of conventional cardiovascular risk factors in patients with chronic heart failure. J Am Coll Cardiol. 2004;43(8):1439–44.

35. Kalantar-Zadeh K, Horwich TB, Oreopoulos A, Kovesdy CP, Younessi H, Anker SD, Morley JE. Risk factor paradox in wasting diseases. Curr Opin Clin Nutr Metab Care. 2007;10(4):433–42.

36. Chlebowski RT, Grosvenor M, Lillington L, Sayre J, Beall G. Dietary intake and counseling, weight maintenance, and the course of HIV infection. J Am Diet Assoc. 1995;95(4):428–32. quiz 433–425.

37. Stevens J, Cai J, Pamuk ER, Williamson DF, Thun MJ, Wood JL. The effect of age on the association between body-mass index and mortality. N Engl J Med. 1998;338(1):1–7.

38. Hanafusa N, Sakurai S, Nangaku M. Heterogeneity of clinical indices among the older dialysis population—a study on Japanese dialysis population. Ren Replace Ther. 2017;3:1.

39. de Mutsert R, Grootendorst DC, Axelsson J, Boeschoten EW, Krediet RT, Dekker FW, Group NS. Excess mortality due to interaction between protein-energy wasting, inflammation and cardiovascular disease in chronic dialysis patients. Nephrol Dial Transplant. 2008;23(9):2957–64.

40. Kim JC, Kalantar-Zadeh K, Kopple JD. Frailty and protein-energy wasting in elderly patients with end stage kidney disease. J Am Soc Nephrol. 2013;24(3):337–51.

41. Nitta K, Tsuchiya K. Recent advances in the pathophysiology and management of protein-energy wasting in chronic kidney disease. Ren Replace Ther. 2016;2:4.

42. Hung MC, Sung JM, Chang YT, Hwang JS, Wang JD. Estimation of physical functional disabilities and long-term care needs for patients under maintenance hemodialysis. Med Care. 2014;52(1):63–70.

43. Inaguma D, Tanaka A, Shinjo H. Physical function at the time of dialysis initiation is associated with subsequent mortality. Clin Exp Nephrol. 2016.

44. Kurella M, Covinsky KE, Collins AJ, Chertow GM. Octogenarians and nonagenarians starting dialysis in the United States. Ann Intern Med. 2007; 146(3):177–83.

45. Lin YT, Wu PH, Kuo MC, Lin MY, Lee TC, Chiu YW, Hwang SJ, Chen HC. High cost and low survival rate in high comorbidity incident elderly hemodialysis patients. PLoS One. 2013;8(9):e75318.

46. Chandna SM, Da Silva-Gane M, Marshall C, Warwicker P, Greenwood RN, Farrington K. Survival of elderly patients with stage 5 CKD: comparison of conservative management and renal replacement therapy. Nephrol Dial Transplant. 2011;26(5):1608–14.

47. An Overview of Regular Dialysis Treatment in Japan (As of December 31, 2008) (in Japanese). http://member.jsdt.or.jp/member/contents/cdrom/2008/Main.html. Accessed 12 Dec 2016.

10

Impact of vascular calcification on cardiovascular mortality in hemodialysis patients: clinical significance, mechanisms and possible strategies for treatment

Takayasu Ohtake[*] and Shuzo Kobayashi

Abstract

Vascular calcification has now been recognized as a major problem in dialysis patients because of its strong influence on the prognosis. Along with the regulatory failure of calcification-inhibitory system, active phenotypic change of vascular smooth muscle cells (VSMCs) to osteoblast-like cells is also involved in the progression of vascular calcification.

Delaying or improving the vascular calcification is thought to be very important to improve the cardiovascular mortality in dialysis patients. Several interventional trials against vascular calcification using non-calcium-containing phosphate binders, low-dose active vitamin D plus cinacalcet, modification of dialysate calcium concentration, and sodium thiosulfate have been done, and some trials including non-calcium-containing phosphate binders showed beneficial effect on delaying vascular calcification in dialysis patients. However, delaying or improving vascular calcification has not been clearly proved to result in improved cardiovascular event and/or mortality rate by prospective interventional randomized controlled trials in dialysis patients. Whether the improvement of vascular calcification could directly lead to the improvement of survival is an urgent issue of clinical trials in dialysis patients.

Keywords: Vascular calcification, Cardiovascular mortality, Phosphate, Phosphate binder, Hemodialysis

Background

As mentioned in a recent review [1], active atherosclerotic process has already begun in the early stages of chronic kidney disease (CKD), and atherosclerotic organ damages deteriorate along with the decreasing renal function. By the time of the initiation of renal replacement therapy (RRT), major atherosclerotic vascular damages have already been completed in many patients. Coronary artery stenosis (CAS) has been shown in almost 50% in patients with end-stage renal failure (ESRD) [2, 3], and almost 80% of diabetic ESRD patients have significant occult CAS at the initiation of RRT in spite of no chest symptom or no previous history of ischemic heart disease [2]. However, as Lindner et al. rung an alarm

42 years ago [4], atherosclerotic process intensively accelerates after the initiation of RRT.

One of the most characteristic features of atherosclerosis seen in dialysis patients is vascular calcification, especially "medial calcification." Medial calcification was initially described in 1903, a hundred years ago by Johann Georg Mönckeberg, a German pathologist. Therefore, medial calcification may be called as "Mönckeberg's mediasclerosis" or "Mönckeberg's mediacalcinosis" [5]. Vascular calcification crossly associates with several target organ damages (TODs) including stroke, ischemic heart disease, and peripheral arterial disease. Vascular calcification causes TODs via the disturbance of vascular function, i.e., "vascular failure."

Vascular calcification affects on the future cardiovascular events and/or mortality in dialysis patients [6–20]. Several clinical trials to aim to improve cardiovascular events and/or mortality in dialysis patients have been planned or reported. Among these trials, the largest

* Correspondence: ohtake@shonankamakura.or.jp
Department of Nephrology, Immunology, and Vascular Medicine, Kidney Disease and Transplant Center, Shonan Kamakura General Hospital, 1370-1 Okamoto, Kamakura 247-8533, Japan

randomized controlled trial (RCT), the LANDMARK study, which compares the effect of non-calcium-containing phosphate binder, lanthanum carbonate, with calcium-containing phosphate binder, is now ongoing in Japan [21]. The result of the LANDMARK study will soon be open.

Here, we want to summarize in the present situation about the clinical significance, mechanisms, and the behavior of vascular calcification by interventional trials and provide update information about clinical trials against vascular calcification in dialysis patients.

Clinical impact of vascular calcification

Several reports have shown the strong relationship between vascular calcification and clinical outcomes including cardiovascular events, and cardiovascular and all-cause mortality.

The number of calcified sites including carotid artery, abdominal aorta, ilio-femoral axis, and legs was a strong predictor of cardiovascular and all-cause mortality in an early study [6]. As to the relationship between coronary artery calcification score (CACS) and clinical outcomes, dialysis patients with higher CACS showed significantly higher rate of cardiovascular and all-cause mortality compared with those with mild or no CACS (Fig. 1) [7–13]. In these reports, cardiovascular events were also significantly correlated with high CACS. Aortic calcification also significantly correlated with cardiovascular and all-cause mortality and was an independent predictor of cardiovascular and all-cause mortality

[14–19]. These associations between vascular calcification and clinical outcomes were independent even after adjusting traditional risk factors such as age, hemodialysis duration, hypertension, diabetes, smoking, and dyslipidemia. Clinical significance in other vascular sites has also been reported. Carotid artery calcification at the initiation of hemodialysis was an independent associating factor for cardiovascular events in incident hemodialysis patients [20]. Furthermore, lower limbs' arterial calcification was crossly associated with the presence and severity of peripheral arterial disease (PAD) in hemodialysis patients [22]. Critical limb ischemia (CLI) strongly impacts on the prognosis of hemodialysis patients, and lower limbs' arterial calcification in CLI patients was extremely high compared with non-PAD or non-CLI patients on hemodialysis (Fig. 2).

Vascular calcification positively correlates with arterial stiffness. Aortic stiffness represented by aortic pulse wave velocity (PWV) was significantly associated with abdominal aortic calcification [23] and CACS [24]. Increased aortic stiffness (increased cardiac afterload) consequently leads to left ventricular hypertrophy (LVH). LVH could be also induced by elevated fibroblast growth factor 23 (FGF23) as proven in an animal experiment [25]. Both calcification-related cardiac ischemia and LVH concomitantly increase the risk of cardiovascular mortality (Fig. 3). Hemodynamic and functional changes associated with vascular calcification have strong clinical impact on morbidity and mortality in dialysis patients. Therefore, clarifying the mechanisms and accelerating

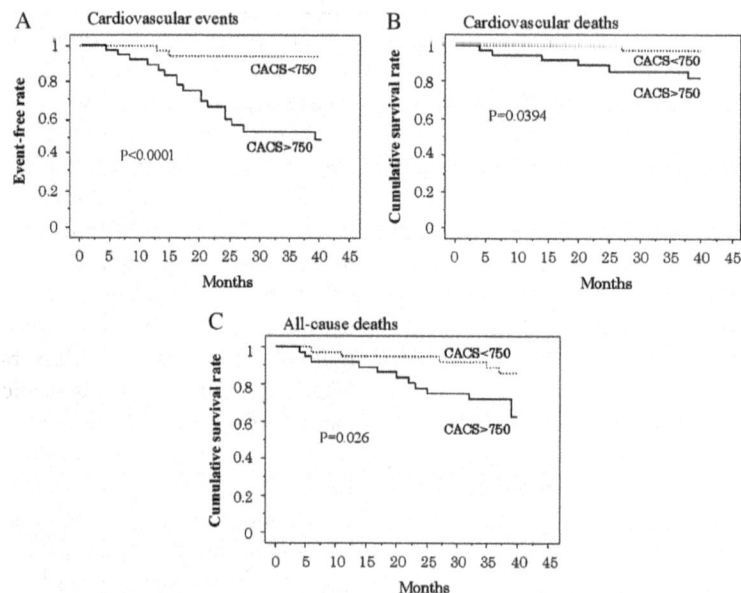

Fig. 1 Impact of CACS on cardiovascular events, cardiovascular mortality, and all-cause mortality [10]. Patients with CACS >750 (N = 37) showed significantly higher cardiovascular event rate, cardiovascular mortality rate, and all-cause mortality rate compared with patients with CACS <750 (N = 37), according to the median value of CACS (748.2) of all 74 patients. **a** Cardiovascular events, **b** cardiovascular mortality, **c** all-cause mortality. *Abbreviation*: CACS coronary artery calcification score

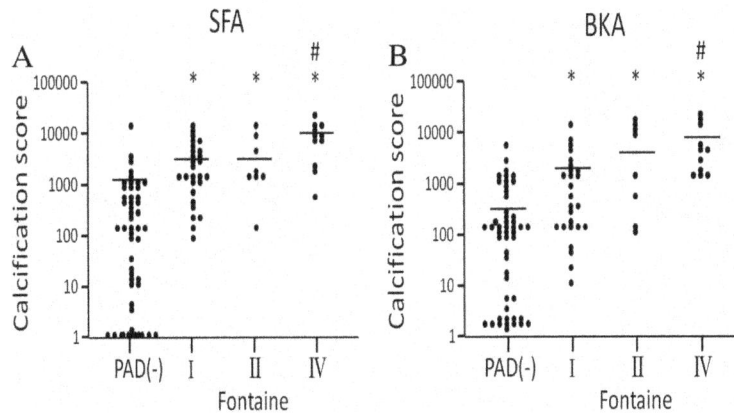

Fig. 2 a, b Lower limbs' arterial calcification score and severity of peripheral arterial disease in hemodialysis patients [22]. Lower limbs' arterial calcification score (above knee, below knee). *$p < 0.01$ vs. PAD(–) group, #$p < 0.01$ vs. PAD Fontaine 1 group. *Abbreviations: SFA* superficial femoral artery, *BKA* below-knee arteries, *PAD* peripheral arterial disease

factors for vascular calcification in dialysis patients is very important.

Mechanisms and associating factors for vascular calcification

Serum levels of both calcium and phosphate in normal physiological condition are tightly regulated in narrow ranges. Formation of hydroxyapatite is limited in bones, and vascular calcification does not occur. Vascular smooth muscle cells (VSMCs) prevent ectopic calcification via inhibitory mechanisms in normal physiological condition. However, extensive and accelerating medial

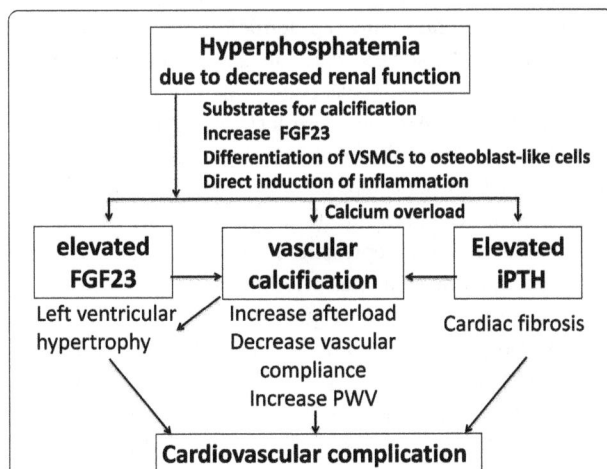

Fig. 3 Clinical aspect of vascular calcification leading to cardiovascular complication. The critical key for vascular calcification is hyperphosphatemia due to decreased renal function. Hyperphosphatemia causes vascular calcification through several mechanisms. Vascular calcification, concomitantly with left ventricular hypertrophy and cardiac fibrosis, causes cardiovascular complication. *Abbreviations: FGF23* fibroblast growth factor 23, *VSMC* vascular smooth muscle cell, *iPTH* intact parathyroid hormone, *PWV* pulse wave velocity

calcification ensues in CKD patients, especially in dialysis patients. Important mechanisms of vascular calcification in dialysis patients are (1) failure of inhibitory systems for vascular calcification and (2) differentiation of VSMCs to osteoblast-like cells (Fig. 4).

Inhibitory factors for vascular calcification include matrix Gla protein (MGP), pyrophosphate (produced in VSMCs), and circulating inhibitor fetuin A. On the other hand, activation of transcription factors "Runx2" and mineralization regulating protein "alkaline phosphatase (ALP)" are important key factors for osteochondrocytic differentiation of VSMCs. Uremic milieu concomitantly inactivates the production of inhibitors and promotes phenotypic changes and/or apoptosis of VSMCs resulting in medial calcification (Fig. 4) [26].

Inhibitory factors (with comment about the risk of warfarin use)

MGP is expressed in VSMCs and loaded in matrix vesicles (scaffold of calcification) around VSMCs, consequently inhibiting their calcification. MGP binds to calcium and pro-osteogenic factor bone morphologic protein 2 (BMP2) and inactivates it in normal condition [27]. However, loading of MGP is decreased in high calcium circumstances, and matrix calcification is promoted [28, 29]. Vitamin K is essential for MGP activation. Therefore, deficiency of vitamin K inhibits MGP activity, thus leading to vascular calcification enhancement. Warfarin, an antagonist to vitamin K, is a strong promoter of arterial calcification via blocking the activation of vitamin K-dependent MGP [30]. Many dialysis patients have cardiovascular complications, including artificial valve replacement, atrial fibrillation, and cardiogenic cerebral embolism, which might necessitate warfarin prescription. However, many cardiologists who prescribe warfarin do not know the profound risk of warfarin as a strong promoter of vascular calcification in

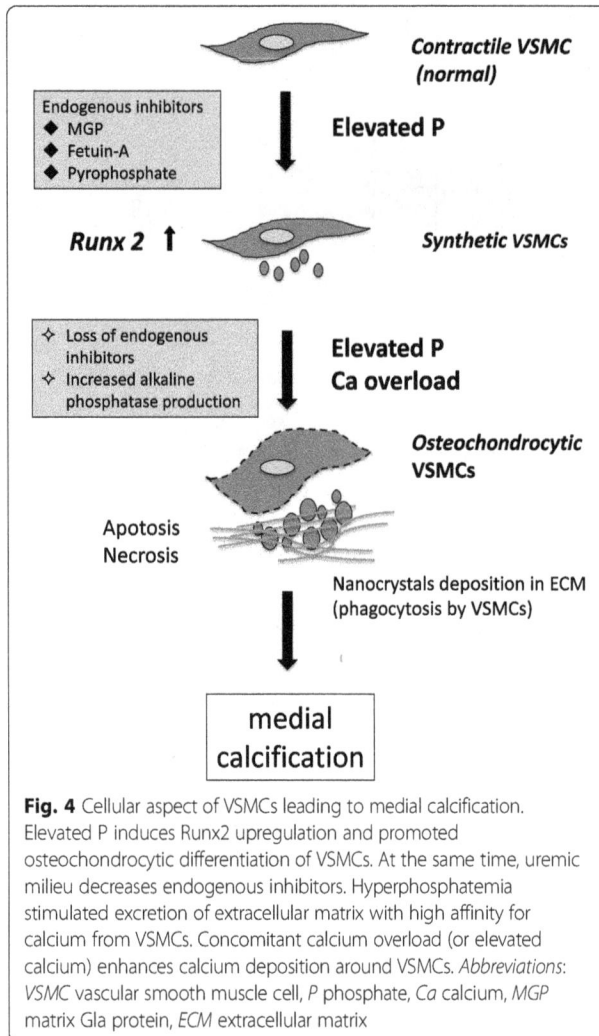

Fig. 4 Cellular aspect of VSMCs leading to medial calcification. Elevated P induces Runx2 upregulation and promoted osteochondrocytic differentiation of VSMCs. At the same time, uremic milieu decreases endogenous inhibitors. Hyperphosphatemia stimulated excretion of extracellular matrix with high affinity for calcium from VSMCs. Concomitant calcium overload (or elevated calcium) enhances calcium deposition around VSMCs. *Abbreviations*: *VSMC* vascular smooth muscle cell, *P* phosphate, *Ca* calcium, *MGP* matrix Gla protein, *ECM* extracellular matrix

dialysis patients. Not only nephrologists but cardiologists should be aware of the profound risk of warfarin use in dialysis patients.

Pyrophosphate binds to hydroxyapatite crystals and inhibits their further growth. ALP, which is upregulated in VSMCs in the early stages of vascular calcification and a key factor for mineralization, degrades pyrophosphate, thereby promoting calcification [31–33]. Osteogenic transcription factor Runx2 is thought to regulate the expression of ALP.

Fetuin A is a circulating inhibitor and forms a complex with calcium and phosphate, forming a calciprotein particle (CPP), thus preventing mineral deposition in vascular walls [34, 35]. Furthermore, fetuin A is taken up by synthetic VSMCs and secreted in a matrix around VSMCs, where it protects from calcification [36]. Therefore, fetuin A has dual inhibitory actions, one in circulation and the other in vascular walls. The levels of fetuin A are reduced in dialysis patients, and it might reflect the excessive CPP formation in dialysis patients [37–40].

Osteoblastic differentiation

Runx2 upregulation and ALP expression in VSMCs is the most important process in the early phase of osteoblast-like cell differentiation of VSMCs [41]. Expression of Runx2 is normally restricted in the bone and cartilage. However, VSMCs express Runx2 via the stimulation of several uremia-related factors including phosphate, oxidative stress [42], and aldosterone [43, 44], among which phosphate is the strongest stimulator of Runx2 upregulation.

Phosphate elevation is the most important and strong key factor for vascular calcification (Fig. 4). An early study by Shigematsu et al. provided that the primary culture of radial artery VSMCs from a dialysis patient showed increased excretion of extracellular matrix with high affinity for calcium when incubated with a high phosphate medium (Pi = 5.4 mg/dl) [45]. They provided the evidence that phosphate overload accelerates vascular calcium deposition in vitro. High phosphate signal around VSMCs was recognized by increased uptake of phosphate by VSMCs via Pit 1 and Pit 2, sodium-dependent phosphate transporters.

As to the implication of calcium, vessel rings from a dialysis patient showed calcium-induced calcification more potently than phosphate (at equivalent calcium-phosphate product) [46]. Higher calcium concentration accelerated calcium deposition more severely than high phosphate concentration in vessel rings. This result suggested calcium has stronger influence on vascular calcification than phosphate. Sustained hyperphosphatemia with episodic increase of calcium or calcium overload is thought to strongly influence the cellular defense mechanism against calcification.

Basic researches and epidemiological observational studies provided several clinical factors that are significantly associated with vascular calcification (Table 1) [10, 22, 45–73]. Among these factors, mineral abnormalities including hyperphosphatemia, hypercalcemia, and elevated Ca × Pi product are the most important key factors for vascular calcification. Our previous study showed micro-inflammation, represented by elevated highly sensitive C-reactive protein, was another strong and independent predictor for CAC progression (Fig. 5) [10]. Other studies also provided the link between micro-inflammation and progression of CAC [24, 74, 75]. It has now been known that hyperphosphatemia itself is an important source of inflammation [76]. Inflammatory cytokine TNF-α upregulates Pit-1 expression and Na-Pi co-transporter and increases phosphate uptake into VSMCs [77]. Both phosphate overload and accompanying inflammation is thought to concomitantly enhance the vascular calcification.

FGF23/*klotho* axis and vascular calcification
Both fibroblast growth factor 23 (FGF23) and *klotho*, the key players in CKD-MBD, have recently attracted great

Table 1 Associating factors for vascular calcification in hemodialysis patients

Inducers	Inhibitors	Target for treatment
Aging	Fetuin A	Phosphate
Phosphate/calcium	MGP	Calcium
Inflammation	Pyrophosphate	Intact PTH
Aldosterone	Osteopontin	Vitamin D
Warfarin use	Osteoprotegerin	Vitamin K
AGEs/diabetes	BMP7	Acidosis
BMP2/4	Adiponectin	Inflammation
Leptin	Collagen IV	Dialysate
oxLDL		
Collagen I/fibronectin		
High blood pressure		

Inducers and inhibitors for vascular calcifications are listed. As shown in the table, several factors associate the pathophysiology of vascular calcification. Several inhibitor systems exist in the human body, and it might mean the importance to protect from ectopic vascular calcification. If the inhibitory system would fail, serious complication might occur. Treatment target which we can intervene are also listed

Abbreviations: AGEs advanced glycation end products, *BMP* bone morphogenic protein, *LDL* low-density lipoprotein, *MGP* matrix Gla protein, *PTH;* parathyroid hormone

concerns in relation to cardiovascular events and vascular calcification in CKD patients. FGF23 was found as a bone-derived (synthesized and excreted by osteoblast) hormone that regulates phosphate and 1,25-hydroxyvitamin D metabolism [78]. FGF23 binds to the FGF receptor with its co-receptor *klotho* and acts to increase renal phosphate excretion. In addition, FGF23 reduces the synthesis of 1,25-hydroxyvitamin D. Furthermore, FGF23 decreases parathyroid hormone synthesis and secretion. FGF23

induces left ventricular hypertrophy [25], and elevated FGF23 is known to associate with vascular calcification in HD patients [60–62].

On the other hand, *klotho*, discovered by Kuro-o et al. in 1997 [79], is expressed in human vascular tissue in addition to its major expression in the kidney and parathyroid [80]. Vascular calcification is a prominent finding in mice with a *klotho* gene deletion, the same as in CKD patients, and *klotho* overexpression by adenoviral delivery to klotho–/– mice reverse the vascular calcification [81]. Suppressive mechanism of *klotho* on vascular calcification is multifactorial. *Klotho* prevents apoptosis of vascular smooth muscle cells [82] and acts as an anti-inflammatory modulator and restricts inflammatory process, thus protecting the vasculature [83].

Elevated FGF23 and hyperphosphatemia (along with *klotho* deficiency) are associated with vascular calcification in many observational studies. However, it should be noted that there is a controversy whether FGF23 is a direct contributor to vascular calcification. Scialla et al. recently reported that the baseline plasma FGF23 level was not associated with the prevalence or severity of coronary artery calcium content in patients with mild to moderate CKD (eGFR 20–70 ml/min/1.73 m^2), suggesting that FGF23 is not associated with arterial calcification [84]. Furthermore, there is no in vitro study that proved direct action of FGF23 on vascular calcification. A major question that remains unresolved is whether FGF23 can directly act on vascular cells to promote or inhibit matrix. Further studies are necessary to investigate the role of FGF23/*klotho* axis on vascular calcification.

Potential tools against vascular calcification
Phosphate binders

The phosphate signal is thought to be an entry gate for the progression of CAC and future cardiovascular complications (Fig. 3). Another important key factor leading to the progression of CAC is calcium overload related to the use of calcium-based phosphate binders [85–88]. Even if levels of serum calcium are within normal ranges, total calcium intake (ingested as phosphate binder) significantly correlated with CAC progression [57]. Therefore, many interventional studies using non-calcium-containing phosphate binders have been performed.

Sevelamer hydrochloride, an available drug as the first non-calcium-containing phosphate binder other than aluminum-containing phosphate binder, has been proved to delay the progression of CAC compared with calcium carbonate [86, 89–92]. Other than binding to phosphate, sevelamer hydrochloride has several pleiotropic effects to lower cholesterol, FGF23, advanced glycation end product, inflammatory markers, and C-reactive protein [86, 90, 93, 94]. Several clinical trials expected the beneficial inhibitory effect of sevelamer hydrochloride on the

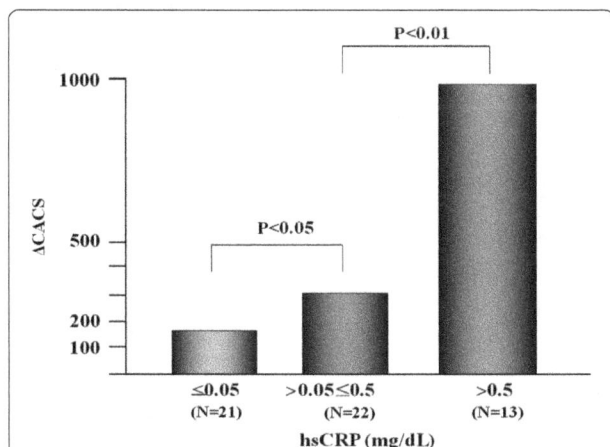

Fig. 5 Stratified hsCRP and the progression of CAC [10]. CACS of 56 patients on maintenance hemodialysis were evaluated repeatedly with 15 months interval, and delta CACS (changes of CACS) were shown according to stratified hsCRP. Progression of CACS was significantly correlated with baseline hsCRP values. *Abbreviations: hsCRP* high sensitive C-reactive protein, *CACS* coronary artery calcification score

progression of vascular calcification. However, one meta-analysis study that analyzed 14 researches containing 3271 patients in total could not provide the effectiveness of sevelamer hydrochloride compared with calcium-based phosphate binders for delaying the progression of CAC [95]. Furthermore, the phosphate-binding capacity of sevelamer hydrochloride is rather weak compared with calcium carbonate and/or lanthanum carbonate [96, 97]. Phosphate-binding capacity is estimated as lanthanum carbonate > calcium carbonate > sevelamer hydrochloride, and the proportion of phosphate-binding capacity is approximately 3:1.5:1 [96, 97]. These might weaken the use of sevelamer hydrochloride in the clinical setting. The important matters to be required as a phosphate binder are good phosphate-binding capacity, good drug adherence, good phosphate control, and drug safety. In this respect, pleiotropic effects might be the next issue to these things.

Compared with sevelamer hydrochloride, lanthanum carbonate, which contains the rare earth element lanthanum, has stronger phosphate-binding capacity and enables good control of serum phosphate [96, 97]. There are several studies that compared the effect of lanthanum carbonate on vascular calcification with calcium-based phosphate binders [98–101]. We performed a prospective randomized interventional study that compared the effect of lanthanum carbonate and calcium carbonate on the progression of CAC (Fig. 6) [98]. Treatment with lanthanum carbonate was more effective compared to calcium carbonate in preventing the progression of CAC in patients on hemodialysis; regression by 6.4% was shown in the lanthanum-treated group vs. 41.2% progression in those receiving calcium carbonate. The serum levels of phosphate and calcium were not different between the two groups. In this study, even if low calcium dialysate (2.5 mEq/l) was used, CACS progressed in hemodialysis patients who are prescribed calcium-based phosphate binders. Meta-analysis, which compared calcium-based and non-calcium-based phosphate binders on survival and vascular calcification in dialysis patients, revealed beneficial effect in non-calcium-based phosphate binders on the progression of CAC [102].

Vascular calcification might be merely one surrogate. The true target is to prevent a cardiovascular event and improve patients' survival. In this regard, recent observational studies provided beneficial effect of lanthanum carbonate on hemodialysis patients' survival [103, 104]. A large RCT, the LANDMARK study, is now ongoing in Japan to evaluate the cardiovascular event and patient survival in the lanthanum carbonate group and calcium carbonate group [21]. As to the safety of lanthanum, side effects and bone toxicity have been evaluated [105–107] and at present, severe side effect or bone toxicity have not been shown. However, because the nature of lanthanum is metal, careful observation for a long period is necessary to conclude the safety of lanthanum carbonate.

Calcimimetic and active vitamin D

Both high and low turnover bone condition could associate with CAC progression [51, 56–59, 70, 85, 89]. Increased release of calcium and phosphate from the bone in patients with high turnover bone and decreased uptake of calcium and phosphate into the bone (disturbed buffer function of the bone) in patients with low turnover bone might cause advanced vascular calcification in such patients. Dialysis patients with intact parathyroid hormone (iPTH) levels >400 pg/ml have, in general, high turnover bone, and those with iPTH levels <150 pg/ml often present adynamic or low turnover bone. Therefore, a control target of iPTH of 150–400 pg/ml might be reasonable from the point of view of preventing vascular calcification.

A randomized interventional study (ADVANCE study) provided that the rate of progression of CAC and aortic valve calcification was reduced when cinacalcet was added to low-dose active vitamin D compared to larger doses of active vitamin D therapy alone [108, 109]. However, significant benefits in overall survival or cardiovascular events by cinacalcet were not observed in a large RCT (EVOLVE trial) in 3883 hemodialysis patients after 5 years' follow-up [110]. Recent manuscripts partly analyzed the data of patients in the EVOLVE trial whose FGF23 decreased more than 30% by cinacalcet within 20 weeks. One showed significant improvement in time to primary endpoint (death or first nonfatal cardiovascular event) compared with placebo [111], and another provided the improved primary composite outcome

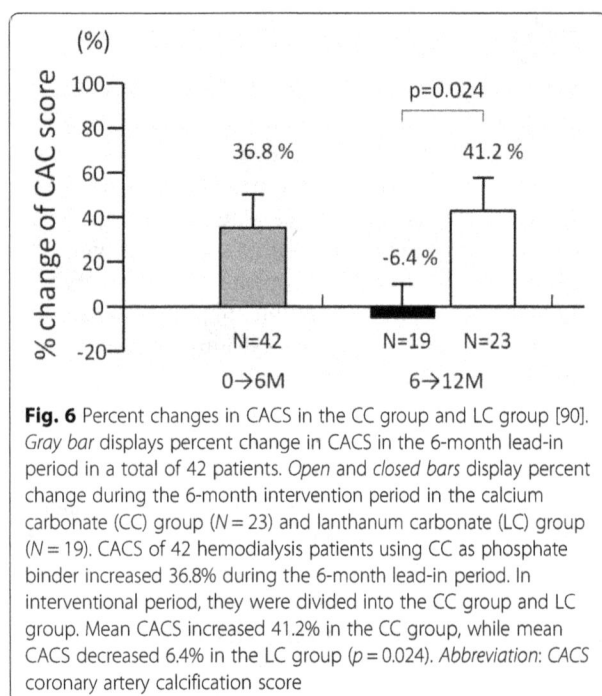

Fig. 6 Percent changes in CACS in the CC group and LC group [90]. *Gray bar* displays percent change in CACS in the 6-month lead-in period in a total of 42 patients. *Open* and *closed bars* display percent change during the 6-month intervention period in the calcium carbonate (CC) group (*N* = 23) and lanthanum carbonate (LC) group (*N* = 19). CACS of 42 hemodialysis patients using CC as phosphate binder increased 36.8% during the 6-month lead-in period. In interventional period, they were divided into the CC group and LC group. Mean CACS increased 41.2% in the CC group, while mean CACS decreased 6.4% in the LC group (*p* = 0.024). *Abbreviation: CACS* coronary artery calcification score

(death and major cardiovascular event) by cinacalcet in patients more than 65 years old [112]. The results of the EVOLVE trial are somewhat inconclusive and should be carefully interpreted.

Increased calcium and phosphate absorption by active vitamin D might influence vascular calcification. However, active vitamin D increased klotho and osteopontin expression in arterial walls while decreasing aortic calcification in CKD mice fed a high phosphate diet [113]. Therefore, low-dose active vitamin D, in the dose that does not increase calcium and phosphate load, might be useful for preventing vascular calcification [80, 114].

Vitamin K

Vitamin K is required as a cofactor in the process of gamma-carboxylation of extracellular matrix protein. Green leaf vegetables contain vitamin K1, and cheese, natto, and animals contain vitamin K2. Coagulation factors require vitamin K1 for their carboxylation process, and MGP requires vitamin K2 for its carboxylation, converting to active form [115]. MGP (in active form) inhibits extracellular matrix calcification and prevents arterial calcification. On the other hand, warfarin, an antagonist to vitamin K, promotes arterial calcification via blocking the activation of MGP as previously described [30]. Furthermore, many hemodialysis patients have vitamin K deficiency. On the basis of these findings, clinical trials intending to prevent vascular calcification by vitamin K1 or K2 supplementation in dialysis patients are now ongoing [116, 117].

Dialysate modification

Calcium overload could occur not only by the use of calcium-containing phosphate binders or high-dose active vitamin D but also by high calcium concentration dialysate. High calcium concentration dialysate (1.75 mmol/l) yields net calcium influx of 978 mg into the body during one hemodialysis session in a patient with serum calcium 9.1 mg/dl [118]. Positive calcium balance excessively inhibits parathyroid function and may cause low turnover bone, which is a known risk factor for vascular calcification.

In a recent randomized controlled study, effect of lowering the dialysate calcium level on the progression of CAC and the histologic bone abnormalities in 425 hemodialysis patients was examined [119]. As a result, progression rate of CAC was significantly lower in the low calcium dialysate (1.25 mmol/l) group than in the high calcium dialysate (1.75 mmol/l) group. Furthermore, the prevalence of histologically diagnosed low turnover bone significantly decreased in the low calcium group (from 85 to 41.8%, $p = 0.001$). Lowering dialysate calcium levels delayed the progression of CAC and

improved bone turnover in patients on hemodialysis with baseline iPTH levels ≤300 pg/ml.

As to other changeable components of dialysate, one recent cross-sectional observational study in our dialysis center provided that pre-dialysis serum bicarbonate levels were significantly associated with coronary CAC score [64]. Acid-base status in dialysis patients associates with vascular calcification, and dialysate bicarbonate could be modifiable. Ultrapure dialysate might be efficacious to delay vascular calcification because micro-inflammation is a strong promoter for vascular calcification [10, 24, 74, 75]. Furthermore, because uremic milieu promotes atherosclerosis in dialysis patients, change of dialysis modality might also affect the progression of vascular calcification. Further interventional study to change dialysate fluid or dialysis modality might bring the benefit for delaying the progression of vascular calcification.

Bisphosphonate

Bisphosphonates are synthetic analogs of inorganic pyrophosphate and suppress bone resorption. Elution of calcium and phosphate (substrate of calcification) from the bone could be decreased or stopped by bisphosphonate. Therefore, bisphosphonates might be beneficial to prevent the progression of vascular calcification. Earlier studies provided the evidence that oral and parenteral etidronate delayed the progression of CAC and aortic calcification [120, 121]. However, this effect was not proven in alendronate [122].

Bisphosphonate use in osteoporotic post-menopausal women increased the risk of calcification in coronary artery and cardiac valves [123]. Furthermore, long-term safety (and efficacy) of bisphosphonate in CKD patients has not been confirmed. Thus, the recent Kidney Disease Improving Global Outcomes (KDIGO) recommendation suggested not to prescribe bisphosphonates in patients with an eGFR <30 ml/min/1.73 m^2 [124], and the Japanese Clinical Practice Guideline for the Management of Chronic Kidney Disease-Mineral and Bone Disorder suggested bisphosphonate use should not be recommended for osteoporosis in dialysis patients [125].

Sodium thiosulfate

Sodium thiosulfate (STS) is a chelating agent and has been applied for calcific uremic arteriolopathy [126, 127]. Calcium-thiosulfate complex is more soluble than calcium oxalate and calcium phosphate, and STS has antioxidant activity [128, 129]. Intravenous infusion of 25% STS solution immediately after hemodialysis for 60 times during 5 months was well tolerated in most patients [126], and calcific uremic arteriolopathy improved in a large observational study [127]. In one study which evaluated the effect of STS on CAC, twice weekly STS infusion post-hemodialysis for 4 months delayed the progression of

CAC compared with non-treated control ($p = 0.03$) [130]. CACS was unchanged in the STS-treated group but increased significantly in the non-treated control group. Considering the chelating and removing nature of STS for precipitated calcium from the vascular walls, long-term use of STS might not only delay the progression of calcification but also decrease the calcification score. Gastrointestinal side effects and subsequent malnutrition and the potential risk of STS to decrease bone mineral density of normal bones should be considered when used for a long period.

Conclusions

Vascular calcification is an independent and important risk factor for cardiovascular events and all-cause mortality in patients on hemodialysis. The mechanism of vascular calcification is multifactorial, and the active process of calcification advances along with dialysis duration. The decrease of three major inhibitory factors of calcification including fetuin A, MGP, and pyrophosphate in the vascular walls and the active osteoblast-like cell differentiation of VSMCs due to Runx2 cascade by phosphate and calcium metabolism abnormality, inflammation, and oxidative stress are involved in vascular calcification.

Several prospective interventional trials against vascular calcification have been performed and are now ongoing. However, no prospective trial has yet proved to improve cardiovascular events and survival in hemodialysis patients. Some observational retrospective studies provided the efficacy of non-calcium-containing phosphate binder. Because vascular calcification strongly influences the outcome of dialysis patients, we wish future interventional RCTs against vascular calcification would clearly provide the beneficial effect on the prognosis of hemodialysis patients.

Acknowledgements
Not applicable.

Funding
Not applicable.

Authors' contributions
TO wrote the whole manuscript, and SK read and advised about the content of the manuscript to the final version. Both authors read and approved the final manuscript.

Competing interests
The authors declare that they have no competing interests.

References

1. Kobayashi S. Cardiovascular events in chronic kidney disease (CKD)—an importance of vascular calcification and microcirculatory impairment. Renal Replacement Therapy. 2016;2:55. doi:10.1186/s41100-016-0062-y.
2. Ohtake T, Kobayashi S, Moriya H, Negishi K, Okamoto K, Maesato K, et al. High prevalence of occult coronary artery stenosis in patients with chronic kidney disease at the initiation of renal replacement therapy: an angiographic examination. J Am Soc Nephrol. 2005;16:1141–8.
3. Joki N, Hase H, Nakamura R, Yamaguchi T. Onset of coronary artery disease prior to initiation of haemodialysis in patients with end stage renal disease. Nephrol Dial Transplant. 1997;12:718–23.
4. Lindner A, Charra B, Sherrard DJ, Scribner BH. Accelerated atherosclerosis in prolonged maintenance hemodialysis. N Engl J Med. 1974;290:697–701.
5. Möncheberg JG. Uber die reine Mediaverkalkung der Extremitätenarterien und ihr verhalten zur Arterosklerose. Virchow Arch Pathol Anat. 1903;171:141–67.
6. Blacher J, Guerin AP, Pannier B, Marchais SJ, London GM. Arterial calcifications, arterial stiffness, and cardiovascular risk in ESRD. Hypertension. 2001;38:938–42.
7. London GM. Cardiovascular calcifications in uremic patients: clinical impact on cardiovascular function. J Am Soc Nephrol. 2003;14:S305–9.
8. Block GA, Raggi P, Bellasi A, Kooienga L, Spiegel DM. Mortality effect of coronary calcification and phosphate binder choice in incident hemodialysis patients. Kidney Int. 2007;71:438–41.
9. Matsuoka M, Iseki K, Tamashiro M, Fujimoto N, Higa N, Touma T, et al. Impact of high coronary artery calcification score (CACS) on survival in patients on chronic hemodialysis. Clin Exp Nephrol. 2004;8:54–8.
10. Ohtake T, Ishioka K, Honda K, Oka M, Maesato K, Mano T, et al. Impact of coronary artery calcification in hemodialysis patients: risk factors and associations with prognosis. Hemodial Int. 2010;14:218–25.
11. Shantouf RS, Budoff MJ, Ahmadi N, Ghaffari A, Flores F, Gopal A, et al. Total and individual coronary artery calcium scores as independent predictors of mortality in hemodialysis patients. Am J Nephrol. 2010;31:419–25.
12. Shimoyama Y, Tsuruta Y, Niwa T. Coronary artery calcification score is associated with mortality in Japanese hemodialysis patients. J Ren Nutr. 2012;22:139–42.
13. Wilkieson T, Rahman MO, Gangii AS, Voss M, Ingram AJ, Ranganath N, et al. Coronary artery calcification, cardiovascular events, and death: a prospective cohort study of incident patients on hemodialysis. Canadian J Kidney Disease. 2015;2:29.
14. Okuno S, Ishimura E, Kitatani K, Fujino Y, Kohno K, Maeno Y, et al. Presence of abdominal aortic calcification is significantly associated with all-cause and cardiovascular mortality in maintenance hemodialysis patients. Am J Kidney Dis. 2007;49:417–25.
15. Verbeke F, Van Biesen W, Honkanen E, Wikstrom B, Jensen PB, Krzesinski JM, et al. CORD study investigators: prognostic value of aortic stiffness and calcification for cardiovascular events and mortality in dialysis patients: outcome of the Calcification Outcome in Renal Disease (CORD) study. Clin J Am Soc Nephrol. 2011;6:153–9.
16. Noordzij M, Cranenburg EM, Engelsman LF, Hermans MM, Boeschoten EW, Brandenburg VM, Bos WJ, et al. NECOSAD study group: progression of aortic calcification is associated with disorders of mineral metabolism and mortality in chronic dialysis patients. Nephrol Dial Transplant. 2011;26:1662–9.
17. Inoue T, Ogawa T, Ishida H, Ando Y, Nitta K. Aortic arch calcification evaluated on chest X-ray is a strong independent predictor of cardiovascular events in chronic hemodialysis patients. Heart Vessels. 2012;27:135–42.
18. Ohya M, Otani H, Kimura K, Saika Y, Fujii R, Yukawa S, et al. Vascular calcification estimated by aortic calcification area index is a significant predictive parameter of cardiovascular mortality in hemodialysis patients. Clin Exp Nephrol. 2011;15:877–83.
19. Komatsu M, Okazaki M, Tsuchiya K, Kawaguchi H, Nitta K. Aortic arch calcification predicts cardiovascular and all-cause mortality in maintenance hemodialysis patients. Kidney Blood Press Res. 2014;39:658–67.
20. Nakayama M, Ura Y, Nagata M, Okada Y, Sumida Y, Nishida K, et al. Carotid artery calcification at the initiation of hemodialysis is a risk factor for cardiovascular events in patients with end-stage renal disease: a cohort study. BMC Nephrol. 2011;12:56.

21. Ogata H, Fukagawa M, Hirakata H, Kaneda H, Kagimura T, Akizawa T, LANDMARK study group: design and baseline characteristics of the LANDMARK study. Clin Exp Nephrol. 2016. in press.

22. Ohtake T, Oka M, Ikee R, Mochida Y, Ishioka K, Moriya H, et al. Impact of lower limbs' arterial calcification on the prevalence and severity of PAD in patients on hemodialysis. J Vasc Surg. 2011;53:676–83.

23. Raggi P, Bellasi A, Ferramosca E, Islam T, Muntner P, Block GA. Association of pulse wave velocity with vascular and valvular calcification in hemodialysis patients. Kidney Int. 2007;71:802–7.

24. Haydar AA, Covic A, Colhoun H, Rubens M, Goldsmith DJ. Coronary artery calcification and aortic pulse wave velocity in chronic kidney disease patients. Kidney Int. 2004;65:1790–4.

25. Faul C, Amaral AP, Oskouei B, Hu MC, Sloan A, Isakova T, et al. FGF23 induces left ventricular hypertrophy. J Clin Invest. 2011. doi:10.1172/JCI46122.

26. Shanahan CM. Mechanisms of vascular calcification in CKD-evidence for premature ageing? Nat Rev Nephrol. 2013;9:661–70.

27. Yao Y, Bennett BJ, Wang X, Rosenfeld ME, Giachelli C, Lusis AJ, et al. Inhibition of bone morphogenic protein protects against atherosclerosis and vascular calcification. Circ Res. 2010;107:485–94.

28. Reynolds JL, Joannides AJ, Skepper JN, McNair R, Schurgers LJ, Proudfoot D, et al. Human vascular smooth muscle cells undergo vesicle-mediated calcification in response to changes in extracellular calcium and phosphate concentrations: a potential mechanism for accelerated vascular calcification in ESRD. J Am Soc Nephrol. 2004;15:2857–67.

29. Kapustin AN, Davies JD, Reynolds JL, McNair R, Jones GT, Sidibe A, et al. Calcium regulates key components of vascular smooth muscle cell-derived matrix vesicles to enhance mineralization. Circ Res. 2011;109:e1–e212.

30. Palaniswamy C, Sekhri A, Aronow WS, Kalra A, Peterson SJ. Association of warfarin use with valvular and vascular calcification: a review. Clin Cardiol. 2011;34:74–81.

31. Lomashvili KA, Garg P, Narisawa S, Millan JL, O'Neill WC. Upregulation of alkaline phosphatase and pyrophosphate hydrolysis: potential mechanism for uremic vascular calcifications. Kidney Int. 2008;73:1024–30.

32. Narisawa S, Harmey D, Yadav MC, O'Neill WC, Hoylaerts MF, Millan JL. Novel inhibitors of alkaline phosphatase suppress vascular smooth muscle cell calcification. J Bone Miner Res. 2007;22:1700–10.

33. O'Neill WC. Pyrophosphate, alkaline phosphatase, and vascular calcification. Circ Res. 2006;99, e2.

34. Kuro-o M. A phosphate-centric paradigm for pathophysiology and therapy of chronic kidney disease. Kidney Int Suppl. 2013;3:420–6.

35. Schinke T, Amendt C, Trindl A, Pöschke O, Müller-Esterl W, Jahnen-Dechent W. The serum protein alpha2-HS glycoprotein/fetuin inhibits apatite formation in vitro and in mineralizing calvaria cells. A possible role in mineralization and calcium homeostasis. J Biol Chem. 1996;271:20789–96.

36. Reynolds JL, Skepper JN, McNair R, Kasama T, Gupta K, Weissberg PL, et al. Multifunctional roles for serum protein fetuin-a in inhibition of human vascular smooth muscle cell calcification. J Am Soc Nephrol. 2005;16:2920–30.

37. Ketteler M, Bongartz P, Westenfeld R, Wildberger JE, Mahnken AH, Böhm R, et al. Association of low fetuin-A (AHSG) concentrations in serum with cardiovascular mortality in patients on dialysis: a cross-sectional study. Lancet. 2003;361:827–33.

38. Smith ER, Cai MM, McMahon LP, Pedegogos E, Toussaint ND, Brumby C, et al. Serum fetuin-A concentration and fetuin-A-containing carciprotein particles in patients with chroic inflammatory disease and renal failure. Nephrology (Carlton). 2013;18:215–21.

39. Smith ER, Ford ML, Tomlinson LA, Rajkumar C, McMahon LP, Holt SG. Phosphorylated fetuin-A-containing carciprotein particles are associated with aortic stiffness and a procalcific milieu in patients with pre-dialysis CKD. Nephrol Dial Transplant. 2012;27:1957–66.

40. Hamano T, Matsui I, Mikami S, Tomida K, Fujii N, Imai E, et al. Fetuin-mineral complex reflects extraosseous calcification stress in CKD. J Am Soc Nephrol. 2010;21:1998–2007.

41. Lyemere VP, Proudfoot D, Weissberg PL, Shanahan CM. Vascular smooth muscle cell phenotypic plasticity and the regulation of vascular calcification. J Intern Med. 2006;260:192–210.

42. Byon CH, Javed A, Dai Q, Kappes JC, Clemens TL, Darley-Usmar VM. Oxidative stress induces vascular calcification through modulation of the osteogenic transcription factor Runx2 by AKT signaling. J Biol Chem. 2008;283:15319–27.

43. Li X, Giachelli CM. Sodium-dependent phosphate cotoransporters and vascular calcification. Curr Opin Nephrol Hypertens. 2007;16:325–8.

44. Voelkl J, Alesutan I, Leibrock CB, Quintanilla-Martinez L, Kuhn V, Feger M, et al. Spironolactone ameliorates PIT1-dependent vascular osteoinduction in klotho-hypomorphic mice. J Clin Invest. 2013;123:812–22.

45. Shigematsu T, Kono T, Satoh K, Yokoyama K, Yoshida T, Hosoya T, et al. Phosphate overload accelerates vascular calcium deposition in end-stage renal disease patients. Nephrol Dial Trasplant. 2003;18 Suppl 3:iii86–9.

46. Shroff RC, McNair R, Skepper JN, Figg N, Schurgers LJ, Deanfield J, et al. Chronic mineral dysregulation promotes vascular smooth muscle cell adaptation and extracellular matrix calcification. J Am Soc Nephrol. 2010;21:103–12.

47. Nitta K, Akiba T, Uchida K, Kawashima A, Yumura W, Kabaya T, et al. The progression of vascular calcification and serum osteoprotegerin levels in patients on long-term hemodialysis. Am J Kidney Dis. 2003;42:303–9.

48. Taki K, Takayama F, Tsuruta Y, Niwa T. Oxidative stress, advanced glycation end product, and coronary artery calcification in hemodialysis patients. Kidney Int. 2006;70:218–24.

49. McCullough PA, Soman S. Cardiovascular calcification in patients with chronic renal failure: are we on target with this risk factor? Kidney Int Suppl. 2004;90:S18–24.

50. McCullough PA. Effect of lipid modification on progression of coronary calcification. J Am Soc Nephrol. 2005;16 Suppl 2:S115–9.

51. Shantouf R, Kovesdy CP, Kim Y, Ahmadi N, Luna A, Luna C, et al. Association of serum alkaline phosphatase with vascular artery calcification in maintenance hemodialysis patients. Clin J Am Soc Nephrol. 2009;4:1106–14.

52. Barreto DV, Barreto Fde C, Carvalho AB, Cuppari L, Draibe SA, Dalboni MA, et al. Association of changes in bone remodeling and coronary artery calcification in hemodialysis patients: a prospective study. Am J Kidney Dis. 2008;52:1139–50.

53. Kirkpantur A, Altun B, Hazirolan T, Akata D, Arici M, Kirazli S, et al. Association among serum fetuin-A level, coronary artery calcification, and bone mineral densitometry in maintenance hemodialysis patients. Art Organs. 2009;33:844–54.

54. Moe SM, Reslerova M, Ketteler M, O'Neill K, Duan D, Koczman J, et al. Role of calcification inhibitors in the pathogenesis of vascular calcification in chronic kidney disease (CKD). Kidney Int. 2005;67:2295–304.

55. Mehrotra R, Westenfeld R, Christenson P, Budoff M, Ipp E, Takasu J, et al. Serum fetuin-A in nondialyzed patients with diabetic nephropathy: relationship with coronary artery calcification. Kidney Int. 2005;67:1070–7.

56. Kim SC, Kim HW, Oh SW, Tang HN, Kim MG, Jo SK, et al. Low iPTH can predict vascular and coronary calcifications in patients undergoing peritoneal dialysis. Nephron Clin Prac. 2011;117:c113–9.

57. London GM, Marty C, Marchais SJ, Guerin AP, Metivier F, de Vernejoul MC. Arterial calcifications and bone histomorphometry in end-stage renal disease. J Am Soc Nephrol. 2004;15:1943–51.

58. Adragao T, Herberth J, Monier-Faugere MC, Branscum AJ, Ferreira A, Frazao JM, et al. Low bone volume—a risk factor for coronary calcification in hemodialysis patients. Clin J Am Soc Nephrol. 2009;4:450–5.

59. Coen G, Ballanti P, Mantilla D, Manni M, Lippi B, Pierantozzi A, et al. Bone turnover, osteopenia and vascular calcifications in hemodialysis patients. Am J Nephrol. 2009;29:145–52.

60. Kahn AM, Chirinos JA, Litt H, Yang W, Rosas SE. FGF-23 and the progression of coronary arterial calcification in patients new to dialysis. Clin J Am Soc Nephrol. 2012;7:2017–22.

61. Ozkok A, Kekik C, Karahan GE, Sakaci T, Ozel A, Unsal A, et al. FGF-23 associated with the progression of coronary artery calcification in hemodialysis patients. BMC Nephrol. 2013;14:241.

62. Nasrallah MM, El-Shehaby AR, Salem MM, Osman NA, El Sheikh E, Sharaf El Din UA. Fibroblast growth factor-23 (FGF-23) is independently correlated to aortic calcification in haemodialysis patients. Nephrol Dial Transplant. 2010;25:2679–85.

63. Jean G, Bresson E, Terrat JC, Vanel T, Hurot JM, Lorriaux C, et al. Peripheral vascular calcification in long-hemodialysis patients: associated factors and survival consequences. Nephrol Dial Transplant. 2009;24:948–55.

64. Oka M, Ohtake T, Mochida Y, Ishioka K, Maesato K, Moriya H, et al. Correlation of coronary artery calcification with pre-hemodialysis bicarbonate levels in patients on hemodialysis. Ther Apher Dial. 2012;16:267–71.

65. Qunibi WY. Dyslipidemia and progression of cardiovascular calcification (CVC) in patients with end-stage renal disease (ESRD). Kidney Int Suppl. 2005;95:S43–50.

66. Greif M, Arnoldt T, von Ziegler F, Ruemmler J, Becker C, Wakili R, et al. Lipoprotein (a) is independently correlated with coronary artery calcification. Eur J Intern Med. 2013;24:75–9.

67. Ozkok A, Caliskan Y, Sakaci T, Erten G, Karahan G, Ozel A, et al. Osteoprotegerin/RANKL axis and progression of coronary artery calcification in hemodialysis patients. Clin J Am Soc Nephrol. 2012;7:965–73.

68. Barreto DV, Barreto FC, Carvalho AB, Cuppari L, Cendoroglo M, Draibe SA, et al. Coronary calcification in hemodialysis patients: the contribution of traditional and uremia-related risk factors. Kidney Int. 2005;67:1576–82.

69. Morena M, Dupuy AM, Jaussent I, Vernhet H, Gahide G, Klouche K, et al. A cut-off value of plasma osteoprotegerin level may predict the presence of coronary artery calcifications in chronic kidney disease patients. Nephrol Dial Transplant. 2009;24:3389–97.

70. Malluche HH, Blomquist G, Monier-Faugere MC, Cantor TL, Davenport DL. High parathyroid hormone level and osteoporosis predict progression of coronary artery calcification in patients on dialysis. J Am Soc Nephrol. 2015;26:2534–44.

71. Wang YN, Sun Y, Wang Y, Jia YL. Serum S100A12 and progression of coronary artery calcification over 4 years in hemodialysis patients. Am J Nephrol. 2015;42:4–13.

72. Zhang H, Wang LJ, Si DL, Wang C, Yang JC, Jiang P, et al. Correlation between osteocalcin-positive endothelial progenitor cells and spotty calcification in patients with coronary artery disease. Clin Exp Pharmacol Physiol. 2015;42:734–9.

73. Wang M, Li H, You L, Yu X, Zhang M, Zhu R, et al. Association of serum phosphate variability with coronary artery calcification among hemodialysis patients. PLoS One. 2014;9, e93360.

74. Jung HH, Kim SW, Han H. Inflammation, mineral metabolism and progressive coronary artery calcification in patients on haemodialysis. Nephrol Dial Transplant. 2006;21:1915–20.

75. Stompór T, Pasowicz M, Sullowicz W, Dembinska-Kiec A, Janda K, Wójcik K, et al. An association between coronary artery calcification score, lipid profile, and selected markers of chronic inflammation in ESRD patients treated with peritoneal dialysis. Am J Kidney Dis. 2003;41:203–11.

76. Izumi M, Morita S, Nishian Y, Miyamoto T, Kasumoto H, Oue M, et al. Switching from calcium carbonate to sevelamer hydrochloride has suppressive effects on the progression of aortic calcification in hemodialysis patients: assessment using plain chest X-ray films. Ren Fail. 2008;30:952–8.

77. Koleganova N, Piecha G, Ritz E, Schirmacher P, Müller A, Meyer HP, et al. Arterial calcification in patients with chronic kidney disease. Nephrol Dial Transplant. 2009;24:2488–96.

78. Riminucci M, Collins MT, Fedarko NS, Cherman N, Corsi A, White KE, et al. FGF-23 in fibrous dysplasia of bone and its relationship to renal phosphate wasting. J Clin Invest. 2003;112:683–92.

79. Kuro-o M, Matsumura Y, Aizawa H, Kawaguchi H, Suga T, Utsugi T, et al. Mutation of the mouse klotho gene leads to a syndrome resembling ageing. Nature. 1997;390:45–51.

80. Lim K, Lu TS, Molostvov G, Lee C, Lam FT, Zehnder D, et al. Vascular klotho deficiency potentiates the development of human artery calcification and mediates resistance to fibroblast growth factor 23. Circulation. 2012;125:2243–55.

81. Shiraki-Iida T, Iida A, Nabeshima Y, Anazawa H, Nishikawa S, Noda M, et al. Improvement of multiple pathophysiological phenotypes of klotho (kl/kl) mice by adenovirus-mediated expression of the klotho gene. J Gene Med. 2000;2:233–42.

82. Nakano-Kurimoto R, Ikeda K, Uraoka M, Nakagawa Y, Yutaka K, Koide M, et al. Replicative senescence of vascular smooth muscle cells enhances the calcification through initiating the osteoblastic transition. Am J Physiol Heart Circ Physiol. 2009;297:H1673–84.

83. Zhao Y, Banerjee S, Dey N, LeJeune WS, Sarkar PS, Brobey R, et al. Klotho depletion contributes to increased inflammation in kidney of the db/db mouse model of diabetes via Re1A (Serine)[536] phosphorylation. Diabetes. 2011;60:1907–16.

84. Scialla JJ, Lau WL, Reilly MP, Isakova T, Yang HY, Crouthamel MH, et al. Fibroblast growth factor 23 is not associated with and does not induce arterial calcification. Kidney Int. 2013;83:1159–68.

85. Chertow GM, Raggi P, Chasan-taber S, Bommer J, Holzer H, Burke SK. Determinants of progressive vascular calcification in hemodialysis patients. Nephrol Dial Transplant. 2004;19:1489–96.

86. Chertow GM, Burke SK, Raggi P. Sevelamer attenuates the progression of coronary and aortic calcification in hemodialysis patients. Kidney Int. 2002;62:245–52.

87. Goodman WG, Goldin J, Kuizon BD, Yoon C, Gales B, Sider D, et al. Coronary artery calcification in young adults with end-stage renal disease who are undergoing dialysis. N Engl J Med. 2000;342:1478–83.

88. Guerin AP, London GM, Marchais SJ, Metivier F. Arterial stiffness and vascular calcifications in end-stage renal disease. Nephrol Dial Transplant. 2000;15:1014–21.

89. Block GA, Spiegel DM, Ehrlich J, Mehta R, Lindbergh J, Dreisbach A, et al. Effects of sevelamer and calcium on coronary artery calcification in patients new to hemodialysis. Kidney Int. 2005;68:1815–24.

90. Kakuta T, Tanaka R, Hyodo T, Suzuki H, Kanai G, Nagaoka M, et al. Effect of sevelamer and calcium-based phosphate binders on coronary artery calcification and accumulation of circulating advanced glycation end products in hemodialysis patients. Am J Kidney Dis. 2011;57:422–31.

91. Shantouf R, Ahmadi N, Flores F, Tiano J, Gopal A, Kalantar-Zadeh K, et al. Impact of phosphate binder type on coronary artery calcification in hemodialysis patients. Clin Nephrol. 2010;74:12–8.

92. Asmus HG, Braun J, Krause R, Brunkhorst R, Holzer H, Schulz W, et al. Two year comparison of sevelamer and calcium carbonate effects on cardiovascular calcification and bone density. Nephrol Dial Transplant. 2005;20:1653–61.

93. Vlassara H, Uribarri J, Cai W, Goodman S, Pyzik R, Post J, et al. Effects of sevelamer on HbA1c, inflammation, and advanced glycation end products in diabetic kidney disease. Clin J Am Soc Nephrol. 2012;7:934–42.

94. Guida B, Cataldi M, Riccio E, Grumetto L, Pota A, Borrelli S, et al. Plasma p-cresol lowering effect of sevelamer in peritoneal dialysis patients: evidence from a Cross-Sectional Observational Study. PLoS One. 2013;8, e73558.

95. Zhang Q, Li M, Lu Y, Li H, Gu Y, Hao C, et al. Meta-analysis comparing sevelamer and calcium-based phosphate binders on cardiovascular calcification in hemodialysis patients. Nephron Clin Pract. 2010;115:c259–67.

96. Akizawa T. Importance of serum phosphate management and feature of phosphate binder in hemodialysis patients. Therapeutic Research. 2014;35:285–91 (in Japanese).

97. Daugirdas JT, Finn WF, Emmett M, Chertow GM. Frequent Hemodialysis Network Trial Group. The phosphate binder equivalent dose. Semin Dial. 2011;24:41–9.

98. Ohtake T, Kobayashi S, Oka M, Furuya R, Iwagami M, Tsutsumi D, et al. Lanthanum carbonate delays progression of coronary artery calcification compared with calcium-based phosphate binders in patients on hemodialysis: a pilot study. J Cardiovasc Pharm Ther. 2013;18:439–46.

99. Toussaint ND, Lau KK, Polkinghorne KR, Kerr PG. Attenuation of aortic calcification with lanthanum carbonate versus calcium-based phosphate binders in haemodialysis: a pilot randomized controlled trial. Nephrology. 2011;16:290–8.

100. Kalil RS, Flanigan M, Stanford W, Haynes WG. Dissociation between progression of coronary artery calcification in hemodialysis patients: a prospective pilot study. Clin Nephrol. 2012;78:1–9.

101. Wada K, Wada Y. Evaluation of aortic calcification with lanthanum carbonate vs. calcium-based phosphate binders in maintenance hemodialysis patients with type 2 diabetes mellitus: an open-label randomized controlled trial. Ther Apher Dial. 2014;18:353–60.

102. Jamal SA, Vandermeer B, Raggi P, Mendelssohn DC, Chatterley T, Dorgan M, et al. Effect of calcium-based versus non-calcium-based phosphate binders on mortality in patients with chronic kidney disease: an updated systematic review and meta-analysis. Lancet. 2013;382:1268–77.

103. Komaba H, Kakuta T, Suzuki H, Hida M, Suga T, Fukagawa M. Survival advantage of lanthanum carbonate for hemodialysis patients with uncontrolled hyperphosphatemia. Nephrol Dial Transplant. 2015;30:107–14.

104. Tsuchida K, Nagai K, Yokota N, Minakuchi J, Kawashima S. Impact of lanthanum carbonate on prognosis of chronic hemodialysis patients: a retrospective cohort study (Kawashima Study). Ther Apher Dial. 2016;20:142–8.

105. Shigematsu T. Lanthanum Carbonate Research Group: three-year extension study of lanthanum carbonate therapy in Japanese hemodialysis patients. Clin Exp Nephrol. 2010;14:589–97.

106. Shigematsu T, Nakashima Y, Ohya M, Tatsuta K, Koreeda D, Yoshimoto W, et al. The management of hyperphosphatemia by lanthanum carbonate in chronic kidney disease patients. Int J Nephrol Renovasc Dis. 2012;5:81–9.

107. Shigematsu T, Ohya M, Negi S, Matsumoto AR, Nakashima YM, Iwatani Y, et al. Safety and efficacy evaluation of lanthanum carbonate in end-stage renal disease patients. Contrib Nephrol. 2015;185:42–55.

108. Raggi P, Chertow GM, Torres PU, Csiky B, Naso A, Nossuli K, et al. The ADVANCE study: a randomized study to evaluate the effect of cinacalcet plus low-dose vitamin D on vascular calcification in patients on hemodialysis. Nephrol Dial Transplant. 2011;26:1327–39.

109. Urena-Torres P, Bridges I, Christiano C, Counoyer SH, Cooper K, Farouk M, et al. Efficiency of cinacalcet with low-dose vitamin D in incidental hemodialysis subjects with secondary hyperparathyroidism. Nephrol Dial Transplant. 2013;28:1241–54.

110. Chertow GM, Block GA, Correa-Rotter R, Drüeke TB, Floege J, Goodman WG, et al. Effect of cinacalcet on cardiovascular disease in patients undergoing dialysis. N Engl J Med. 2012;367:2482–94.

111. Moe SM, Chertow GM, Parfrey PS, Kubo Y, Block GA, Correa-Rotter R, et al. Cinacalcet, fibroblast growth factor 23, and cardiovascular disease in hemodialysis: the evaluation of cinacalcet HCL therapy to lower cardiovascular events (EVOLVE) trial. Circulation. 2015;132:27–39.

112. Parfrey P, Drüeke TB, Block GA, Correa-Rotter R, Floege J, Herzog CA, et al. The effects of cinacalcet in older and younger patients on hemodialysis: the evaluation of cinacalcet HCL therapy to lower cardiovascular events (EVOLVE) trial. Clin J Am Soc Nephrol. 2015;10:791–9.

113. Lau WL, Leaf EM, Hu MC, Takeno MM, Kuro-o M, Moe OW, et al. Vitamin D receptor agonists increase klotho and osteopontin while decreasing aortic calcification in mice with chronic kidney disease fed a high phosphate diet. Kidney Int. 2012;82:1261–70.

114. Mathew S, Lund RJ, Chaudhary LR, Geurs T, Hruska KA. Vitamin D receptor activators can protect against vascular calcification. J Am Soc Nephrol. 2008;19:1509–19.

115. Price PA. Gla-containing proteins of bone. Connect Tissue Res. 1989;21:51–7.

116. Holden RM, Booth SL, Day AG, Clase CM, Zimmerman D, Moist L, et al. Inhibiting the progression of arterial calcification with vitamin K in hemodialysis patients (iPACK-HD) trial: rationale and study design for a randomized trial of vitamin K in patients with end stage kidney disease. Can J Kidney Health Dis. 2015;2:17.

117. Caluwé R, Pyfferoen L, De Boeck K, De Vriese AS. The effects of vitamin K supplementation and vitamin K antagonists on progression of vascular calcification: ongoing randomized controlled trials. Clin Kideny J. 2016;9:273–9.

118. Hou SH, Zhao J, Ellman CF, Hu J, Griffin Z, Spiegel DM, et al. Calcium and phosphate fluxes during hemodialysis with low calcium dialysate. Am J Kidney Dis. 1991;18:217–24.

119. Ok E, Asci G, Bayraktaroglu S, Toz H, Ozkahya M, Yilmaz M, et al. Reduction of dialysate calcium level reduces progression of coronary artery calcification and improves low bone turnover in patients on hemodialysis. J Am Soc Nephrol. 2016;27:2475–86.

120. Nitta K, Akiba T, Suzuki K, Uchida K, Watanabe R, Majima K, et al. Effects of cyclic intermittent etidronate therapy on coronary artery calcification in patients receiving long-term hemodialysis. Am J Kideny Dis. 2004;44:680–8.

121. Hashiba H, Aizawa S, Tamura K, Shigematsu T, Kogo H. Inhibitory effects of etidronate on the progression of vascular calcification in hemodialysis patients. Ther Apher Dial. 2004;8:241–7.

122. Toussaint ND, Lau KK, Strauss BJ, Polkinghorne KR, Kerr PG. Effect of alendronate on vascular calcification n CKD stages 3 and 4: a pilot randomized controlled trial. Am J Kidney Dis. 2010;56:57–68.

123. Elmarish S, Delaney JA, Bluemke DA, Budoff MJ, O'Brien KD, Fuster V, et al. Associations of LV hypertrophy with prevalent and incident valve calcification: multi-ethnic study of atherosclerosis. JACC Cardiovasc Imaging. 2012;5:781–8.

124. Wheeler DC, Becker GJ. Summary of KDIGO guideline. What do we really know about management of blood pressure in patients with chronic kidney disease? Kidney Int. 2013;83:377–83.

125. Fukagawa M, Yokoyama K, Koiwa F, Taniguchi M, Shoji T, Kazama JJ, et al. Clinical practice guideline for the management of chronic kidney disease-mineral and bone disorder. Ther Apher Dial. 2013;17:247–88.

126. Mathews SJ, de Las FL, Podaralla P, Cabellon A, Zheng S, Bierhals A, et al. Effects of sodium thiosulfate on vascular calcification in end-stage renal disease: a pilot study of feasibility, safety and efficacy. Am J Nephrol. 2011;33:131–8.

127. Nigwekar SU, Brunelli SM, Meade D, Wang W, Hymes J, Lacson E. Sodium thiosulfate therapy for calcific uremic arteriolopathy. Clin J Am Soc Nephrol. 2013;8:1162–70.

128. Pasch A, Schffner T, Huynh-Do U, Frey BM, Frey FJ, Farese S. Sodium thiosulfate prevents vascular calcification in uremic rats. Kidney Int. 2008;74:1444–53.

129. Schlieper G, Brandenburg V, Ketteler M, Floege J. Sodium thiosulfate in the treatment of calcific uremic arteriolopathy. Nat Rev Nephrol. 2009;5:539–43.

130. Adirekkiat S, Sumethkul V, Ingsathit A, Domrongkitchaiporn S, Phakdeekitcharoen B, Kantachuvesiri S, et al. Sodium thiosulfate delays the progression of coronary artery calcification in haemodialysis patients. Nephrol Dial Transplant. 2010;25:1923–9.

11

Relationship between serum calcium level at dialysis initiation and subsequent prognosis

Daijo Inaguma[*], Shigehisa Koide, Kazuo Takahashi, Hiroki Hayashi, Midori Hasegawa, Yukio Yuzawa and For the Aichi Cohort Study of Prognosis in Patients Newly Initiated Into Dialysis (AICOPP)

Abstract

Background: In patients on maintenance dialysis, increased serum calcium levels are known to be associated with a poor prognosis. However, it is not known whether serum calcium levels at dialysis initiation have an impact on subsequent prognosis.

Methods: The subjects were patients who were newly initiated dialysis at the 17 Aichi Cohort Study of Prognosis in Patients Newly Initiated into Dialysis (AICOPP) group centers. The study included 1524 patients who were at least 20 years old, had CKD, and provided written consent. We excluded one patient whose serum adjusted calcium was not assessed and six patients whose outcomes were unknown. Thus, we enrolled 1517 subjects into the study. The patients were divided into the following five groups: (1) G1 with a serum adjusted calcium level <7.0 mg/dL, (2) G2 with 7.0 to <8.0 mg/dL, (3) G3 with 8.0 to <9.0 mg/dL, (4) G4 with 9.0 to <10.0 mg/dL, and (5) G5 with ≥10.0 mg/dL. The study outcomes included: (1) comparisons of all-cause mortality rates in the five groups; (2) extraction of factors influencing all-cause mortality.

Results: There were 268 deaths during the follow-up period (G1, 9 cases; G2, 30 cases; G3, 91 cases; G4, 110 cases; G5, 28 cases). Significant differences were observed between the five groups' cumulative survival rates (Logrank test $p = 0.005$) by using Kaplan-Meier method. There were significant differences in the incidence of either aortic or cardiac valve calcification among the five groups (aortic calcification: $p = 0.006$, cardiac valve calcification: $p = 0.008$). Moreover, lower Barthel Index, which evaluated activities of daily living, were associated with higher serum adjusted calcium levels ($p < 0.001$). Multivariate Cox proportional hazard analysis using the stepwise method indicated that increasing serum adjusted calcium was associated with all-cause mortality (every 1 mg/dL increase, HR = 1.267, 95% CI = 1.092 − 1.470, $p = 0.002$). In addition, high mortality was associated with advanced age, male gender, low systolic blood pressure, history of cardiovascular disease, and no prior use of calcium carbonate.

Conclusions: Serum adjusted calcium levels at dialysis initiation were demonstrated to be associated with all-cause mortality after dialysis initiation.

Keywords: Dialysis initiation, Serum calcium, All-cause mortality, Chronic kidney disease

* Correspondence: daijo@fujita-hu.ac.jp
Department of Nephrology, Fujita Health University, Toyoake, Aichi, Japan

Background

In patients newly starting dialysis, advanced age and concurrent cardiovascular diseases (CVDs) are major problems which are strongly associated with survival prognosis. The concept of chronic kidney disease-mineral and bone disorders (CKD-MBD) focuses on survival prognosis rather than bone lesions, and management of serum phosphorus and calcium levels is considered to be especially important [1]. In patients on dialysis, serum phosphorus levels have been shown to have a U-shaped association with mortality [2–7]. As for serum calcium levels, although it is not clear whether low levels are detrimental, high levels are known to be associated with a poor prognosis [3, 4, 8]. Given these background conditions, each guideline provides target values for serum phosphorus and calcium levels when managing patients on dialysis [1, 9].

Increased serum calcium levels reportedly cause vascular calcification and carry a risk of CVD [10–12]. However, serum calcium levels often tend to decrease during the predialysis stage of CKD including the period immediately before dialysis initiation [13]. Although secondary hyperparathyroidism has already manifested in this stage, it rarely progresses to nodular hyperplasia and is unlikely to cause hypercalcemia. Doi et al. documented a serum calcium level >8.5 mg/dL at dialysis initiation to be associated with outcomes at one year after dialysis initiation [14], but only a few other reports have described similar findings. Whether the association observed in patients on maintenance dialysis between serum calcium levels and survival prognosis is also present in patients starting dialysis merits investigation.

Thus, the present study aimed to elucidate the association between serum calcium levels at dialysis initiation and subsequent prognosis.

Methods

Subjects

The subjects were patients who were newly initiated dialysis at the 17 Aichi Cohort Study of Prognosis in Patients Newly Initiated into Dialysis (AICOPP) group centers from October 2011 to September 2013 [15]. Patients who were withdrawn from dialysis while hospitalized, died while hospitalized, or did not agree to be registered were excluded. The study included 1524 patients who were at least 20 years old, had CKD, and provided written consent. We excluded one patient whose serum adjusted calcium was not assessed and six patients whose outcomes were unknown, as determined by a survey conducted at the end of March 2015. Thus, we enrolled 1517 subjects into the study.

Patient characteristics and data when dialysis was initiated (baseline)

Body mass index (BMI) was measured at the first dialysis session. Diabetes was defined as a fasting blood glucose ≥126 mg/dL, casual blood glucose ≥200 mg/dL, HbA1c (NGSP) ≥6.5%, use of insulin, or use of oral hypoglycemic agents. History of cardiovascular disease (CVD) was defined as a history of heart failure requiring hospitalization, coronary artery disease requiring coronary artery intervention or heart bypass surgery, stroke, aortic disease requiring surgery, or peripheral artery disease requiring hospitalization. The period of nephrology care was established, based on patients' medical records, as the period from referral to the nephrologist until the initiation of dialysis. Medication use referred to the drugs taken at dialysis initiation. Blood tests were performed on samples taken before the first dialysis session. Blood pressure was measured before the first dialysis session.

Group assignment according to serum adjusted calcium levels

The serum calcium levels at dialysis initiation of patients with a serum albumin level <4.0 g/dL were adjusted employing the Payne formula. According to adjusted serum calcium levels, the patients were divided into the following 5 groups: (1) G1 with a serum adjusted calcium level <7.0 mg/dL, (2) G2 with 7.0 to <8.0 mg/dL, (3) G3 with 8.0 to <9.0 mg/dL, (4) G4 with 9.0 to <10.0 mg/dL, and (5) G5 with ≥10.0 mg/dL.

Assessment of aortic and cardiac valve calcification

Aortic calcification was assessed according to the presence or absence of aortic arch calcification on plain frontal chest radiographs taken immediately before dialysis initiation. Cardiac valve calcification was assessed according to the presence or absence of a calcified aortic or mitral valve determined by B-mode echocardiography during the 1-month periods before and after dialysis initiation.

Assessment of activities of daily living with the Barthel index

The BI is composed of 10 items: (1) eating, (2) transferring between the bed and wheelchair, (3) grooming, (4) using the toilet, (5) bathing, (6) walking on a flat surface, (7) climbing and descending stairs, (8) dressing, (9) controlling bowel movements, and (10) controlling urination. Each item is evaluated on a 2-point (0 and 5) to 4-point (0, 5, 10, and 15) scale, and the total score (0–100 in increments of 5) is used for assessment [16]. In the present study, experienced nurses assessed the patients to determine the BI on discharge for dialysis initiation.

Survey of survival prognosis

Survival prognosis as of March 31, 2015 was determined by surveying medical records. For patients who were transferred to other institutions, information was obtained by mailing out survey forms.

Outcomes

The study outcomes included (1) comparisons of all-cause mortality rates in the five groups as categorized by serum adjusted calcium level; (2) extraction of factors, which included serum adjusted calcium, influencing all-cause mortality.

Statistical processing

The easy R (EZR) was used for statistical processing [17]. Comparisons of characteristics and baseline data between the five groups of patients were performed using the analysis of variance (ANOVA) for continuous variables and chi-square test for nominal variables. All-cause mortality rates were compared using the log-rank test for the Kaplan-Meier curves. Factors contributing to the all-cause mortality rates were examined using univariate Cox proportional hazard regression analysis. In addition to the serum adjusted calcium level, factors that were significant in the univariate analysis served as explanatory variables for the multivariate Cox proportional hazard analysis using the stepwise method (i.e., serum adjusted calcium, age, gender, BMI, SBP, DBP, CTR, history of CVD, use of calcium carbonate, hemoglobin, serum albumin, eGFR, PTH, and CRP). In stratified analyses, all-cause mortality rates were compared by Cox proportional hazard models adjusted for the factors used

Table 1 Patient characteristics at baseline by serum adjusted calcium levels

Variables	All $n = 1517$	G1 $n = 114$	G2 $n = 241$	G3 $n = 530$	G4 $n = 522$	G5 $n = 110$	p trend
Age (years old)	67.5 + 13.1	60.4 + 14.0	63.8 + 13.4	69.2 + 12.5	68.8 + 12.7	68.2 + 11.9	<0.001
Female gender[a]	491 (32.4)	43 (37.7)	61 (25.3)	167 (31.5)	176 (33.7)	44 (40.0)	0.033
BMI (kg/m^2)	23.5 + 4.4	23.5 + 4.2	24.7 + 4.9	23.5 + 4.4	23.1 + 4.1	23.1 + 4.4	<0.001
SBP (mmHg)	151 + 26	154 + 24	154 + 28	152 + 25	150 + 26	148 + 28	0.129
DBP (mmHg)	77 + 15	82 + 14	80 + 17	77 + 15	76 + 15	74 + 15	<0.001
Diabetes Mellitus[a]	774 (51.0)	39 (34.2)	125 (51.9)	275 (51.9)	275 (52.7)	60 (54.5)	0.007
Cancer-bearing	93 (6.1)	5 (4.4)	16 (6.6)	32 (6.0)	32 (6.1)	8 (7.3)	0.914
History of CVD	681 (44.9)	29 (25.4)	98 (40.6)	248 (46.8)	251 (48.1)	55 (50.0)	<0.001
Barthel index score[b]	100 (90-100)	100 (100-100)	100 (100-100)	100 (90-100)	100 (80-100)	100 (50-100)	<0.001
Use of ACEIs or ARBs[a]	913 (60.2)	64 (56.1)	146 (60.6)	323 (60.9)	315 (60.3)	65 (59.1)	0.896
Use of beta blockers[a]	525 (34.6)	32 (28.1)	89 (36.9)	197 (37.2)	182 (34.9)	25 (22.7)	0.025
Use of VDRAs[a]	412 (27.2)	30 (26.3)	58 (24.1)	142 (26.8)	143 (27.4)	39 (35.5)	0.290
Use of calcium carbonate[a]	531 (35.0)	45 (39.5)	91 (37.8)	194 (36.6)	165 (31.6)	36 (32.7)	0.254
Use of thiazide[a]	347 (22.9)	18 (15.8)	62 (25.7)	134 (25.3)	109 (20.9)	24 (21.8)	0.117
Use of ESAs[a]	1303 (85.9)	92 (80.7)	203 (84.2)	476 (89.8)	449 (86.0)	83 (75.5)	<0.001
Hemoglobin (g/dL)	9.4 + 1.6	8.8 + 1.8	9.4 + 1.5	9.5 + 1.5	9.4 + 1.6	9.4 + 1.4	0.002
Serum albumin (g/dL)	3.20 + 0.60	3.44 + 0.45	3.25 + 0.58	3.29 + 0.54	3.10 + 0.62	2.89 + 0.67	<0.001
BUN (mg/dL)	91.8 + 30.4	105.3 + 34.3	96.9 + 31.7	90.7 + 27.5	88.1 + 29.5	89.1 + 36.0	<0.001
eGFR (ml/min/1.73 m2)	5.44 + 2.22	4.21 + 1.36	4.92 + 1.95	5.44 + 1.92	5.77 + 2.28	6.30 + 3.48	<0.001
Serum creatinine (mg/dL)	8.98 + 3.22	11.53 + 4.52	9.97 + 3.21	8.75 + 2.83	8.35 + 2.73	8.23 + 3.72	<0.001
Serum adjusted calcium (mg/dL)	8.62 + 1.06	6.37 + 0.52	7.50 + 0.29	8.51 + 0.28	9.34 + 0.27	10.45 + 0.59	<0.001
Serum phosphorus (mg/dL)	6.36 + 1.88	7.89 + 2.24	7.01 + 1.95	6.22 + 1.62	5.97 + 1.77	5.97 + 1.92	<0.001
Alkaline phosphatase (IU/L)	265 + 173	291 + 137	272 + 144	260 + 164	259 + 202	265 + 155	0.441
PTH (pg/mL)[b]	292 (186-432)	440 (329-625)	375 (274-518)	307 (208-429)	231 (147-360)	150 (71-230)	<0.001
CRP (mg/dl)[b]	0.30 (0.10-1.34)	0.31 (0.09-1.36)	0.32 (0.10-1.24)	0.20 (0.09-0.99)	0.30 (0.10-1.53)	0.62 (0.18-5.41)	<0.001
Duration of NC[b]	588 (160-1307)	576 (77-1226)	579 (195-1107)	636 (208-1295)	573 (132-1509)	465 (80-1161)	0.517

Mean ± SD, [a]value (%), [b]median (inter-quartile range)

G1 with a serum adjusted calcium level <7.0 mg/dL, G2 with 7.0 to <8.0 mg/dL, G3 with 8.0 to <9.0 mg/dL, G4 with 9.0 to <10.0 mg/dL, and G5 with ≥10.0 mg/dL

BMI body mass index, *SBP* systolic blood pressure, *DBP* diastolic blood pressure, *CTR* cardiothoracic rate, *CVD* cardiovascular disease, *ACEI* angiotensin converting enzyme inhibitor, *ARB* angiotensin-1 receptor blocker, *VDRA* vitamin D receptor activator, *ESA* erythropoiesis stimulating agent, *BUN* blood urea nitrogen, *eGFR* estimated glomerular filtration rate, *PTH* parathyroid hormone, *CRP* C reactive protein, *NC* nephrologist care

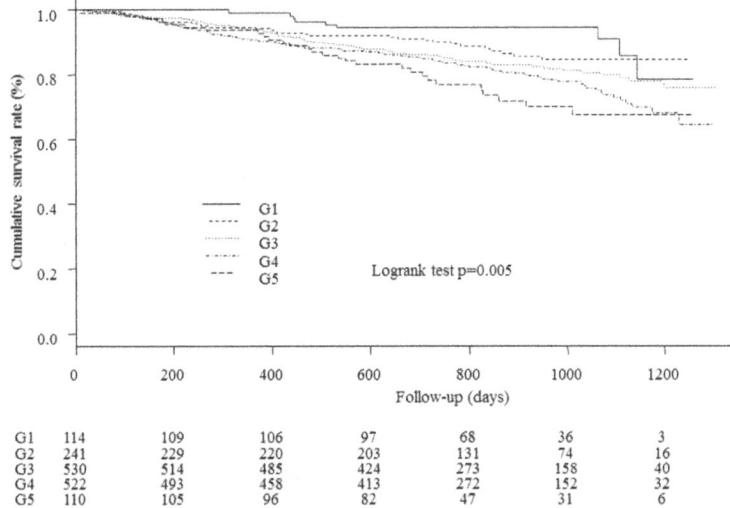

Fig. 1 Comparison of all-cause mortality among the five groups. Significant differences were observed between the five groups' cumulative survival rates ($p = 0.005$). G1 with a serum-adjusted calcium level <7.0 mg/dL, G2 with 7.0 to <8.0 mg/dL, G3 with 8.0 to <9.0 mg/dL, G4 with 9.0 to <10.0 mg/dL, and G5 with ≥10.0 mg/dL)

in the above-described step-wise analysis. Comparisons of aortic or cardiac valve calcification between the five groups of patient were performed using the chi-square test. Comparisons of Barthel index score between the five groups of patient were performed the analysis of variance (ANOVA). *P* values less than 5% were considered statistically significant.

Results

Comparison of patient characteristics and baseline data

Table 1 shows the patient characteristics and baseline data in the five groups. Significant differences between the five groups were observed in age, gender, BMI, DBP, prevalence of diabetes mellitus, history of CVD, BI, rate of beta blockers use, rate of ESAs use, hemoglobin level, serum albumin level, blood urea nitrogen (BUN) level, eGFR, serum creatinine level, serum phosphorus level, serum PTH level, and C-reactive protein (CRP) level.

Comparison of all-cause mortality

Figure 1 shows Kaplan-Meier curves for the cumulative survival rates of the five groups. There were 268 deaths during the follow-up period (G1, 9 cases; G2, 30 cases; G3, 91 cases; G4, 110 cases; G5, 28 cases). Significant differences were observed between the five groups' cumulative survival rates ($p = 0.005$).

Factors affecting all-cause mortality

The results of univariate Cox proportional hazard regression analysis are presented in Table 2. The increase in serum adjusted calcium levels was associated with the survival prognosis (every 1 mg/dL increase, hazard ratio [HR] = 1.332, 95% confidence interval [CI] = 1.185 – 1.498,

$p < 0.001$). In addition, high mortality was associated with advanced age, male gender, low BMI, low blood pressure, presence of cardiomegaly, history of CVD, no prior use of renin angiotensin system (RAS) inhibitors, no prior use of vitamin D receptor activator (VDRA), no prior use of calcium carbonate, no prior ESA use, presence of anemia, presence of hypoalbuminemia, high BUN level, high eGFR, low serum creatinine level, low serum phosphorus level, low PTH level, and high CRP level.

The results of multivariate Cox proportional hazard analysis using the stepwise method are shown in Table 3. Increasing serum adjusted calcium was associated with survival prognosis (every 1 mg/dL increase, HR = 1.267, 95% CI = 1.092–1.470, $p = 0.002$). In addition, high mortality was associated with advanced age, male gender, low systolic blood pressure, history of CVD, and no prior use of calcium carbonate.

Association of serum adjusted calcium levels with aortic and cardiac valve calcification

The five groups based on serum adjusted calcium levels at dialysis initiation were compared for aortic and cardiac valve calcification. There were significant differences in the incidence of either aortic or cardiac valve calcification among the five groups (aortic calcification $p = 0.006$, cardiac valve calcification $p = 0.008$). The incidence of calcification was especially low for G1 (Fig. 2).

Association between serum adjusted calcium levels and the Barthel index

BI scores were compared among the five groups based on serum adjusted calcium levels at dialysis initiation.

Table 2 Associations of variables with all-cause mortality according to the univariate Cox proportional hazard regression analysis

Variables	HR	95% CI	p value
Serum adjusted calcium	1.332	1.185–1.498	<0.001
Age	1.057	1.045–1.070	<0.001
Female gender	0.685	0.521–0.901	0.007
BMI	0.912	0.882–0.943	<0.001
SBP (/10 mmHg)	0.922	0.892–0.953	<0.001
DBP (/10 mmHg)	0.837	0.789–0.888	<0.001
CTR	1.034	1.017–1.051	<0.001
Diabetes Mellitus	1.018	0.801–1.294	0.882
History of CVD	2.435	1.896–3.128	<0.001
Use of ACEIs or ARBs	0.732	0.576–0.931	0.011
Use of beta blockers	1.182	0.924–1.512	0.183
Use of VDRAs	0.708	0.529–0.949	0.021
Use of calcium carbonate	0.405	0.298–0.551	<0.001
Use of ESAs	0.657	0.482–0.896	0.008
Hemoglobin	0.883	0.818–0.953	0.001
Serum albumin	0.642	0.529–0.779	<0.001
BUN (/10 mg/dL)	1.041	1.004–1.080	0.032
eGFR	1.117	1.078–1.157	<0.001
Serum creatinine	0.868	0.826–0.912	<0.001
Serum phosphorus	0.927	0.865–0.993	0.032
PTH (/10 pg/mL)	0.994	0.988–0.999	0.034
CRP	1.036	1.017–1.056	<0.001
Duration of NC (/100 days)	0.989	0.978–1.001	0.066

BMI body mass index, *SBP* systolic blood pressure, *DBP* diastolic blood pressure, *CTR* cardiothoracic rate, *CVD* cardiovascular disease, *ACEI* angiotensin converting enzyme inhibitor, *ARB* angiotensin-1 receptor blocker, *VDRA* vitamin D receptor activator, *ESA* erythropoiesis stimulating agent, *BUN* blood urea nitrogen, *eGFR* estimated glomerular filtration rate, *PTH* parathyroid hormone, *CRP* C reactive protein, *NC* nephrologist care

Table 3 Associations of variables with all-cause mortality according to the multivariate Cox proportional hazard regression analysis using the stepwise method

Variables	HR	95% CI	P value
Serum adjusted calcium	1.267	1.092-1.470	0.002
Age	1.045	1.030-1.060	<0.001
Female gender	0.656	0.471-0.912	0.012
SBP (/10 mmHg)	0.918	0.877-0.960	<0.001
History of CVD	1.656	1.229-2.231	<0.001
Use of calcium carbonate	0.580	0.409-0.822	0.002

Adjusted for serum adjusted calcium, age, gender, BMI, SBP, DBP, CTR, history of CVD, use of calcium carbonate, hemoglobin, serum albumin, eGFR, PTH, and CRP
BMI body mass index, *SBP* systolic blood pressure, *DBP* diastolic blood pressure, *CTR* cardiothoracic rate, *CVD* cardiovascular disease, *eGFR* estimated glomerular filtration rate, *PTH* parathyroid hormone, *CRP* C reactive protein

Lower BI scores were associated with higher serum adjusted calcium levels ($p < 0.001$) (Fig. 3).

Stratified analysis

The association between serum adjusted calcium levels and all-cause mortality was assessed with stratification by age, gender, history of CVD, BI score, VDRA use, calcium carbonate use, eGFR, and the PTH level. A significant association between serum adjusted calcium levels and all-cause mortality was observed in male patients age 70 years and older, a history of CVD, the full score of BI, VDRA use, no prior use of calcium carbonate, and an eGFR ≥ 5 mL/min/1.73 m^2 (Fig. 4).

Discussion

The present results revealed serum adjusted calcium levels at dialysis initiation to be associated with all-cause mortality after dialysis initiation. Moreover, multivariate analysis identified a high serum adjusted calcium level as an independent risk factor for poor survival prognosis. Severe hypocalcemia is highly likely to occur during the early period after dialysis initiation. On the other hand, we found that high serum adjusted calcium levels were associated with poor outcomes. In other words, pathological conditions that inhibit the decrease in serum adjusted calcium levels might have been associated with poor survival prognosis.

We considered that renal function at dialysis initiation influenced serum adjusted calcium levels. As the glomerular filtration rate (GFR) decreases, serum phosphorus and fibroblast growth factor 23 levels increase, followed by a decrease in the serum activated vitamin D level. As a consequence, the serum calcium level decreases. Thus, if dialysis is initiated in patients with a high GFR, their serum calcium may still be elevated. Regarding the association between renal function at dialysis initiation and survival prognosis, there is reports describing the survival prognosis as being rather poor when dialysis is initiated in patients with a high eGFR [18, 19]. This is considered to be attributable to many patients who begin dialysis in the early stage being elderly, and also to early initiation of dialysis being inevitable in some patients because of concurrent CVDs. The present study also showed higher adjusted serum calcium levels at dialysis initiation to be associated with higher eGFR, more advanced age, and/or a greater likelihood of concurrent CVDs. Because stratified analysis by eGFR revealed high serum adjusted calcium levels to be associated with poor survival prognosis, regardless of renal function level at dialysis initiation, higher serum adjusted calcium levels with respect to renal function might be a clinical issue. Common causes of hypercalcemia include (1) hyperparathyroidism, (2) malignancy, (3) chronic granulomatous disease, (4) drugs (e.g., activated vitamin D preparations,

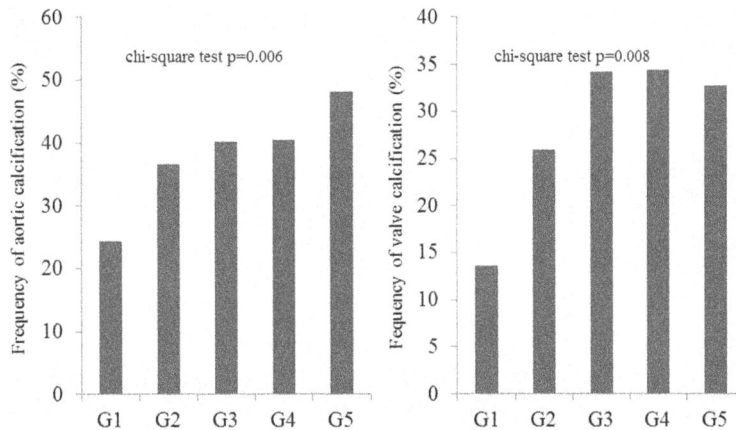

Fig. 2 Comparison of aortic and cardiac valve calcification among the five groups. Significant differences were observed between the five groups' frequency of aortic and cardiac valve calcification ($p = 0.006$ and $p = 0.008$). G1 with a serum adjusted calcium level <7.0 mg/dL, G2 with 7.0 to <8.0 mg/dL, G3 with 8.0 to <9.0 mg/dL, G4 with 9.0 to <10.0 mg/dL, and G5 with ≥10.0 mg/dL

thiazide diuretics, and teriparatide), (5) hyperthyroidism, (6) adrenal insufficiency, (7) immobility, (8) total parenteral nutrition, and (9) milk-alkali syndrome [20]. We considered that among above causes of hypercalcemia, drugs or immobility led to increase in serum adjusted calcium level inconsistent with renal function. Because many reports have recently indicated that the use of calcium-containing phosphate binders in patients with dialysis worsens survival prognosis [21–23], we additionally examined drugs affecting serum calcium levels. The rate of using thiazide diuretics, VDRA, or calcium-containing phosphate binders did not differ significantly among the groups. After the patients were stratified based on the use of VDRA or calcium-containing phosphate binders, the effects of these drugs on survival

prognosis were assessed. Regardless of the use of these drugs, high serum adjusted calcium levels were generally associated with poor survival prognosis. Thus, when these serum calcium-elevating drugs are used, it would apparently be important to maintain the serum adjusted calcium concentration at "a level commensurate with renal function". The use of calcium carbonate was unexpectedly associated with better prognosis in the present study. Comparison of serum adjusted calcium and phosphorus levels between use and no use of calcium carbonate groups showed no significant differences (Additional file 1: Figure S1). In other word, patients who took more amount of phosphorus intake were likely administered calcium carbonate. We suspected that those of patients probably took sufficient dietary protein

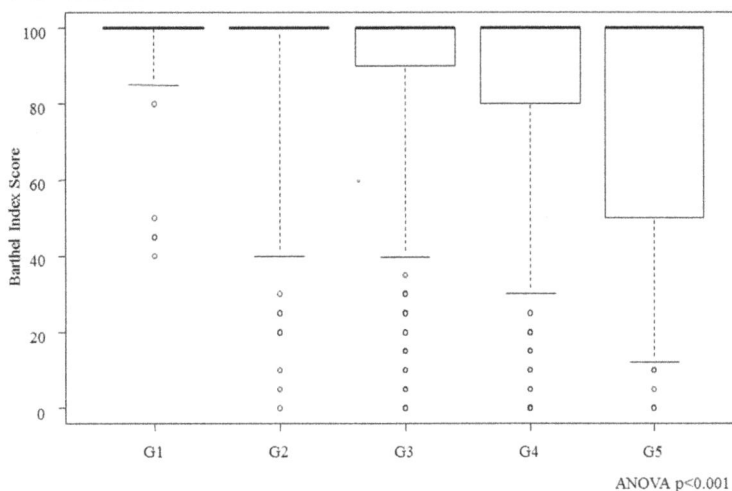

Fig. 3 Comparison of Barthel index score among the five groups. Significant differences were observed between the five groups' Barthel index score ($p < 0.001$). G1 with a serum adjusted calcium level <7.0 mg/dL, G2 with 7.0 to <8.0 mg/dL, G3 with 8.0 to <9.0 mg/dL, G4 with 9.0 to <10.0 mg/dL, and G5 with ≥10.0 mg/dL. ANOVA, analysis of variance

	HR	95%CI
Age<70	1.050	0.792-1.393
Age≥70	1.356	1.120-1.641
Male gender	1.274	1.039-1.563
Female gender	1.230	0.912-1.659
No history of CVD	1.249	0.964-1.619
History of CVD	1.251	1.002-1.575
Barthel index=100	1.323	1.048-1.670
Barthel index<100	1.166	0.917-1.485
No use of VDRA	1.166	0.966-1.408
Use of VDRA	1.394	1.006-1.931
No use of CC	1.233	1.015-1.499
Use of CC	1.302	0.944-1.795
eGFR<5	1.206	0.921-1.580
5≤eGFR<10	1.242	1.005-1.552
10≤eGFR	2.023	1.009-3.540
PTH<300	1.214	0.966-1.525
PTH≥300	1.167	0.904-1.508

Elevated serum adjusted calcium is associated with poorer prognosis

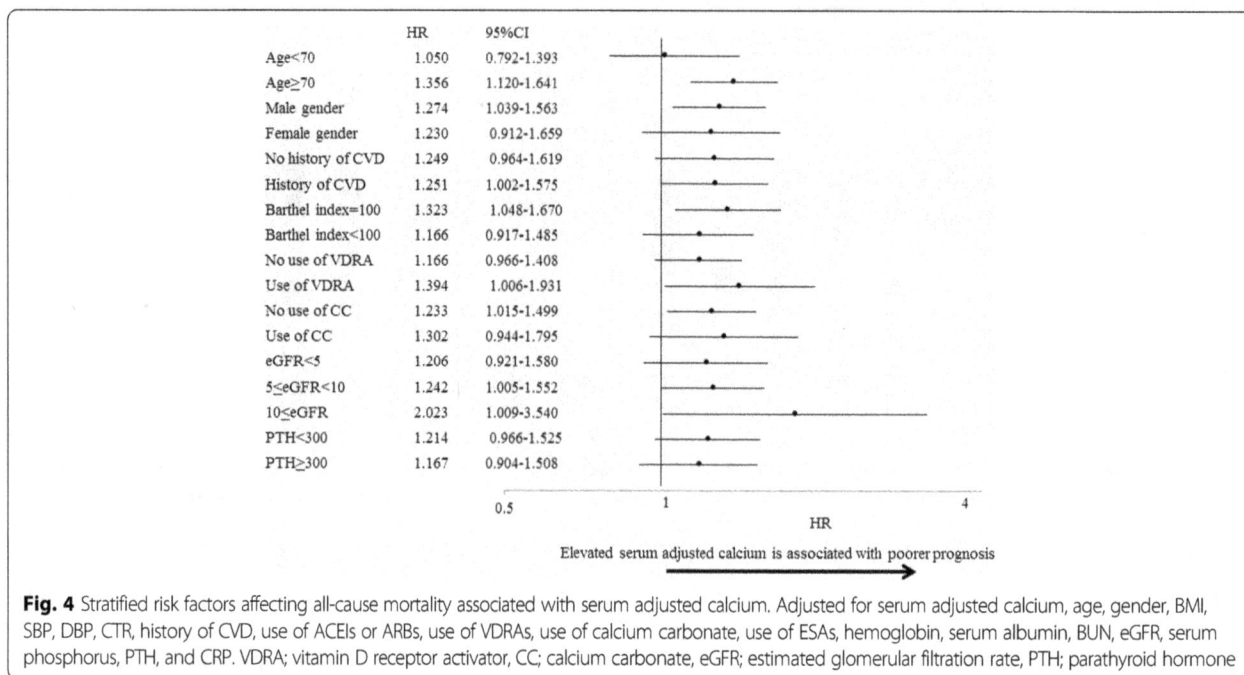

Fig. 4 Stratified risk factors affecting all-cause mortality associated with serum adjusted calcium. Adjusted for serum adjusted calcium, age, gender, BMI, SBP, DBP, CTR, history of CVD, use of ACEIs or ARBs, use of VDRAs, use of calcium carbonate, use of ESAs, hemoglobin, serum albumin, BUN, eGFR, serum phosphorus, PTH, and CRP. VDRA; vitamin D receptor activator, CC; calcium carbonate, eGFR; estimated glomerular filtration rate, PTH; parathyroid hormone

after dialysis initiation. Therefore, good nutritional status led to better prognosis during the relatively short term follow up period.

In the present study, patients with a high serum adjusted calcium level at dialysis initiation included many elderly as well as those with a low BI score, which reflects ADL. Thus, increased serum calcium levels due to immobility, one of the above-described causes of hypercalcemia, might have contributed to our results. Immobility promotes bone resorption via mobilization of calcium from bone, which in turn causes hypercalcemia [24, 25]. Consequently, PTH levels are suppressed. In the present study, PTH levels decreased as serum adjusted calcium levels rose. This result appears to be consistent with the known effects of immobility.

Elevated serum calcium is known to be a factor promoting vascular calcification [26]. Moreover, vascular calcification is an important pathological condition that affects survival prognosis [27]. The results of the present study revealed the prevalence of aortic and cardiac valve calcification to be higher in patients with higher serum-adjusted calcium levels. This suggests that the poor survival prognosis in patients with higher serum adjusted calcium levels might be attributable to advanced organ dysfunction due to vascular calcification. However, it is also possible that such ectopic calcification is strongly associated with age-related factors.

The present study has the following limitations. First, because of the observational study design, there were differences in patient characteristics and baseline data among the groups, although the data were adjusted for several of these factors. We could not exclude the bias because several factors including age, gender, BMI, diabetes, and history of CVD were strongly associated mortality in general. Second, there was difference in the number of patients among the five groups. Hence, we conducted comparison of all-cause mortality between five groups classified by quintile of serum adjusted calcium. We considered that the bias was at minimum because the results were similar (Additional file 2: Figure S2). Third, the extent to which low BI scores reflect bone resorption due to immobility is unknown. The subjects of the present study were limited to patients who could be discharged to home or transferred to another facility after dialysis initiation. Thus, there were only a few patients with very low ADL who were bedridden 24 h a day. In this situation, it is not certain whether the physical activity levels of the patients can be regarded as "immobility." Fourth, neither vascular nor cardiac valve calcification was assessed quantitatively. As the severity calcification was not considered, i.e., cases with mild to severe calcifications were handled equally in performing the analyses, this study lacks sufficient objectivity to identify calcification as a cause of poor prognosis.

Conclusions

Serum-adjusted calcium levels at dialysis initiation were demonstrated to be associated with all-cause mortality after dialysis initiation.

Acknowledgements

We acknowledge the support provided by the following investigators and members of the Aichi Cohort study of Prognosis in Patients Newly Initiated Into Dialysis (AICOPP), who participated in this study: Akihito Tanaka, Minako Murata, Hibiki Shinjo, Yasuhiro Otsuka, Asami Takeda (Japanese Red Cross Nagoya Daini Hospital), Hirofumi Tamai (Anjo Kosei Hospital), Tomohiko Naruse (Kasugai Municipal Hospital), Kei Kurata (Tosei General Hospital), Hideto Oishi (Komaki City Hospital), Isao Aoyama (Japanese Community Healthcare Organization Chukyo Hospital), Hiroshi Ogawa (Shinseikai Daiichi Hospital), Hiroko Kushimoto (Chita City Hospital), Hideaki Shimizu (Chubu-Rosai Hospital), Junichiro Yamamoto (Tsushima City Hospital), Hisashi Kurata (Toyota Kosei Hospital), Taishi Yamakawa (Toyohashi Municipal Hospital), Takaaki Yaomura (Nagoya Medical Center), Hirotake Kasuga (Nagoya Kyouritsu Hospital), Shizunori Ichida (Japanese Red Cross Nagoya Daiichi Hospital), Shoichi Maruyama (Nagoya University Graduate School of Medicine), Seiichi Matsuo (Nagoya University Graduate School of Medicine), and Noritoshi Kato (Nagoya University Graduate School of Medicine).

Funding

Not applicable.

Authors' contributions

DI participated in the design of the study and interpretation of the data. DI, SK, and HH participated in writing the manuscript. All authors were involved in drafting, reviewing, and approving the final manuscript.

Competing interests

The authors declare that they have no competing interests.

References

1. Kidney Disease: Improving Global Outcomes (KDIGO) CKD-MBD Work Group. KDIGO clinical practice guideline for the diagnosis, evaluation, prevention, and treatment of Chronic Kidney Disease-Mineral and Bone Disorder (CKD-MBD). Kidney Int Suppl. 2009;113:S1–130.
2. Block GA, Klassen PS, Lazarus JM, Ofsthun N, Lowrie EG, Chertow GM. Mineral metabolism, mortality, and morbidity in maintenance hemodialysis. J Am Soc Nephrol. 2004;15(8):2208–18.
3. Stevens LA, Djurdjev O, Cardew S, Cameron EC, Levin A. Calcium, phosphate, and parathyroid hormone levels in combination and as a function of dialysis duration predict mortality: evidence for the complexity of the association between mineral metabolism and outcomes. J Am Soc Nephrol. 2004;15(3):770–9.
4. Taniguchi M, Fukagawa M, Fujii N, Hamano T, Shoji T, Yokoyama K, Nakai S, Shigematsu T, Iseki K, Tsubakihara Y, Committee of Renal Data Registry of the Japanese Society for Dialysis Therapy. Serum phosphate and calcium should be primarily and consistently controlled in prevalent hemodialysis patients. Ther Apher Dial. 2013;17(2):221–8.
5. Kalantar-Zadeh K, Kuwae N, Regidor DL, Kovesdy CP, Kilpatrick RD, Shinaberger CS, McAllister CJ, Budoff MJ, Salusky IB, Kopple JD. Survival predictability of time-varying indicators of bone disease in maintenance hemodialysis patients. Kidney Int. 2006;70(4):771–80.
6. Floege J, Kim J, Ireland E, Chazot C, Drueke T, de Francisco A, Kronenberg F, Marcelli D, Passlick-Deetjen J, Schernthaner G, Fouqueray B, Wheeler DC, ARO Investigators. Serum iPTH, calcium and phosphate, and the risk of mortality in a European hemodialysis population. Nephrol Dial Transplant. 2011;26(6):1948–55.
7. Tentori F, Blayney MJ, Albert JM, Gillespie BW, Kerr PG, Bommer J, Young EW, Akizawa T, Akiba T, Pisoni RL, Robinson BM, Port FK. Mortality risk for dialysis patients with different levels of serum calcium, phosphorus, and PTH: the Dialysis Outcomes and Practice Patterns Study (DOPPS). Am J Kidney Dis. 2008;52(3):519–30.
8. Lin YC, Lin YC, Hsu CY, Kao CC, Chang FC, Chen TW, Chen HH, Hsu CC, Wu MS, Taiwan Society of Nephrology. Effect Modifying Role of Serum Calcium on Mortality-Predictability of PTH and Alkaline Phosphatase in Hemodialysis Patients: An Investigation Using Data from the Taiwan Renal Registry Data System from 2005 to 2012. PLoS One. 2015;10(6):e0129737.
9. Fukagawa M, Yokoyama K, Koiwa F, Taniguchi M, Shoji T, Kazama JJ, Komaba H, Ando R, Kakuta T, Fujii H, Nakayama M, Shibagaki Y, Fukumoto S, Fujii N, Hattori M, Ashida A, Iseki K, Shigematsu T, Tsukamoto Y, Tsubakihara Y, Tomo T, Hirakata H, Akizawa T, CKD-MBD Guideline Working Group; Japanese Society for Dialysis Therapy. Clinical practice guideline for the management of chronic kidney disease-mineral and bone disorder. Ther Apher Dial. 2013;17(3):247–88.
10. Moldovan D, Rusu C, Kacso IM, Potra A, Patiu IM, Gherman-Capioara M. Mineral and bone disorders, morbidity and mortality in end-stage renal failure patients on chronic dialysis. Clujul Med. 2016;89(1):94–103.
11. Chen NX, Moe SM. Pathophysiology of Vascular Calcification. Curr Osteoporos Rep. 2015;13(6):372–80.
12. Ossareh S. Vascular calcification in chronic kidney disease: mechanisms and clinical implications. Iran J Kidney Dis. 2011;5(5):285–99.
13. Hutchison AJ. Predialysis management of divalent ion metabolism. Kidney Int Suppl. 1999;73:S82–4.
14. Doi T, Yamamoto S, Morinaga T, Sada KE, Kurita N, Onishi Y. Risk Score to Predict 1-Year Mortality after Hemodialysis Initiation in Patients with Stage 5 Chronic Kidney Disease under Predialysis Nephrology Care. PLoS One. 2015;10(6):e0129180.
15. Hishida M, Tamai H, Morinaga T, Maekawa M, Aoki T, Tomida H, Komatsu S, Kamiya T, Maruyama S, Matsuo S, Inaguma D. Aichi cohort study of the prognosis in patients newly initiated into dialysis (AICOPP): baseline characteristics and trends observed in diabetic nephropathy. Clin Exp Nephrol. 2016 Feb 23. [Epub ahead of print]
16. Mahoney FI, Barthel DW. Functional Evaluation: The Barthel Index. Md State Med J. 1965;14:61–5.
17. Kanda Y. Investigation of the freely available easy-to-use software 'EZR' for medical statistics. Bone Marrow Transplant. 2013;48(3):452–8.
18. Hwang SJ, Yang WC, Lin MY, Mau LW, Chen HC, Taiwan Society of Nephrology. Impact of the clinical conditions at dialysis initiation on mortality in incident hemodialysis patients: a national cohort study in Taiwan. Nephrol Dial Transplant. 2010;25(8):2616–24.
19. Rosansky SJ, Eggers P, Jackson K, Glassock R, Clark WF. Early start of hemodialysis may be harmful. Arch Intern Med. 2011;171(5):396–403.
20. Khairallah W, Fawaz A, Brown EM, El-Hajj FG. Hypercalcemia and diabetes insipidus in a patient previously treated with lithium. Nat Clin Pract Nephrol. 2007;3(7):397–404.
21. Borzecki AM, Lee A, Wang SW, Brenner L, Kazis LE. Survival in end stage renal disease: calcium carbonate vs. sevelamer. J Clin Pharm Ther. 2007;32(6):617–24.
22. Block GA, Raggi P, Bellasi A, Kooienga L, Spiegel DM. Mortality effect of coronary calcification and phosphate binder choice in incident hemodialysis patients. Kidney Int. 2007;71(5):438–41.
23. Jamal SA, Vandermeer B, Raggi P, Mendelssohn DC, Chatterley T, Dorgan M, Lok CE, Fitchett D, Tsuyuki RT. Effect of calcium-based versus non-calcium-based phosphate binders on mortality in patients with chronic kidney disease: an updated systematic review and meta-analysis. Lancet. 2013;382(9900):1268–77.
24. Stewart AF, Adler M, Byers CM, Segre GV, Broadus AE. Calcium homeostasis in immobilization: an example of resorptive hypercalciuria. N Engl J Med. 1982;306(19):1136–40.
25. Alborzi F, Leibowitz AB. Immobilization hypercalcemia in critical illness following bariatric surgery. Obes Surg. 2002;12(6):871–3.
26. Razzaque MS. The dualistic role of vitamin D in vascular calcifications. Kidney Int. 2011;79(7):708–14.
27. Blacher J, Guerin AP, Pannier B, Marchais SJ, London GM. Arterial calcifications, arterial stiffness, and cardiovascular risk in end-stage renal disease. Hypertension. 2001;38(4):938–42.

12

A new polymethylmetacrylate membrane improves the membrane adhesion of blood components and clinical efficacy

Ikuto Masakane[1], Shiho Esashi[1], Asami Yoshida[1], Tetsuro Chida[1], Hiroaki Fujieda[2*], Yoshiyuki Ueno[2] and Hiroyuki Sugaya[2]

Abstract

Background: Hemodialysis with polymethylmetacrylate (PMMA) membrane dialyzers allows unique protein adsorption. New PMMA dialyzers should demonstrate equivalent protein adsorption, but improved hemocompatibility.

Methods: Platelet adhesion and activation and protein adsorption were determined for the new PMMA membrane dialyzer Filtryzer® NF (NF) and conventional Filtryzer® BG (BG) in vitro. In clinical study, six subjects were treated with NF and BG for 3 months each in a crossover design. Three months after the use of each dialyzer, solute removal, hemocompatibility, peripheral circulation by skin perfusion pressure (SPP), and other dialysis-related side effects were also compared.

Results: Protein adsorption pattern was similar on NF and BG, but platelet adhesion and activation were much lower on NF in vitro. Clinically, NF and BG removed equivalent amounts of small molecule solutes and low-molecular-weight proteins. The platelet count and peripheral circulation were stable during dialysis with NF, whereas both were decreased during dialysis with BG. The percent changes in SPP were significantly smaller with NF compared with BG. Data on the dialysis-related side effects were no significant differences in any individual items or in the mean total score for the two groups, but the mean score of the seven items tended to be lower with NF. Protein adsorption by the membranes is considered one factor associated with clinically improvements. But activated platelets induce the aggregation of platelets, leukocytes, and erythrocytes, which can interfere with peripheral circulation during dialysis. Decreased peripheral circulation causes dialysis-related side effects. Therefore reduced platelet activation during dialysis by NF may be significant in improving the prognosis of patients, as well as reducing the frequency of side effects.

Conclusions: The new PMMA membrane dialyzer NF shows substantially improved hemocompatibility. We expect this product will improve the condition of chronic dialysis patients.

Keywords: Dialysis, PMMA membrane, Protein adsorption, Hemocompatibility

* Correspondence: Hiroaki_Fujieda@nts.toray.co.jp
[2]Advanced Materials Research Labs, Toray Industries, Inc., 2-2 Sonoyama 3-chome, Otsu, Shiga, Japan
Full list of author information is available at the end of the article

Background

Hemodialysis with polymethylmetacrylate (PMMA) dialyzers allows unique protein adsorption [1, 2]. Clinically, hemodialysis with PMMA dialyzers is associated with the relief of dialysis-induced itching [3, 4] and improvement of nutrition [5]. A new PMMA dialyzer was developed to improve hemocompatibility while maintaining the amount of protein adsorption. The present study aimed to determine the basic properties of the new membrane and its performance in solute removal and peripheral circulation under standard clinical conditions.

Methods

Subjects

We evaluated the new PMMA dialyzer; "Filtryzer® NF" (NF) and compared it with the conventional PMMA dialyzer; "Filtryzer® BG" (BG). The performance of the dialyzers were compared in experimental and clinical studies. For the testing in vitro, hollow fiber membranes were cut from the dialyzers and used as samples. For the clinical testing, dialyzers with a 1.6 m^2 membrane surface area were used. Technical data on BG and NF are summarized in Table 1.

Membrane analysis

Blood component adhesion

The hollow fiber membranes were longitudinally cut to expose the inner surface and then incubated with fresh human whole blood containig 50 U/mL of heparin (Heparin Sodium Injection, Ajinomoto, Tokyo, Japan) for 1 h at 37 ℃ with continuous agitation. After washing with phosphate-buffered saline (PBS), the samples were fixed with 25% glutaraldehyde (Sigma-Aldrich) and observed by field emission scanning electron microscopy (S-800, Hitachi High-Tech Fielding Corp., Tokyo, Japan) to count the number of adhered

Table 1 Technical data on BG and NF

		BG	NF
Ultrafiltration rate[a] [mL/h mmHg]		38	35
Clearance[b] [mL/min]	Urea	191	193
	Creatinine	174	180
	Phosphate	164	172
	Vitamin B_{12}	114	126
Negative charge[c] [meq/g]		110	80

[a]Ultrafiltration rate was measured with bovine blood (hematocrit, 30 ± 3%; total protein, 6.0 ± 0.5 g/dl; blood flow rate, 200 ± 4 mL/min; transmembrane pressure, 13.3 ± 1.3 kPa; temp., 37 ± 1 °C
[b]Clearance was measured with aqueous solution. Blood flow rate, 200 ± 4 mL/min; dialyzate flow rate, 500 ± 10 mL/min, filtration rate, 10 ± 2 mL/min; temp., 37 ± 1 °C
[c]Negative charge on the membranes was determined from the evaluation of the triiodide complex. It was created by the reaction of iodine and iodide ions after dried hollow fiber membrane immersed in a solution of 5% potassium iodide in methanol for 24 h

platelets. The blood was obtained from volunteers after ethical review and approval by Toray Industries, Inc.

Activation of platelets

We prepared the mini modules of NF, BG. The mini-module had a length of 120 mm and a diameter of 5 mm, and contained 48 hollow fibers. Membrane surface area of mini module was 3619 mm2. 6.5 mL of fresh human blood, including the 15% acid citrate dextrose solution (ACD) as an anti-coagulant, was circulated to it at 1.0 mL/min for 30 min. The collected blood was allowed to stand in ice water for 15 min and centrifuged at 2000g at 4 °C for 30 min. The β-thromboglobulin (β-TG) concentration in the resulting plasma was determined by the enzyme immunoassay (EIA) method.

Electrophoresis of the adsorbed proteins

We prepared the mini modules of polysulfone membrane dialyzer "Toraylight® NV-U" as a reference, in addition to NF and BG. 6.5 mL of human serum (Human Serum type AB, Sigma-Aldrich) was circulated to it at 1.0 mL/min for 4 h. After circulation, the column was washed with 20 mL of PBS. The hollow fiber membranes were removed and cut into 5-mm-long pieces, which were then immersed in 50% acetic acid (017-00251, Wako Pure Chemical Industries, Ltd., Osaka, Japan) for 24 h to extract the adsorbed proteins. The extracted samples were freeze-dried and dissolved in PBS. We determined the quantity of protein in the samples using the BCA Assay (Pierce BCA Protein Assay Kit, Takara Bio, Otsu, Japan). Next, the samples were processed into aliquots with 0.2 g of protein each in the same volume of sample buffer (Tris-aspartic acid sample buffer, TEFCO, Aomori, Japan) and were heated at 95 °C for 5 min. The samples were electrophoresed through a gel (4–12% LS-PAGE mini, TEFCO) at 100 V for 1 h in Tris-aspartic acid running buffer (TEFCO). The gels were stained with Coomassie Brilliant Blue (PhastGel Blue R 40Tablets, Pharmacia Biotech, Uppsala, Sweden) and silver staining (Silver Staining II Kit, Wako) and then imaged.

Clinical study

Subjects

Six anuric patients (five males and one female) with no inflammatory signs who were on maintenance dialysis were enrolled. Subject characteristics included a mean age of 69 ± 16 years and a mean duration of dialysis therapy of 9.1 ± 2.5 years. Underlying conditions were glomerulonephritis in two patients, nephrosclerosis in two, diabetic nephropathy in one, and unknown in one. All subjects had undergone hemodialysis with Filtryzer ® BK (BK) before enrolling in the study. All patients were confirmed to have no clinical findings or data on the ankle-brachial pressure index (ABI), which is indicative of arterial stenosis or obstruction of the lower extremities, or a past history of arteriosclerosis obliterans. This clinical study was approved by the ethical committee of Yabuki Hospital (Authorization No. 30), and documented informed consent was obtained from each patient.

Methods

As shown in Fig. 1, the six subjects were treated with NF and BG for 3 months each in a crossover design. The last dialysis treatment using each dialyzer for 3 months, the amount of solute removal, percent changes in platelet count during dialysis, changes in peripheral circulation, and any dialysis-related complaints from the patients were evaluated. The prescription dialysis was performed with a blood flow rate of 270 mL/min, dialyzate flow rate of 500 mL/min, and dialysis time of 4 h. The solute removal capacity was evaluated based on the percent reduction of the blood concentrations of urea nitrogen, creatinine, uric acid, inorganic phosphorus, β_2 microglobulin (β_2MG), and α_1 microglobulin (α_1MG) and the total amounts of albumin in the effluent dialyzate. The peripheral circulation was evaluated with PAD-3000® (Kaneka Medix, Osaka, Japan). The skin perfusion pressure (SPP) of the sole of the right foot [6] was measured before dialysis and at every hour during dialysis, and the rate of change was evaluated based on the value before dialysis. SPP measurement was performed twice a week with each dialyzer. In addition, at the same time of SPP measurement, systolic blood pressure was also measured.

Dialysis-related side effects, including itching, distraction, malaise, headache, hypotension, fatigue after dialysis, and appetite, were evaluated for each dialyzer. Each side effect was evaluated on a 5-grade scale (0–4), with lower scores meaning fewer complaints.

Statistical analysis

Student's t tests were used to compare activation of platelets in vitro and laboratory results from the clinical study between groups. Results of the investigation of unidentified complaints were tested with Friedman's test. The analytical data are shown as the mean ± standard deviation. P values <0.05 were considered statistically significant.

Results

Membrane analysis

The number of adhered platelets in vitro was at least 100-fold lower on NF than on BG (Fig. 2). When the β-TG level, as a platelet activation marker, was evaluated in vitro, that of NF was 30% lower than BG (Fig. 3). The molecular weights of the proteins adsorbed on NF and BG were nearly equivalent, as assessed by electrophoresis (Fig. 4).

Clinical study

The percent reduction of small molecules and low-molecular-weight proteins in the blood before and after dialysis is shown in Fig. 5, and the total amount of albumin in the effluent dialyzate is shown in Fig. 6. There were no significant differences in any of these parameters between NF and BG.

During dialysis, the percent changes in platelet count were (for NF and BG, respectively) 97.1 and 86.1% after 15 min of dialysis, 96.5 and 85.1% after 30 min, 97.3 and 88.3% after 1 h, and 99.6 and 90.1% after 4 h. The changes in platelet count during dialysis were significantly smaller with NF than with BG (Fig. 7).

The systolic blood pressure during dialysis was shown in Fig. 8a. There were no significant difference between NF and BG, and no cases of intradialytic hypotension which required intervention.

Peripheral circulation was evaluated through changes in SPP during dialysis and compared between groups. The SPP values were 69.6 + 12.2 mmHg before the start of dialysis, 69.8 ± 11.5 mmHg after 1 h (percent change, +0.6 ± 7.7%), 70.4 ± 10.0 mmHg (+1.7 ± 9.7%) after 2 h, 67.7 ± 14.4 mmHg (−2.8 ± 11.8%) after 3 h, and 64.6 ± 14.5 mmHg (−7.7 ± 11.1%) after 4 h with NF, indicating that the SPP was maintained and did not significantly change during dialysis. With BG, the SPP values were 77.7 ± 10.4 mmHg before the start of dialysis, 71.4 ± 14.2 mmHg (−7.6 ± 16.5%) after 1 h, 66.9 ± 12.7 mmHg (−13.4 ± 15.6%) after 2 h, 65.4 ± 10.4 mmHg (−15.7 ± 9.9%) after 3 h, and 63.6 ± 9.6 mmHg

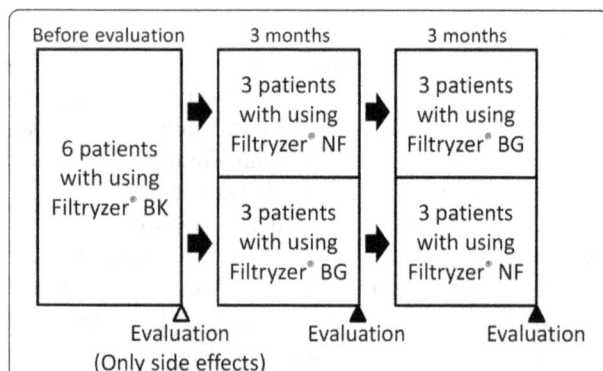

Fig. 1 The design of clinical study

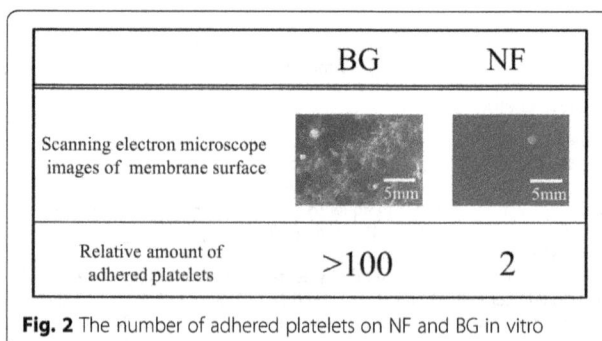

Fig. 2 The number of adhered platelets on NF and BG in vitro

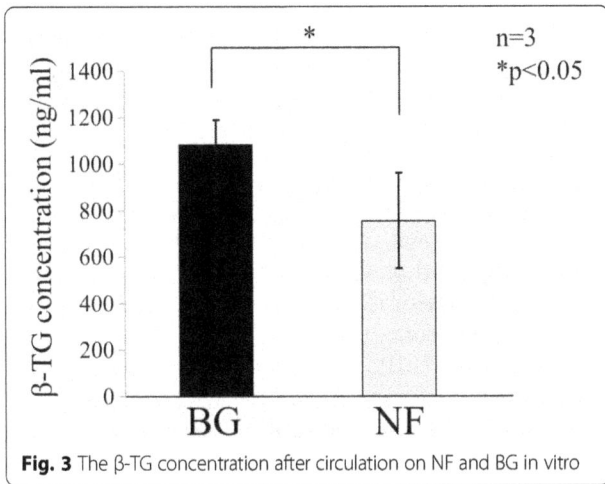

Fig. 3 The β-TG concentration after circulation on NF and BG in vitro

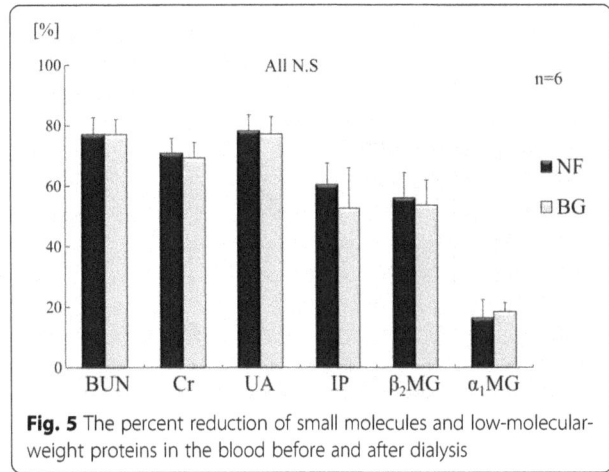

Fig. 5 The percent reduction of small molecules and low-molecular-weight proteins in the blood before and after dialysis

(−17.9 ± 9.4%) after 4 h, indicating significant decreases in the SPP after 3 and 4 h compared with before starting dialysis. The percent changes in SPP were significantly smaller at 2 and 3 h with NF compared with BG (Fig. 8b).

Data on the dialysis-related side effects are shown in Fig. 9. There were no significant differences in any individual items or in the mean total score for the two groups, but the mean score of the seven items tended to be lower with NF.

Discussion

The number of adhered platelets on NF was at least 100-fold lower than that on BG (Fig. 2), and the platelet activation of NF was 30% lower than that of BG (Fig. 3). On the other hand, no substantial differences were found in the amount of adsorbed proteins or their molecular weight between NF and BG. These results indicate that protein adsorption pattern by the hollow fiber NF was similar to that of BG (Fig. 4). (Although the used blood in this electrophoresis experiment was not of

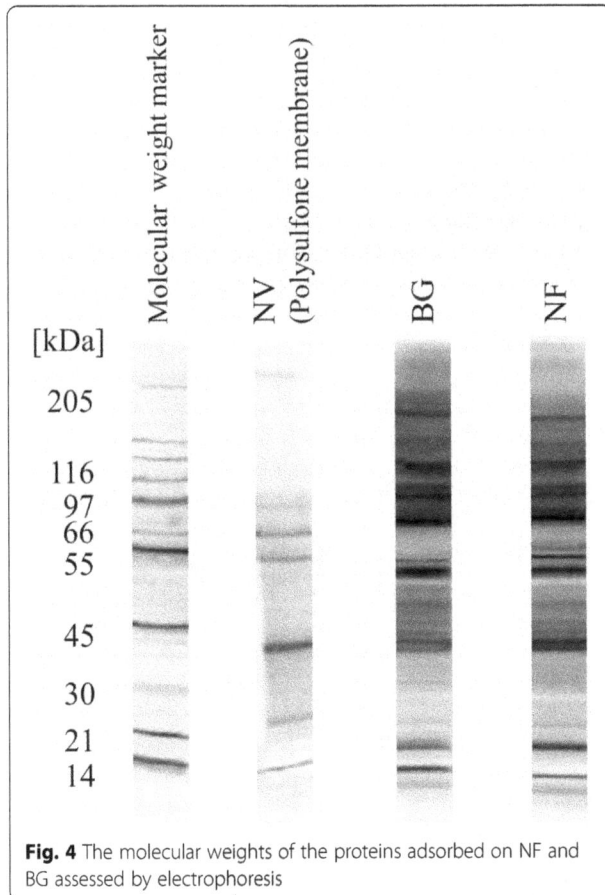

Fig. 4 The molecular weights of the proteins adsorbed on NF and BG assessed by electrophoresis

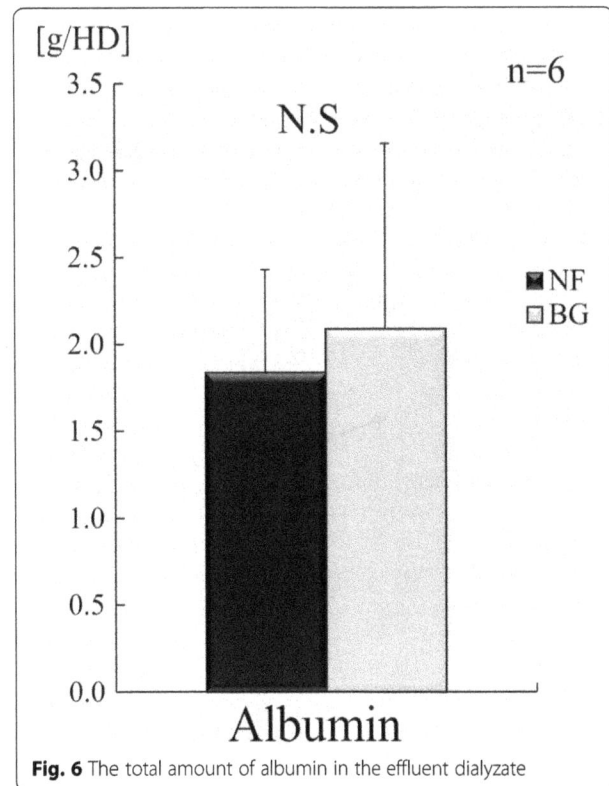

Fig. 6 The total amount of albumin in the effluent dialyzate

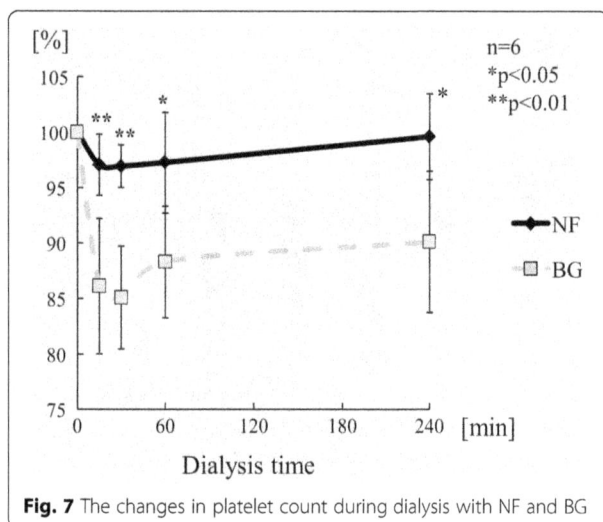

Fig. 7 The changes in platelet count during dialysis with NF and BG

In this study, we evaluated peripheral circulation by SPP which is a method measuring non-invasively dermal microcirculation by using Laser Doppler imaging-based methods because there are many reports describing them being useful to evaluate peripheral circulation disturbance such as lower limb ischemia in hemodialysis patients [7, 8]. Evaluation of the SPP suggested that peripheral circulation was more stable during dialysis with NF (Fig. 8). Additionally, dialysis-related side effects tended to be reduced in patients who continued using NF for 3 months (Fig. 9). Previous articles have reported the improvements of various clinical symptoms with the conventional PMMA dialyzers [3–5, 9–19]. Protein adsorption by PMMA membranes is considered one factor associated with these improvements. However, on BG, platelets also tend to adhere and be activated. Activated platelets induce the aggregation of platelets alone, platelets and leukocytes together, and platelets, leukocytes, and erythrocytes, which can interfere with peripheral circulation during dialysis [20, 21]. Deteriorated peripheral circulation causes dialysis-related side effects, including muscle cramps and abdominal pain during and after dialysis and fatigue after dialysis. Recently, the problem of dialysis-related side effects as factors affecting the prognosis of dialysis patients has gained attention from researchers [22–24], who have tried to identify the importance of dialysis prescriptions for reducing side effects [5]. On the other hand, in dialysis patients, aggregates of platelets and leukocytes remain in the serum even after dialysis and are associated with poor prognosis of these patients [25]. Improved platelet activation in NF may be significant in improving the prognosis of patients, as well as reducing the frequency of side effects.

hemodialysis patients, NF and BG would have approximately the same adsorption pattern even when the same experiment is performed on the blood of hemodialysis patients.) Comparing NF to BG in the clinical setting, the two dialyzers showed equivalent solute removal (Figs. 5 and 6). However, changes in the platelet count during dialysis confirmed reduced platelet adhesion to NF (Fig. 7). It was considered that BG and NF have almost the same adsorption and fractionation characteristics, which suggested that the membrane structure of BG and NF are equivalent. The difference between the two membranes is only the electrostatic charge (Table 1). Since NF has a less negative charge than BG, the electrostatic interaction between NF and platelets might be reduced. This is considered to be the reason why platelet adhesion and activation was suppressed significantly on NF.

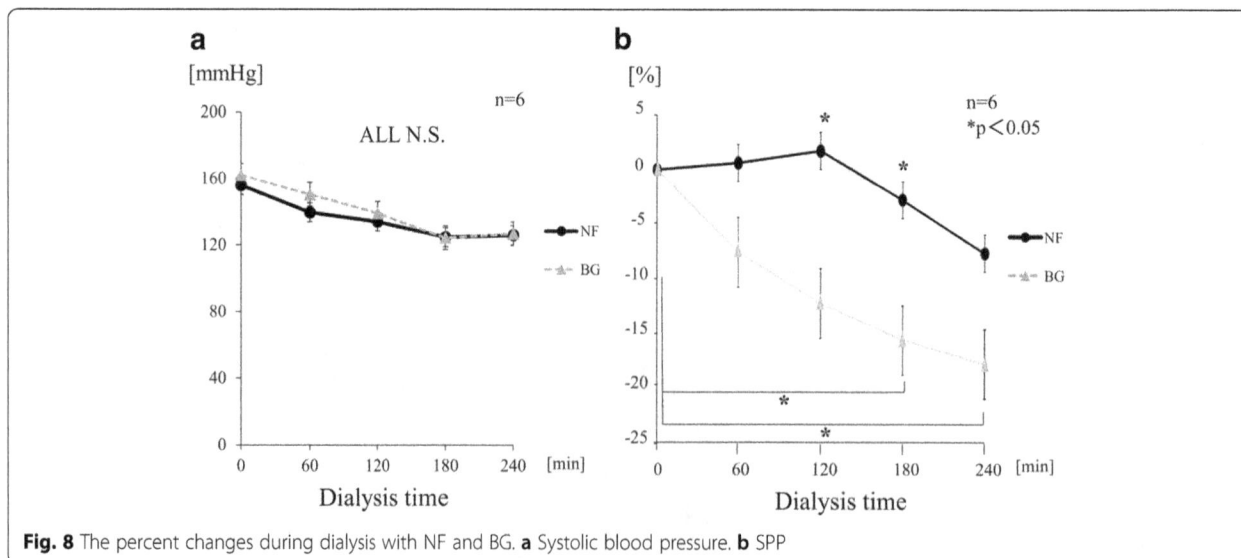

Fig. 8 The percent changes during dialysis with NF and BG. **a** Systolic blood pressure. **b** SPP

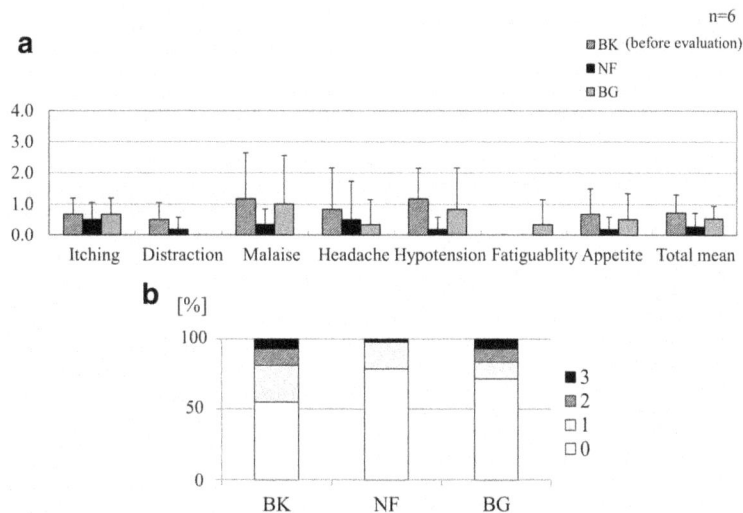

Fig. 9 The results of investigation of dialysis-related side effects under using PMMA dialyzers. **a** Score by item (mean ± SD). **b** Frequency by score

Conclusions

The new PMMA dialyzer NF shows substantially improved hemocompatibility. We expect this product will improve the condition of chronic dialysis patients.

Acknowledgements
Not applicable.

Funding
IM received research funds from Toray Industries, Inc.

Authors' contributions
HF, YU, and HS performed the evaluations in vitro. IM, SE, AY, and TC performed the clinical study. IM was a major contributor in writing the manuscript. All authors read and approved the final manuscript.

Competing interests
Three of the authors (HF, YU and HS) are employees of Toray Industries, Inc. Four of the authors (IM, SE, AY, TC) are employees of Yabuki Hospital.

Author details
[1]Yabuki Hospital, Yamagata, Japan. [2]Advanced Materials Research Labs, Toray Industries, Inc., 2-2 Sonoyama 3-chome, Otsu, Shiga, Japan.

References
1. Birk HW, Kistner A, Wizemann V, Schutterle G. Protein adsorption by artificial membrane materials under filtration conditions. Artif Organs. 1995;19(5):411–5.
2. Tomisawa N, Yamashita AC. Amount of adsorbed albumin loss by dialysis membranes with protein adsorption. J Artif Organs. 2009;12:194–9.
3. Kato A, Takita T, Furuhashi M, Takahashi T, Watanabe T, Maruyama Y, Hishida A. Polymethylmethacrylate efficacy in reduction of renal itching in hemodialysis patients: crossover study and role of tumor necrosis factor-α. Artif Organs. 2001;25(6):441–7.
4. Lin HH, Liu YL, Liu JH, Chou CY, Yang YF, Kuo HL, Huang CC. Uremic pruritus, cytokines, and polymethylmethacrylate artificial kidney. Artif Organs. 2008;32(6):468–72.
5. Masakane I. High-quality dialysis: a lesson from the Japanese experience. NDT Plus. 2010;3(Suppl 1):i28–35.
6. Adera HM, James K, Castronuovo Jr JJ, et al. Prediction of amputation wound healing with skin perfusion pressure. J Vasc Surg. 1995;21:823–8.
7. Shimazaki M, Matsuki T, Yamauchi K, Iwata M, Takahashi H, Genda S, Ohata J, Nakamura Y, Inaba Y, Yokouchi S, Kikuiri T, Ashie T. Assessment of lower limb ischemia with measurement of skin perfusion pressure in patients on hemodialysis. Ther Apher Dial. 2007;11:196–201.
8. Hiratsuka M, Koyama K, Yamamoto J, Narita A, Sasakawa Y, Shimogushi H, Ogawa A, Kimura T, Mizuguchi K, Mizuno M. Skin perfusion pressure and the prevalence of atherothrombosis in hemodialysis patients. Ther Apher Dial. 2016;20:40–5.
9. Biasioli S, Schiavon R, Petrosino L, Cavallini L, Cavalcanti G, Fanti E, Zambello A, Borin D. Role of cellulosic and noncellulosic membranes in hyperhomocysteinemia and oxidative stress. ASAIO J. 2000;46:625–34.
10. Galli F, Benedetti S, Buoncristiani U, Piroddi M, Conte C, Canestrari F, Buoncristiani E, Floridi A. The effect of PMMA-based protein-leaking dialyzers on plasma homocysteine levels. Kidney Int. 2003;64:748–55.
11. Galli F, Benedetti S, Floridi A, Canestrari F, Piroddi M, Buoncristiani E, Buoncristiani U. Glycoxidation and inflammatory markers in patients on treatment with PMMA-based protein-leaking dialyzers. Kidney Int. 2005;67:750–9.
12. Niwa T, Asada H, Tsutsui S, Miyazaki T. Efficient removal of albumin-bound furancarboxylic acid by protein-leaking hemodialysis. Am J Nephrol. 1995;15:463–7.
13. Cohen G, Rudnicki M, Schmaldienst S, Horl WH. Effect of dialysis on serum/plasma levels of free immunoglobulin light chains in end-stage renal disease patients. Nephrol Dial Transplant. 2002;17:879–83.

14. Hata H, Nishi K, Oshihara W, Arai J, Shimizu K, Kawakita T, Nkamura M, Mitsuya H. Adsorption of Bence-Jones protein to polymethylmethacrylate membrane in primary amyloidosis. Amyloid. 2009;16(2):108–10.

15. Contin C, Lacraz A, Precigout V. Potential role of the soluble form of CD40 in deficient immunological function of dialysis patients: new findings of its amelioration using polymethylmethacrylate (PMMA) membrane. NDT Plus. 2010;3(Suppl 1):i20–7.

16. Duranti E, Duranti D. Polymethylmethacrylate strengthens antibody response hemodialysis patients not responding to hepatitis vaccine: preliminary data. MINERVA MED. 2011;102:1–2.

17. Kuramochi G, Shima K. Reduction of hepatitis C virus by dialysis membrane. J Artif Organs. 2001;4:146–9.

18. Kreusser W, Reiermann S, Vogelbusch G, Bartual J, Schulze E. Effect of different synthetic membranes on laboratory parameters survival in chronic haemodialysis patients. NDT Plus. 2010;3(Suppl 1):i12–9.

19. Aoike I. Clinical significance of protein adsorbable membranes-Long-term clinical effects and analysis using a proteomic technique. Nephrol Dial Transplant. 2007;22(Suppl 5):v13–9.

20. Sirolli V, Ballone E, Amoroso L, Liberato L, Mascio R, Cappelli P, Albertazzi A, and Bonomini M. Leukocyte adhesion molecules and leukocyte-platelet interactions during hemodialysis: effects of different synthetic membranes. Int J Artif Organs. 1999;22:536-542.

21. Sato M, Morita H, Ema H, Yamaguchi S, Amano I. Effect of different dialyzer membranes on cutaneous microcirculation during hemodialysis. Clin Nephrol. 2006;66:426–32.

22. Lopes AA, Albert JM, Young EW, et al. Screening for depression in hemodialysis patients: associations with diagnosis, treatment, and outcomes in the DOPPS. Kidney Int. 2004;66:2047–53.

23. Elder SJ, Pisoni RL, Akizawa T, Fissell R, Andreucci VE, Fukuhara S, Kurokawa K, Rayner HC, Furniss AL, Port FK, Saran R. Sleep quality predicts quality of life and mortality risk in haemodialysis patients: results from the Dialysis Outcomes and Practice Patterns Study (DOPPS). Nephrol Dial Transplant. 2008;23:998–1004.

24. Pisoni R, Wikstrom B, Elder SJ, Akizawa T, Asano Y, Keen ML, Saran R, Mendelssohn DC, Young EW, Port FK. Pruiritus in haemodialysis patients: international results from the Dialysis Outcomes and Practice Patterns Study (DOPPS). Nephrol Dial Transplant. 2006;21:3495–505.

25. Kobayashi S, Miyamoto M, Kurumatani H, Oka M, Maesato K, Mano T, Ikee R, Moriya H, Ohtake T. Increased leukocyte aggregates are associated with atherosclerosis in patients with hemodialysis. Hemodial Int. 2009;13:286–92.

13

Survival rates and causes of death in Vietnamese chronic hemodialysis patients

Bach Nguyen[1*] and Fumiko Fukuuchi[2]

Abstract

Background: Thirty years have passed since hemodialysis therapy first started in Vietnam. However, there have been no reports on information such as the survival rate, mortality, and cause of death of hemodialysis patients on a national level. The aim of this study is to retrospectively analyze the data on hemodialysis patients from the flagship hospital in Ho Chi Minh City and to shed light on the status of hemodialysis patients in Vietnam.

Methods: The patients in this report were all 18 years or older who underwent hemodialysis at the Thong Nhat Hospital between April 1997 and December 2014. There were a total of 349 patients, with 225 males and 124 females. Data was collected on the age, sex, primary causes of end-stage renal diseases, starting date of hemodialysis, vascular access, hemodialysis therapy prescription, hemodialysis dose, coexisting conditions, clinical test data, and cause of death. IBM's statistical analysis software SPSS Statistics 23.0 was used.

Results: The survival time after hemodialysis introduction was 5.27 ± 0.31 years (mean ± standard deviation). The factors which impacted the survival rate included being 60 years of age or older at the initiation of hemodialysis, being male, coexisting conditions, and vascular access apart from an artery venous fistula. The prognosis of diabetic patients suffering from renal failure was poor when compared to that of patients without diabetes; however, there was no statistical significance. The most common cause of death was cardiovascular disease (46.1%), followed by other causes (11.8%) and unknown causes (23.6%).

Conclusions: Our data shows that mean survival time was shorter than that in other countries. One-year and 5-year survival rates were not so different. However, a 10-year survival rate was very low. Significant risk factors were not so special, but we have a problem in medical cost in Vietnam. To improve the long-term survival rate, we are trying to change the situation.

Keywords: Survival rate, Maintenance hemodialysis, Vietnamese adults

Background

There is no national data available for the survival rate and cause of death in hemodialysis patients in Vietnam. While this data is only for a single hospital, we hope to gain an understanding of the situation regarding hemodialysis patients in Vietnam and we started with this investigation.

There are aspects with the hemodialysis patients in Vietnam that are different from those in other countries. First, the starting point for hemodialysis therapy is delayed. There is a tendency to prolong the starting point of hemodialysis as long as possible. The economic situation also plays a role in this tendency. The cost of one session of hemodialysis is US$20, which is cheap when compared to that in other countries. Note that the government's health insurance generally covers the reuse of a dialyzer for up to six times. If a patient wishes to extend the treatment further, the patient must pay for the expense himself or herself. There is also an insurance system that provides assistance for the poor; however, there is not enough money to introduce hemodialysis. Hemodialysis is only used when patient's circumstances take a turn for the worse including increased risk and the situation calls for it. In addition, there is also a variance in the proportion of diseases similar to other Asian countries. The Doi Moi Policy

* Correspondence: nguyenbach69@gmail.com
[1]Department of Nephrology and Dialysis, Thong Nhat Hospital, 01 Ly Thuong Kiet Street, Tan Binh Dist, Ho Chi Minh City, Vietnam
Full list of author information is available at the end of the article

introduced economic reforms in 1986, and the number of infections decreased, which had previously accounted for more than 50% of all deaths. This figure dropped to below 20% in 2005. On the other hand, a change in lifestyle most likely caused an increase in circulatory diseases and diabetes. The number of deaths caused by non-infectious diseases, including malignant neoplasms or growths, exceeds 62%.

Based on this medical data and the conditions in Vietnam, we shall perform an analysis on the survival rate and cause of death in hemodialysis patients.

Methods

Patients

All patients in this study were 18 years or older who underwent hemodialysis at the Thong Nhat Hospital between April 1997 and December 2014. This is the first class, governmental, and teaching hospital with 700 beds in 1997 and upgraded 1200 beds in 2014. There were only 10 hemodialysis machines sponsored by a Japanese donor in 1997 and increased to 25 machines in 2014. Hemodialysis center is open 24 h per day with four sections and serves around 360 new patients annually. Some of stable patients were transferred back to provincial hospitals around Ho Chi Minh City for chronic hemodialysis.

All patients included in this study met the following conditions: (1) patients who received the appropriate hemodialysis prescription (the standard for hemodialysis was $kt/v > 1.2$), (2) patients who underwent hemodialysis for more than 1 month, and (3) patients that have all patient data available. The following patients were excluded: (1) cases in which the patient could have suffered from acute kidney injury or could have withdrawn from hemodialysis therapy and (2) patients who are undergoing or underwent hemodialysis at other hospitals.

The standard for introducing hemodialysis therapy to patients was a creatinine clearance that is less than 10 mL/min for non-diabetic patients and a creatinine clearance of 15 mL/min for diabetic patients. In terms of the hemodialysis conditions, a bicarbonate dialysate was used, and the dialysate flow rate was 500 mL/min. The blood flow rate (mL/min) was $5 \times$ DW (dry weight) and 250–300 mL/min in average. A standard heparin was used as an anticoagulant. All the patients were dialyzed three times per week, and the average duration per dialysis session was 4 h with Nipro and Nikkiso Machines. The dialyzer was selected based on the financial status of the patient. The dialyzer was reused on average up to six times. The target hemoglobin level for anemia treatment was 10 g/dL or greater.

Coexisting conditions included cardiovascular diseases (myocardial infarction, congestive heart failure, atherosclerosis, cerebrovascular accident, cardiac arrhythmia, and thoracic or abdominal artery aneurysm), cirrhosis, malignant tumors, tuberculosis, gastric ulcers, malnutrition, cognitive disorders, hematologic diseases, and chronic obstructive pulmonary disease. The causes of death were divided into six categories: (1) myocardial infarction, (2) heart failure, (3) infections, (4) stroke, (5) others, and (6) unknown cause of death.

Table 1 Baseline characteristics of the chronic hemodialysis patients ($n = 349$)

Baseline characteristics of the patients	Number of patient (%)
Age at the initiation of hemodialysis ($\overline{X}$ ±SD, years)	65.24 ± 12.56 (22–96)
Age group at the start of hemodialysis	
<60	85 (24.4)
60–69	129 (37)
70–79	97 (27.8)
≥80	38 (77.55)
Male	225 (64.5)
Primary causes of end-stage renal disease	
Diabetes	153 (43.8)
Hypertension	109 (31.2)
Chronic glomerulonephritis	35 (10)
Unknown	52 (14.9)
Coexisting conditions	180 (51.6)
Cardiovascular diseases[a]	109 (31.2)
Tuberculosis	10 (3.72)
Liver cirrhosis	20 (5.73)
Dementia	19 (5.44)
Malignancy	15 (4.29)
Chronic obstructive pulmonary disease	7 (2.01)
Serum albumin ≥35 g/dL	279 (79.94)
Erythropoietin use (subcutaneous route)	349 (100)
Hemoglobin ≥10 g/dL	198 (56.73)
The initiation of chronic hemodialysis with sudden change	330 (94.56)
Hemodialyzed by a high-flux dialyzer	192 (55.01)
Reuse of a dialyzer	324 (92.84)
Follow-up period of patients (month)	
Median (25–75%)	25(10–51.5)
Minimum–maximum	1–172

[a]Cardiovascular diseases (myocardial infarction, congestive heart failure, cerebrovascular accident, arrhythmia, thoracic or abdominal artery aneurysm, and coronary artery diseases)

Survival Function

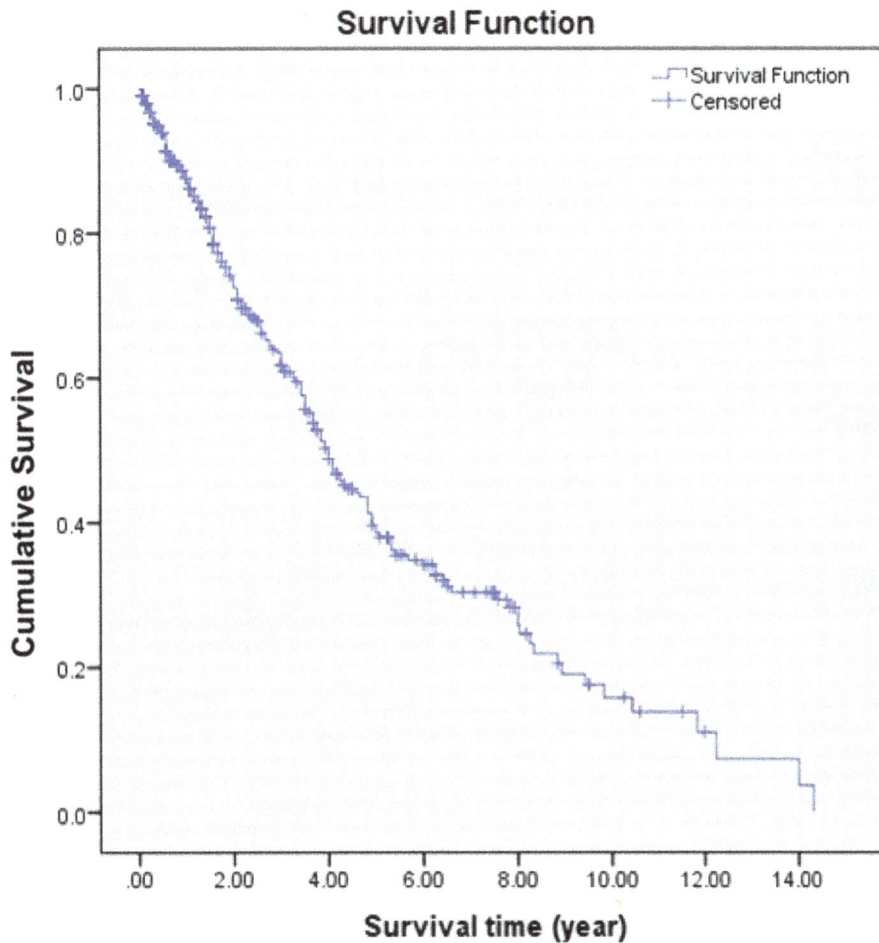

Fig. 1 Kaplan–Meier survival curves of chronic hemodialysis

Methods

This was a retrospective, observational study to evaluate the survival rate and causes of death in chronic hemodialysis patients at the Thong Nhat Hospital.

Statistical analysis

IBM's statistical analysis software SPSS Statistics 23.0 was used. The percentage and mean ± SD of the mean were used to describe categorical and continuous variables, respectively. The Kaplan–Meier method was used to calculate the cumulative survival rate, and the log-rank test, for extracting the factors that impacted the survival rate, was used to examine the data. In addition, the Cox proportional hazards model or regression analysis was used to calculate the hazard rate. For univariate analysis, a cross tabulation was created for one factor/variable and a chi-squared (χ^2) test was performed. Any factor that was determined significant in the univariate analysis was used in the multivariate analysis. In the two-tailed test, the statistical significance was computed as $p < 0.05$.

Table 2 Factors affecting survival time

Factors	Mean survival time (year)	χ^{2a}	p
Age group at the initiation of hemodialysis			
≥60	3.64	11.496	0.0007
<60	8.27		
End-stage renal disease caused by diabetes			
Yes	3.53	2.754	0.097
No	4.62		
Sex			
Male	3.74	4.821	0.028
Female	5.07		
Coexisting conditions			
Yes	3.37	13.896	0.0002
No	6.01		
Vascular access			
Arteriovenous fistula	4.47	87.10	0.0032
Arteriovenous graft, tunnel permanent catheter	2.82		

aLog-rank test

Results

Table 1 shows the patient background or baseline characteristics. The total number of patients was 349. The average age at the initiation of hemodialysis was 65.25 ± 12.56 years (mean $\pm$ standard deviation). There were 225 males and 124 females. Eighty-five patients (24.4%) started hemodialysis before 60 years of age. The most common primary disease was diabetes, found in 43.8% of the patients. Chronic glomerulonephritis was found in 10% of the patients. The primary disease was unknown in 14.9% of the patients. The introduction of hemodialysis due to a sudden change in the patient's condition occurred in 94.56% of the patients. These patients were admitted to the hospital because of acute complications of ESRD such as pulmonary edema, hyperkalemia, severe metabolic acidosis, and severe congestive heart failure. The introduction of hemodialysis was scheduled or planned for only 19 patients (5.44%). The poor management of chronic kidney diseases in primary health care system is responsible for this problem. Coexisting conditions were found in 51.6% of the patients, and the most common coexisting conditions were cardiovascular

complications, existing in 31.2% of the patients. Erythropoietin is generally administered as a subcutaneous injection. A high-flux dialyzer was used in 55.01% of the patients and was only single use in 7.16% of the patients. The average follow-up time was 25 months.

Figure 1 shows the cumulative survival rate for all the patients. The average survival time is 5.27 ± 0.31 years (mean $\pm$ standard deviation). Eighty-five percent of the patients had a 1-year survival rate, 58% had a 5-year survival rate, and 20% had a 10-year survival rate. The cumulative survival rate calculated using the Kaplan–Meier method is displayed according to each factor, and the log-rank test is used to compare those factors (Table 2). First, the patients were compared dividing the age at the initiation of hemodialysis into two groups (Fig. 2): under 60 years old and 60 years of age or older. There was a significant decrease in the survival rate for the 60 years of age and older group.

After comparing the survival times between the diabetic patients and the non-diabetic patients, the non-diabetic patient group had an average survival time of 5.71 ± 0.41 years

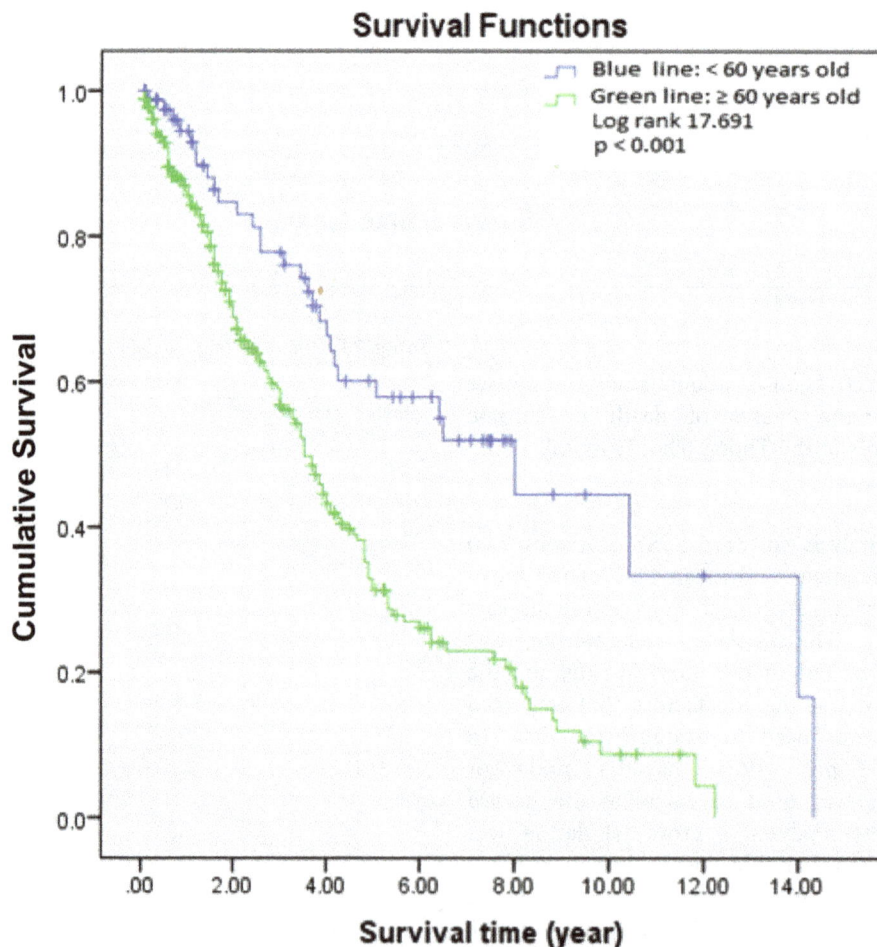

Fig. 2 Factor (60 years of age or older at initiation of hemodialysis) added to Kaplan–Meier and log-rank test

(mean ± standard deviation), and the diabetic patient group had an average survival time of 4.45 ± 0.36 years (Fig. 3). The diabetic patient group had a lower survival rate; however, there was no statistical significance. When comparing the males and females, the females had a significantly higher survival rate. The average survival time for males was 4.77 ± 0.348 years, and the average for females was 6.00 ± 0.500 years (Fig. 4). There was also a significant difference seen even between the patient group with coexisting conditions and the group without them. The survival time for the patient group with coexisting conditions was 6.91 ± 0.598 years, and it was 4.285 ± 0.327 years for the patient group without coexisting conditions (Fig. 5). In addition, there was a significant difference seen even with the vascular access. Compared to the patient group with an arteriovenous fistula, the patient group using an arteriovenous graft or tunnel permanent catheter had a significantly lower survival time (Fig. 6). A multivariate analysis was performed using a Cox proportional hazards model on those factors that showed a significant difference. The vascular access problems affected the survival rate with a hazard rate

of 1.395. The survival curve for the covariate average values approaches the survival curve computed using the Kaplan–Meier method (Table 3). In the cause of death analysis, cardiovascular deaths were the most common at 46.1%, and infections were next in line at 18.5%. Cirrhosis, malignant tumors, tuberculosis, and traffic accident deaths all together accounted for 11.8%. Unknown cause of death accounted for 23.6% (Table 4). The patients with an unknown cause of death were cases in which the patients died at home.

In a multivariate analysis using the Cox proportional hazards model, a univariate chi-squared (χ^2) test was performed on the three factors (sex, age at the initiation of hemodialysis, coexisting conditions) with a hazard rate of less than 1 and on the presence of diabetes. There was no significance with the presence of diabetes; however, being male, being 60 years of age or older at the initiation of hemodialysis, and having coexisting conditions had a significant impact on the survival time (Table 3). A logistic regression analysis was carried out using these factors. Patients having coexisting conditions had the most impact with a 3.174 odds ratio. Being male and being 60 years of

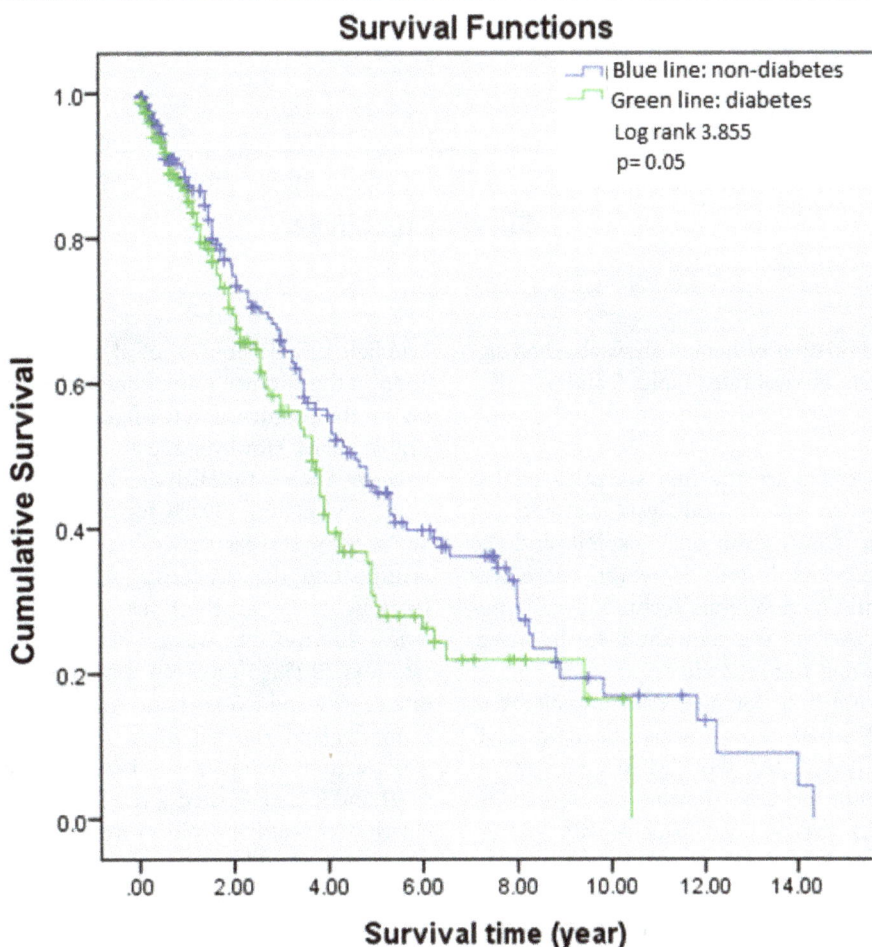

Fig. 3 Factors (primary disease and diabetic nephropathy) added to Kaplan–Meier and log-rank test

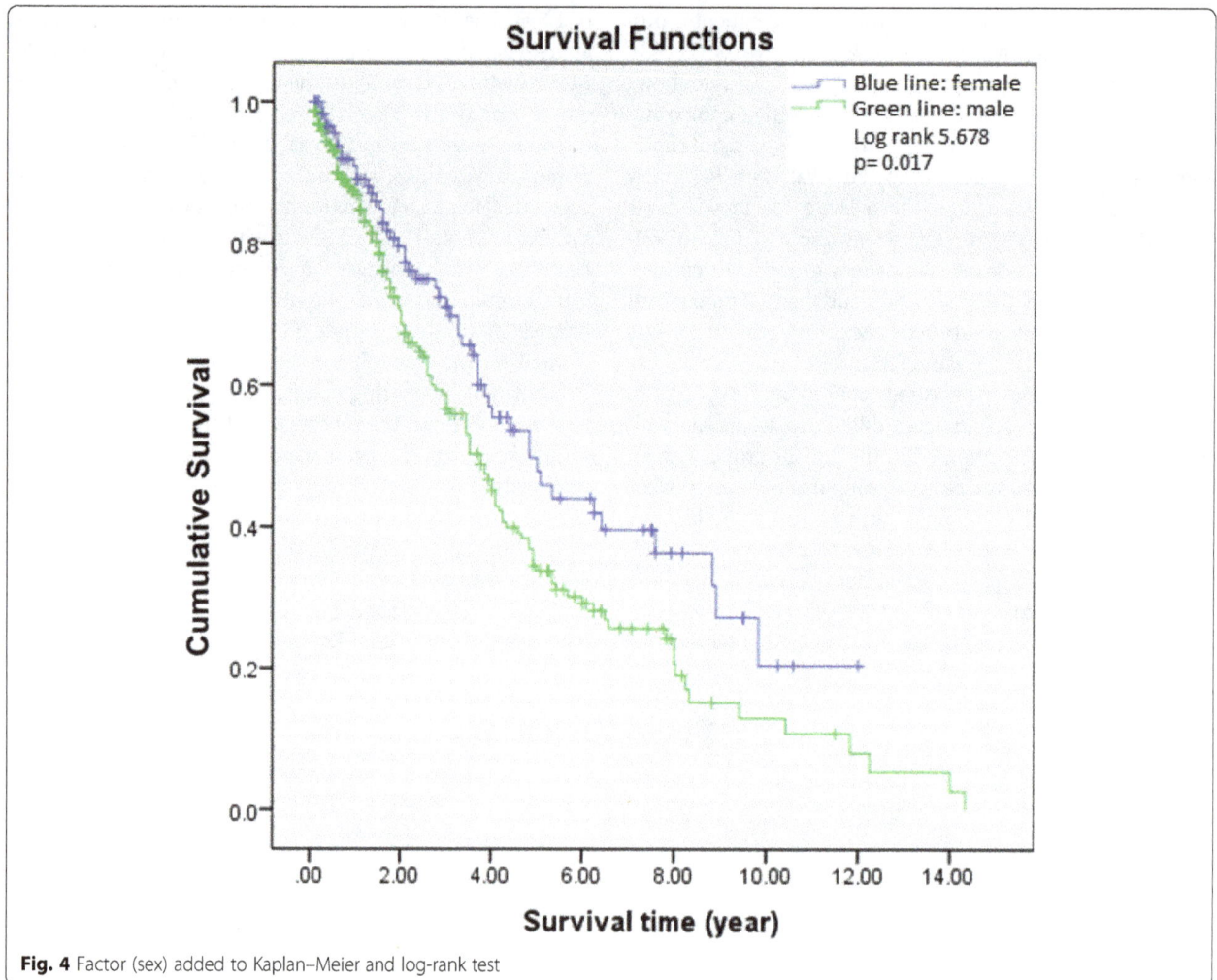

Fig. 4 Factor (sex) added to Kaplan–Meier and log-rank test

age or older at the initiation of hemodialysis also had significant impact on the survival rate (Tables 5 and 6).

Discussion

Our investigation results are the first statistics related to the survival rate of hemodialysis patients in Vietnam. The data is only from one hospital, and the total number of patients is low. However, there was little variation in the hemodialysis technique and prescription, and the therapy regimen could be followed, thereby also increasing the reliability.

The average survival time for hemodialysis patients in this study was 5.27 ± 0.31 years (mean $\pm$ standard deviation). These time periods are short when compared to those in a report from the USA showing female patients with an average of 7.1 years and male patients with an average of 7.2 years [1]. With regard to the survival rate, 85% of the patients had a 1-year survival rate, 58% had a 5-year survival rate, and 20% had a 10-year survival rate. Survival time of our patients was better than that of Sawhney S et al. in British Columbia and Scotland [2] and Seyed

Seifollah Beladi Mousavi et al. in Iran [3]. There is variation in the survival rate of hemodialysis patients depending on the country, and the figures cannot be compared in simple terms. However, the annual statistics report by The Japanese Society for Dialysis Therapy shows 87.6% for a 1-year survival rate, 59.8% for a 5-year survival rate, and 36.3% for a 10-year survival rate in 2013 [4]. In a report investigating the prognosis of hemodialysis patients in Japan by Iseki et al., the 1-year survival rate was 87.4%, the 5-year survival rate was 60.9%, and the 10-year survival rate was 39.1% [5]. Korean data showed a 1-year survival rate of 94% and a 5-year survival rate of 66% [6]. A report from England showed improvement between 1997 and 2006, with a change in the 1-year survival rate from 85.9 to 91.5%. It also showed a rise in the survival rate for the elderly (65 years and older) from 63.8 to 72.9% [7]. Our investigation results are comparable to the data from these countries for the 1- and 5-year survival rates, but the 10-year survival rate is lower. Improvements need to be made for the prognosis of hemodialysis patients with respect to long-term care.

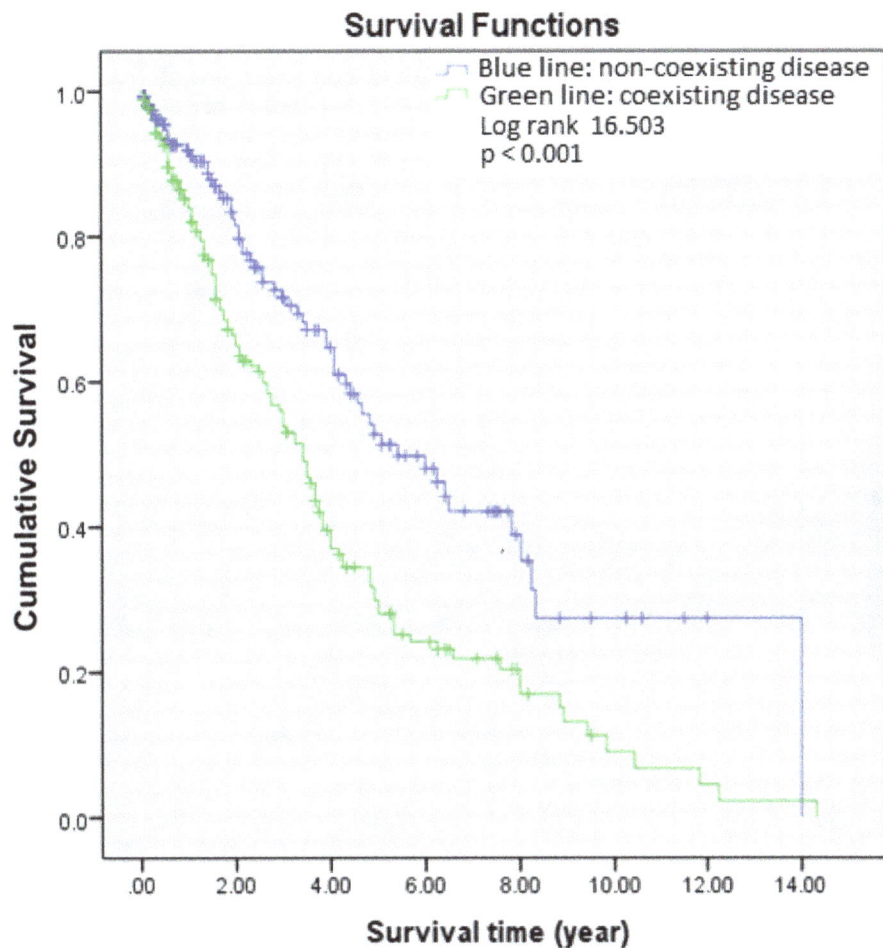

Fig. 5 Factor (coexisting conditions) added to Kaplan–Meier and log-rank test

Vascular access problems, being 60 years of age or older at the initiation of hemodialysis, being male, and having coexisting conditions were reported as factors that impact the survival rate. Using a catheter or arteriovenous graft can adversely impact the prognosis, which is consistent with other investigation results. Shunt clotting can be attributed to the impact from diabetes or arteriosclerosis [8, 9]. Other investigations as well have indicated that female hemodialysis patients tend to have a better prognosis [1]. There were no new risk factors that were specifically identified in this investigation. As noted in the results from this investigation, the aging of patients at the initiation of hemodialysis is becoming a problem in other countries as well [10, 11]. The report from England indicates that the age of patients at the initiation of hemodialysis greatly influences the prognosis. When comparing the 5-year survival rates, the survival rate is 70% for patients who are between 45 and 54 years old at the initiation of hemodialysis and only 30% when the patient is between 65 and 74 years old [12]. In addition, a report by Uchida et al. shows a 65% 3-year survival rate for the

patient group who have an age of 61.7 ± 14.4 years at the initiation of hemodialysis [13]. The average age at the initiation of hemodialysis for the patient groups of our investigation was 65.24 ± 12.56 years, with a 5-year survival rate of 58%, but there is nothing that can really be done about this. Although it must be considered that almost hemodialysis introduction has been done in emergency in Vietnam, emergency hemodialysis introduction is very hard for old patients. We know that it is better to do planned hemodialysis introduction, but it is impossible in Vietnam now. It is caused by poor management of chronic kidney disease (CKD) and economical problem. It is very difficult for us to do adequate treatment in time. We are short of doctors and medical system to follow up CKD patients. We are trying better in the future.

Similarly, to other countries, the number one cause of death was cardiovascular death. After that, what is distinctive about our investigation is infections. Death caused by infection was primarily pneumonia-related. Even in Vietnam, the country is in a transitional phase, moving from developing status to developed status; the

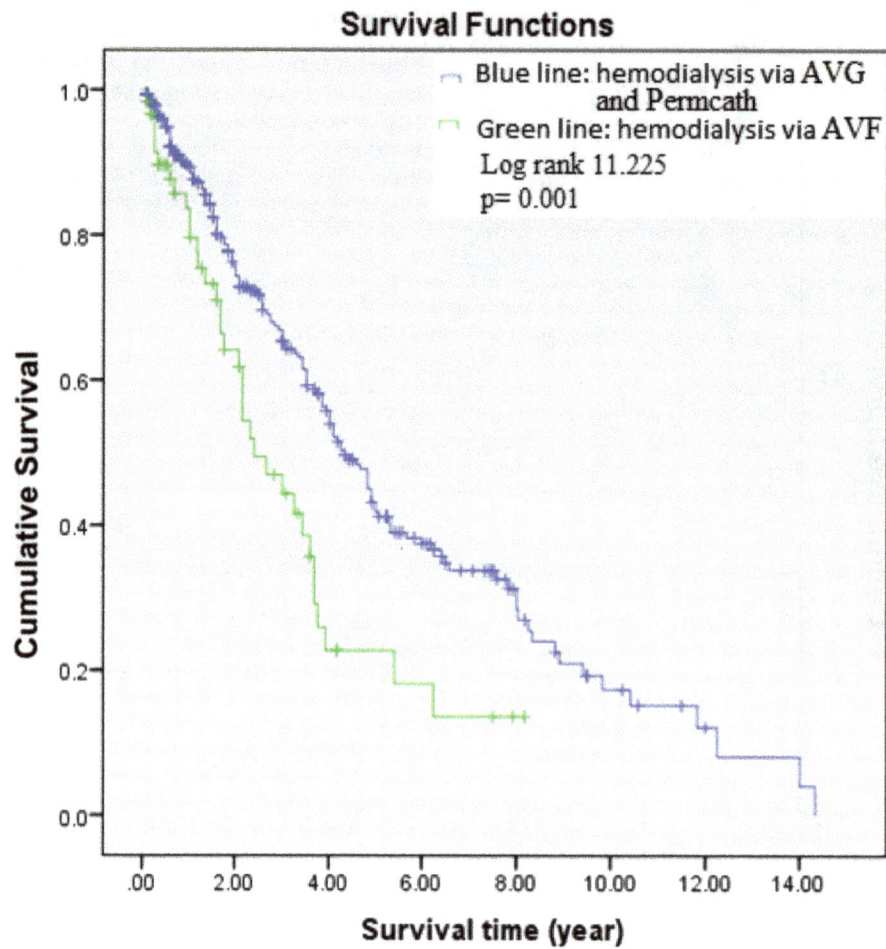

Fig. 6 Factor (vascular access) added to Kaplan–Meier and log-rank test

Table 3 Multivariate analysis: Cox proportional hazards model including factors predicting mortality

Factors	B	SE	x^2	p	Hazard ratio	CI 95% for HR
Age group at the initiation of hemodialysis ≥60	−0.701	0.210	11.080	0.001	0.496	0.423–0.793
Male	−0.545	0.176	9.626	0.002	0.580	0.411–0.818
Coexisting conditions	−0.546	0.161	11.578	0.001	0.579	0.423–0.793
Vascular access via arteriovenous graft, tunnel permanent catheter	−0.772	0.204	14.374	<0.001	0.462	0.310–0.689

Table 4 Causes of death (n = 178)

Causes of death	Number of patient	Percentage (%)
Stroke	43	24.2
Heart failure	28	15.7
Myocardial infarction	11	6.2
Infections with etiologies from	33	18.5
Respiratory system	16	
Gastrology	6	
Urology	3	
Others	8	
Other causes[a]	21	11.8
Unknown causes	42	23.6

[a]Liver cirrhosis, malignancy, tuberculosis, and transportation accident

Table 5 Univariate comparison of factors between patients alive and dead

Factors	Alive (n = 171)	Dead (n = 178)	p
Male, n (%)	98 (57.31)	127 (71.35)	0.004
End-stage renal disease caused by diabetes, n (%)	74 (43.27)	79 (44.38)	0.460
Age at the initiation of hemodialysis ($\bar{X}$ ± SD)	61.74 ± 13.68	68.61 ± 10.12	<0.001
Age group at the initiation of hemodialysis			
<60	55 (32.16)	30 (23.62)	
60–69	64 (37.43)	65 (36.52)	0.002
70–79	39 (22.81)	58 (32.58)	
≥80	13 (7.6)	27 (15.16)	
Coexisting conditions, n (%)	62 (36.26)	118 (66.29)	<0.001

diet has become more westernized. As a result, conditions attributed to lifestyle and diet as well as diabetic patients are also increasing. It is known that diabetic patients undergoing hemodialysis are more susceptible to infection. It is likely that improvements in the sanitary conditions in Vietnam have had a positive impact on the prognosis of hemodialysis patients.

We hope to see improvements not only in the sanitary conditions but in the current low-cost hemodialysis as well. The current cost of hemodialysis for a single session in Vietnam is approximately US$20. In order to achieve this low cost, the dialyzer is reused up to six times. The same blood circuit or access is also reused depending on the circumstances. A high-flux dialyzer and single-use application can be effective for the prognosis of hemodialysis patients for long-term care, but it is quite difficult to achieve this immediately. However, we would like to strive toward making this a reality.

Limitations to the study
This study has several limitations like the lack of longitudinal data on all the risk factors such as serum calcium, phosphate, serum albumin, glucose control, lipid profile, and dialyzers, and causes of death might be incorrect, especially in dialysis patients who died at home.

Table 6 Multinominal logistic regression of factor predicting mortality

Factors	B	SE	χ^2	p	Hazard ratio	CI 95% for HR
Age ≥60 years old	−0.337	0.124	7.390	0.007	0.714	0.560–0.910
Male	−0.536	0.240	5.498	0.019	0.570	0.356–0.912
Coexisting conditions	−1.142	0.230	24.554	<0.001	0.319	0.230–0.510

Conclusions
This is the first published statistics related to the survival rate of hemodialysis patients in Vietnam, although the data is only from one hospital. We hope this paper is useful to improve the long-term survival rate in hemodialysis patients in Vietnam.

Abbreviations
AVF: Arteriovenous fistula; AVG: Arteriovenous graft; CHD: Chronic hemodialysis; ESRD: End-stage renal disease; HD: Hemodialysis; Permcath: Permanent catheter (tunnel permanent catheter)

Acknowledgements
We thank the directors of the Thong Nhat Hospital, Prof Nguyen Manh Phan and Prof Nguyen Duc Cong for their encouragements, Ms Vu Thi Hoa and Ms Hua To Hoa for assisting us in collecting the data.

Funding
This study has not received any grants.

Authors' contributions
BN carried out the design of the study and collected the data. FF participated in the design of the study, performed the statistical analysis, and edited the draft. Both authors read and approved the final manuscript.

Competing interests
The authors declare that they have no competing interests.

Author details
[1]Department of Nephrology and Dialysis, Thong Nhat Hospital, 01 Ly Thuong Kiet Street, Tan Binh Dist, Ho Chi Minh City, Vietnam. [2]Department of Nephrology and Dialysis, Hayama Heart Center, Hayama, Japan.

References
1. United States Renal Data System. 2008 Annual Data Report. Am J Kidney Dis. 2009;53(1 Suppl):S1-374. doi:10.1053/j.ajkd.2008.10.005.
2. Sawhney S, Djurdjev O, Simpson K, et al. Survival and dialysis initiation: comparing British Columbia and Scotland registries. Nephrol Dial Transplant. 2009;24(10):3186–92.
3. Seyed S, Beladi M, Fatemeh H, et al. Comparison of survival in patients with end-stage renal disease. Receiving hemodialysis versus peritoneal dialysis. Saudi J Kidney Dis Transpl. 2015;26(2):392-7.
4. An overview of regular dialysis treatment in Japan as of 31 December 2003. Patient Registration Committee, Japanese Society for Dialysis Therapy, Tokyo, Japan. et al. Ther Apher Dial. 2005.
5. Iseki K, Shinzato T, Nagura Y, Akiba T. Factors influencing long-term survival in patients on chronic dialysis. Clin Exp Nephrol. 2004;8(2):89–97.
6. Jin DC. Current status of dialysis therapy in Korea. Korean J Intern Med. 2011;26:123–31.
7. Ansell D, Roderick P, Hodsman A, Ford D, Steenkamp R, Tomson C. UK Renal Registry 11th Annual Report (December 2008): Chapter 7 survival and causes of death of UK adult patients on renal replacement therapy in 2007: national and centre-specific analyses. Nephron Clin Pract. 2009;111 Suppl 1: c113–39.
8. Wolfe RA. The standardized mortality ratio revisited; improvements; innovations. Am J Kidney Dis. 1994;24:290–7.

9.   Wolfe RA, Sheraon TE, Ashby VB, Messana JM. Decreases in catheter uses are associated with decreases in mortality for dialysis facilities during 2000-03. Abstract Renal Week 2005, SA-FC063

10.   Choi J-Y, Jang HM, Jongha P, et al. Survival Advantage of Peritoneal Dialysis Relative to Hemodialysis in the Early Period of Incident Dialysis Patients: A Nationwide Prospective Propensity- Matched Study in Korea. PLoS One. 2013;8(12):e84257. doi:10.1371/journal.pone.0084257. eCollection 2013.

11.   Browne OT , Allgar V, Bhandari S. Analysis of factors predicting mortality of new patients commencing renal replacement therapy 10 years of follow-up. BMC Nephrol. 2014;15:20. doi:10.1186/1471-2369-15-20.

12.   Levy J, Brown E, Daley C, Lawrence A. Death in dialysis patient. Principles of dialysis. Oxford Handbook of Dialysis. 3th Edition. Oxford University Press; 2009. pp 566–8.

13.   Uchida K, Shoda J, Sugahara S, et al. Comparison and survival of patients receiving hemodialysis and peritoneal dialysis in a single center. Adv Perit Dial. 2007;23:144–17.

14

Histopathological findings in transplanted kidneys

Ai Katsuma, Takafumi Yamakawa, Yasuyuki Nakada, Izumi Yamamoto[*] and Takashi Yokoo

Abstract

Improvements in immunosuppression have reduced acute kidney allograft rejection and clinicians are now seeking ways to prolong allograft survival to 20 years and beyond. The primary cause of kidney allograft loss is still chronic rejection, followed by death with a functioning allograft and primary kidney disease recurrence. Thus, overcoming kidney allograft rejection remains the most important issue. Kidney allograft rejection can be classified into two types: T cell- and antibody-mediated rejection. Both are diagnosed pathologically based on the Banff 2013 classification. Other important pathological features in addition to rejection include calcineurin inhibitor toxicity, polyomavirus nephropathy, and recurrence of the primary kidney disease. Here, we review the diagnosis and representative features of histopathological findings in transplanted kidneys.

Keywords: Transplant kidney pathology, Antibody-mediated rejection, T cell-mediated rejection, Calcineurin inhibitor (CNI) nephrotoxicity, Polyoma virus nephropathy, Recurrence of primary kidney disease

Background

Kidney transplantation enhances the quality of life and patient survival in end-stage renal disease (ESRD). The total number of kidney transplantations has increased 1.6-fold over the past decade in Japan. The Japanese Society for Clinical Renal Transplantation (JSCRT) reported that the total number of renal transplantations in 2015 was 1661 versus 994 in 2005. JSCRT data obtained since 2000 showed that the 10-year patient and graft survival times were 93.8 and 80.2%, respectively (http://www.asas.or.jp/jst/pdf/factbook/factbook/2015.pdf).

Reasons for graft loss were primarily chronic rejection (47%), followed by acute rejection (6.2%), and recurrence of the original kidney disease (1.8%) (http://www.asas.or.jp/jst/pdf/factbook/factbook2015.pdf). These data clearly suggest that the diagnosis and treatment of kidney allograft rejection remains the most important issue. Rates of acute rejection in the first year post-transplant have improved consistently since 2008 and remain similar for deceased- and living-donor recipients. For the period 2012–2013, only 8.5% of patients with deceased-donor kidneys and 8.1% with living-donor kidneys experienced

acute rejection (T cell- or antibody-mediated) by 1 year after kidney transplantation [1]. Risk factors for acute rejection—T cell- and/or antibody-mediated—include the degree of histocompatibility between the donor and recipient, the level of presensitization [previous graft, pregnancy, blood transfusion], immunosuppressive drug regimens, and the level of patient adherence with daily therapy [2]. Current immunosuppressive drug protocols with calcineurin inhibitors (CNIs), steroids, and mycophenolate mofetil (MMF) have reduced the frequency of acute T cell-mediated rejection (TCMR) considerably [3].

Kidney allograft rejection can be classified into two types: T cell- and antibody-mediated rejection (ABMR). Both are diagnosed pathologically based on the Banff 2013 classification. The Banff meeting, firstly started in 1991 by Prof. Kim Solez of University of Alberta, is a consensus meeting regarding allograft pathology that has been held every 2 years. The latest version of the Banff classification was prepared in 2013. The Banff classification consists of the following six categories: (1) normal, (2) ABMR, (3) borderline changes, (4) TCMR, (5) interstitial fibrosis and tubular atrophy (IF/TA), and (6) other. It should be noted that not only rejection but also additional histopathological findings, such as CNI toxicity and polyomavirus nephropathy, may overlap [4]. Here, we introduce

* Correspondence: izumi26@jikei.ac.jp
Division of Nephrology and Hypertension, Department of Internal Medicine, The Jikei University School of Medicine, 3-25-8, Nishi-Shimbashi, Minato-ku, Tokyo 105-8461, Japan

details of the classification and discuss representative histopathological findings from transplanted kidneys.

Kidney allograft rejection

ABMR

ABMR was first recognized in 1996 in the form of hyperacute rejection in patients with pre-transplant donor-specific antibodies (DSAs) [5]. DSAs, largely reactive to human leukocyte antigens (HLAs), are now recognized as a significant cause of ABMR [6]. In the Banff classification, ABMR is divided into two types: acute/active ABMR (acute ABMR) and chronic/active ABMR (chronic ABMR).

Acute ABMR occurs in patients who develop a threshold level of antidonor antibodies after transplantation or who were presensitized and transplanted after desensitization. Acute ABMR occurs most commonly 1–3 weeks after transplantation, particularly in desensitized patients, but can develop suddenly at any time. The primary risk factor for acute ABMR is presensitization [blood transfusion, pregnancy, prior transplant], as judged by a historical positive cross-match or high levels of panel-reactive antibody (PRA), flow cytometry cross-match, or LABScreen methods [6, 7].

In contrast, chronic ABMR typically presents insidiously, several years after transplantation. Chronic ABMR develops through a number of stages over many months to years [8]. The mechanism for the development of chronic ABMR consists of four steps:(1) de novo DSA production, (2) interaction of de novo DSA with the microvascular endothelium, resulting in C4d positivity, (3) specific histopathological changes, such as transplant glomerulopathy and peritubular capillary basement membrane multilayering accompanied by microvascular inflammation, and (4) increased serum creatinine. This sequence is based on several observations. For example, in non-presensitized patients, de novo DSA preceded the onset of proteinuria by an average of 9 months and the onset of elevated serum creatinine by 12 months [9]. Additionally, Regele et al. showed that, in the first year post-transplant, patients with C4d+ biopsies had a higher frequency of transplant glomerulopathy (TG) and representative histopathology of chronic ABMR in later biopsies [10].

In the past decade, it has become clear that late-graft failure is often due to chronic ABMR [9, 11]. Indeed, ~60% of late-graft failure is due to chronic ABMR [12]. The histological features of acute ABMR are not absolutely specific and are thus insufficient alone for a definitive diagnosis. The Banff 2013 classification included a scheme for ABMR that required both pathological and clinical laboratory elements, as follows: (1) characteristic histological manifestations of both acute and chronic ABMR, (2) DSA-induced endothelial cell injury, represented by C4d positivity, microvascular inflammation

(MVI), or the expression of activated endothelial gene transcripts (ENDATs), and (3) DSA positivity (Table 1).

Characteristic histological manifestations of acute ABMR

Histological evidence of acute ABMR has been divided into four types, based on light microscopy: (1) MVI with neutrophils and mononuclear cells in capillaries (i.e., transplant glomerulitis and peritubular capillaritis) (Fig. 1a, b), (2) intimal or transmural arteritis (Fig. 1c), (3) acute thrombotic microangiopathy (TMA) (Fig. 1d), and (4) acute tubular injury in the absence of any other cause. Transplant glomerulitis is characterized histologically by glomerular MVI and the enlargement of endothelial cells. Glomerular capillaries have neutrophils in 10–55% and mononuclear glomerulitis in 19–90% [13, 14] of cases (Fig. 1a). In the Banff 2013 classification, determination of the numerical transplant glomerulitis (g) score was still based on the percentage of glomeruli involved [15]: 1–25, 26–50, and >50% for g1, g2, and g3, respectively (Table 2). Indeed, the scoring of glomerulitis based on these fractions of involved glomeruli using the definition above was superior to scoring based on numbers of leukocytes per glomerulus, even when CD68 staining was added. In addition to these conventional criteria, endothelial swelling and capillary occlusion were adopted as a definition of transplant glomerulitis at the Banff 2013 meeting [16].

Peritubular capillaritis shows findings of dilated peritubular capillaries (PTCs) containing three to four more inflammatory cells per cross section in more than 10% of PTCs in non-atrophic cortex. Determination of the peritubular capillaritis (ptc) score is based on the number of inflammatory cells involved: 3–4, 5–10, and >10 for ptc1, ptc2, and ptc3, respectively (Fig. 1b). The scores refer to the highest number of cells in a single PTC (Table 2). Diffuse capillaritis in early protocol biopsies showed a significant negative prognostic impact in terms of glomerular filtration rate 2 years later. Subsequent work on the specificity and sensitivity of capillaritis, by Sis et al. in 329 indication biopsies [17], revealed peritubular capillaritis in not only 75% of acute and chronic ABMR biopsies but also in acute TCMR and acute tubular necrosis. The authors concluded that the g-score + the ptc-score sum, the MVI, was the best predictor of DSA, followed by time post-transplant in late-graft biopsies. We suggested that lymphatic vessels should be excluded by podoplanin staining to score ptc in confusing cases [18].

Intimal or transmural arteritis, defined by the infiltration of mononuclear cells under enlarged and "activated" arterial endothelial cells (primarily arcuate caliber vessels or interlobular arteries, and less often arterioles), has been scored according to the degree of luminal narrowing: <25%, ≥25%, and transmural necrosis for v1, v2, and v3, respectively (Table 2) (Fig. 1c). Intimal or transmural arteritis has long been categorized as a typical lesion of acute TCMR;

Table 1 The Banff 2013 classification

1. Normal

2. Antibody-mediated

   Acute/active ABMR; all three features must be present for diagnosis

   1. Histologic evidence of acute tissue injury, including one or more of the following:

      Microvascular inflammation (g > 0 and/or ptc > 0)

      Intimal or transmural arteritis (v > 0)

      Acute thrombotic microangiopathy, in the absence of any other cause

   2. Evidence of current/recent antibody interaction with vascular endothelium, including at least one of the following:

      Linear C4d staining in peritubular capillaries (C4d2 or C4d3 by IF on frozen sections, or C4d > 0 by IHC on paraffin sections)

      At least moderate microvascular inflammation ([g +ptc] > 2)

      Increased expression of gene transcripts in the biopsy tissue indicative of endothelial injury if thoroughly validated

   3. Serologic evidence of donor-specific antibodies (DSAs) (HLAor other antigens)

   Chronic, active ABMR; all three features must be present for diagnosis

   1. Morphologic evidence of chronic tissue injury, including one or more of the following:

      Transplant glomerulopathy (TG) (eg > 0), if no evidence of chronic thrombotic microangiopathy Severe peritubular capillary basement membrane multilayering (requires EM)

      Arterial intimal fibrosis of new onset, excluding other causes

   2. Evidence of current/recent antibody interaction with vascular endothelium, including at least one of the following:

      Linear C4d staining in peritubular capillaries (C4d2 or C4d3 by IF on frozen sections, or C4d > 0 by IHC on paraffin sections)

      At least moderate microvascular inflammation ([g +ptc] > 2)

      Increased expression of gene transcripts in the biopsy tissue indicative of endothelial injury, if thoroughly valiated

   3. Serologic evidence of DSAs (HLA or other antigens)

   C4d staining without evidence of rejection; all three features must be present for diagnosis

   1. Linear C4d staining in peritubular capillaries (C4d2 or C4d3 by IF on frozen sections, or C4d > 0 by IHC on paraffin sections)

   2. g = 0, ptc = 0, eg = 0 (by light microscopy and by EM if available), v = 0; no TMA, no peritubular capillary basement membrane multilayering, no acute tubular injury (in the absence of another apparent cause for this)

   3. No acute cell-mediated rejection (Banff 97 type 1A or greater) or borderline changes

3. Borderline changes: 'Suspicious' for acute T-cell mediated rejection (may coincide with categories 2 and 5, and 6)

   This category is used when no intimal arteritis is present, but there are foci of tubulitis (t1, t2, or t3) with minor interstitial infiltration (i0, or i1) or interstitial infiltration (i2, i3) with mild (t1) tubulitis

4. T cell mediated rejection (TCMR, may coincide with categories 2 and 5 and 6)

Table 1 The Banff 2013 classification (Continued)

   Acute T-cell mediated rejection (Type/Grade:)

   I A. Cases with significant interstitial infiltration (>25% of parenchyma affected, i2 or i3) and foci of moderate tubulitis (t2)

   I B. Cases with significant interstitial infiltration (>25% of parenchyma affected, i2 or i3) and foci of severe tubulitis (t3)

   II A. Cases with mild to moderate intimal arteritis (v1)

   II B. Cases with sever intimal arteritis comprising >25% of the luminal area (v2)

   III. Cases with 'transmural' arteritis and/or arterial fibrinoid change and necrosis of medial smooth muscle cells with accompanying lymphocytic inflammation (v3)

   Chronic active T-cell mediated rejection

   'chronic allograft aiteriopathy' (arterial intimal fibrosis with mononuclear cell infiltration in fibrosis, formation of neo-intima)

5. Interstitial fibrosis and tubular atrophy, no evidence of any specific etiology

   (may include nonspecific vascular and glomerular sclerosis, but severity graded by tubulointerstitial features)

   I. Mild interstitial fibrosis and tubular atrophy (>25% of cortical area)

   II. Moderate interstitial fibrosis and tubular atrophy (26-50% of cortical area)

   III. Sever interstitial fibrosis and tubular atrophy/loss (>50% of cortical area)

6. Other: Changes not considered to be due to rejection-acute and/or chronic

   (For diagnoses see table 14 in (Banff 97 KI -1999:)[15]); may include isolated g, eg, or cv lesions and coincide with categories 2, 3,4, and 5)

Modified Table of ref. [16]
cg Banff chronic glomerulopathy score, *EM* electron microscopy, *ENDAT* endothelial activation and injury transcript, *g* Banff glomerulitis score, *GBM* glomerular basement membrane, *IF* immunofluorescence, *IHC* immunohistochemistry, *ptc* peritubular capillary, *TCMR* T cell-mediated rejection, *v* Banff arteritis score

however, recent observations showed that the occurrence of intimal or transmural arteritis was more often observed in cases with acute ABMR (21%) than TCMR (9%), and the grade of intimal arteritis in acute ABMR was 52% in v1, followed by 30% in v2, and 19% in v3. [19]. These pathological features correlated historically with increased graft loss in acute rejection with fibrinoid necrosis of the arteries (type III), with ~25% graft survival at 1 year [20, 21].

Recently, isolated endarteritis in kidney transplants has become an increasingly recognized and reported entity [22], but identification of the mechanisms underlying the arterial lesions remains problematic. Salazar ID et al. [23] suggested that after 1-year post-transplant, isolated v lesions usually indicate rejection. Many such cases are DSA-positive and have acute ABMR, but some may reflect TCMR, particularly at less than 5 years post-transplant. Although it has not yet been established about the need and the contents of the antirejection treatment to isolated v lesion, a recent report showed the efficacy of antirejection

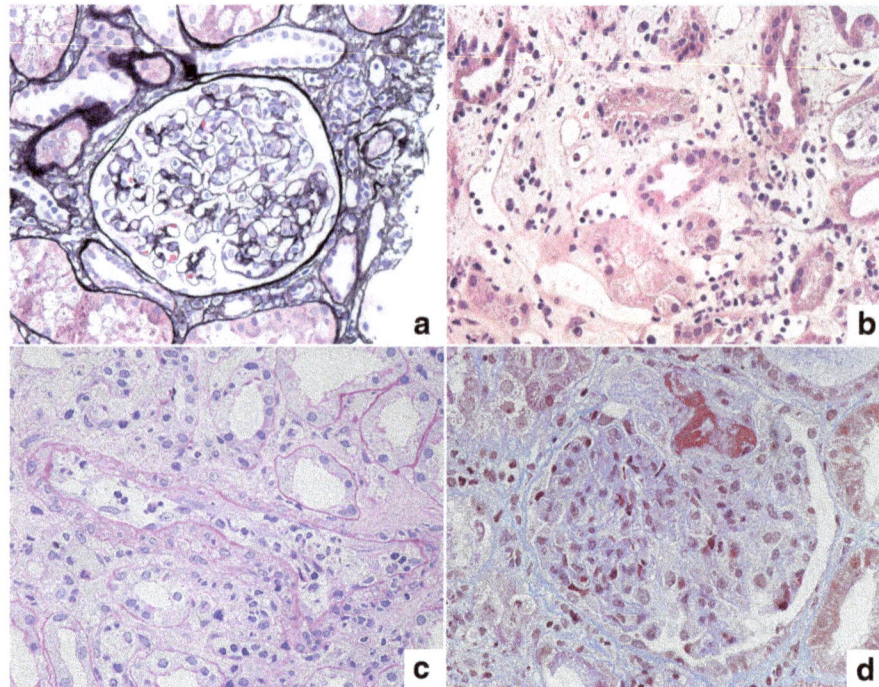

Fig. 1 Pathological findings of acute antibody-mediated rejection. **a** Transplant glomerulitis (Banff classification; g) in a patient with ABMR. Most of the endothelial cells were swelling and inflammatory cells including mononuclear cells and neutrophils were present with focal occlusion in glomerular capillaries. [PAM, ×400]. **b** Peritubular capillaritis (Banff classification; ptc) in a patient with antibody-mediated rejection (ABMR). Peritubular capillaries (PTCs) were markedly dilated, and inflammatory cells including mononuclear cells and neutrophils were present in PTCs [HE, ×400]. **c** Transplant endoarteritis (Banff classification; v) in a patient with ABMR. Endothelial cells of interlobular artery were swelling and marked inflammatory cells infiltration narrowed the lumen [PAS, ×400]. **d** Thrombotic microangiopathy in a patient with ABMR. The dilated capillary lumen was occluded by a fibrin thrombus in glomerulus focally, and the fragment red blood cells were present in mesangial lesion. Endothelial cells were swelling and capillary walls were dilated with subendothelial widening [Masson Trichrome, ×400]

Table 2 Pathological features and Banff score

Feature	Banff term	Banff Score			
		0	1	2	3
Interstitial inflammation (% of nonfibrotic cortex)	i	<10%	10–25%	26–50%	>50%
Total inflammation (% all cortex)	ti	<10%	10–25%	26–50%	>50%
Tubulitis (maximum mononuclear cells/tubule)	t	0	1–4	5–10	>10
Arterial inflammation (% lumen endarteritis)	V	None	<25%	>25%	Transmural or necrosis
Glomerulitis (% glomeruli involved)	g	None	<25%	26–50%	>50%
Capillaritis (cells per cortical PTC, requires >10% of PTC to be affected for scoring)	ptc	<10%	<5/PTC	5–10/PTC	>10/PTC
C4d deposition in PTC (% positive)	C4d	0%	I–9%	10–50%	>50%
Interstitial fibrosis (% of cortex)	ci	<5%	6–25%	26–50%	>50%
Tubular atrophy (% cortex)	ct	0%	<25%	26–50%	>50%
Arterial intimal thickening (% narrowing lumen of most severely affected glomerulus)	cv	0%	<25%	26–50%	>50%
Transplant glomerulopathy (% of capillaries with duplication in most severely affected glomerulus)	cg	0%	<25%	26–50%	>50%
Arteriolar hyalinosis (number with focal or circumferential hyaline)	ah	None	1 focal	>1 focal	1 circumferential >50%
Mesangial matrix increase (% affected glomeruli)	mm	0%	<25%	26–50%	>50%

treatment including high-dose steroids and sometimes followed by antithymocyte globulin [23].

Acute TMA, characterized by endothelial swelling and subendothelial widening, fibrin thrombi in capillary lumens, mesangiolysis, and fragmented red blood cells in the subendothelium and mesangium, occurs in several diseases (Fig. 1d). Acute ABMR has emerged as a significant cause of TMA, based on the occurrence of TMA being higher in cases that were PTC C4d$^+$ (13.6%) versus PTC C4d$^-$ (3.6%). Moreover, plasma exchange was effective in TMA cases with PTC C4d positivity [24]. An acute tubular necrosis-like histology with minimal inflammation can also occur in cases with acute ABMR.

Characteristic histological manifestations of chronic ABMR

Histological evidence of chronic ABMR includes three types: (1) TG type, (2) severe PTC basement membrane multilayering type, and (3) arterial intimal fibrosis of new onset type. The most characteristic feature of chronic ABMR is TG, defined as the widespread duplication or multilayering of glomerular basement membrane (GBM) in the absence of specific de novo or recurrent glomerular disease or evidence of TMA (Fig. 2a). TG develops in stages, best seen by electron microscopy

(EM), and these stages have been related to chronic ABMR recently [25].

In addition to these chronic features, signs of activity are often present, with prominent mononuclear cells in capillary loops with endothelial swelling (transplant glomerulitis) [26]. The cells are primarily monocytes, with few T cells. There is no known specific tubular or interstitial lesion in chronic ABMR. The median time of diagnosis for TG by indication biopsies is 5–8 years [27, 28]. The risk of TG is increased by the presence of higher levels of class II DSA [29], particularly those reactive to HLA-DQ which was refractory to conventional therapy [30, 31]. A history of acute ABMR and presensitization also increases the risk [29].

TG has a poor prognosis, particularly when accompanied by PTC C4d deposition [29, 32]. Lesage et al. showed recently that TG was associated with a poor prognosis, independent of the level of graft dysfunction and other chronic histological changes [33]. Notably, the early diagnosis of, and therapy for, TG within 3 months may be important for graft survival [25]. Based on these observations, the Banff 2013 meeting focused on the early diagnosis of TG. The Banff cg0 was defined as no double contours by light microscopy

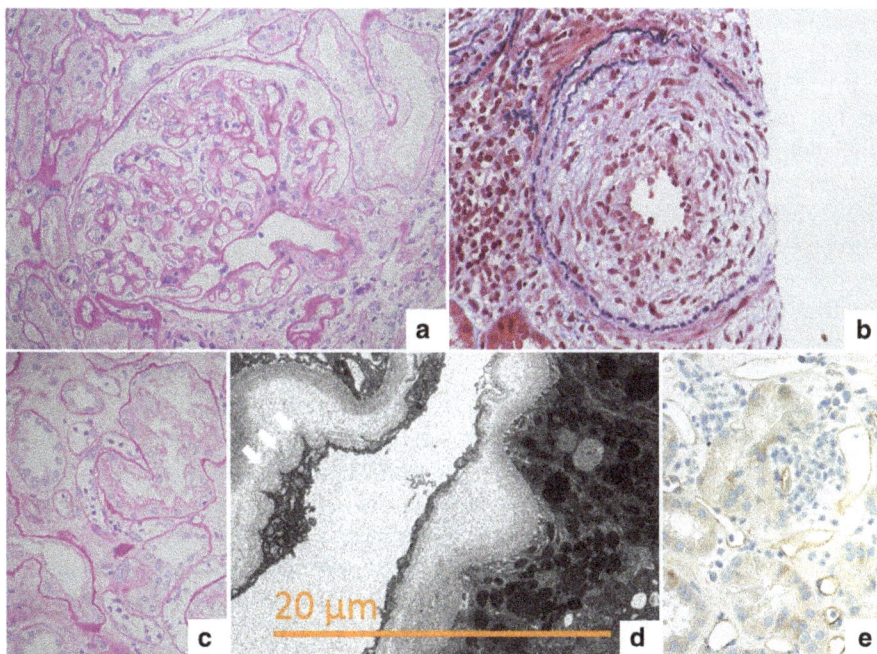

Fig. 2 Pathological findings of chronic antibody-mediated rejection. **a** Transplant glomerulopathy (Banff classification; cg). Glomerular capillary walls were duplicated diffusely and narrowed capillary lumens were markedly present with endothelial cell swelling and few inflammatory cells [PAS, ×400]. **b** Transplant arteriopathy (Banff classification;cv) The intima in interlobular arteries showed a neointima formation without prominent elastic fibers, in which a few mononuclear inflammatory cells were included [Masson Trichrome, ×400]. **c** Transplant capillaropathy, multilayering of the basement membrane in PTCs (*arrow*). Light microscopic findings showed PTCs in chronic ABMR. Basement membranes of PTCs were thick as same as tubular basement membranes [PAS, ×400]. **d** Electron microscopy findings showed multilayering of the PTCs basement membrane outside (*arrow*). Mononuclear cells were present in PTCs and endothelial cell was swelling. **e** Positive C4d immunostaining in PTCs of ABMR. C4d immunostaining in dilated PTCs was linearly positive with inflammatory cells presentation in the capillary lumens

or EM. Regarding cg1, two subcategories were newly defined: cg1a indicates double contours associated with subendothelial widening detected only by EM, whereas cg1b corresponds to one or more glomerular capillaries with double contours in non-sclerotic glomeruli, observed by light microscopy [16]. The duplicated GBM, best seen with periodic acid–Schiff (PAS) or silver staining in light microscopy, is involved segmentally or globally and may show mesangial cell interposition. The TG (cg) score is still based on the most severely affected glomeruli: 1–25, 26–50, and >50% for cg1, cg2, and cg3, respectively (Table 2).

Multilayering of the basement membrane in PTCs has been associated with chronic ABMR [10]. Each ring of basement membrane surrounding a PTC probably represents the residue of one previous episode of endothelial injury, from oldest (outer) to most recent (inner) (Fig. 2d). Ivanyi found that biopsies with three or more PTCs with seven or more circumferential layers were found only in patients with other features of chronic rejection [34]. A subsequent comprehensive study by Liapis et al. compared native and transplanted kidneys [35]. In this study, higher threshold levels were set to define severe PTC lamination (15 PTCs examined, with the three most-affected used for scoring: severe PTC lamination defined as ≥7 layers in one capillary and ≥5 layers in the remaining two capillaries). Based on these observations, severe peritubular basement membrane multilayering was defined by seven or more layers in one cortical PTC and five or more in two additional PTCs using EM. Aita et al. demonstrated that thickening and lamination of the basement membrane may be seen by light microscopy in favorable PAS- or silver-stained sections. When the thickness is similar to or thicker than non-atrophic tubular basement membrane (TBM), it correlates well with multilayering on EM [36]. Although these light microscopic observations of peritubular basement membrane multilayering might be useful, it is not incorporated in the current Banff criteria.

The molecular mechanisms involving the endothelium of the GC and PTC in patients with chronic ABMR are not fully understood. We previously reported that PV-1 and caveolin-1 expression were a distinct feature of chronic rejection-induced transplant glomerulopathy and capillaropathy, respectively [37–39]. More recent data showed that three markers of endothelial-to-mesenchymal transition (EndMT), fascin1, vimentin, and heat shock protein 47 provide a sensitive and reliable diagnostic tool for detecting endothelial activation during ABMR [40].

Arterial intimal fibrosis is a typical feature of rejection in late grafts. These lesions are thought to be caused by antibodies, T cells, or both. Intimal changes are most prominent in the larger arteries, but extend from the main renal artery to the interlobular arteries. The intima shows pronounced fibrous thickening without prominent elastic fiber accumulation, in contrast to the multilayering of elastic typical of hypertensive and involutive arteriosclerosis (Fig. 2b) Arterial intimal thickening (cv) scores are still based on the most severely affected artery: 1–25, 26–50, and > 50% for cv1, cv2, and cv3, respectively. The elastic interna generally remains intact. The media generally shows no obvious abnormality, aside from the focal loss of smooth muscle.

Arterial lesions are common in allografts caused by chronic rejection (including ABMR and TCMR), hypertension, and donor disease. Transplant arteriopathy is associated with DSA in kidney transplants. DSA may also promote arteriosclerosis, as judged by progression of severity in allografts from patients with DSA. Loupy et al. recently suggested that circulating antibodies are major determinants of severe arteriosclerosis and major adverse cardiovascular events, independent of traditional cardiovascular risk factors [41].

C4d positivity, MVI, and ENDAT

To determine DSA-induced endothelial cell injury, the clinician must confirm one of the following: (1) C4d positivity in PTC, (2) MVI, or (3) expression of activated ENDATs. C4d positivity in PTCs has been a cardinal feature for the diagnosis of both acute and chronic ABMR since its adoption into the Banff 2005 classification [42]. However, previous report showed the evidence of ABMR without complement activation demonstrated by transcriptome analysis using ENDATs [43], and now C4d staining has been considered as one of the criteria to suggest evidence of endothelial activation triggered by DSA interaction. Of note, positive C4d deposition in PTCs without graft dysfunction in ABO-incompatible kidney transplantation may present accommodation since they do not appear to be injurious to the renal allografts [44, 45].

In the 2013 Banff classification [16], the threshold for C4d positivity was modified. In a four-tiered grading system that ranged from 0 to 3+ (1–9, 10–50, and > 50% for c4d1, c4d2, and c4d3, respectively; Table 2), C4d positivity was defined originally as 3+ in both frozen (immunofluorescence, IF) and paraffin (immunohistochemistry, IHC) sections [46]. The criteria for C4d positivity were revised to 2+ or 3+ in frozen sections (IF) and > 0 in paraffin wax sections (IHC) [16] (Fig. 2e) However, 1+ in frozen sections was not approved unanimously as a criterion for C4d positivity. The pattern tends to be linear and circumferential, similar to that in acute ABMR; however, fewer positive capillaries are found and the "widespread" pattern is not common. In chronic ABMR, PTC C4d deposition was found in ~50% of the grafts with transplant arteriopathy or glomerulopathy [27, 47]. Cases with little or no C4d (C4d0-1) but demonstrating other features of chronic ABMR (e.g., DSA, capillaritis, TG) are referred to as C4d-negative chronic ABMR [48] according to the Banff 2013 classification [16].

The MVI score was defined as the total of the Banff g + ptc scores. Recent data showed that the threshold for moderate MVI (g + ptc ≥ 2) was associated with the development of overt TG in the presence of DSA, even in C4d$^-$ cases [17, 49]. Gupta et al. showed that MVI scores of 2 or more were significantly associated with a histological diagnosis of acute and chronic ABMR using microarrays [50], confirming the validity of the MVI score.

The Alberta Transplant Applied Genomics Center (ATAGC) team at the University of Alberta developed a "molecular microscope" approach to kidney transplant biopsies and has provided a system for distinguishing TCMR from ABMR by the expression of activated ENDATs. They proposed new rules to integrate molecular tests and histology into a precise diagnostic system that can reduce errors, ambiguity, and inter-pathologist disagreement [51, 52]. Reeve et al. showed that histological assessments can be improved by placing more emphasis on i and t lesions and incorporating new algorithms for diagnosis [53]. Halloran et al. recently showed that ABMR presented distinct subphenotypes—early "pg (peritubular capillaries and/or glomerulitis lesion)-dominant," late "cg (GBM double contour)-dominant," and combined "pgcg phenotype"—differing in time, molecular features, accompanying TCMR, HLA antibodies, and the probability of non-adherence, using a microarray assessment [54]. This combined approach will help in developing new diagnostic tools and will lead to new disease classifications. But it has not yet been prevailing in clinical setting in the present time.

DSA positivity

DSAs may be directed against HLAs or other endothelial cell antigens, and their presence is required for the diagnosis of acute and chronic, active ABMR [55]. DSAs bind to HLAs on endothelium and complement activation is accelerated through the C1 complex. The complement cascade proceeds through C4, C2, C3, and C5, finally leading to the membrane-attack complex (MAC) resulting in endothelial cell lysis.

There is growing evidence supporting risk stratification according to anti-HLA DSA phenotypes, as follows: (1) preformed/de novo, (2) mean fluorescence intensity (MFI), (3) C1q/C3d binding, and (4) immunoglobulin G (IgG) subclass. Preformed and de novo DSAs are independent risk factors for acute and chronic ABMR and graft loss [56–58]. Wiebe et al. [9] followed 365 non-presensitized patients prospectively with protocol biopsies and serum samples for DSAs. Overall, 15% developed de novo DSAs,

at a mean time of 4.6 years post-transplant. Most patients developed DSAs to HLA class II (94%); only 6% had antibodies to donor HLA class I alone.

Most of the graft loss in the DSA-positive patients was due to chronic ABMR (84%). Wiebe also showed in a subsequent study [58] that, in recipients with de novo DSAs, the rate of estimated glomerular filtration rate (eGFR) decline increased significantly prior to de novo DSA onset and accelerated post-de novo DSAs, suggesting that de novo DSAs were both a marker and contributor to ongoing alloimmunity. Another report supported the evidence that the risk of acute ABMR and poor outcome were correlated with the level of MFI of the DSAs in Luminex assays [59]. Importantly, not all DSAs fix complement or cause ABMR and, conversely, not all episodes of acute graft injury with capillary inflammation and C4d deposition are associated with DSAs detectable with standard assays. For example, Loupy et al. demonstrated that C1q-binding DSAs showed worse graft survival than non-C1q-binding DSA (HR = 9.23, 95% CI: 5.99–14.23, $p < 0.001$). Moreover, the existence of C1q-binding DSA correlated with MVI, PTC C4d deposition, TG, and IF/TA [60]. Sicard et al. demonstrated that C3d-binding DSAs showed worse graft survival than non-C3d-binding DSA [log-rank test, $p = 0.0003$]. Additionally, the existence of C3d-binding DSAs showed better sensitivity (84.7%) and specificity (73.3%) than C1q-binding DSAs or PTC C4d positivity [61]. Lefaucheur et al. suggested the clinical relevance of IgG DSA subclasses and their association with the phenotype of antibody-mediated injury [62].

Recent studies have focused on DSA other than anti-HLA antibodies: i.e., non-HLA antibodies. Non-HLA antibodies existed in 2.3% of ABMR cases occurring within 7 days after kidney transplantation [63, 64]. Representative non-HLA antibodies included MICA, MICB, and angiotensin type 1 receptor [AT1R] antibodies [65–68]. Among these, AT1R antibodies were the most investigated. Banasik et al. reported that 27 of 117 (23%) patients were positive for anti-AT1R antibodies prior to surgery and 4 (3.4%) developed acute rejection [67]. Importantly, Dragun et al. found that 11 of 16 patients with acute rejection resulting from anti-AT1R antibodies were C4d$^-$ [65]. Beyond this observation, Reinsmoen et al. evaluated 63 patients with acute rejection; six cases resulted from anti-AT1R antibodies and four of them were PTC C4d$^-$ [69]. Additionally, Scornik et al. found no correlation between antibodies to HLA-DP, MICA, or AT1R and C4d$^+$ rejection [69]. Recently, antivascular endothelial cell antibodies (AECAs: XM-ONE) [70], and reagents for identification of non-HLAs, non-MICA antibodies, have become available. Moreover, Jackson et al. discovered four new non-HLA antibodies: endoglin, Fms-like tyrosine kinase-3 ligand, EGF-like repeats and discoidin I-like domains 3, and intercellular adhesion molecule 4. All four AECAs were detected in 24% of pre-transplant sera, and they were associated with post-transplant DSA, ABMR, and early TG [71].

Treatment of ABMR

The treatment of acute ABMR is still evolving; however, randomized controlled trials of therapies are rare [72]. The most common strategies are based on the quick reduction of antibody titers with plasmapheresis (PE), intravenous immunoglobulin (IVIG), and thymoglobulin to treat any concurrent TCMR. The best evidence supporting the use of PE and IVIG shows various immuno-modulatory effects, especially on B cells, antibodies, and complement. Rituximab, an anti-CD20 monoclonal antibody, reacts with CD20 on pre- and mature B cells and leads to transient B-cell depletion, with B-cell recovery after 6–9 months. Bortezomib, a proteasome inhibitor used in the treatment of multiple myeloma for plasma cell depletion, has been tried in a small cohort with acute ABMR, with some evidence of success [73, 74]. Eculizumab, an antibody to C5 that blocks the terminal complement pathway, has shown some efficacy in non-randomized pilot trials and isolated cases. The efficacy of eculizumab in the prevention of ABMR was also assessed in renal transplant recipients with a positive cross-match [75]. In this study, the authors concluded that despite decreasing acute clinical ABMR rates, eculizumab-treated (EC)-positive cross-match kidney transplants did not prevent chronic ABMR in recipients with persistently high B flow cytometric cross-matches [76].

Treatment of chronic ABMR remains to be established. Strategies have included IVIG and rituximab [77] and bortezomib [78]. Whether complement inhibition will be useful remains to be determined. Regular monitoring of DSAs and appropriate surveillance biopsies are recommended [6, 79]. The best intervention is prevention, which remains elusive.

TCMR

TCMR was long believed to be the central process in allograft rejection. Consequently, therapies to prevent and treat allograft rejection were directed primarily against T cells before ABMR was recognized. In the Banff 2013 classification, T cell-mediated rejection (TCMR) included categories 3 (borderline changes) and 4 (acute/chronic TCMR) (Table 1). TCMR can be divided into two types: acute TCMR and chronic TCMR. Acute TMCR (Banff category 4, types I–III) is the form of rejection that develops most commonly in the first several months after transplantation. TCMR can occur as early as 6 days, and as late as decades, post-transplantation [1]. The clinical manifestations of severe acute TCMR include an abrupt increase in serum creatinine, a decline in urine output, fever, graft tenderness, and swelling, but these symptoms are often absent in patients under modern immunosuppression.

Characteristic histological manifestations of acute TCMR

Acute TCMR is characterized by tubulitis with interstitial inflammatory cells infiltration and arteritis in more severe form. In the former, the infiltration of activated T lymphocytes and macrophages occurs into a mildly edematous interstitial lesion and into the tubules, so-called tubulointerstitial cellular rejection (Banff category 4, type I) (Fig. 3a, b). In the latter, another major finding is the infiltration of mononuclear cells in the enlarged and activated arterial endothelial cells, so-called transplant endarteritis (Banff category 4, type II or III). The approximate frequencies of the different patterns of acute TCMR are 45–70% tubulointerstitial, 30–55% arteritis, and 2–4% glomerular (not used specifically for the categorization of rejection in the Banff 2013 classification). Notably, ~20–40% of acute TCMR cases show C4d positivity along with PTC; that is, evidence of concurrent antibody-mediated injury [80]. Mixed ABMR and acute TCMR episodes are more severe and constitute an independent risk factor for graft failure [19, 81].

Regarding the detailed morphological features of tubulointerstitial cellular rejection, T cells and macrophages invade tubules and insinuate between tubular epithelial cells inside the basement membrane, a process termed "tubulitis" (Fig. 3a, b). Tubulitis is usually recognized by increased numbers of small, dark nuclei, often arranged along the inner aspect of the TBM and occasionally surrounded by small clear spaces/halos. In the Banff 2013 classification, determination of the numerical tubulitis (t) score is based on the maximum number of mononuclear cells in the most affected tubuli: 1–4, 5–10, and >10 for t1, t2, and t3, respectively (Table 2). Tubulitis affects mostly distal tubular segments in the cortex; proximal tubules are often spared and collecting ducts in the medulla are hardly involved [82]. Tubulitis in distal segment should be excluded infection which are commonly extended from proximal site. Contrary to this, tubulitis in proximal segments means extended inflammation from distal by rejection. Tubulitis in atrophic tubules (<50% of the original diameter and markedly thickened TBMs) is currently considered to be a non-diagnostic sign of parenchymal scarring; presently, this feature is not used to establish a diagnosis of acute TCMR. However, this view may change in the future because there is increasing evidence that all tubulitis (in atrophic and non-atrophic tubules) and all interstitial inflammation (in scarred and non-scarred regions) is a sign of TCMR [83].

Mononuclear cell interstitial inflammation was defined by a pleomorphic interstitial infiltrate of mononuclear cells

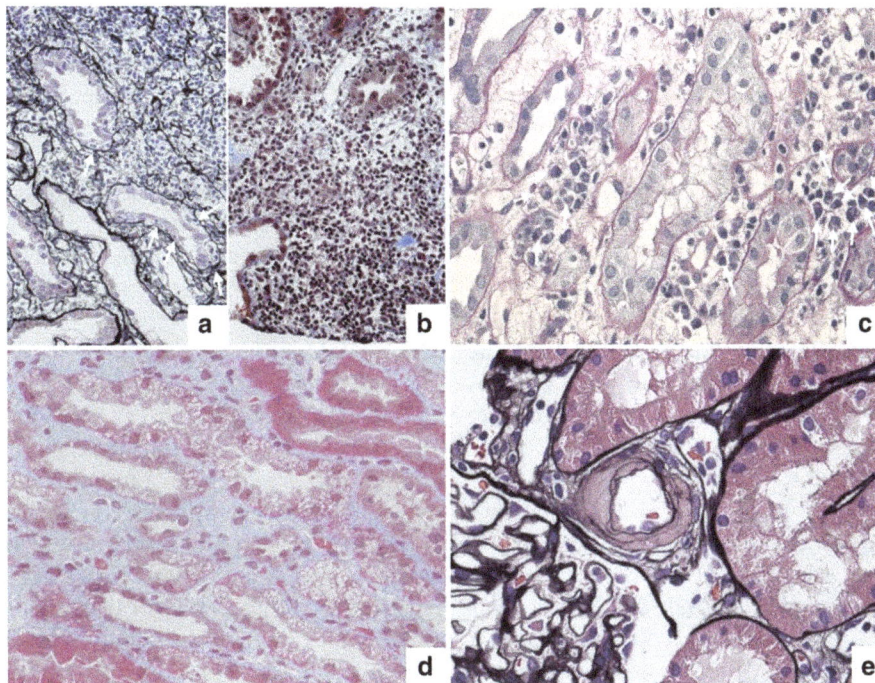

Fig. 3 Pathological findings of T cell-mediated rejection, plasma cell-rich rejection, and acute and chronic CNI nephrotoxicity. **a** Focal aggressive tubulointerstitial rejection with moderate tubulitis. (Banff classification; i and t) Inflammatory cells were present in the edematous interstitial lesions and inside of tubular basement membrane staying between tubular epithelial cells (*arrow*). **b** Diffuse aggressive tubulointerstitial rejection with severe tubulitis. (Banff classification; i and t) Massive inflammatory cells were occupied in the interstitium. Partial dissolution and rupture of the tubular basement membrane were evident (*arrow*) [Masson Trichrome, ×400]. **c** Plasma cell-rich acute rejection (PCAR). Tubulointerstitial inflammatory cells infiltration, which are predominantly plasma cells (*arrow*) [PAS, ×400]. **d** Acute CNI nephrotoxicity. The straight portion of proximal tubular epithelial cells showed isometric vacuolization. **e** Chronic CNI nephrotoxicity. Arteriole were surrounded by the amorphous materials substitute for the medial smooth muscle cells

(lymphocytes, macrophages) and occasionally scattered polymorphonuclear leukocytes in areas of severe tubular injury. In the Banff 2013 classification, determination of the numerical interstitial inflammation (i) score is based on the parenchymal area affected by inflammatory cells: <10–25, 25–50, and >50% for i1, i2, and i3, respectively (Table 2). Using these t and i scores, tubulointerstitial cellular rejection includes type IA (i2, 3 with t2) and type IB (i2, 3 with t3 or at least two areas of TBM destruction and moderate tubulitis elsewhere).

In acute TCMR, MHC class II/HLA-DR antigens and intercellular adhesion molecules are expressed, stimulated by the release of interferon-γ in inflamed regions [84, 85]. The detection of MHC class II in the cytoplasm of tubular epithelial cells by IF in frozen tissue samples may be used as an adjunct marker to establish a diagnosis of acute TCMR.

Regarding the detailed morphological features of transplant endarteritis, infiltration of mononuclear cells under enlarged and activated arterial endothelial cells, mainly arcuate-caliber vessels or interlobular arteries, and less often arterioles, is often observed [endarteritis figure IIA(v1), IIB(v2), II(v3)] (Table 2). The importance of this lesion has been emphasized for many years and is accepted widely as a feature of acute TCMR, particularly if transplant endarteritis is accompanied by tubulointerstitial cellular rejection. However, a considerable proportion of acute TCMR with transplant endarteritis also shows concurrent acute ABMR [19]. Endarteritis has been reported in 18–56% of renal biopsies with acute TCMR [20, 21, 86]. The prevalence of endarteritis in biopsies is affected by the sample size, timing of the biopsy, HLA matching, and the level of immunosuppression. Endarteritis tends to affect larger arteries preferentially [87]. If biopsy samples are small and do not contain arcuate arteries or interlobular arteries, such transplant endarteritis may remain undetected. In cases of endarteritis, endothelial cells are usually activated, with basophilic cytoplasms, and show lifting from the supporting elastic intern by infiltrating inflammatory cells. One inflammatory cell under the arterial endothelium is considered to be sufficient for the diagnosis of transplant endarteritis. Mononuclear inflammatory cells that are solely adherent to the lumina surface of endothelial cells are insufficient for making a diagnosis of transplant endarteritis.

Usually, elastic tissue staining allows for easy detection because hypertension-induced arterial intimal fibroelastosis gives an intense staining reaction that is lacking in cases of chronic vascular rejection. In transplant endarteritis, inflammation is typically limited to the intima/subendothelial zone, sparing the medial smooth muscle layer. Transmural inflammation, involving all layers of the arterial walls, including segmental fibrinoid necrosis, can occur in severe cases of acute TCMR (Banff category 4, type III rejection). However, this feature is more often seen in biopsies with concurrent acute AMR and C4d positivity [88]. Infiltration of mononuclear cells into the wall of the veins or lymphatics is found in ~10% of biopsies with acute TCMR. This is a sign of inflammatory cell trafficking in areas of inflammation with no direct diagnostic significance [89].

The so-called isolated v lesion is characterized by endarteritis with minimal interstitial inflammation ($i \leq 1$) and tubulitis ($t \leq 1$) [22]. The Banff working group reported that the risk for renal allograft failure was 3.51-fold higher in patients with isolated v lesions versus a patient having no diagnostic rejection, concluding that isolated v lesions should be diagnosed and treated as acute rejection to prevent long-term kidney transplant failure [90].

Characteristic histological manifestations of chronic TCMR

In the Banff 2013 classification, chronic TCMR was defined by sclerosing transplant arteriopathy. This lesion is characterized by intimal widening due to the de novo accumulation of collagens I and III, lack of elastosis, and varying degrees of intimal inflammation with mononuclear inflammatory cells. In sclerosing transplant arteriopathy, the intima usually contains varying numbers of myofibroblasts, occasional foam cells, and, in active disease stages, scattered, often clustered mononuclear inflammatory cells that may be most prominent along the inner elastic lamina. Endothelial cells are often enlarged with reactive nuclei sometimes overlying an ill-defined ring of smooth muscle cells: that is, so-called neomedia formation.

Treatment of TCMR

The first-line treatment for acute cellular rejection (i.e., rejection in the absence of C4d staining and/or circulating DSA) is bolus steroids for up to 3 days. This therapeutic approach works well in patients with T cell-mediated tubulointerstitial rejection (i.e., Banff category 4, type I). In patients who do not respond, primarily those with transplant endarteritis and glomerulitis, the standard rescue therapy is thymoglobulin. Certain pathological features of acute cellular rejection have prognostic significance. The most important predictors of outcome are arterial lesions. Endarteritis, which defines type II rejection, has an adverse effect on prognosis compared with tubulointerstitial rejection with no arterial involvement [21]. The intensity of the interstitial infiltrate, or tubulitis, for that matter, has no correlation with the severity of the rejection episode [86, 91]. Many, but not all, "borderline" cases are, indeed, rejection. Untreated borderline cases can progress to frank rejection during follow-up [92]. If there is any evidence that favors rejection, a diagnosis of rejection should be made and therapy initiated.

Subclinical rejection

Rejection episodes detected in allografts with stable function are referred to as "subclinical". Subclinical rejection is defined as the presence of histological evidence of acute rejection on a protocol or surveillance biopsy with no elevation in the serum creatinine level. Most previous reports of subclinical rejection involved cellular rejection [93–95]. However, there are reports of allografts with histological manifestations of ABMR in the absence of functional deterioration of kidney function [30, 96–99]. Loupy et al. suggested that subclinical TCMR was not associated with a significant effect on allograft outcome but triggered the appearance of de novo DSAs and progression to TG in a subset of patients. They also showed that subclinical ABMR detected at the 1-year screening biopsy carried prognostic value independent of initial DSA status, previous immunological events, current eGFR, and proteinuria [100]. Further studies with longer follow-up are required to determine whether surveillance biopsies, combined with enhanced immunosuppression, administered for the treatment of subclinical rejection, improve long-term outcomes.

Plasma cell-rich acute rejection (PCAR)

PCAR is a morphological type of acute rejection with prominent plasma cells, which normally account for >10% of interstitial mononuclear cells [101–104] (Fig. 3c). The histological diagnosis of PCAR requires consideration of post-transplant lymphoproliferative disorder (PTLD), viral infection, and drug toxicity. In previous studies, the response to antirejection therapy in PCAR, such as steroids, was less than satisfactory, with poor graft survival rates [105]. Some reports support the hypothesis that an antibody-mediated component participates in the graft injury of PCAR because it can be associated with both C4d staining and DSAs [99, 103, 106]. If there appears to be rapid progression of allograft dysfunction in the setting of significant plasma cell infiltration, then treatment modalities targeting both cellular and antibody-mediated pathways can be considered, although there are no data to support this line of treatment. In the setting of a significant plasma cell infiltrate with slow progression of allograft dysfunction, it is unclear whether therapies used in the setting of ABMR are of any benefit, and augmentation of the maintenance immunosuppressive regimen may be the best approach. Abbas et al. reported that PCAR occurs late after transplantation and in many cases associated with DSAs. Graft outcome was poor when PCAR was associated with DSAs [107]. Due to the rarity of PCAR, its incorporation into the Banff classification is still awaited. Recognition of this entity, description of more cases in the literature, and further molecular approaches would help in determining its clinical features and appropriate therapeutic approaches. The differential diagnosis of PCAR includes polyomavirus allograft nephropathy (PVN), PTLD, and cytomegalovirus infection. Therefore, SV40 staining, light chain (kappa and lambda) staining, and EBER (Epstein-Barr encoded early RNAs) were useful to diagnose PCAR.

CNI nephrotoxicity

CNIs are fundamental maintenance immunosuppressants but, ironically, these drugs can cause renal toxicity by several mechanisms. The histological features can be divided into two types, acute and chronic nephrotoxicity, and the target lesions involve the glomeruli, arterioles, and tubulo-interstitium. Acute CNI nephrotoxicity include TMA, afferent arteriolar vasoconstriction, and isometric vacuolization of tubules, whereas chronic CNI nephrotoxicity includes glomerulosclerosis, arteriolar hyaline thickening, and IF/TA [108]. CNI nephrotoxicity also affects recipients with non-renal organ transplantation. Indeed, the risk of chronic renal failure at 10 years after transplantation of a non-renal organ was reported to be ~20% [107]. However, end-stage renal failure caused by CNIs is uncommon, at 3.2–4.8% [109, 110]. For kidney transplantation, the actual occurrence rates at 5 and 10 years after kidney transplantation were 66 and 100%, respectively [111].

Characteristic histological manifestations of acute CNI nephrotoxicity

Early histopathological changes in glomerular capillaries include fibrin thrombi and endothelial cell swelling. These TMA-like changes range from mild to severe, and mild changes occur sometimes with no clinical sign. Afferent arterioles are likely to be affected by CNI nephrotoxicity and the histopathology shows smooth muscle cell swelling and ballooning in early changes. Regarding tubular injury, the straight portions of proximal tubules are likely to be affected. An isometric

vacuolization, characterized by small vacuoles filled to normal-size tubular epithelial cells, is an early change in CNI nephrotoxicity [112] (Fig. 3d).

Characteristic histological manifestations of chronic CNI nephrotoxicity

Late histopathological changes in glomerular capillaries include the thickening and duplication GBM. These changes are believed to result from the remodeling action induced by chronic CNI endothelial cell injury [113]. The nodular hyaline deposits, which are replaced by the necrotic smooth muscle cells of the media, are distinct features of late changes in CNI nephrotoxicity (Fig. 3e) [114]. In chronic tubular injury, IF/TA may occur but such changes are non-specific.

Therapy for CNI nephrotoxicity

To reduce CNI nephrotoxicity, the clinician should try to control serum CNI concentrations to lower levels, but such methodologies may induce rejection episodes. Recent data from CTOT-9 (Clinical Trial of Transplantation) investigated a CNI withdrawal regimen in cases with an immunologically low risk of rejection. However, 6 of 14 cases of CNI withdrawal experienced acute rejection [115]. Also, ZEUS study reported by Budde et al. demonstrated the development of de novo DSA production after conversion from cyclosporine to everolimus [116]. Additionally, Gallon et al. investigated the conversion from CNI to sirolimus. It was concluded that renal function was equal between the groups but the sirolimus group showed activation of IL6 and IFN-γ, suggesting indirect alloreactive T cell activation [117].

Polyomavirus infection

Polyomavirus allograft nephropathy (PVN), typically associated with BK virus, is caused by re-activation of latent intragraft polyomaviruses under immunosuppression. PVN was first described by Mackenzie in 1978 [118], and subsequent reports described the importance of PVN in patients with kidney transplantation. Approximately 30–50% of recipients demonstrate viruria by cytology or polymerase chain reaction within the first 3 months after kidney transplantation and PVN can occur at the average time of 10–14 months, but as early as 6 days and as late as 6 years, after kidney transplantation [119]. The prevalence of PVN was reportedly 1–10 and 20% of PVN cases showed graft failure [120].

The key to diagnosing PVN is the histological features of the epithelial cells: the so-called ground-glass intranuclear inclusion body, cell lysis, necrosis, shedding into the tubular lumen, denudation of tubular basement membrane, interstitial inflammation, tubulitis, IF/TA, and the positivity of these cells for SV40 staining [121]. Clinicopathological features of PVN include a high rate of false-negative biopsies, difficulties in distinguishing TCMR, the presence of CMV infection, and persistence, for months to years [122–126].

Characteristic histological manifestations of polyomavirus infection

The target lesions in PVN are epithelial cells of the collecting duct, tubules, and Bowman's capsule (parietal epithelial cells). PVN may spread from the urothelium and medulla to the ascending parts of the tubules and Bowman's capsule. Thus, if the foci of parenchymal involvement are smaller, there may be a higher rate of false-negative biopsies. To diagnose early PVN, it is important to pay attention to the depth zones of the kidney samples (medullary ray and medulla). The distinctive histological findings of PVN consist of four types. The most common type is (1) the ground-glass intranuclear inclusion body, followed by (2) a central intranuclear inclusion body surrounded by a halo, (3) nuclear enlargement and fine granular and vesicular changes, and (4) clumped changes [122] (Fig. 4a). The positivity of SV40 T antigen staining is also helpful and indicates polyomavirus replication [124] (Fig. 4b). Banff Polyomavirus Working Group has performed multicenter retrospective study to develop the histological staging system of this disease. AST (American Society of Transplantation) staging system focuses on interstitial inflammation and fibrosis [127], and Banff Working Proposal 2009 focused on tubular cell shedding and fibrosis

[22]. Both systems did not show significant predictive value in a single center study [121]. In 2013, Banff Working Group proposed a new staging system consists of in situ viral load (pvl score) and interstitial fibrosis and now under consideration to incorporate official Banff criteria [128].

Treatment of polyomavirus infection

Specific antiviral drugs for polyomavirus infections are not yet available; thus, patient screening and early diagnosis remain important. Therapeutic methods consist primarily of reduced maintenance immunosuppression proposed in AST guideline [127]. However, clinicians should be aware that about one-quarter of patients experience acute rejection during such a reduction in immunosuppressive therapy [126]. Beyond serum CNI concentrations, mycophenolic acid monitoring is also useful in the clinical setting [129]. In terms of a preventive protocol, low-dose maintenance tacrolimus showed decreased PVN [130]. Of note, Johnston et al. reported the effect of cidofovir and leflunomide for PVN in meta-analysis [131].

Recurrent disease

Graft loss due to recurrent native kidney disease had been thought to be rare and the prevalence was estimated at 1.8% in Japan (http://www.asas.or.jp/jst/pdf/factbook/factbook2015.pdf). However, several recent reports suggest that recurrent kidney disease could contribute more than had been estimated previously. To

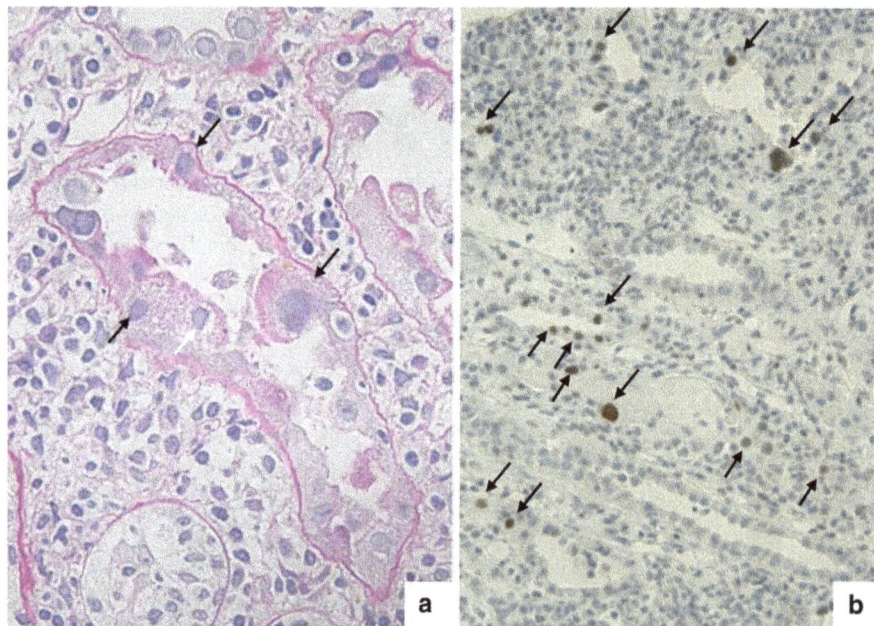

Fig. 4 Pathological findings of BK virus nephropathy. **a** Tubular epithelial cells were swelling and showed ground-glass intranuclear inclusion body (*black arrow*) or intranuclear inclusion body surrounded by a halo (*white arrow*) in a patient with BK virus nephropathy. **b** SV40 immunostaining in a patient with BK virus nephropathy. Distal tubular epithelial cells showed scattered nuclear SV 40 positivity (*arrow*)

diagnose recurrent disease, we should confirm the diagnosis of the native kidney biopsy together with the kidney allograft biopsy. Importantly, the timing or criteria for episode or protocol biopsies differ by institution; these differences can affect the rate and period of the recurrent disease. In most cases, estimations of the recurrence rate for native kidney disease based on protocol biopsies showed higher recurrence rates (Table 3).

Immunoglobulin A neuropathy/immunoglobulin A (IgAN/IgA) vasculitis

The reported recurrence rates of IgAN after transplantation vary between 30 and 35%. The diagnosis of IgAN recurrence requires the presence of mesangial deposits and hyperplasia in the graft, as well as known primary IgAN. IgAN recurrence occurs typically more than 3 years after transplantation. The risk of graft loss due to IgAN recurrence ranged from 3 to 5% [132]. Compared with IgAN, relatively little is known about recurrent IgA vasculitis in renal allografts. The recurrence rate ranges from 15 to 53%, and graft loss due to recurrent IgA vasculitis was 7.5–28.6% in different observation periods [133–135]. A large case-controlled study of 318 patients from one center showed no difference in 10-year graft survival between patients with IgAN recurrence and non-IgAN matched controls: 75% versus 82% [136]. However, it is possible that IgAN recurrence represents a risk factor for graft loss over the long term.

Predictors of active IgAN recurrence include young age, rapid progression of the original disease, and high serum levels of galactose-deficient IgA1 and IgA-IgG complexes [137–139]. Risk factors associated with recurrent IgA vasculitis include shorter duration of the original disease, a living related donor, and necrotizing/crescent glomerulonephritis of the native kidneys [140]. No specific therapy for IgAN and IgA vasculitis recurrence is available; guidelines recommend using angiotensin-converting enzyme inhibitors/angiotensin receptor blockers (ACEI/ARBs) [141]. No immunosuppressive regimen has been shown to be superior [142]. There are some reports that a tonsillectomy followed by steroid pulse therapy resulted in

decreased proteinuria and improved renal function and pathological findings of recurrent IgAN and IgA vasculitis in a renal allograft [143–146].

FSGS

The reported risk of recurrence of focal segmental glomerulosclerosis (FSGS) in the first graft ranges from 30 to 60%, whereas the rate approaches 100% in subsequent grafts [147]. Clinical features of FSGS recurrence include the early and acute onset of massive proteinuria (hours to days after transplantation). Risk factors for recurrence include childhood onset, age <15 years, progression to ESRD within 3 years of onset, diffuse increases in mesangial cells in the native kidney, development of recurrent FSGS in a previous allograft kidney, white race, and receiving a kidney from an elderly donor [148, 149].

The existence of circulating permeability factors, proposed by Savin's group, may be a notable predictor of FSGS recurrence [150]. Circulating urokinase receptor (suPAR), which has been reported as a cause of FSGS, may also be a predictor of FSGS recurrence [151]. However, the significance of suPAR is still controversial [152]. In addition, novel candidates such as CLC-1, anti-CD40 Ab, and vasodilator-stimulated phosphoprotein are proposed [153]. The pathological significance of variant transition remains unknown. IJpelaar et al. [154] evaluated variants of primary and recurrent FSGS for both native and transplanted kidneys and found that 81% of patients showed variant consistency between native and allograft kidneys. They also found collapsing variant and cellular variant (CELL) to be distinct disease entities that did not change after transplantation [154]. In contrast, Canaud et al. [155] reported several transitions between variants in recurrent FSGS after transplantation. PE and immunoadsorption (IA) are effective treatments for recurrent FSGS [148]. Ponticelli reported that partial or complete remission was achievable using PE or IA in 63% of adult patients [148]. Rituximab is also known to be an effective treatment for FSGS and was more effective with PE [156, 157]. However, other reports have noted that rituximab showed an intermediate, or no, response [158].

MN

Recurrence rates of membranous nephropathy (MN) after kidney transplantation have been reported to be 30–45%. The disease usually occurs 2–3 years after transplantation, negatively impacting graft survival with a 10–50% rate of graft loss at 10 years [159]. Determination of the IgG subtypes within the immune deposits in MN may be helpful in the differential diagnosis. IgG4 is the predominant subtype in idiopathic MN and recurrent MN, which did not change over time in recurrent MN [160]. Phospholipase A2 receptor (PLA2R) staining

Table 3 Recurrence rate and consequent graft loss risk of glomerular disease

	Recurrence rate	Graft loss risk
IgAN	30–35%	3–5%
IgA vasculitis (HSPN)	15–53%	7.5–21%
FSGS	30–60%	~50%
MN	30–45%	10–50%
MPGN type I	30–50%	~15%
MPGN type II (DDD)	66–100%	34–66%

IgAN IgA nephroathy, *HSPN* Henoch Schonlein purpura nephritis, *FSGS* focal segmental glomerulosclerosis, *MN* membranous nephropathy, *MPGN* membranoproliferative glomerulonephritis, *DDD* dense deposit disease

in kidney biopsy specimens is useful to distinguish between recurrent and de novo MN. Larsen and Walker reported that recurrent MN was correlated closely with PLA2R positivity, with a sensitivity of 83% and a specificity of 92% for recurrent MN [161]. Circulating anti-PLA2R antibodies at the time of transplantation seems to be a potential risk factor for MN recurrence [162]. Symptomatic treatment with diuretics, ACEI/ARBs, and anticoagulants may be useful in recurrent MN with nephritic syndrome. Some cases of complete responses to therapy with steroids and cyclophosphamide have been reported [163, 164]. Rituximab showed responses more frequently in several, but not all, cases of MN recurrence [165, 166].

MPGN

The traditional classification of membranoproliferative glomerulonephritis (MPGN) was based on the location and type of electron-dense deposits: type I was characterized by subendothelial deposits, type II by intramembranous electron-dense deposits, and type III by subendothelial and subepithelial deposits. The current classification recognizes the importance of IF microscopy in further dividing MPGN into immune complex-mediated MPGN, with glomerular immunoglobulins and complement deposition, and MPGN with abnormalities in alternative complement pathway regulation, resulting in isolated C3 deposits with little or no immunoglobulin by IF(C3 glomerulopathy). MPGN type II is currently designated as dense deposit disease (DDD) and is recognized as a variant of C3 glomerulopathy. C3 glomerulonephritis (C3GN) refers to cases of C3 glomerulopathy in which the electron-dense deposits do not have classic appearance like DDD. The recurrence rate of DDD is 66–100% and has the worst prognosis in MPGN. The rates of graft loss due to recurrence ranges between 34 and 66% [167, 168]. A few patients may respond to plasma exchange [169]. Good results have been reported with eculizumab in DDD patients [170, 171]. Fourteen of 21 (66.7%) patients with C3GN developed recurrence at 28 months (median) after transplantation. Graft failure occurred in 50% of patients with recurrent C3GN after 77 months (median). The remaining 50% of patients had functioning grafts, with a median follow-up of 73.9 months [172]. MPGN type I shows a high recurrence rate, of ~30–50% after transplantation. Risk factors for recurrence include young recipient age, aggressive disease in the native kidneys, and persistently low complement levels. Recurrence occurs early, usually in the first year post-transplantation. The risk for graft loss is ~15% at 10 years [132].

Information on recurrence rates for MPGN type III is limited. Little et al. [167] showed recurrence of MPGN type III in 4 of 12 patients [33%]. Risk factors for recurrent MPGN type III were younger age at initial diagnosis

and the presence of crescents on the original biopsy [167].

Conclusions

The combination of molecular and conventional data will provide new diagnostic criteria in the near future, but conventional histopathology remains the gold standard for the specific diagnosis of allograft dysfunction. Because kidney allografts show considerable diversity, understanding the basics of rejection, CNI nephrotoxicity, PVN, and native kidney disease recurrence is essential for better kidney allograft survival.

Acknowledgements

We thank Department of Urology and Pathology of The Jikei University School of Medicine for their collaboration. We thank Dr. Hiroyasu Yamamoto (Atsugi City Hospital, Kanagawa, Japan) for critical reading of this manuscript. We thank figures courtesy of Dr. Masayoshi Okumi, Department of Urology, Tokyo Women's Medical University, Tokyo, Japan.

Funding

None.

Authors' contributions

AK designed and wrote the manuscript. TY designed and wrote the manuscript. YN designed and helped to draft the manuscript. IY designed and wrote the manuscript and performed the manuscript review. TY performed manuscript review. All authors read and approved the final manuscript.

Competing interests

The authors declare that they have no competing interests.

References

1. Hart A, Smith JM, Skeans MA, Gustafson SK, Stewart DE, Cherikh WS, et al. Kidney. Am J Transplant. 2016;16(S2):11–46.
2. Morrissey PE, Reinert S, Yango A, Gautam A, Monaco A, Gohh R. Factors contributing to acute rejection in renal transplantation: the role of noncompliance. Transplant Proc. 2005;37(5):2044–7.
3. Kasiske BL, Gaston RS, Gourishankar S, Halloran PF, Matas AJ, Jeffery J, et al. Long-term deterioration of kidney allograft function. Am J Transplant. 2005;5(6):1405–14.
4. Nickeleit V. Pathology: donor biopsy evaluation at time of renal grafting. Nat Rev Nephrol. 2009;5(5):249–51.
5. Kissmeyer-Nielsen F, Olsen S, Petersen VP, Fjeldborg O. Hyperacute rejection of kidney allografts, associated with pre-existing humoral antibodies against donor cells. Lancet. 1966;2(7465):662–5.
6. Tait BD, Susal C, Gebel HM, Nickerson PW, Zachary AA, Claas FH, et al. Consensus guidelines on the testing and clinical management issues associated with HLA and non-HLA antibodies in transplantation. Transplantation. 2013;95(1):19–47.
7. Lorenz M, Regele H, Schillinger M, Exner M, Rasoul-Rockenschaub S, Wahrmann M, et al. Risk factors for capillary C4d deposition in kidney allografts: evaluation of a large study cohort. Transplantation. 2004;78(3):447–52.

8. Colvin RB. Antibody-mediated renal allograft rejection: diagnosis and pathogenesis. J Am Soc Nephrol. 2007;18(4):1046–56.

9. Wiebe C, Gibson IW, Blydt-Hansen TD, Karpinski M, Ho J, Storsley LJ, et al. Evolution and clinical pathologic correlations of de novo donor-specific HLA antibody post kidney transplant. Am J Transplant. 2012;12(5):1157–67.

10. Regele H, Bohmig GA, Habicht A, Gollowitzer D, Schillinger M, Rockenschaub S, et al. Capillary deposition of complement split product C4d in renal allografts is associated with basement membrane injury in peritubular and glomerular capillaries: a contribution of humoral immunity to chronic allograft rejection. J Am Soc Nephrol. 2002;13(9):2371–80.

11. Gaston RS, Cecka JM, Kasiske BL, Fieberg AM, Leduc R, Cosio FC, et al. Evidence for antibody-mediated injury as a major determinant of late kidney allograft failure. Transplantation. 2010;90(1):68–74.

12. Einecke G, Sis B, Reeve J, Mengel M, Campbell PM, Hidalgo LG, et al. Antibody-mediated microcirculation injury is the major cause of late kidney transplant failure. Am J Transplant. 2009;9(11):2520–31.

13. Regele H, Exner M, Watschinger B, Wenter C, Wahrmann M, Osterreicher C, et al. Endothelial C4d deposition is associated with inferior kidney allograft outcome independently of cellular rejection. Nephrol Dial Transplant. 2001;16(10):2058–66.

14. Mauiyyedi S, Crespo M, Collins AB, Schneeberger EE, Pascual MA, Saidman SL, et al. Acute humoral rejection in kidney transplantation: II. Morphology, immunopathology, and pathologic classification. J Am Soc Nephrol. 2002;13(3):779–87.

15. Racusen LC, Solez K, Colvin RB, Bonsib SM, Castro MC, Cavallo T, et al. The Banff 97 working classification of renal allograft pathology. Kidney Int. 1999;55(2):713–23.

16. Haas M, Sis B, Racusen LC, Solez K, Glotz D, Colvin RB, et al. Banff 2013 meeting report: inclusion of c4d-negative antibody-mediated rejection and antibody-associated arterial lesions. Am J Transplant. 2014;14(2):272–83.

17. Sis B, Jhangri GS, Riopel J, Chang J, de Freitas DG, Hidalgo L, et al. A new diagnostic algorithm for antibody-mediated microcirculation inflammation in kidney transplants. Am J Transplant. 2012;12(5):1168–79.

18. Yamamoto I, Yamaguchi Y, Yamamoto H, Hosoya T, Horita S, Tanabe K, Fuchinoue S, Teraoka S, Toma H. A pathological analysis of lymphatic vessels in early renal allograft. Transplant Proc. 2006;38(10):3300–3.

19. Lefaucheur C, Loupy A, Vernerey D, et al. Antibody-mediated vascular rejection of kidney allografts: a population-based study. Lancet. 2013;381(9863):313–9.

20. Nickeleit V, Vamvakas EC, Pascual M, Poletti BJ, Colvin RB. The prognostic significance of specific arterial lesions in acute renal allograft rejection. J Am Soc Nephrol. 1998;9(7):1301–8.

21. Bates WD, Davies DR, Welsh K, Gray DW, Fuggle SV, Morris PJ. An evaluation of the Banff classification of early renal allograft biopsies and correlation with outcome. Nephrol Dial Transplant. 1999;14(10):2364–9.

22. Sis B, Mengel M, Haas M, Colvin RB, Halloran PF, Racusen LC, et al. Banff '09 meeting report: antibody mediated graft deterioration and implementation of Banff working groups. Am J Transplant. 2010;10(3):464–71.

23. Salazar ID, Merino Lopez M, Chang J, Halloran PF. Reassessing the significance of intimal arteritis in kidney transplant biopsy specimens. J Am Soc Nephrol. 2015;26(12):3190–8.

24. Satoskar AA, Pelletier R, Adams P, et al. De novo thrombotic microangiopathy in renal allograft biopsies-role of antibody-mediated rejection. Am J Transplant. 2010;10(8):1804–11.

25. Haas M, Mirocha J. Early ultrastructural changes in renal allografts: correlation with antibody-mediated rejection and transplant glomerulopathy. Am J Transplant. 2011;11(10):2123–31.

26. Hara S, Matsushita H, Yamaguchi Y, Kawaminami K, Horita S, Furusawa M. Allograft glomerulitis: histologic characteristics to detect chronic humoral rejection. Transplant Proc. 2005;37(2):714–6.

27. Sijpkens YW, Joosten SA, Wong MC, Dekker FW, Benediktsson H, Bajema IM, et al. Immunologic risk factors and glomerular C4d deposits in chronic transplant glomerulopathy. Kidney Int. 2004;65(6):2409–18.

28. Sis B, Campbell PM, Mueller T, Hunter C, Cockfizeld SM, Cruz J, et al. Transplant glomerulopathy, late antibody-mediated rejection and the ABCD tetrad in kidney allograft biopsies for cause. Am J Transplant. 2007;7(7):1743–52.

29. Issa N, Cosio FG, Gloor JM, Sethi S, Dean PG, Moore SB, et al. Transplant glomerulopathy: risk and prognosis related to anti-human leukocyte antigen class II antibody levels. Transplantation. 2008;86(5):681–5.

30. Fujimoto T, Nakada Y, Yamamoto I, Kobayashi A, Tanno Y, Yamada H, et al. A refractory case of subclinical antibody-mediated rejection due to anti-HLA-DQ antibody in a kidney transplant patient. Nephrology (Carlton). 2015;20 Suppl 2:81–5.

31. Willicombe M, Brookes P, Sergeant R, Santos-Nunez E, Steggar C, Galliford J, et al. De novo DQ donor-specific antibodies are associated with a significant risk of antibody-mediated rejection and transplant glomerulopathy. Transplantation. 2012;94(2):172–7.

32. Kieran N, Wang X, Perkins J, Davis C, Kendrick E, Bakthavatsalam R, et al. Combination of peritubular c4d and transplant glomerulopathy predicts late renal allograft failure. J Am Soc Nephrol. 2009;20(10):2260–8.

33. Lesage J, Noel R, Lapointe I, Cote I, Wagner E, Desy O, et al. Donor-specific antibodies, C4d and their relationship with the prognosis of transplant glomerulopathy. Transplantation. 2015;99(1):69–76.

34. Ivanyi B, Fahmy H, Brown H, Szenohradszky P, Halloran PF, Solez K. Peritubular capillaries in chronic renal allograft rejection: a quantitative ultrastructural study. Hum Pathol. 2000;31(9):1129–38.

35. Liapis G, Singh HK, Derebail VK, Gasim AM, Kozlowski T, Nickeleit V. Diagnostic significance of peritubular capillary basement membrane multilaminations in kidney allografts: old concepts revisited. Transplantation. 2012;94(6):620–9.

36. Aita K, Yamaguchi Y, Horita S, Ohno M, Tanabe K, Fuchinoue S, et al. Thickening of the peritubular capillary basement membrane is a useful diagnostic marker of chronic rejection in renal allografts. Am J Transplant. 2007;7(4):923–9.

37. Yamamoto I, Horita S, Takahashi T, Tanabe K, Fuchinoue S, Teraoka S, Hattori M, Yamaguchi Y. Glomerular expression of plasmalemmal vesicle-associatedprotein-1 in patients with transplant glomerulopathy. Am J Transplant. 2007;7(8):1954–60.

38. Yamamoto I, Horita S, Takahashi T, Kobayashi A, Toki D, Tanabe K, Hattori M, Teraoka S, Aita K, Nagata M, Yamaguchi Y. Caveolin-1 expression is a distinct feature of chronic rejection-induced transplant capillaropathy. Am J Transplant. 2008;8(12):2627–35.

39. Nakada Y, Yamamoto I, Horita S, Kobayashi A, Mafune A, Katsumata H, Yamakawa T, Katsuma A, Kawabe M, Tanno Y, Ohkido I, Tsuboi N, Yamamoto H, Okumi M, Ishida H, Yokoo T, Tanabe K, Japan Academic Consortium of Kidney Transplantation [JACK]. The prognostic values of Caveolin-1 immunoreactivity in peritubular capillaries in patients with kidney transplantation. Clin Transplant. 2016. doi:10.1111/ctr.12833. [Epub ahead of print]

40. Xu-Dubois YC, Peltier J, Brocheriou I, Suberbielle-Boissel C, Djamali A, Reese S, Mooney N, Keuylian Z, Lion J, Ouali N, Levy PP, Jouanneau C, Rondeau E, Hertig A. Markers of endothelial-to-mesenchymal transition: evidence for antibody-endothelium interaction during antibody-mediated rejection in kidney recipients. J Am Soc Nephrol. 2016;27(1):324–32.

41. Loupy A, Vernerey D, Viglietti D, Aubert O, Duong Van Huyen JP, Empana JP, et al. Determinants and outcomes of accelerated arteriosclerosis: major impact of circulating antibodies. Circ Res. 2015; 117(5):470–82.

42. Solez K, Colvin RB, Racusen LC, Sis B, Halloran PF, Birk PE, et al. Banff '05 Meeting Report: differential diagnosis of chronic allograft injury and elimination of chronic allograft nephropathy ['CAN']. Am J Transplant. 2007;7(3):518–26.

43. Sis B, Jhangri GS, Bunnag S, Allanach K, Kaplan B, Halloran PF. Endothelial gene expression in kidney transplants with alloantibody indicates antibody-mediated damage despite lack of C4d staining. Am J Transplant. 2009;9(10):2312–23.

44. Setoguchi K, Ishida H, Shimmura H, et al. Analysis of renal transplant protocol biopsies in ABO-incompatible kidney transplantation. Am J Transplant. 2008;8(1):86–94.

45. Haas M, Rahman MH, Racusen LC, et al. C4d and C3d staining in biopsies of ABO- and HLA-incompatible renal allografts: correlation with histologic findings. Am J Transplant. 2006;6(8):1829–40.

46. Solez K, Colvin RB, Racusen LC, Haas M, Sis B, Mengel M, et al. Banff 07 classification of renal allograft pathology: updates and future directions. Am J Transplant. 2008;8(4):753–60.

47. Toki D, Inui M, Ishida H, Okumi M, Shimizu T, Shirakawa H, et al. Interstitial fibrosis is the critical determinant of impaired renal function in transplant glomerulopathy. Nephrology (Carlton). 2016;1:20–5.

48. Loupy A, Hill GS, Jordan SC. The impact of donor-specific anti-HLA antibodies on late kidney allograft failure. Nat Rev Nephrol. 2012;8(6):348–57.

49. Haas M. An updated Banff schema for diagnosis of antibody-mediated rejection in renal allografts. Curr Opin Organ Transplant. 2014;19(3):315–22.

50. Gupta A, Broin PO, Bao Y, Pullman J, Kamal L, Ajaimy M, et al. Clinical and molecular significance of microvascular inflammation in transplant kidney biopsies. Kidney Int. 2016;89(1):217–25.

51. Reeve J, Sellares J, Mengel M, Sis B, Skene A, Hidalgo L, et al. Molecular diagnosis of T cell-mediated rejection in human kidney transplant biopsies. Am J Transplant. 2013;13(3):645–55.

52. Halloran PF, Pereira AB, Chang J, Matas A, Picton M, De Freitas D, et al. Microarray diagnosis of antibody-mediated rejection in kidney transplant biopsies: an international prospective study [INTERCOM]. Am J Transplant. 2013;13(11):2865–74.

53. Reeve J, Chang J, Salazar ID, Lopez MM, Halloran PF. Using molecular phenotyping to guide improvements in the histologic diagnosis of T cell-mediated rejection. Am J Transplant. 2016;16(4):1183–92.

54. Halloran PF, Merino Lopez M, Barreto PA. Identifying subphenotypes of antibody-mediated rejection in kidney transplants. Am J Transplant. 2016;16(3):908–20.

55. Mengel M, Sis B, Haas M, Colvin RB, Halloran PF, Racusen LC, et al. Banff 2011 Meeting report: new concepts in antibody-mediated rejection. Am J Transplant. 2012;12(3):563–70.

56. Mohan S, Palanisamy A, Tsapepas D, Tanriover B, Crew RJ, Dube G, et al. Donor-specific antibodies adversely affect kidney allograft outcomes. J Am Soc Nephrol. 2012;23(12):2061–71.

57. Bentall A, Cornell LD, Gloor JM, Park WD, Gandhi MJ, Winters JL, et al. Five-year outcomes in living donor kidney transplants with a positive crossmatch. Am J Transplant. 2013;13(1):76–85.

58. Wiebe C, Gibson IW, Blydt-Hansen TD, Pochinco D, Birk PE, Ho J, et al. Rates and determinants of progression to graft failure in kidney allograft recipients with de novo donor-specific antibody. Am J Transplant. 2015;15(11):2921–30.

59. Lefaucheur C, Loupy A, Hill GS, Andrade J, Nochy D, Antoine C, et al. Preexisting donor-specific HLA antibodies predict outcome in kidney transplantation. J Am Soc Nephrol. 2010;21(8):1398–406.

60. Loupy A, Lefaucheur C, Vernerey D, et al. Complement-binding anti-HLA antibodies and kidney-allograft survival. N Engl J Med. 2013;369(13):1215–26.

61. Sicard A, Ducreux S, Rabeyrin M, et al. Detection of C3d-binding donor-specific anti-HLA antibodies at diagnosis of humoral rejection predicts renal graft loss. J Am Soc Nephrol. 2015;26(2):457–67.

62. Lefaucheur C, Viglietti D, Bentlejewski C, van Huyen JP D, Vernerey D, Aubert O, et al. IgG donor-specific anti-human HLA antibody subclasses and kidney allograft antibody-mediated injury. J Am Soc Nephrol. 2016;27(1):293–304.

63. Park H, Lim Y, Han B, et al. Frequent false-positive reactions in pronase-treated T-cell flow cytometric cross-match tests. Transplant Proc. 2012;44(1):87–90.

64. Amico P, Honger G, Bielmann D, et al. Incidence and prediction of early antibody-mediated rejection due to non-human leukocyte antigen-antibodies. Transplantation. 2008;85:1557–63.

65. Duska D, Dominik NM, Jan HB, et al. Angiotensin II type 1-receptor activating antibodies in renal-allograft rejection. N Engl J Med. 2005;352:558–69.

66. Jurcevic S, Ainsworth ME, Pomerance A, et al. Anti-vimentin antibodies are an independent predictor of transplant-associated coronary artery disease after cardiac transplantation. Transplantation. 2001;71:886–92.

67. Banasik M, Boratynska M, Koscielska-Kasprzak K, et al. The influence of non-HLA antibodies directed against angiotensin II type 1 receptor [AT1R] on early renal transplant outcomes. Transpl Int. 2014. doi:10.1111/tri.12371 [Epub ahead of print].

68. Reinsmoen NL, Lai CH, Heidecke H, et al. Anti-angiotensin type 1 receptor antibodies associated with antibody-mediated rejection in donor HLA antibody-negative patients. Transplantation. 2010;90:1473–7.

69. Scornik JC, Guerra G, Schold JD, et al. Value of posttransplant antibody tests in the evaluation of patients with renal graft dysfunction. Am J Transplant. 2007;7:1808.

70. Breimer ME, Rydberg L, Jackson AM, et al. Multicenter evaluation of a novel endothelial cell crossmatch test in kidney transplantation. Transplantation. 2009;87(4):549–56.

71. Jackson AM, Sigdel TK, Delville M, Hsieh SC, Dai H, Bagnasco S, Montgomery RA, Sarwal MM. Endothelial cell antibodies associated with novel targets and increased rejection. J Am Soc Nephrol. 2015;26(5):1161–71.

72. Roberts DM, Jiang SH, Chadban SJ. The treatment of acute antibody-mediated rejection in kidney transplant recipients-a systematic review. Transplantation. 2012;94(8):775–83.

73. Schmidt N, Alloway RR, Walsh RC, Sadaka B, Shields AR, Girnita AL, et al. Prospective evaluation of the toxicity profile of proteasome inhibitor-based therapy in renal transplant candidates and recipients. Transplantation. 2012;94(4):352–61.

74. Walsh RC, Everly JJ, Brailey P, Rike AH, Arend LJ, Mogilishetty G, et al. Proteasome inhibitor-based primary therapy for antibody-mediated renal allograft rejection. Transplantation. 2010;89(3):277–84.

75. Stegall MD, Diwan T, Raghavaiah S, Cornell LD, Burns J, Dean PG, et al. Terminal complement inhibition decreases antibody-mediated rejection in sensitized renal transplant recipients. Am J Transplant. 2011;11(11):2405–13.

76. Cornell LD, Schinstock CA, Gandhi MJ, Kremers WK, Stegall MD. Positive crossmatch kidney transplant recipients treated with eculizumab: outcomes beyond 1 year. Am J Transplant. 2015;15(5):1293–302.

77. Fehr T, Rusi B, Fischer A, Hopfer H, Wuthrich RP, Gaspert A. Rituximab and intravenous immunoglobulin treatment of chronic antibody-mediated kidney allograft rejection. Transplantation. 2009;87(12):1837–41.

78. Schwaiger E, Regele H, Wahrmann M, Werzowa J, Haidbauer B, Schmidt A, et al. Bortezomib for the treatment of chronic antibody-mediated kidney allograft rejection: a case report. Clin Transpl. 2010:391-396.

79. O'Leary JG, Samaniego M, Barrio MC, Potena L, Zeevi A, Djamali A, et al. The Influence of Immunosuppressive Agents on the Risk of De Novo Donor-Specific HLA Antibody Production in Solid Organ Transplant Recipients. Transplantation. 2016;100(1):39–53.

80. Herzenberg AM, Gill JS, Djurdjev O, Magil AB. C4d deposition in acute rejection: an independent long-term prognostic factor. J Am Soc Nephrol. 2002;13(1):234–41.

81. Matignon M, Muthukumar T, Seshan SV, Suthanthiran M, Hartono C. Concurrent acute cellular rejection is an independent risk factor for renal allograft failure in patients with C4d-positive antibody-mediated rejection. Transplantation. 2012;94(6):603–11.

82. Ivanyi B, Hansen HE, Olsen S. Segmental localization and quantitative characteristics of tubulitis in kidney biopsies from patients undergoing acute rejection. Transplantation. 1993;56(3):581–5.

83. Mannon RB, Matas AJ, Grande J, Leduc R, Connett J, Kasiske B, et al. Inflammation in areas of tubular atrophy in kidney allograft biopsies: a potent predictor of allograft failure. Am J Transplant. 2010;10(9):2066–73.

84. Hall BM, Bishop GA, Duggin GG, Horvath JS, Philips J, Tiller DJ. Increased expression of HLA-DR antigens on renal tubular cells in renal transplants: relevance to the rejection response. Lancet. 1984;2(8397):247–51.

85. Gonzalez-Posada JM, Garcia-Castro MC, Tamajon LP, Torres A, Hernandez D, Losada M, et al. HLA-DR class II and ICAM-1 expression on tubular cells taken by fine-needle aspiration biopsy in renal allograft dysfunction. Nephrol Dial Transplant. 1996;11(1):148–52.

86. Colvin RB, Cohen AH, Saiontz C, Bonsib S, Buick M, Burke B, et al. Evaluation of pathologic criteria for acute renal allograft rejection: reproducibility, sensitivity, and clinical correlation. J Am Soc Nephrol. 1997;8(12):1930–41.

87. Bellamy CO, Randhawa PS. Arteriolitis in renal transplant biopsies is associated with poor graft outcome. Histopathology. 2000;36(6):488–92.

88. Nickeleit V, Zeiler M, Gudat F, Thiel G, Mihatsch MJ. Detection of the complement degradation product C4d in renal allografts: diagnostic and therapeutic implications. J Am Soc Nephrol. 2002;13(1):242–51.

89. Torbenson M, Randhawa P. Arcuate and interlobular phlebitis in renal allografts. Hum Pathol. 2001;32(12):1388–91.

90. Sis B, Bagnasco SM, Cornell LD, Randhawa P, Haas M, Lategan B, et al. Isolated endarteritis and kidney transplant survival: a multicenter collaborative study. J Am Soc Nephrol. 2015;26(5):1216–27.

91. Gaber LW, Moore LW, Gaber AO, Tesi RJ, Meyer J, Schroeder TJ. Correlation of histology to clinical rejection reversal: a thymoglobulin multicenter trial report. Kidney Int. 1999;55(6):2415–22.

92. Meehan SM, Siegel CT, Aronson AJ, Bartosh SM, Thistlethwaite JR, Woodle ES, et al. The relationship of untreated borderline infiltrates by the Banff criteria to acute rejection in renal allograft biopsies. J Am Soc Nephrol. 1999;10(8):1806–14.

93. Rush D, Nickerson P, Gough J, McKenna R, Grimm P, Cheang M, et al. Beneficial effects of treatment of early subclinical rejection: a randomized study. J Am Soc Nephrol. 1998;9(11):2129–34.

94. Rush D, Arlen D, Boucher A, Busque S, Cockfield SM, Girardin C, et al. Lack of benefit of early protocol biopsies in renal transplant patients receiving TAC and MMF: a randomized study. Am J Transplant. 2007;7(11):2538–45.

95. Kurtkoti J, Sakhuja V, Sud K, Minz M, Nada R, Kohli HS, et al. The utility of 1- and 3-month protocol biopsies on renal allograft function: a randomized controlled study. Am J Transplant. 2008;8(2):317–23.

96. Haas M, Montgomery RA, Segev DL, Rahman MH, Racusen LC, Bagnasco SM, et al. Subclinical acute antibody-mediated rejection in positive crossmatch renal allografts. Am J Transplant. 2007;7(3):576–85.

97. Loupy A, Suberbielle-Boissel C, Hill GS, Lefaucheur C, Anglicheau D, Zuber J, et al. Outcome of subclinical antibody-mediated rejection in kidney transplant recipients with preformed donor-specific antibodies. Am J Transplant. 2009;9(11):2561–70.

98. Yamamoto T, Watarai Y, Takeda A, Tsujita M, Hiramitsu T, Goto N, et al. De Novo Anti-HLA DSA Characteristics and Subclinical Antibody-Mediated Kidney Allograft Injury. Transplantation. 2016;100(10):2194–202.

99. Katsuma A, Yamamoto I, Komatsuzaki Y, Niikura T, Kawabe M, Okabayashi Y, et al. Subclinical antibody-mediated rejection due to anti-human-leukocyte-antigen-DR53 antibody accompanied by plasma cell-rich acute rejection in a patient with cadaveric kidney transplantation. Nephrology (Carlton). 2016;21 Suppl 1:31–4.

100. Loupy A, Vernerey D, Tinel C, Aubert O, Duong van Huyen JP, Rabant M, et al. Subclinical rejection phenotypes at 1 year post-transplant and outcome of kidney allografts. J Am Soc Nephrol. 2015;26(7):1721–31.

101. Charney DA, Nadasdy T, Lo AW, Racusen LC. Plasma cell-rich acute renal allograft rejection. Transplantation. 1999;68(6):791–7.

102. Meehan SM, Domer P, Josephson M, Donoghue M, Sadhu A, Ho LT, et al. The clinical and pathologic implications of plasmacytic infiltrates in percutaneous renal allograft biopsies. Hum Pathol. 2001;32(2):205–15.

103. Desvaux D, Le Gouvello S, Pastural M, Abtahi M, Suberbielle C, Boeri N, et al. Acute renal allograft rejections with major interstitial oedema and plasma cell-rich infiltrates: high gamma-interferon expression and poor clinical outcome. Nephrol Dial Transplant. 2004;19(4):933–9.

104. Gartner V, Eigentler TK, Viebahn R. Plasma cell-rich rejection processes in renal transplantation: morphology and prognostic relevance. Transplantation. 2006;81(7):986–91.

105. Chang A, Moore JM, Cowan ML, Josephson MA, Chon WJ, Sciammas R, et al. Plasma cell densities and glomerular filtration rates predict renal allograft outcomes following acute rejection. Transpl Int. 2012;25(10):1050–8.

106. Furuya M, Yamamoto I, Kobayashi A, Nakada Y, Sugano N, Tanno Y, et al. Plasma cell-rich rejection accompanied by acute antibody-mediated rejection in a patient with ABO-incompatible kidney transplantation. Nephrology (Carlton). 2014;19 Suppl 3:31–4.

107. Abbas K, Mubarak M, Zafar MN, Aziz T, Abbas H, Muzaffar R, et al. Plasma cell-rich acute rejections in living-related kidney transplantation: a clinicopathological study of 50 cases. Clin Transplant. 2015;29(9):835–41.

108. Naesens M, Kuypers DR, Sarwal M. Calcineurin inhibitor nephrotoxicity. Clin J Am Soc Nephrol. 2009;4(2):481–508.

109. Ojo AO, Held PJ, Port FK, Wolfe RA, Leichtman AB, Young EW, Arndorfer J, Christensen L, Merion RM. Chronic renal failure after transplantation of a nonrenal organ. N Engl J Med. 2003;349(10):931–40.

110. English RF, Pophal SA, Bacanu SA, Fricker J, Boyle GJ, Ellis D, Harker K, Sutton R, Miller SA, Law YM, Pigula FA, Webber SA. Long-term comparison of tacrolimus- and cyclosporine-induced nephrotoxicity in pediatric heart-transplant recipients. Am J Transplant. 2002;2(8):769–73.

111. Nankivell BJ, Borrows RJ, Fung CL, O'Connell PJ, Allen RD, Chapman JR. The natural history of chronic allograft nephropathy. N Engl J Med. 2003;349(24):2326–33.

112. Mihatsch MJ, Thiel G, Ryffel B. Cyclosporine nephrotoxicity. Adv Nephrol Necker Hosp. 1988;17:303–20.

113. Mihatsch MJ, Morozumi K, Strøm EH, Ryffel B, Gudat F, Thiel G. Renal transplant morphology after long-term therapy with cyclosporine. Transplant Proc. 1995;27(1):39–42.

114. Yamaguchi Y, Teraoka S, Yagisawa T, Takahashi K, Toma H, Ota K. Ultrastructural study of cyclosporine-associated arteriolopathy in renal allografts. Transplant Proc. 1989;21(1 Pt 2):1517–22.

115. Formica R, Nickerson P, Poggio E, et al. Immune monitoring and tacrolimus [Tac] withdrawal in low risk recipients of kidney transplants—results of CTOT09. Am J Transplant. 2014;14:225.

116. Budde K, Lehner F, Sommerer C, et al. Conversion from cyclosporine to everolimus at 4.5 months posttransplant: 3-year results from the randomized ZEUS study. Am J Transplant. 2012;12(6):1528–40.

117. Gallon L, Gehrau R, Leventhal J, et al. Chronic immune activation after sirolimus conversion in kidney transplant recipients. Am J Transplant. 2014;14:112.

118. Mackenzie EF, Poulding JM, Harrison PR, Amer B. Human polyoma virus [HPV]—a significant pathogen in renal transplantation. Proc Eur Dial Transplant Assoc. 1978;15:352–60.

119. Sachdeva MS, Nada R, Jha V, Sakhuja V, Joshi K. The high incidence of BK polyoma virus infection among renal transplant recipients in India. Transplantation. 2004;77(3):429–31.

120. Brennan DC, Agha I, Bohl DL, Schnitzler MA, Hardinger KL, Lockwood M, Torrence S, Schuessler R, Roby T, Gaudreault-Keener M, Storch GA. Incidence of BK with tacrolimus versus cyclosporine and impact of preemptive immunosuppression reduction. Am J Transplant. 2005;5(3):582–94. Erratum in: Am J Transplant. 2005 Apr;5[4 Pt 1]:839.

121. Masutani K, Shapiro R, Basu A, Tan H, Wijkstrom M, Randhawa P. The Banff 2009 Working Proposal for polyomavirus nephropathy: a critical evaluation of its utility as a determinant of clinical outcome. Am J Transplant. 2012;12(4):907–18.

122. Nickeleit V, Mihatsch MJ. Polyomavirus nephropathy in native kidneys and renal allografts: an update on an escalating threat. Transpl Int. 2006;19(12):960–73.

123. Mafune A, Tanno Y, Yamamoto H, Kobayashi A, Saigawa H, Yokoo T, Hayakawa H, Miyazaki Y, Yokoyama K, Yamaguchi Y, Hosoya T. A case of BK virus nephropathy and cytomegalovirus infection concurrent with plasma cell-rich acute rejection. Clin Transplant. 2012;26 Suppl 24:49–53.

124. Nickeleit V, Hirsch HH, Zeiler M, Gudat F, Prince O, Thiel G, Mihatsch MJ. BK-virus nephropathy in renal transplants-tubular necrosis, MHC-class II expression and rejection in a puzzling game. Nephrol Dial Transplant. 2000;15(3):324–32.

125. Nickeleit V, Hirsch HH, Binet IF, Gudat F, Prince O, Dalquen P, Thiel G, Mihatsch MJ. Polyomavirus infection of renal allograft recipients: from latent infection to manifest disease. J Am Soc Nephrol. 1999;10(5):1080–9.

126. Bohl DL, Brennan DC. BK virus nephropathy and kidney transplantation. Clin J Am Soc Nephrol. 2007;2 Suppl 1:S36–46.

127. Hirsch HH, Randhawa P, AST Infectious Diseases Community of Practice. BK virus in solid organ transplant recipients. Am J Transplant. 2009;9 Suppl 4:S136–46.

128. Hara S. Banff 2013 update: pearls and pitfalls in transplant renal pathology. Nephrology (Carlton). 2015;20 Suppl 2:2–8.

129. Kobayashi A, Yamamoto I, Nakada Y, Kidoguchi S, Matsuo N, Tanno Y, Ohkido I, Tsuboi N, Yamamoto H, Yokoyama K, Yokoo T. Successful treatment of BK virus nephropathy using therapeutic drug monitoring of mycophenolic acid. Nephrology (Carlton). 2014;19 Suppl 3:37–41.

130. Cosio FG, Amer H, Grande JP, Larson TS, Stegall MD, Griffin MD. Comparison of low versus high tacrolimus levels in kidney transplantation: assessment of efficacy by protocol biopsies. Transplantation. 2007;83(4):411–6.

131. Johnston O, Jaswal D, Gill JS, et al. Treatment of polyomavirus infection in kidney transplant recipients: a systematic review. Transplantation. 2010;89(9):1057–70.

132. Ponticelli C, Moroni G, Glassock RJ. Recurrence of secondary glomerular disease after renal transplantation. Clin J Am Soc Nephrol. 2011;6(5):1214–21.

133. Samuel JP, Bell CS, Molony DA, et al. Long-term outcome of renal transplantation patients with Henoch–Schönlein purpura. Clin J Am Soc Nephrol. 2011;6(8):2034–40.

134. Meulders Q, Pirson Y, Cosyns JP, et al. Course of Henoch–Schönlein nephritis after renal transplantation. Report on ten patients and review of the literature. Transplantation. 1994;58(11):1179–86.

135. Kawabe M, Yamamoto I, Komatsuzaki Y, Japan Academic Consortium of Kidney Transplantation [JACK], et?al. Recurrence and graft loss after renal transplantation in adults with IgA vasculitis. Clin Exp Nephrol. 2016. [Epub ahead of print] PubMed PMID: 27677884.

136. Wang AY, Lai FM, Yu AW, et al. Recurrent IgA nephropathy in renal transplant allografts. Am J Kidney Dis. 2001;38(3):588–96.

137. Sato K, Ishida H, Uchida K, et al. Risk factors for recurrence of immunoglobulin a nephropathy after renal transplantation: single center study. Ther Apher Dial. 2013;17(2):213–20.

138. Soler MJ, Mir M, Rodriguez E, et al. Recurrence of IgA nephropathy and Henoch–Schönlein purpura after kidney transplantation: risk factors and graft survival. Transplant Proc. 2005;37(9):3705–9.

139. Berthelot L, Robert T, Vuiblet V, et al. Recurrent IgA nephropathy is predicted by altered glycosylated IgA, autoantibodies and soluble CD89 complexes. Kidney Int. 2015;88(4):815–22.

140. Moroni G, Gallelli B, Diana A, et al. Renal transplantation in adults with Henoch–Schönlein purpura: long-term outcome. Nephrol Dial Transplant. 2008;23:3010–6.

141. Oka K, Imai E, Moriyama T, et al. A clinicopathological study of IgA nephropathy in renal transplant recipients: beneficial effect of angiotensin-converting enzyme inhibitor. Nephrol Dial Transplant. 2000;15(5):689–95.

142. Floege J. Recurrent IgA nephropathy after renal transplantation. Semin Nephrol. 2004;24(3):287–91.

143. Tanno Y, Yamamoto H, Yamamoto I, et al. Recurrence of Henoch-Schoenlein purpura nephritis superimposed on severe pre-eclampsia in a kidney transplant recipient. Clin Transplant. 2007;21 Suppl 18:36–9.

144. Yaginuma T, Yamamoto H, Mitome J, et al. Successful treatment of nephritic syndrome caused by recurrent IgA nephropathy with chronic active antibody-mediated rejection three years after kidney transplantation. Clin Transplant. 2011;Suppl 23:28–33. doi:10.1111/j.1399-0012.2011.01456.x.

145. Hotta K, Fukasawa Y, Akimoto M, et al. Tonsillectomy ameliorates histological damage of recurrent immunoglobulin A nephropathy after kidney transplantation. Nephrology. 2013;18(12):808–12.

146. Yamakawa T, Yamamoto I, Komatsuzaki Y, et al. Successful treatment of recurrent Henoch–Schönlein purpura nephritis in a renal allograft with tonsillectomy and steroid pulse therapy. Nephrology [Carlton]. 2016. [Epub ahead of print]

147. Messina M, Gallo E, Mella A, et al. Update on the treatment of focal segmental glomerulosclerosis in renal transplantation. World J Transplant. 2016;6(1):54–68.

148. Ponticelli C. Recurrence of focal segmental glomerular sclerosis [FSGS] after renal transplantation. Nephrol Dial Transplant. 2010;25:25–31.

149. Morozumi K, Takeda A, Otsuka Y, et al. Recurrent glomerular disease after kidney transplantation: an update of selected areas and the impact of protocol biopsy. Nephrol. 2014;19 Suppl 3:6–10.

150. McCarthy ET, Sharma M, Savin VJ. Circulating permeability factors in idiopathic nephrotic syndrome and focal segmental glomerulosclerosis. Clin J Am Soc Nephrol. 2010;5:2115–21.

151. Wei C, Hindi SE, Li J, et al. Circulating urokinase receptor as a cause of focal segmental glomerulosclerosis. Nat Med. 2011;17:952–60.

152. Spinale JM, Mariani LH, Kapoor S, et al. NephroticSyndrome Study Network. A reassessment of soluble urokinase-type plasminogen activator receptor in glomerular disease. Kidney Int. 2015;87(3):564–74.

153. Messina M, Gallo E, Mella A, Pagani F, Biancone L. Update on the treatment of focal segmental glomerulosclerosis in renal transplantation. World J Transplant. 2016;6(1):54–68.

154. IJpelaar DH, Farris AB, Goemaere N, et al. Fidelity and evolution of recurrent FSGS in renal allografts. J Am Soc Nephrol. 2008;19:2219–24.

155. Canaud G, Dion D, Zuber J, et al. Recurrence of nephritic syndrome after transplantation in a mixed population of children and adults: course of glomerular lesions and value of the Columbia classification of histological variants of focal and segmental glomerulosclerosis [FSGS]. Nephrol Dial Transplant. 2010;25:1321–8.

156. Garrouste C, Canaud G, Büchler M, Rivalan J, Colosio C, Martinez F, et al. Rituximab for Recurrence of Primary Focal Segmental Glomerulosclerosis After Kidney Transplantation: Clinical Outcomes. Transplantation. 2016. [Epub ahead of print].

157. Cravedi P, Kopp JB, Remuzzi G. Recent progress in the pathophysiology and treatment of FSGS recurrence. Am J Transplant. 2013;13:266–74.

158. Yabu JM, Ho B, Scandling JD, Vincenti F. Rituximab failed to improve nephrotic syndrome in renal transplant patients with recurrent focal segmental glomerulosclerosis. Am J Transplant. 2008;8:222–7.

159. Moroni G, Gallelli B, Quaglini S, Leoni A, Banfi G, Passerini P, Montagnino G, Messa P. Long-term outcome of renal transplantation in patients with idiopathic membranous glomerulonephritis [MN]. Nephrol Dial Transplant. 2010;25(10):3408–15.

160. Kattah AG, Alexander MP, Angioi A, et al. Temporal IgG subtype changes in recurrent idiopathic membranous nephropathy. Am J Transplant. 2016;XX:1–9.

161. Larsen CP, Walker PD. Phospholipase A2 receptor [PLA2R] staining is useful in the determination of de novo versus recurrent membranous glomerulopathy. Transplant. 2013;95:1259–62.

162. Kattah A, Ayalon R, Beck Jr LH, et al. Anti-phospholipase A[2] receptor antibodies in recurrent membranous nephropathy. Am J Transplant. 2015;15:1349–59.

163. Carneiro-Roza F, Walker PD. Phospholipase A2 receptor [PLA2R] staining is useful in the determination of de novo versus recurrent membranous glomerulopathy. Transplant Proc. 2006;38:3491–7.

164. Larsen CP, Walker PD. Phospholipase A2 receptor [PLA2R] staining is useful in the determination of de novo versus recurrent membranous glomerulopathy. Transplantation. 2013;95(10):1259–62.

165. El-Zoghby ZM, Grande JP, Fraile MG, et al. Recurrent idiopathic membranous nephropathy: early diagnosis by protocol biopsies and treatment with anti-CD20 monoclonal antibodies. Am J Transplant. 2009;9(12):2800–7.

166. Sprangers B, Lefkowitz GI, Cohen SD, et al. Beneficial effect of rituximab in the treatment of recurrent idiopathic membranous nephropathy after kidney transplantation. Clin J Am Soc Nephrol. 2010;5:790–7.

167. Little MA, Dupont P, Campbell E, et al. Severity of primary MPGN, rather than MPGN type, determines renal survival and post-transplantation recurrence risk. Kidey Int. 2006;69:504–11.

168. Ivanyi B. A primer on recurrent and de novo glomerulonephritis in renal allografts. Nat Clin Pract Nephrol. 2008;4:446–57.

169. Haffner K, Michelfelder S, Pohl M. Successful therapy of C3Nef-positive C3 glomerulopathy with plasma therapy and immunosuppression. Pediatr Nephrol. 2015;30:1951–9.

170. Sanchez-Moreno A, De la Cerda F, Cabrera R, et al. Eculizumab in dense-deposit disease after renal transplantation. Pediatr Nephrol. 2014;29:2055–9.

171. Oosterveldt M, Garrelfs MR, Hoppe B, et al. Eculizumab in pediatric dense deposit disease. Clin J Am Soc Nephrol. 2015;10:1773–82.

172. Zand L, Lorenz EC, Cosio FG. Clinical findings, pathology, and outcomes of C3GN after kidney transplantation. J Am Soc Nephrol. 2014;25:1110–7.

15

Urinary excretion of liver-type fatty acid-binding protein reflects the severity of sepsis

Eiichi Sato[1*], Atsuko Kamijo-Ikemori[2,4], Tsuyoshi Oikawa[3], Aya Okuda[3], Takeshi Sugaya[3,4], Kenjiro Kimura[5], Tsukasa Nakamura[1,4] and Yugo Shibagaki[4]

Abstract

Sepsis due to microbial invasion often causes multiple organ failure (MOF), including acute kidney injury (AKI), with high mortality rates in serious cases. Hence, there is an urgent need for diagnostic biomarkers that can be used to rapidly, accurately, and easily detect sepsis to identify the condition early and guide the selection of appropriate treatment. Liver-type fatty acid-binding protein (L-FABP), which localizes in renal proximal tubules, is excreted into the urine in response to oxidative stress-induced tubular injury. Because of this mechanism, L-FABP has been reported to be a useful urinary biomarker not only for renal disease but also for the severity of sepsis. Based on this concept, we developed a new L-FABP point-of-care (POC) assay kit that can be used to rapidly measure human L-FABP in the urine to further improve the usefulness of this biomarker in clinical settings. In this review, we describe the molecular mechanisms of L-FABP, its clinical usefulness, and the performance of the POC assay kit.

Keywords: L-FABP, POC, Sepsis, AKI, Oxidative stress, Biomarker

Background

Sepsis is a severe inflammatory response to microbial invasion of the bloodstream and causes multiple organ failure (MOF), including acute kidney injury (AKI). Serious cases of sepsis have a high mortality rate. The initial definition of sepsis was proposed in 1991 [1] and then revised in 2001 [2] and 2016 [3] by the sepsis definition task-force. The most recent definition emphasized the severity of organ failure, although previous definitions mainly focused on inflammation. Sepsis was defined as "life-threatening organ dysfunction caused by a dysregulated host response to infection" in the most recent revision [3]. Moreover, Systemic Inflammatory Response Syndrome (SIRS) criteria were excluded, and a new clinical score for multiple organ failure was proposed, named the quick sepsis-related organ failure assessment (qSOFA) criteria, which comprise the following: a high respiratory rate (≥22/min), altered mentation, and low systolic blood pressure (≤100 mmHg). With the qSOFA criteria, a blood test is not necessary, and the scoring is very simple and intuitive compared with the SIRS criteria. Thus, all medical staff can identify patients with infections who are likely to have a poor outcome by using the qSOFA at the bedside, and the patients can receive appropriate treatment at an early stage.

Therefore, diagnostic biomarkers that can be used to rapidly detect sepsis and MOF and predict its progression are needed. These biomarkers could guide early decisions regarding the appropriate treatment for sepsis. To date, more than 170 biomarkers for sepsis have been evaluated [4]. Among these biomarkers, C-reactive protein (CRP) and procalcitonin (PCT) are reported that these have been most widely used, but these biomarkers require broader validation before they can be incorporated into the clinical criteria describing sepsis [3]. Hence, there is an urgent need for diagnostic biomarkers that can be used to rapidly, accurately, and easily detect the severity of sepsis to identify the condition early and guide the selection of appropriate treatment.

Liver-type fatty acid-binding protein (L-FABP), which localizes in renal proximal tubules, is excreted into the urine during the response to tubular injury in renal disease [5]. L-FABP has been shown to be a useful urinary biomarker for the diagnosis of renal disease in the following clinical conditions: diabetic nephropathy [6–9], anemia [10], acute kidney injury (AKI) [11–16], pediatric

* Correspondence: satou@db4.so-net.ne.jp
[1]Division of Nephrology, Department of Medicine, Shinmatsudo Central General Hospital, 1-380 Shinmatsudo, Matsudo, Chiba 270-0034, Japan
Full list of author information is available at the end of the article

AKI [17], contrast medium-induced nephropathy [18, 19], IgA nephropathy [20], human immunodeficiency virus (HIV)-associated nephropathy [21, 22], and reduced graft function in renal transplantation [23, 24]. Numerous AKI cohort studies have reported increased urinary levels of L-FABP in patients with septic shock-induced AKI [25–28]. In this review, we describe the molecular mechanisms of L-FABP in response to ischemic and oxidative stress, the clinical usefulness of urinary L-FABP for sepsis, and a new method for detecting L-FABP using a POC assay kit.

Molecular characteristics of L-FABP

Fatty acid-binding proteins (FABPs) are members of the intracellular lipid-binding protein family and are expressed as 14–15 kDa proteins; they reversibly bind to hydrophobic ligands such as fatty acids and function as intracellular transporters [29]. To date, nine human FABPs have been identified: L-FABP (or FABP1), intestinal FABP (I-FABP or FABP2), heart FABP (H-FABP or FABP3), adipocyte FABP (A-FABP or FABP4), epidermal FABP (E-FABP or FABP5), ileal FABP (Il-FABP or FABP6), brain FABP (B-FABP or FABP7), myelin FABP (M-FABP or FABP8), and testis FABP (T-FABP, FABP9). The structure of L-FABP includes ten stranded β-barrel structures that form interior hydrophobic ligand binding pockets and two α-helixes as cap domains [30] (Fig. 1). The *l-fabp* gene has binding domains for the following transcriptional factors: hypoxia inducible factor (HIF-1α and HIF-2α), caudal-related homeobox (CDX), CCAAT/enhancer-binding protein (C/EBP), forkhead box A (FOXA), GATA, hepatocyte nuclear factor (HNF-1 and HNF-4), and peroxisome proliferator-activated receptor (PPAR), which are related to cell proliferation, cell differentiation, and lipid metabolism [31–33]. Hence, it was concluded that L-FABP transports free fatty acids to organelles such as the mitochondria and lysosomes for β-oxidation for use in these cellular processes [34].

Ischemic and oxidative stress induces the excretion of L-FABP into the urine

Hypoxic regulation induces *l-fabp* gene expression by HIF-1α and HIF-2α [33]. To evaluate the response of L-FABP to hypoxic stress, the gene expression of *l-fabp* was measured in the LLC-PK1 porcine cell line, which was derived from proximal tubules, after the cells were cultured in hypoxic conditions using an anaerobic chamber. The results indicated that the expression level of *l-fabp* was increased by hypoxic stress (Fig. 2), demonstrating that L-FABP was a hypoxic-induced protein in proximal tubular cells [35].

It was also reported that L-FABP was excreted into the urine following ischemic stress in vivo. Yamamoto T. and colleagues studied the association of peritubular

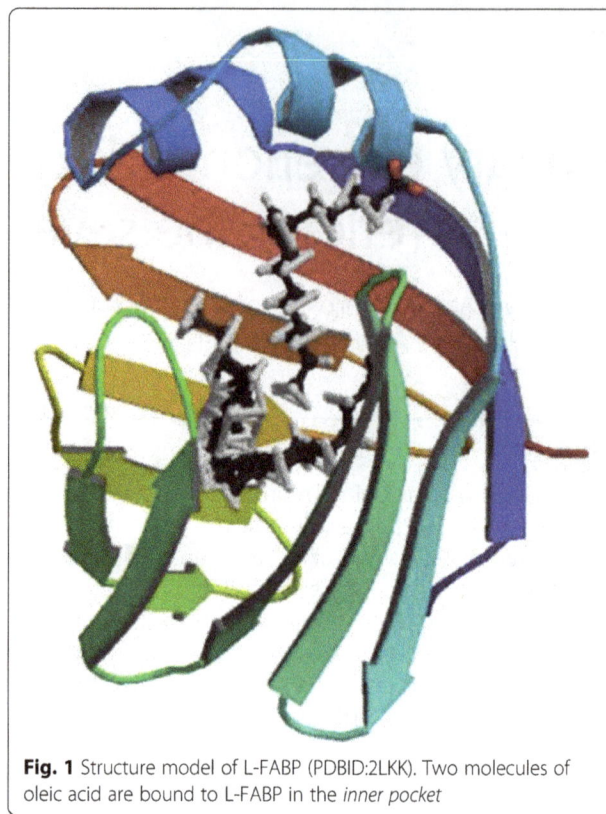

Fig. 1 Structure model of L-FABP (PDBID:2LKK). Two molecules of oleic acid are bound to L-FABP in the *inner pocket*

capillary blood flow with the urinary excretion of L-FABP during reperfusion after living donor kidney transplantation [36]. They found that urinary L-FABP was inversely correlated with peritubular capillary blood flow (Fig. 3). This finding indicates that L-FABP is excreted into the proximal tubular lumen in response to ischemic and oxidative stress [36].

Antioxidative effect of L-FABP

The findings regarding the response of L-FABP to ischemic and oxidative stress led to the hypothesis that L-FABP itself has an antioxidative role. Hence, the association of reactive oxygen species (ROS) generation with *l-fabp* gene expression was evaluated, and it was found that L-FABP itself has an antioxidative property that is independent of the activities of superoxide dismutase (SOD), glutathione peroxidase (GPx), and catalase (CAT) [37, 38]. The antioxidative capacity was also demonstrated using an animal model in which the human *l-fabp* gene was expressed in the proximal tubules of transgenic mice (Tg-mice) [39]. Administration of aristolochic acid [40] and aldosterone [41], which induced ROS generation, promoted tubular injury and the urinary excretion of L-FABP. However, the oxidative markers Nε-hexanoyl lysine (HEL) and 2-thiobarbituric acid reactive substances (TBARS) were lower in the Tg-mice than in the wild type controls, indicating that the

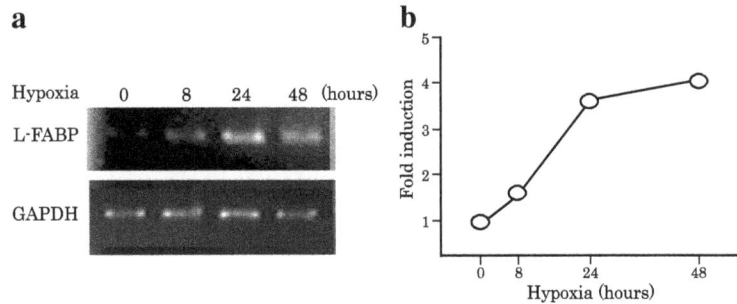

Fig. 2 Expression of the *l-fabp* gene following hypoxic stress. Glyceraldehyde-3-phosphate dehydrogenase (GAPDH) was used as the housekeeping gene. The results of the RT-PCR analysis are shown in (**a**), and the quantified the expression levels are shown in (**b**) [35]

tubulointerstitial injury caused by ischemic and oxidative stress was attenuated by the antioxidative effect of L-FABP. The kidney contains a large amount of fatty acids, which can easily form lipid peroxides (LOOH), through peroxidation. Because L-FABP has high selectivity for fatty acids possessing long alkyl chains or carbon double bonds, or fatty acid peroxides [42–44] (Table 1), suggesting that L-FABP might protect the kidney by removing LOOH from the proximal tubules as shown in Fig. 4.

Urinary L-FABP reflects the severity of sepsis

As mentioned above, L-FABP has an antioxidant capacity and is excreted into the urine in response to ischemic and oxidative stress. It has also been reported that endotoxin-induced oxidative stress in sepsis induces AKI in patients [45], suggesting that L-FABP would be excreted into the urine in these cases. Indeed, it was shown that the urinary L-FABP level was higher in patients with sepsis than in healthy controls [25, 26] (Table 2). It was noted that urinary L-FABP levels differed significantly among patients with septic shock, severe sepsis, or AKI and healthy subjects (as well as patients with an infectious disease or a non-infectious disease). An endotoxin removal cartridge (Toraymyxin) composed of a poly-myxin B-immobilized fiber (PMX-F) was developed to

apply to patients with endotoxemia or suspected gram-negative infection [46]. Our group also showed that PMX-F hemoperfusion decreased the plasma endotoxin level, urinary L-FABP level, and urinary 8-hydroxy-2'-deoxyguanosine (8-OHdG) level [25, 47]. Doi K et al. were also reported that in patients treated with PMX, the urinary L-FABP and blood endotoxin levels decreased in survivors but not in non-survivors [48].These reports suggested that the urinary L-FABP level might reflect the severity of the oxidative state in patients with sepsis and have value as an indicator of whether the treatment is successful.

Predicting poor outcomes

Several studies have reported the clinical significance of urinary L-FABP as a predictor of and risk factor for poor outcomes. Urinary L-FABP can predict the onset of AKI after cardiac surgery [13, 49, 50], pediatric cardiopulmo-nary bypass [17], stem cell transplantation [12], and endovascular and open-abdominal aortic aneurysm repair [16] as well as in intensive care unit populations [15]. Additionally, L-FABP can also predict the progression to end-stage renal disease (ESRD), the onset of cardiovascular disease (CVD), or death for patients with AKI [14, 51], type 2 diabetes [8, 52], or chronic kidney

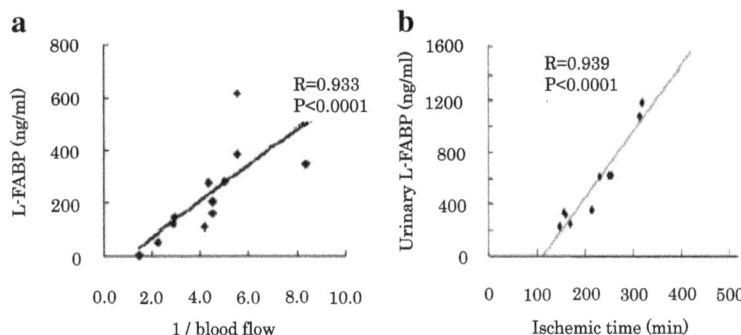

Fig. 3 Correlation between ischemic stress and urinary L-FABP. **a** Correlation between peritubular capillary blood flow and urinary L-FABP. **b** Correlation between ischemic time and urinary L-FABP. *R* indicates correlation coefficient [36]

Table 1 Affinity of fatty acids for L-FABP

Fatty acids		K_d (µM)	Refs.
Palmitic acid	16:0	4.02	[42]
Oleic acid	18:1, n-9	0.89	
Arachidonic acid	20:4, n-6	0.44	
Eicosapentaenoic acid	20:5, n-3	0.2	[43]
Docosapentaenoic acid	22:5, n-3	0.067	
Docosahexaenoic acid	22:6, n-3	0.14	
Tetracosapentaenoic acid	24:5, n-3	0.066	
Tetracosahexaenic acid	24:6, n-3	0.18	
Arachidonic acid	20:4, n-6	0.11	
Adrenic acid	22:4, n-6	0.11	
Tetracosatetraenoic acid	24:4, n-6	0.054	
Tetracosapentaenoic acid	24:5, n-6	0.007	
Oleic acid	18:1, n-9	1.2	[44]
Arachidonic acid	20:4, n-6	1.7	
15-Hydroperoxy-5, 8, 11, 13-eicosatetraenoic acid (15-HPETE)		0.076	
5-Hydroxy-6, 8, 11, 14-eicosatetraenoic acid (5-HETE)		0.175	
15-Hydroxy-5, 8, 11, 13-eicosatetraenoic acid (15-HETE)		1.8	

disease (CKD) [53] or those who have undergone cardiac catheterization [54, 55] or renal transplantation [56, 57]. Clinical prospective observation studies to predict mortality in sepsis using urinary L-FABP have been conducted with both adult patients and pediatric patients (Table 3) [27, 28]. A significant difference in the urinary L-FABP level in the first urine sample was observed between survivors and non-survivors in each study. In the ROC curve analysis, the area under the curve (AUC) values were 0.993 (95% CI, 0.956–0.999) for adult patients and 0.647 (95% CI, 0.500–0.795) for pediatric patients. Further improvement would be required before using L-FABP as a predictor of mortality in pediatric patients with sepsis, but it might be useful for adult patients because the AUC-ROC of urinary L-FABP was significantly higher than the acute physiology and chronic health evaluation (APACHE) II score (0.927) and sepsis-related organ failure assessment (SOFA) score (0.813) (Fig. 5) [27].

Animal models of sepsis

Animal models that mimic human sepsis have been developed, and their usefulness was reviewed by Doi K. et al. [58]. The diagnostic value of urinary L-FABP for sepsis has been evaluated in animal models of sepsis [27]. In this study, sepsis was induced by cecal ligation puncture (CLP) or intratracheal lipopolysaccharide (LPS) injection, causing mild tubular damage with vacuolization, an increase in bronchoalveolar lavage fluid protein, and leukocyte infiltration in the interstitial space of the

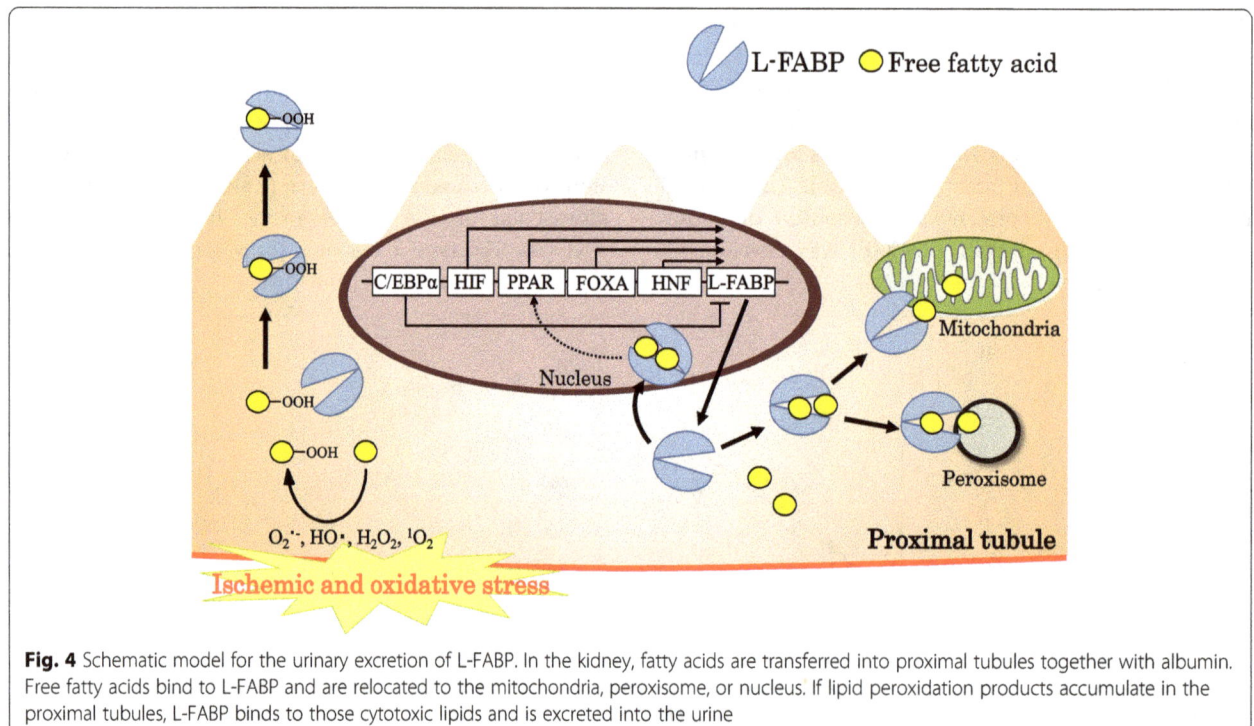

Fig. 4 Schematic model for the urinary excretion of L-FABP. In the kidney, fatty acids are transferred into proximal tubules together with albumin. Free fatty acids bind to L-FABP and are relocated to the mitochondria, peroxisome, or nucleus. If lipid peroxidation products accumulate in the proximal tubules, L-FABP binds to those cytotoxic lipids and is excreted into the urine

Table 2 Urinary L-FABP levels in patients with sepsis

	Number	Urinary L-FABP concentration	Refs.
Septic shock			
PMX-F treatment	40	1860 ± 1260 µg/g Cr	[25]
Nom-PMX-F treatment	10	1740 ± 1140 µg/g Cr	
Severe sepsis	20	248 ± 100 µg/g Cr*	
AKI	20	120 ± 84 µg/g Cr*†	
Healthy subjects	30	4.2 ± 2.4 µg/g Cr*†	
Sepsis (severe sepsis/septic shock)	25	2054 ± 8839 ng/ml	[26]
SIRS	13	598 ± 1939 ng/ml	
Infectious disease	20	33 ± 57 ng/ml	
Non-infectious disease	22	9.0 ± 10.4 ng/ml	

Values are presented as the mean ± SD
*$P < 0.001$ vs. septic shock; †$P < 0.01$ vs. severe sepsis
Cr indicates creatinine

lung. Urinary L-FABP was higher in the severe group than in the less severe group and sham-operated animals, suggesting it can indicate the severity of sepsis.

These reports indicate that urinary L-FABP might not only detect the severity of sepsis but also predict poor outcomes. Although, to date, there have been several reports on diagnosing sepsis using urinary L-FABP, additional studies are required to elucidate the usefulness of urinary L-FABP within the context of the new definition of sepsis.

POC assay kit for urinary L-FABP

In many studies, L-FABP was measured using the enzyme-linked immunosorbent assay (ELISA) method. However, this assay requires several hours, specialized equipment, and highly trained personnel to obtain reliable results. If L-FABP is to be used to diagnose sepsis, the method must be rapid, accurate, and easy to perform at the bedside. Therefore, we developed the L-FABP POC assay kit, which can rapidly measure human L-FABP in the urine.

Clinical significance of the POC assay for urinary L-FABP

The principles of the POC assay kit are shown as Fig. 6. The POC assay kit utilizes an immuno-chromatography method, and the result is obtained within 15 min. The POC assay and ELISA (CMIC HOLDINGS Co., Ltd., Tokyo, Japan) were performed on urine samples from two groups of patients: 35 patients who were admitted to the intensive care unit (ICU) at Shinmatsudo Central General Hospital (Chiba, Japan) as critically ill patients with sepsis (186 points) and 80 patients who were outpatients with CKD at St. Marianna University School of Medicine Hospital (Kanagawa, Japan) (106 points). When the ELISA and POC assay results were compared, the result of POC assay was assessed using three-score method, score 1; <12.5 ng/ml, score 2; ≥12.5 ng/ml and <100 ng/ml, or score 3; ≥ 100 ng/ml (Fig. 7). It is important to measure the higher range near 100 ng/ml for ICU patients because it was suggested that upper levels of urinary L-FABP than 100 µg/g Cr may be specific to septic shock [25]. Additionally, it is also important to measure the range near 12.5 ng/ml for CKD patients because it was reported that levels of urinary L-FABP above the

Table 3 Urinary L-FABP levels in patients with sepsis

	Number	Urinary L-FABP concentration			Refs.
Septic shock					
Non-survivors	68	4366 ± 192 µg/g Cr*			[27]
Survivors	77	483 ± 71 µg/g Cr			
Pediatric sepsis		First urine	Day 1	Day 2	
Non-survivors	22	715 ng/ml** (61.4–2470)	370 ng/ml (67.0–2047)	580 ng/ml† (38.8–2053)	[28]
Survivors	83	107 ng/ml (35.1–303)	152 ng/ml (40.1–627)	68.2 ng/ml (21.6–231)	

Urine samples were obtained at the time of admission to the ICU except as otherwise noted. Values are presented as the mean ± SEM [27] or median (interquartile range) [28]
*$P < 0.05$ vs. survivors; **$P = 0.034$ vs. survivors; †$P = 0.016$ vs. survivors
Cr indicates creatinine

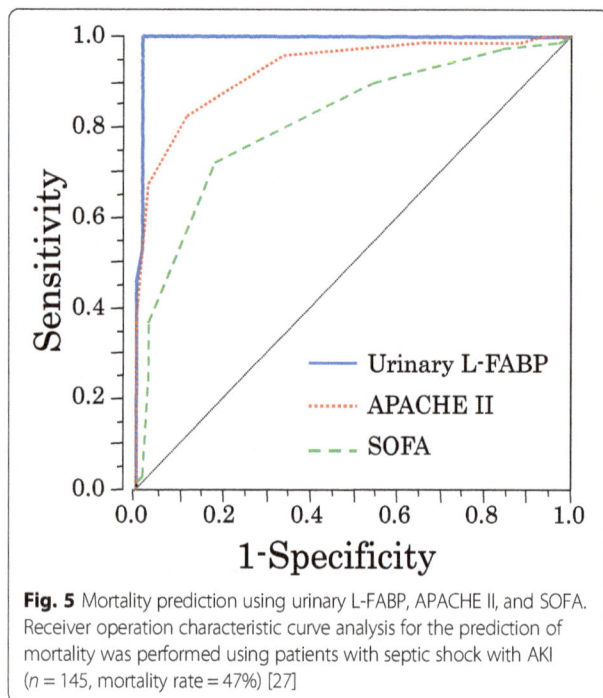

Fig. 5 Mortality prediction using urinary L-FABP, APACHE II, and SOFA. Receiver operation characteristic curve analysis for the prediction of mortality was performed using patients with septic shock with AKI (*n* = 145, mortality rate = 47%) [27]

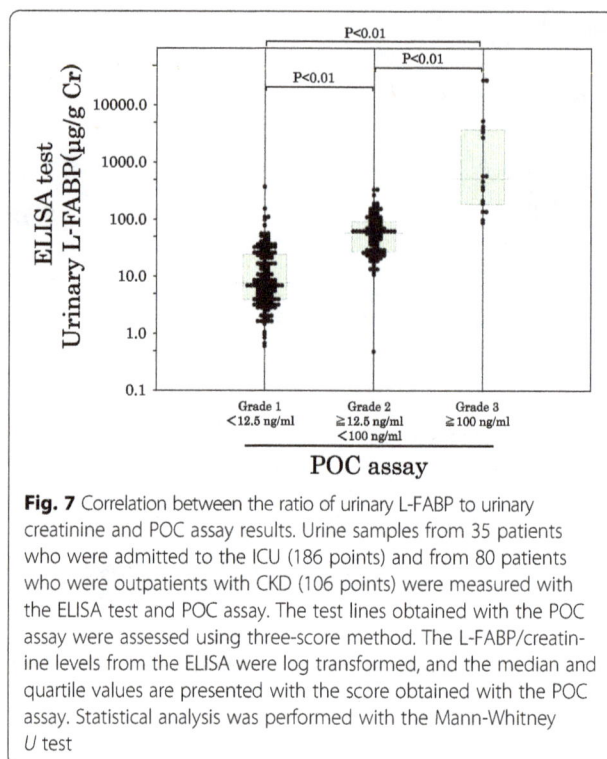

Fig. 7 Correlation between the ratio of urinary L-FABP to urinary creatinine and POC assay results. Urine samples from 35 patients who were admitted to the ICU (186 points) and from 80 patients who were outpatients with CKD (106 points) were measured with the ELISA test and POC assay. The test lines obtained with the POC assay were assessed using three-score method. The L-FABP/creatinine levels from the ELISA were log transformed, and the median and quartile values are presented with the score obtained with the POC assay. Statistical analysis was performed with the Mann-Whitney *U* test

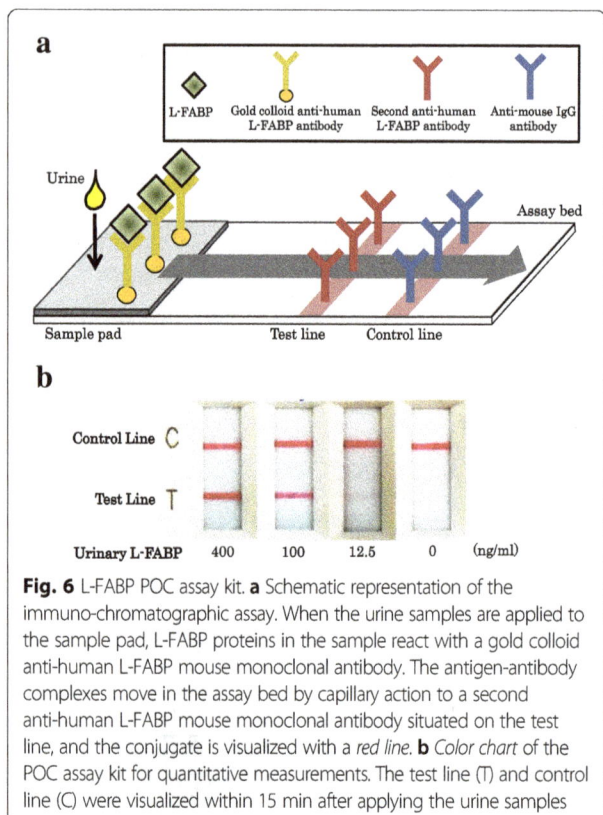

Fig. 6 L-FABP POC assay kit. **a** Schematic representation of the immuno-chromatographic assay. When the urine samples are applied to the sample pad, L-FABP proteins in the sample react with a gold colloid anti-human L-FABP mouse monoclonal antibody. The antigen-antibody complexes move in the assay bed by capillary action to a second anti-human L-FABP mouse monoclonal antibody situated on the test line, and the conjugate is visualized with a *red line*. **b** *Color chart* of the POC assay kit for quantitative measurements. The test line (T) and control line (C) were visualized within 15 min after applying the urine samples

upper limit of the reference value (8.4 μg/g Cr [6]) are a risk factor for the progression to ESRD, the onset of cardiovascular disease CVD, and death [53]. When we reanalyzed reference value to L-FABP concentration, the reference value which converted to L-FABP concentration was 10.1 ng/ml. Therefore, the assessment of the upper level of 12.5 ng/ml in POC assay indicated that urinary L-FABP/creatinine level was at least the upper level of 8.4 μg/g Cr.

The correlation between the ratio of urinary L-FABP to urinary creatinine and POC assay results and the accuracy of the L-FABP POC assay for diagnosis of the patients with sepsis or CKD was evaluated for clinical use. The ratio of urinary L-FABP to urinary creatinine for the ICU patients and the outpatients were determined and compared with the POC assay results. The results showed multi-group comparisons revealed significant differences in the L-FABP/creatinine levels between the results of the POC assay (Fig. 7). Additionally, it was found that the specificity (true negative ratio) and sensitivity (true positive ratio) to assess the reference value (8.4 μg/g Cr) were 99% (87/88) and 61% (125/204), respectively. Recently, Asada T. and colleagues reported that concentration of urinary L-FABP above the upper limit of the reference value (100 ng/ml) were defined as a risk factor of AKI in ICU patients [59]. This report supports the validity of the higher cutoff value of L-FABP (100 ng/ml) for diagnosis of AKI. Further evaluation is necessary to confirm the cutoff values of L-

FABP. Moreover, Sato R. and colleagues reported that urinary L-FABP levels in ICU patients including those with sepsis were also measured using the POC assay [26]. They found a positive correlation between serum creatinine levels and POC assay score, suggesting that the L-FABP POC assay might be alternative method for assessing creatinine levels, which are widely used. These results indicate the potential of the POC assay for use in diagnosing sepsis-induced AKI and CKD in patients rapidly.

Clinical evaluation of POC assay for urinary L-FABP in PMX intervention

Clinical evaluation of the L-FABP POC assay kit was performed in PMX intervention.

The POC assay and ELISA (CMIC HOLDINGS Co., Ltd., Tokyo, Japan) were performed on urine samples from three patients who were admitted to the ICU at Shinmatsudo Central General Hospital (Chiba, Japan) as critically ill patient with sepsis. The lactate level which was described as the new criteria of sepsis in third international consensus definition for sepsis and septic shock (sepsis-3) was also evaluated at pre- and post-PMX intervention by the blood gas analyzer. In the result, the patient who is 84-year-old man had septic shock with transverse colon cancer after surgery suture failure. The lactate (mg/dl) and

urinary L-FABP/creatinine (µg/g Cr) were decreased after PMX intervention. Moreover, the patient who is 93-year-old woman had septic shock with iliopsoas abscess. Similarly, the lactate and urinary L-FABP/creatinine were decreased after PMX intervention. The results of POC assay were assessed as score 3; ≥100 ng/ml at pre-1st PMX intervention and as score 1; <12.5 ng/ml at post-2nd PMX intervention in the patients (Fig. 8a, b). Urinary creatinine excretion was 78.6 and 112.7 mg/dl in pre-PMX and 117.3 and 220.1 mg/dl in post-PMX in two patients. These patients discharged from the hospital. In contrast, the patient who is a 75-year-old woman has septic shock with acute obstructive suppurative cholangitis. In the patient after PMX intervention, the lactate was decreased slightly, whereas the urinary L-FABP was increased. Also, the result of POC assay was assessed as score 2; ≥ 12.5 and <100 ng/ml at pre-PMX intervention, and as score 3; ≥100 ng/ml at post-PMX intervention (Fig. 8c). Urinary creatinine excretion was 78.6 mg/dl in pre-PMX and 19.1 mg/dl in post-PMX. The patient died after 3 days of PMX intervention. In this case, serum lactate and urinary L-FABP levels were sustained abnormal level in each point. In this sense, neither lactate value nor urine L-FABP value decreased by PMX intervention. Furthermore, another group developed a new algorithm by combining urinary

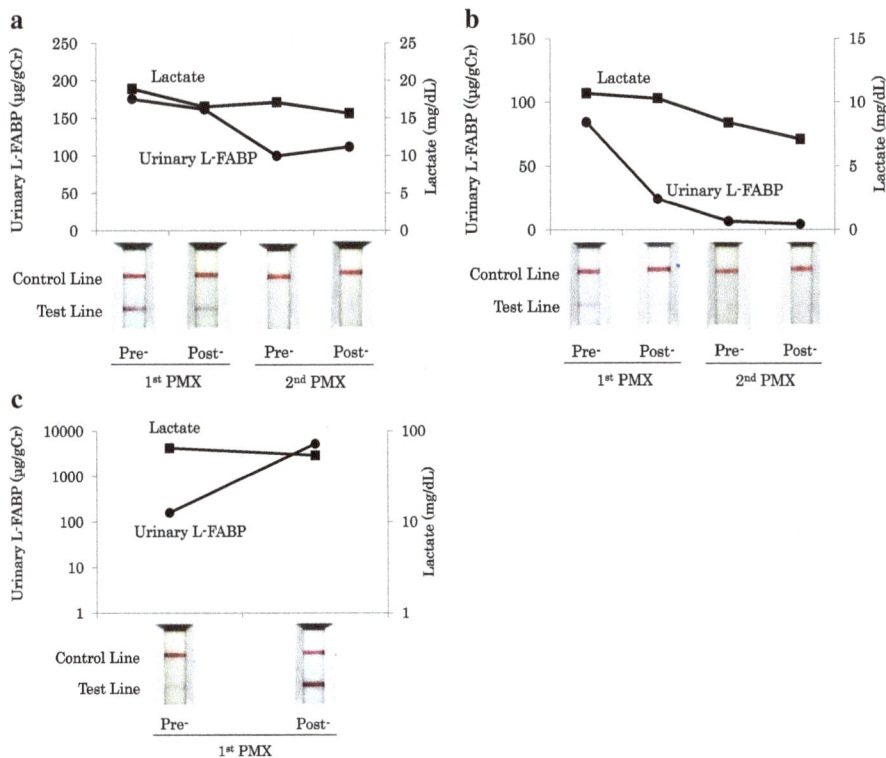

Fig. 8 Correlation between the ratio of urinary L-FABP to urinary creatinine, POC assay results and lactate levels in PMX-treated patients. Urine samples from three patients who were admitted to the ICU were measured with the ELISA test and POC assay. The test lines obtained with the POC assay kit were scored using three-score method. Lactate levels measured by the blood gas analyzer. Two patients had discharged from the hospital (**a**, **b**). Another patient died after 3 days of PMX intervention (**c**)

NGAL and L-FABP with stratification by the APACHE II score, presence of sepsis and blood lactate levels to improve their AKI predictive performance [59]. From this report, it is also considered that there are cases in which it is difficult to make a prognostic prediction only by changes in urine L-FABP in a high concentration range. As a whole, when the score of POC assay for urinary L-FABP and lactate level were decreased in the patients after PMX intervention, the patient tended to improve the condition. On the other hand, when the score of POC assay and lactate were sustained high level in the patient even after PMX intervention, the patient tended to deteriorate the condition. Therefore, these results suggested that POC assay for urinary L-FABP may be useful to evaluate therapeutic efficacy of PMX intervention in sepsis patient.

Conclusions

In conclusion, endotoxin induces oxidative stress and the excretion of L-FABP into the urine in patients with sepsis-induced AKI. If urinary L-FABP can be measured in these patients, it is possible to diagnose the severity of sepsis. However, to date, there is little evidence for the clinical usefulness of urinary L-FABP for sepsis. Further studies are required to elucidate the reliability of diagnostic methods using urinary L-FABP and to determine the cutoff values for predicting poor outcomes. The L-FABP POC assay kit is expected to be useful for its rapidness and simplicity. Our study was performed at a single center. Our findings should be confirmed in a large multicenter trial. Future studies need to be conducted.

Abbreviations

A-FABP/FABP4: Adipocyte-type fatty acid-binding protein; AKI: Acute kidney injury; APACHE: Acute physiology and chronic health evaluation; AUC: Area under the curve; B-FABP/FABP7: Brain-type fatty acid binding protein; CAT: Catalase; CDX: Caudal-related homeobox; C/EBP: CCAAT/enhancer-binding protein; CKD: Chronic kidney disease; CLP: Cecal ligation puncture; Cr: Creatinine; CRP: C-reactive protein; CVD: Cardiovascular disease; E-FABP/FABP5: Epidermal-type fatty acid-binding protein; ELISA: Enzyme-linked immunosorbent assay; ESRD: End-stage renal disease; FABPs: Fatty acid-binding proteins; FOXA: Forkhead box A; GPx: Glutathione peroxidase; HEL: Nε-hexanoyl lysine; HIF: Hypoxia inducible factor; HIV: Human immunodeficiency virus; H-FABP/FABP3: Heart-type fatty acid-binding protein; HNF: Hepatocyte nuclear factor; ICU: Intensive care unit; I-FABP/FABP2: Intestinal-type fatty acid-binding protein; Il-FABP/FABP6: Ileal-type fatty acid binding protein; L-FABP/FABP1: Liver-type fatty acid-binding protein; LOOH: Lipid peroxides; M-FABP/FABP8: Myelin-type fatty acid-binding protein; MOF: Multiple organ failure; 8-OHdG: 8-Hydroxy-2'-deoxyguanosine; PCT: Procalcitonin; PPAR: Peroxisome proliferator-activated receptor; POC: Point-of-care; PMX-F: Polymyxin B-immobilized fiber; qSOFA: Quick sepsis-related organ failure assessment; ROC: Receiver operatographic characteristic; ROS: Reactive oxygen species; SIRS: Systemic inflammatory response syndrome; SOD: Superoxide dismutase; SOFA: Sepsis-related organ failure assessment; TBARS: 2-Thiobarbituric acid reactive substances; T-FABP/FABP9: Testis-type fatty acid-binding protein; Tg-mice: Transgenic mice

Acknowledgements

We also would like to thank Editage (http://www.editage.jp/) for English language editing.

Funding

There is no funding to be disclosed.

Authors' contributions

ES, AK-I, TS, KK, TN, and YS contributed to the study design. AO, TO, AK-I, and ES performed the data collection. ES, TO, and TS participated in the data analysis. ES, AK-I, TO, TS, and TN interpreted the data. ES and TO carried out the literature search and generation of figures. ES and TO wrote the manuscript. All authors gave their final approval of the submitted version.

Competing interests

T. Sugaya is the Director and Senior scientist, and T. Oikawa and A. Okuda are the scientist of CMIC HOLDINGS Co., Ltd., the company that produced the ELISA and POC assay for L-FABP analysis.
None of the other authors have competing interest or financial disclosures of any relevance to the present study.

Author details

[1]Division of Nephrology, Department of Medicine, Shinmatsudo Central General Hospital, 1-380 Shinmatsudo, Matsudo, Chiba 270-0034, Japan. [2]Department of Anatomy, St. Marianna University School of Medicine, Sugao, Miyamae-Ku, Kawasaki, Kanagawa 216-8511, Japan. [3]CMIC HOLDINGS Co., Ltd., Hamamatsucho Bldg., 1-1-1 Shibaura, Minato-ku, Tokyo 105-0023, Japan. [4]Department of Nephrology and Hypertension, Department of Internal Medicine, St. Marianna University School of Medicine, Sugao, Miyamae-Ku, Kawasaki, Kanagawa 216-8511, Japan. [5]Department of Internal Medicine, Japan Community Health Care Organization, Tokyo Takanawa Hospital, Tokyo, Japan.

References

1. Bone R, Balk R, Cerra F, et al. Definitions for sepsis and organ failure and guidelines for the use of innovative therapies in sepsis. The ACCP/SCCM consensus conference committee. American college of chest physicians/society of critical care medicine. Chest. 1992;101(6):1644–55.
2. Levy MM, Fink MP, Marshall JC, et al. 2001 SCCM/ESICM/ACCP/ATS/SIS international sepsis definitions conference. Intensive Care Med. 2003;29(4):530–8.
3. Singer M, Deutschman CS, Seymour CW, et al. The third international consensus definitions for sepsis and septic shock (Sepsis-3). JAMA. 2016;315(8):801–10.
4. Pierrakos C, Vincent JL. Sepsis biomarkers: a review. Crit Care. 2010;14(1):R15.
5. Kamijo A, Kimura K, Sugaya T, et al. Urinary fatty acid-binding protein as a new clinical marker of the progression of chronic renal disease. J Lab Clin Med. 2004;143(1):23–30.
6. Kamijo-Ikemori A, Sugaya T, Yasuda T, et al. Clinical significance of urinary liver-type fatty acid-binding protein in diabetic nephropathy of type 2 diabetic patients. Diabetes Care. 2011;34(3):691–6.
7. Nielsen SE, Sugaya T, Tarnow L, et al. Tubular and glomerular injury in diabetes and the impact of ACE inhibition. Diabetes Care. 2009;32(9):1684–8.
8. Fufaa GD, Weil EJ, Nelson RG, et al. Association of urinary KIM-1, L-FABP, NAG and NGAL with incident end-stage renal disease and mortality in American Indians with type 2 diabetes mellitus. Diabetologia. 2015;58(1):188–98.

9. Fu WJ, Wang DJ, Deng RT, et al. Urinary liver-type fatty acid-binding protein change in gestational diabetes mellitus. Diabetes Res Clin Pract. 2015;109(3):e36–8.

10. Imai N, Yasuda T, Kamijo-Ikemori A, et al. Distinct roles of urinary liver-type fatty acid-binding protein in non-diabetic patients with anemia. PLoS ONE. 2015;10(5):e0126990.

11. Matsui K, Kamijo-Ikemori A, Sugaya T, et al. Usefulness of urinary biomarkers in early detection of acute kidney injury after cardiac surgery in adults. Circ J. 2012;76(1):213–20.

12. Shingai N, Morito T, Najima Y, et al. Urinary liver-type fatty acid-binding protein linked with increased risk of acute kidney injury after allogeneic stem cell transplantation. Biol Blood Marrow Transplant. 2014;20(12):2010–4.

13. Portilla D, Dent C, Sugaya T, et al. Liver fatty acid-binding protein as a biomarker of acute kidney injury after cardiac surgery. Kidney Int. 2008;73(4):465–72.

14. Parr SK, Clark AJ, Bian A, et al. Urinary L-FABP predicts poor outcomes in critically ill patients with early acute kidney injury. Kidney Int. 2014;87(3):640–8.

15. Doi K, Negishi K, Ishizu T, et al. Evaluation of new acute kidney injury biomarkers in a mixed intensive care unit. Crit Care Med. 2011;39(11):2464–9.

16. Obata Y, Kamijo-Ikemori A, Ichikawa D, et al. Clinical usefulness of urinary liver-type fatty-acid-binding protein as a perioperative marker of acute kidney injury in patients undergoing endovascular or open-abdominal aortic aneurysm repair. J Anesth. 2016;30(1):89–99.

17. Krawczeski CD, Goldstein SL, Woo JG, et al. Temporal relationship and predictive value of urinary acute kidney injury biomarkers after pediatric cardiopulmonary bypass. J Am Coll Cardiol. 2011;58(22):2301–9.

18. Manabe K, Kamihata H, Motohiro M, et al. Urinary liver-type fatty acid-binding protein level as a predictive biomarker of contrast-induced acute kidney injury. Eur J Clin Invest. 2012;42(5):557–63.

19. Nakamura T, Sugaya T, Node K, et al. Urinary excretion of liver-type fatty acid-binding protein in contrast medium-induced nephropathy. Am J Kidney Dis. 2006;47(3):439–44.

20. Nakamura T, Sugaya T, Ebihara I, et al. Urinary liver-type fatty acid-binding protein: discrimination between IgA nephropathy and thin basement membrane nephropathy. Am J Nephrol. 2005;25(5):447–50.

21. Jablonowska E, Wojcik K, Piekarska A. Urine liver-type fatty acid-binding protein and kidney injury molecule-1 in HIV-infected patients receiving combined antiretroviral treatment based on tenofovir. AIDS Res Hum Retroviruses. 2014;30(4):363–9.

22. Peralta C, Scherzer R, Grunfeld C, et al. Urinary biomarkers of kidney injury are associated with all-cause mortality in the Women's Interagency HIV Study (WIHS). HIV Med. 2014;15(5):291–300.

23. Parikh CR, Hall IE, Bhangoo RS, et al. Associations of perfusate biomarkers and pump parameters with delayed graft function and deceased-donor kidney allograft function. Am J Transplant. 2016;16(5):1526–39.

24. Koo TY, Jeong JC, Lee Y, et al. Pre-transplant evaluation of donor urinary biomarkers can predict reduced graft function after deceased donor kidney transplantation. Medicine (Baltimore). 2016;95(11):e3076.

25. Nakamura T, Sugaya T, Koide H. Urinary liver-type fatty acid-binding protein in septic shock: effect of polymyxin B-immobilized fiber hemoperfusion. Shock. 2009;31(5):454–9.

26. Sato R, Suzuki Y, Takahashi G, et al. A newly developed kit for the measurement of urinary liver-type fatty acid-binding protein as a biomarker for acute kidney injury in patients with critical care. J Infect Chemother. 2014;21(3):165–9.

27. Doi K, Noiri E, Maeda-Mamiya R, et al. Urinary l-type fatty acid-binding protein as a new biomarker of sepsis complicated with acute kidney injury. Crit Care Med. 2010;38(10):2037–42.

28. Yoshimatsu S, Sugaya T, Hossain MI, et al. Urinary L-FABP as a mortality predictor among <5-year-old children with septic children in Bangladesh. Pediatr Int. 2016;58(3):185–91.

29. Furuhashi M, Hotamisligil GS. Fatty acid-binding proteins: role in metabolic diseases and potential as drug targets. Nat Rev Drug Discov. 2008;7(6):489–503.

30. Cai J, Lucke C, Chen Z, et al. Solution structure and backbone dynamics of human liver fatty acid binding protein: fatty acid binding revisited. Biophys J. 2012;102(11):2585–94.

31. Divine JK. McCaul SP. Simon T. C. HNF-1alpha and endodermal transcription factors cooperatively activate fabpl: MODY3 mutations abrogate cooperativity. Am J Physiol Gastrointest Liver Physiol. 2003;285(1):G62-72.

32. Schachtrup C, Scholzen TE, Grau V, et al. L-FABP is exclusively expressed in alveolar macrophages within the myeloid lineage: evidence for a PPARalpha-independent expression. Int J Biochem Cell Biol. 2004;36(10):2042–53.

33. Jadoon A, Cunningham P, McDermott LC. Regulation of fatty acid binding proteins by hypoxia inducible factors 1alpha and 2alpha in the placenta: relevance to pre-eclampsia. Prostaglandins Leukot Essent Fatty Acids. 2015;93:25–9.

34. Veerkamp JH, Zimmerman AW. Fatty acid-binding proteins of nervous tissue. J Mol Neurosci. 2001;16(2-3):133–42. discussion 151-7.

35. Okazaki M, Oikawa T, Sugaya T. The biomarker for CKD: urinary L-FABP-from molecular function to clinical significance. Nihon Yakurigaku Zasshi. 2015;146(1):27–32.

36. Yamamoto T, Noiri E, Ono Y, et al. Renal L-type fatty acid-binding protein in acute ischemic injury. J Am Soc Nephrol. 2007;18(11):2894–902.

37. Wang G, Gong Y, Anderson J, et al. Antioxidative function of L-FABP in L-FABP stably transfected chang liver cells. Hepatology. 2005;42(4):871–9.

38. Rajaraman G, Wang GQ, Yan J, et al. Role of cytosolic liver fatty acid binding protein in hepatocellular oxidative stress: effect of dexamethasone and clofibrate treatment. Mol Cell Biochem. 2007;295(1-2):27–34.

39. Kamijo A, Sugaya T, Hikawa A, et al. Urinary excretion of fatty acid-binding protein reflects stress overload on the proximal tubules. Am J Pathol. 2004;165(4):1243–55.

40. Matsui K, Kamijo-Ikemorif A, Sugaya T, et al. Renal liver-type fatty acid binding protein (L-FABP) attenuates acute kidney injury in aristolochic acid nephrotoxicity. Am J Pathol. 2011;178(3):1021–32.

41. Ichikawa D, Kamijo-Ikemori A, Sugaya T, et al. Human liver-type fatty acid-binding protein protects against tubulointerstitial injury in aldosterone-induced renal injury. Am J Physiol Renal Physiol. 2014;308(2):F114–121.

42. Zimmerman AW, van Moerkerk HT, Veerkamp JH. Ligand specificity and conformational stability of human fatty acid-binding proteins. Int J Biochem Cell Biol. 2001;33(9):865–76.

43. Norris AW, Spector AA. Very long chain n-3 and n-6 polyunsaturated fatty acids bind strongly to liver fatty acid-binding protein. J Lipid Res. 2002;43(4):646–53.

44. Raza H, Pongubala JR, Sorof S. Specific high affinity binding of lipoxygenase metabolites of arachidonic acid by liver fatty acid binding protein. Biochem Biophys Res Commun. 1989;161(2):448–55.

45. Kalakeche R, Hato T, Rhodes G, et al. Endotoxin uptake by S1 proximal tubular segment causes oxidative stress in the downstream S2 segment. J Am Soc Nephrol. 2011;22(8):1505–16.

46. Shoji H. Extracorporeal endotoxin removal for the treatment of sepsis: endotoxin adsorption cartridge (Toraymyxin). Ther Apher Dial. 2003;7(1):108–14.

47. Nakamura T, Fujiwara N, Sato E, et al. Effect of polymyxin B-immobilized fiber hemoperfusion on serum high mobility group box-1 protein levels and oxidative stress in patients with acute respiratory distress syndrome. ASAIO J. 2009;55(4):395–9.

48. Doi K, Noiri E, Sugaya T. Urinary l-type fatty acid-binding protein as a new renal biomarker in critical care. Curr Opin Crit Care. 2010;16(6):545–9.

49. Ho J, Tangri N, Komenda P, et al. Urinary, plasma, and serum biomarkers' utility for predicting acute kidney injury associated with cardiac surgery in adults: a meta-analysis. Am J Kidney Dis. 2015;66(6):993–1005.

50. Katagiri D, Doi K, Honda K, et al. Combination of two urinary biomarkers predicts acute kidney injury after adult cardiac surgery. Ann Thorac Surg. 2012;93(2):577–83.

51. Cooper DS, Claes D, Goldstein SL, et al. Follow-up renal assessment of injury long-term after acute kidney injury (FRAIL-AKI). Clin J Am Soc Nephrol. 2016;11(1):21–9.

52. Araki S, Haneda M, Koya D, et al. Predictive effects of urinary liver-type fatty acid-binding protein for deteriorating renal function and incidence of cardiovascular disease in type 2 diabetic patients without advanced nephropathy. Diabetes Care. 2013;36(5):1248–53.

53. Matsui K, Kamijo-Ikemori A, Imai N, et al. Clinical significance of urinary liver-type fatty acid-binding protein as a predictor of ESRD and CVD in patients with CKD. Clin Exp Nephrol. 2016;20(2):195–203.

54. Fujita D, Takahashi M, Doi K, et al. Response of urinary liver-type fatty acid-binding protein to contrast media administration has a potential to predict one-year renal outcome in patients with ischemic heart disease. Heart Vessels. 2015;30(3):296–303.

55. Kamijo-Ikemori A, Hashimoto N, Sugaya T, et al. Elevation of urinary liver-type fatty acid binding protein after cardiac catheterization related to cardiovascular events. Int J Nephrol Renovasc Dis. 2015;8:91–9.

56. Bansal N, Carpenter MA, Weiner DE, et al. Urine injury biomarkers and risk of adverse outcomes in recipients of prevalent kidney transplants: the folic acid for vascular outcome reduction in transplantation trial. J Am Soc Nephrol. 2016;27(7):2109–21.

Efficacy of tonsillectomy for the treatment of immunoglobulin A nephropathy recurrence after kidney transplantation

Hiroshi Nihei[1], Ken Sakai[1*], Seiichiro Shishido[1], Kazutoshi Sibuya[2], Hideo Edamatsu[3] and Atsushi Aikawa[1]

Abstract

Background: Post-transplant recurrent nephritis is the third common complication that leads to graft loss, which affects the long-term graft survival of kidney transplant patients. Immunoglobulin A nephropathy (IgAN) is the most common for recurrent nephritis, with a recurrence rate of 13–53%. In this study, 12 patients diagnosed with recurrent IgAN were divided into two groups, one which underwent tonsillectomy and another which did not, to analyze the effect of treating IgAN recurrent with or without tonsillectomy.

Methods: Urinary findings, estimated GFR (eGFR), and histopathological alteration (Banff and Oxford classifications) were examined for >5 years after kidney transplantation.

Results: We found that tonsillectomy protected graft function and prevented pathological alterations. The levels of urinary proteins increased in the no tonsillectomy group, whereas no difference was observed in the severity of hematuria between two groups. eGFR declined and mesangial hypercellularity score increased in the no tonsillectomy group.

Conclusions: Tonsillectomy not only results in a favorable clinical outcome but also protects against the histological damage caused by recurrent IgAN after kidney transplantation.

Keywords: Immunoglobulin A nephropathy (IgAN), Kidney transplantation, Recurrent nephritis, Tonsillectomy

Background

The recurrence rate of IgAN in renal graft is 13–53% among transplant recipients with IgAN, which affects long-term graft survival [1, 2]. In recent trials of immunosuppression therapy, mycophenolate mofetil was expected to suppress IgAN after transplantation; however, it failed to enhance graft survival [3]. In another study of 532 transplant recipients by Esther et al., graft loss due to IgAN recurrence occurred in as many as 9.7% patients at 10 years. Among these, IgAN accounted for 22% of the total cases of graft loss, IgAN recurrence was the third major cause of graft loss after chronic rejection and death with a functioning graft [4]. Establishing a treatment for recurrent nephritis, particularly recurrent IgAN, is

crucial for improving the renal graft survival. Berger et al. first described IgAN in 1968 [5]; it is now the most frequent form of chronic glomerulonephritis in Japan. In another study, Xie et al. compared patients with primary IgAN that did or did not undergo tonsillectomy, and renal survival rates for the two groups at 240 months were 89.6 and 63.7%, respectively; this difference was statistically significant [6]. Tonsillectomy monotherapy or steroid pulse therapy following tonsillectomy is commonly used to treat primary IgAN in Japan [6–9]. This therapy achieves particularly beneficial effects in the early stages of IgAN. Protocol graft biopsy can reveal important findings regarding the onset and extension of IgAN, which might explain why tonsillectomy has particularly favorable effects on early stage recurrent IgAN. To our knowledge, few reports have assessed the natural progression of recurrent IgAN using protocol graft biopsies.

---

* Correspondence: kensakai@med.toho-u.ac.jp
[1]Department of Nephrology, Faculty of Medicine, Toho University, 6-11-1 Omori-Nishi, Ota-ku, Tokyo 143-8541, Japan
Full list of author information is available at the end of the article

In this study, we evaluated the efficacy of tonsillectomy for the treatment of IgAN recurrence after kidney transplantation.

Methods

Between 1984 and 2008, kidney transplantation was performed on 520 patients at our department. Among these recipients, 76 (14.6%) were diagnosed with primary IgAN that was confirmed pathologically. Among these, 23 (30.3%) had recurrent IgAN in the kidney graft. After excluding individuals who we were unable to follow-up for 5 years or more, 12 patients were included in the final analysis. All 12 patients received immunosuppressive therapy including tacrolimus, cyclosporine, azathioprine, mycophenolate mofetil (MMF), and methylprednisolone during the study period. IgAN recurrence was defined as follows:

1. The confirmation of primary IgAN using a native kidney biopsy.
2. The new appearance of urinary findings (proteinuria and/or hematuria)
3. New-onset histological IgA deposition without previous IgAN deposition at 1-h biopsy.

Tonsillectomy was offered to all 12 patients as a treatment option, and it was only performed on patients who provided consent. After given the informed consent, five patients (tonsillectomy group) underwent tonsillectomy, whereas the remaining seven patients (no tonsillectomy group) did not. Protocol biopsies were routinely performed at 1 h, 3 months, 12 months, 36 months, 60 months, and 84 months after kidney transplantation. One nephrologist and one or two pathologists evaluated the pathological findings using the Banff classification 2007 [10] and the Oxford classification [11, 12]. Informed consent was obtained from all patients regarding the use of their pathological specimens in this study before each graft biopsy.

The degree of urinary findings, histopathological alterations, the decline slope of 1/Cr, and estimated glomerular filtration (eGFR) were analyzed retrospectively in the two patient groups. Microhematuria was defined as five or more erythrocytes per high-power microscopy field (×400) in urinary sediment, according to the Japanese Urological Association guidelines. Proteinuria was evaluated using the protein/creatinine ratio (g/gCr) in a urine sample obtained in the morning at the outpatient clinic. eGFR was calculated using serum creatinine levels on the day or the day before the renal biopsy. Clinical data are expressed as mean ± standard deviations (SDs). Statistical comparisons between the two groups were performed using Wilcoxon rank sum test, and individual pairs of specimens were analyzed using matched-pair t tests. $P < 0.05$ was considered to denote statistical significance in all tests.

This study was approved by the Ethics Committee of Toho University Omori Medical Center, Tokyo, Japan (approval number: 26–60), and was performed in adherence with the Declaration of Helsinki. Informed consent was obtained from all patients.

Results

In the tonsillectomy group, two patients were male and three were female, and the mean age was 33.7 ± 9.7 years at kidney transplantation. The mean period from transplantation to IgAN recurrence was 37.4 ± 25.7 months, and the median time between IgAN recurrence and tonsillectomy was 3.1(1.4–28.9) months. The mean follow-up period after kidney transplantation was 146.8 ± 30.1 months. At the time of the diagnosis of IgAN recurrence, the mean serum creatinine (SCr) levels were 1.15 ± 0.28 mg/dl (eGFR was 47.7 ± 14.6 ml/min/1.73 m^2). Three of the five patients (60%) had hematuria, and the mean proteinuria was 0.33 ± 0.52 g/gCr. All patients were administered antihypertensive agents such as angiotensin-converting enzyme inhibitors (ACE-I) or angiotensin receptor blockers (ARB) after IgAN recurrence was confirmed. The no tonsillectomy group included six males and one female with mean age of 36.6 ± 8.6 years. The mean period from transplant to IgAN recurrence was 31.8 ± 19.3 months, and the mean follow-up period was 193.6 ± 105.1 months. The mean SCr and eGFR at the time of diagnosis of IgAN recurrence was 1.29 ± 0.17 mg/dl and 39.1 ± 5.8 ml/min/1.73 m^2, respectively. Four of seven patients (57%) had hematuria, and the mean proteinuria was 0.07 ± 0.19 g/gCr. ACE-I or ARB therapy was initiated after IgAN recurrence was confirmed in all but one patient. All patients were re-evaluated for IgAN recurrence or not by repetitive protocol biopsy (Table 1).

We showed a recurrence rate in each protocol graft biopsy within all cases: 1 h, 0%; 3 months, 8.3%; 12 months, 25%; 3 years, 41.7%; 5 years, 25%; 7 year, 0%. Among 3 years after transplantation, 66% of recurrence was noted.

The therapeutic response was measured by assessing hematuria and proteinuria in each group. The tonsillectomy group exhibited more proteinuria than did the no tonsillectomy group at recurrence. However, no significant differences were observed in the degree of proteinuria between groups (0.33 ± 0.52 vs. 0.07 ± 0.19 g/gCr, respectively; $p = 0.33$). In the no tonsillectomy group, the mean proteinuria at recurrence was 0.07 ± 0.19 g/gCr, which increased significantly to 0.97 ± 1.09 g/gCr at 60 months after recurrence ($p = 0.043$). However, no significant change was observed in proteinuria in the tonsillectomy group (0.33 ± 0.52 vs. 0.40 ± 0.53 g/gCr, $p = 0.87$) during the same observation period (Fig. 1a, b). No significant differences were observed in the degree of hematuria between groups.

In terms of the histological damage caused by IgAN in the tonsillectomy group, no significant differences were

Table 1 Patient characteristics

	Tonsillectomy ($n = 5$)	No tonsillectomy ($n = 7$)	p
Recipient gender (M/F)	2/3	6/1	0.10
Recipient age at transplantation (mean ± SD)	33.7 ± 9.7	36.6 ± 8.6	0.75
Donor age at transplantation (mean ± SD)	57.7 ± 15.5	53.1 ± 17.1	1.00
Duration of pre-transplant dialysis (months)	41.3 ± 42.1	9.6 ± 3.6	0.10
Living/deceased	5/0	6/1	1.00
ABO compatible/incompatible	3/2	7/0	0.15
Immunosuppressant use (CsA/FK)	3/2	6/1	0.52
SCr at recurrence (mg/dl)	1.15 ± 0.28	1.29 ± 0.17	0.33
eGFR at recurrence (ml/min)	47.7 ± 14.6	39.1 ± 5.8	0.33
Urinary findings at recurrence			
Hematuria	3/5 (60%)	4/7 (57%)	1.00
Proteinuria (g/g·Cr)	0.33 ± 0.52	0.07 ± 0.19	0.39
Use of RASI	5/5 (100%)	6/7 (85.7%)	1.00
Period between transplant and IgAN recurrence (months)	37.4 ± 25.7	31.8 ± 19.3	0.94
Median time between IgAN recurrence and tonsillectomy (months)	3.1(1.4 – 28.9)	–	–
Time between IgAN recurrence and the next protocol biopsy (months)	57.4 ± 10.1	61.4 ± 8.5	0.76
Follow-up period (months)	146.8 ± 30.1	193.6 ± 105.1	0.75

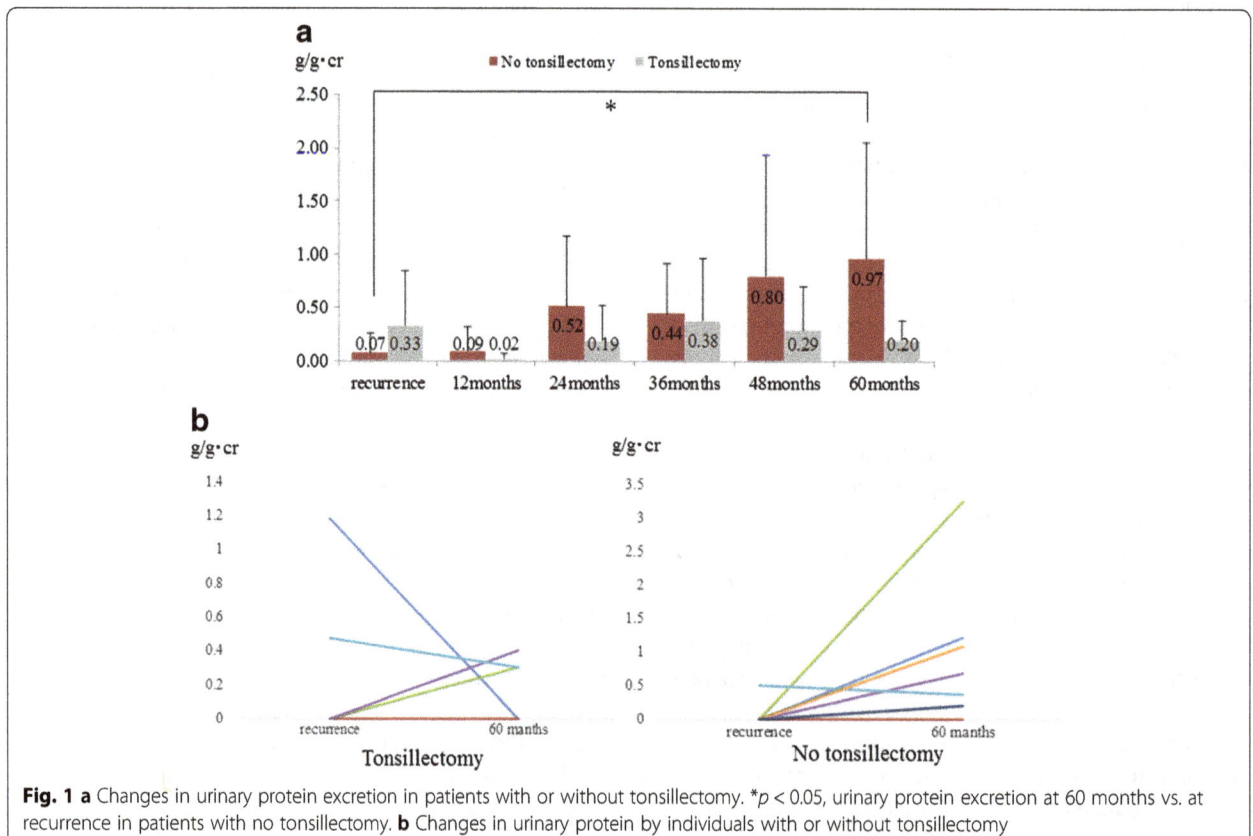

Fig. 1 a Changes in urinary protein excretion in patients with or without tonsillectomy. *$p < 0.05$, urinary protein excretion at 60 months vs. at recurrence in patients with no tonsillectomy. **b** Changes in urinary protein by individuals with or without tonsillectomy

observed in the histopathological alterations before and after tonsillectomy. However, in the no tonsillectomy group, the mesangial matrix score (mm) in the Banff classification 2007 increased from 0.14 ± 0.38 to 2.14 ± 0.69 ($p = 0.002$), the mesangial hypercellularity score (MS) in the Oxford classification increased from 0.20 ± 0.36 to 0.69 ± 0.37 ($p = 0.003$), and the segmental glomeruloscreosis score (SS) in the Oxford classification increased from 0 to 0.57 ± 0.54 ($p = 0.03$) (Table 2). Pathological rejection, except for borderline changes, was not observed during the study period.

Figure 2 shows the change in eGFR between groups. The decreases in eGFR before and 60 months after transplantation were as follows: tonsillectomy group, 47.7 ± 14.6 to 34.8 ± 12.2 ml/min/1.73 m^2 ($p = 0.11$); no tonsillectomy group, 39.1 ± 5.8 to 30.4 ± 10.2 ml/min/1.73 m^2 ($p = 0.03$). In terms of the change in 1/Cr between groups, the decreases in 1/Cr before and 60 months after transplantation were as follows: tonsillectomy group, 0.91 ± 0.21 to 0.73 ± 0.26 mg/dl ($p = 0.14$); no tonsillectomy group, 0.79 ± 0.11 to 0.65 ± 0.22 ml/min/1.73 m^2 ($p = 0.03$). Although eGFR and 1/Cr reduced in both groups, the decline was only significant in the no tonsillectomy group. No patients in the tonsillectomy group experienced renal graft loss, while three (42.3%) patients lost their graft in the no tonsillectomy group (Fig. 3). Among these, the mean graft survival was 11.3 ± 6.8 years, and the reason for graft loss was followed, two patients for IgAN recurrence, one patient for interstitial fibrosis and tubular atrophy (IF/TA).

Discussion

We found that tonsillectomy is an effective treatment for IgAN recurrence after kidney transplantation both clinically and pathologically. Hotta et al. reported that tonsillectomy and steroid pulse therapy had a significant effect in patients with primary IgAN. In addition, patients with early to mid-stage primary IgAN with relatively preserved renal function were more likely to respond satisfactorily [13]. In the current study, the tonsillectomy group exhibited no significant differences in the degree of proteinuria and eGFR. Graft loss did not occur during the observation period, and there were no remarkable changes in mesangial hypercellularity score (MS in the Oxford classification) or matrix expansion (mm score in the Banff classification 2007).

Kennoki et al. conducted a retrospective study of 28 transplant recipients with IgAN recurrence and persistent proteinuria. Of the 16 and 12 patients with or without tonsillectomy during a mean follow-up period of 60 months, proteinuria decreased significantly in all tonsillectomized patients but did not in no tonsillectomy patients. No significant differences were observed in the degree of hematuria and eGFR between the groups [14]. In other study, Ushigome et al. analyzed four transplant

Table 2 Changes in renal pathological findings in patients with or without tonsillectomy according to the Banff classification and the Oxford classification

			At recurrence	Post tonsillectomy	p
Tonsillectomy group					
Banff classification		t	0.60 ± 0.89	0.20 ± 0.45	0.48
		i	0.60 ± 0.89	0.20 ± 0.45	0.48
		v	0	0.20 ± 0.45	0.37
		g	0.20 ± 0.45	0.20 ± 0.45	1.00
		ci	0	0.60 ± 0.55	0.07
		ct	0.40 ± 0.55	0.80 ± 0.45	0.37
		mm	0.40 ± 0.55	0.80 ± 0.45	0.37
		cg	0	0	–
		cv	0.40 ± 0.55	0.40 ± 0.89	1.00
		ah	0.20 ± 0.45	0.60 ± 0.89	0.18
		ptc	0.20 ± 0.45	0.60 ± 0.89	0.48
		Scl (%)	6.20 ± 6.46	18.06 ± 22.02	0.19
Oxford classification		M	0.24 ± 0.21	0.32 ± 0.29	0.59
		S	0.40 ± 0.55	0.40 ± 0.55	1.00
		E	0.20 ± 0.45	0	0.37
		T	0	0.20 ± 0.45	0.37
No tonsillectomy group					
Banff classification		t	0.14 ± 0.38	0.14 ± 0.38	1.00
		i	0.14 ± 0.38	0	0.36
		v	0	0	–
		g	0	0.14 ± 0.38	0.36
		ci	0.14 ± 0.38	0.29 ± 0.49	0.60
		ct	0.43 ± 0.53	0.71 ± 0.49	0.17
		mm	0.14 ± 0.38	2.14 ± 0.69	0.002
		cg	0	0.29 ± 0.49	0.17
		cv	0.43 ± 0.53	0.71 ± 0.76	0.17
		ah	0.29 ± 0.38	0.71 ± 0.49	0.20
		ptc	0.14 ± 0.38	0.14 ± 0.38	1.00
		Scl (%)	6.43 ± 11.43	14.5 ± 13.45	0.25
Oxford classification		M	0.20 ± 0.36	0.69 ± 0.37	0.003
		S	0	0.57 ± 0.54	0.03
		E	0	0.14 ± 0.38	0.36
		T	0.24 ± 0.21	0.14 ± 0.38	0.25

recipients with IgAN recurrence who underwent tonsillectomy. The urinary findings were improved in all patients after tonsillectomy, including a histologically severe case, for a mean period of 13.5 months [15]. Furthermore, Koshino et al. reported date from seven transplant recipients with IgAN recurrence who underwent tonsillectomy. Both of urinary findings and SCr levels improved in the mild-grade recurrent IgAN cases

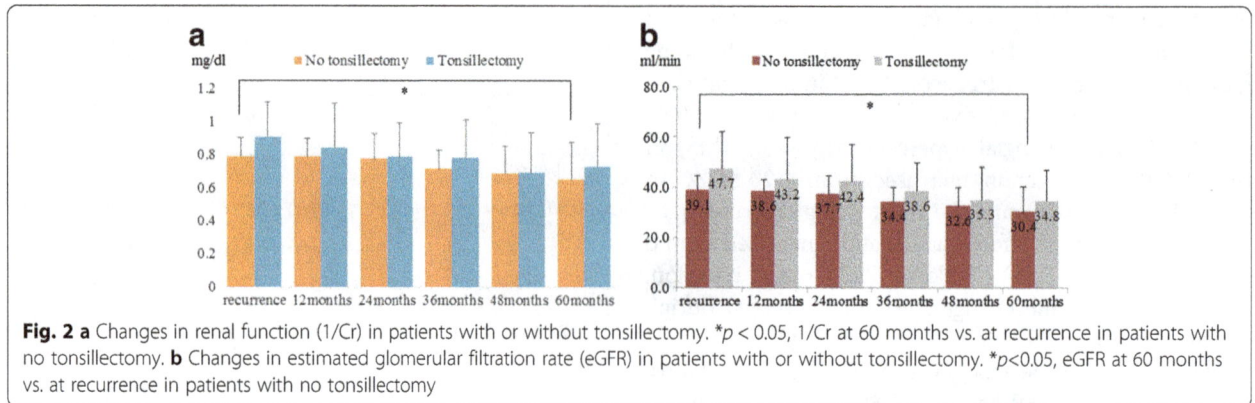

Fig. 2 a Changes in renal function (1/Cr) in patients with or without tonsillectomy. *$p < 0.05$, 1/Cr at 60 months vs. at recurrence in patients with no tonsillectomy. **b** Changes in estimated glomerular filtration rate (eGFR) in patients with or without tonsillectomy. *$p<0.05$, eGFR at 60 months vs. at recurrence in patients with no tonsillectomy

after tonsillectomy over a mean observation period of 48.4 months [16].

In the current study, patients with tonsillectomy group exhibited improved urinary findings, whereas proteinuria increased significantly in the no tonsillectomy group. Consistent with previous studies, tonsillectomy treatment reduced proteinuria. We hypothesize that tonsillectomy alone protects graft function and pathology. In the tonsillectomy group, the slope of eGFR seemed to be greater, but SD was higher in tonsillectomy than no tonsillectomy group, higher SD might result in no statistical different during 60 months observation. We therefore tried to show graft function by other parameter instead of eGFR (Fig. 2a), the slope of 1/Cr was similar as the slope of eGFR. Although the decline of eGFR (from 47.7 to 34.8ml/min) was 27.0% during 60 months (less than 30%) in the tonsillectomy group (Fig. 2b), the most important factor for IgAN progression depends on the amount of proteinuria at the same kidney function [17].

Ohya and Shigematsu et al. showed that the efficacy of tonsillectomy in IgAN in native kidney [18]. Mean age (34.6 years) and levels of serum creatinine (0.9 mg/dl) and proteinuria (0.87 g/dl) were similar to our study

population. They concluded that tonsillectomy resulted in lower relapse after achieving remission compared to steroid therapy alone. In order to reveal the effect of tonsillectomy alone, our results as well as other reports [18] made possible this hypothesis. The mechanism of tonsillectomy is an antigenic stimulation of immune system by the tonsillar mucosa via the mucosa-bone marrow axis [19].

Histological evidence is required to confirm that tonsillectomy exhibits a graft-protecting effect. In the current study, there was no change in mesangial cell proliferation in the tonsillectomy group. In contrast, the mm, MS, and SS scores significantly increased in the no tonsillectomy group. This suggests that tonsillectomy improves mesangial cell proliferation and matrix expansion. Hotta et al. reported that both of urinary findings and graft pathology were improved in 15 transplant recipients with IgAN recurrence who underwent tonsillectomy [20]. Although their results were consistent with those of the current study, they were unable to confirm IgAN as a primary disease in those recipients.

When considering the effects of tonsillectomy, it is necessary to compare a tonsillectomy group to no tonsillectomy group. It is also important to confirm any changes pathologically using protocol graft biopsies. However, several previous studies [14–16, 20] did not perform long-term evaluations using protocol graft biopsies. We can also evaluate rejection according to the Banff classification and aggravation of the IgAN process for long-term observation about 10 years. The Banff classification is a useful tool for standardizing to evaluate rejection, but it is not designed to evaluate the recurrence of nephritis. On the other hand, the Oxford classification was announced in 2009 by a working group of the International IgAN Network and Association of International Kidney Pathology. It analyzes the reproducibility of lesions in IgAN by every pathologist, and it then can be confirmed as the responsible lesion for the prognosis of IgAN. This classification also takes into consideration the mesangial cells proliferation, which is an important reason why this classification system was

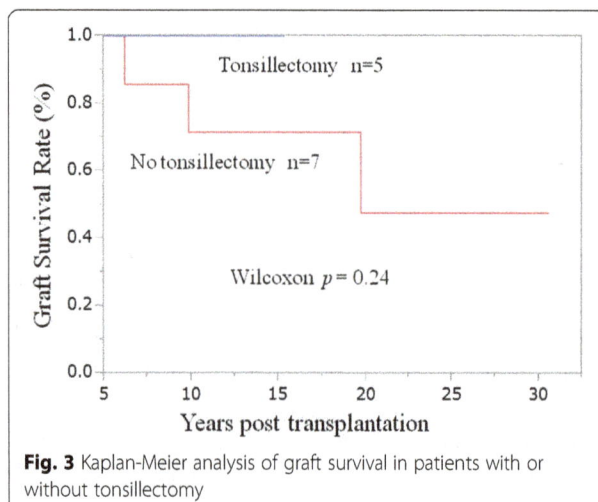

Fig. 3 Kaplan-Meier analysis of graft survival in patients with or without tonsillectomy

Efficacy of tonsillectomy for the treatment of immunoglobulin A nephropathy recurrence after...

145

generated [21]. IgAN recurrence in renal grafts is generally categorized with mild histological findings; therefore, lesions such as cellular crescents, fibrocellular crescents, and intraluminal lesions are usually not considered. Therefore, we utilized the Oxford classification system with the Banff classification to determine IgAN recurrence in the current study. Even if just mild lesion seen at protocal biopsy, tonsillectomy resulted in favorable outcome based on repetitive biopsies in our study.

The effectiveness of tonsillectomy and steroid pulse combined-therapy, for improving mesangial cell proliferation and fibrosis, has been reported previously [13, 22]. However, there is concern that the additional steroid pulse therapy might lead to over-immunosuppression. Therefore, many physicians hesitate steroid pulse therapy in patients with recurrent IgAN after transplantation. Although, the postoperative use of immunosuppressive agents might suppress the development of IgAN, the addition of steroid pulse therapy is doubted for taking a side effect into account. Immunosuppressive therapy might not successfully prevent from IgAN recurrence even in this era after kidney transplantation [23]; therefore, we evaluated the efficacy of tonsillectomy alone in the current study.

Study limitations

This study has three limitations: First, the number of cases was insufficient in both groups. In order to make a diagnosis of recurrent IgAN, both pre- and post-transplant renal biopsy diagnosis is required. Unfortunately, there were few patients who diagnosed IgAN as primary disease. We extensively recruited patients since 1984 because of above reason. Second, more patients with proteinuria were included in the tonsillectomy group; therefore, there is a selection bias in this retrospective study. Third, most of patients introduce our hospital to transplant purpose; we could not take information about IgAN activity in detail.

Conclusions

This study demonstrated that tonsillectomy protected clinical and pathological alteration in patients with IgAN recurrence after kidney transplantation. However, a large sample size and more long-term observation are necessary to determine the effectiveness of tonsillectomy in case of IgAN recurrence after kidney transplantation.

Abbreviations

Ah: Arteriolar hyaline thickening score; Cg: Allograft glomerulopathy score; ci: Interstitial fibrosis score; CsA: Cyclosporin A; Ct: Tubular atrophy score; Cv: Fibrous intimal thickening score; E: Endocapillary hypercellularity score; eGFR: Estimated glomerular filtration rate; g: Early allograft glomerulitis score; i: Mononuclear cell interstitial inflammation score; IgAN: Immunoglobulin A nephropathy; M: Mesangial hypercellularity score; Mm: Mesangial matrix increase score; Ptc: Peritubular capillaritis score; RASI: Renin-angiotensin system inhibitors; S: Segmental glomerulosclerosis score; Scl: Glomerular sclerosis; SCr: Serum creatinine; SD: Standard deviation; T: Tubular atrophy/interstitial fibrosis score; T: Tubulitis score; V: Intimal arteritis score

Acknowledgements
We would like to express our gratitude to Associate Prof. Tetsuo Nemoto at the Department of Surgical Pathology. This work was supported by all the staffs at the Department of Nephrology, Faculty of Medicine, Toho University.

Funding
There was no funding.

Authors' contributions
HN and KS (corresponding author) planned the study, searched the literature, assessed studies, extracted data, analyzed data, and wrote the manuscript. HE assisted the study operation and data collection. SS, KS, and AA assessed studies and assisted in the data analysis. All authors read and approved the final manuscript.

Competing interests
The authors declare that they have no competing interests.

Author details
[1]Department of Nephrology, Faculty of Medicine, Toho University, 6-11-1 Omori-Nishi, Ota-ku, Tokyo 143-8541, Japan. [2]Department of Surgical Pathology, Faculty of Medicine, Toho University, Tokyo, Japan. [3]Department of Otolaryngology, Faculty of Medicine, Toho University, Tokyo, Japan.

References
1. Choy BY, Chan TM, Lai KN. Recurrent glomerulonephritis after kidney transplantation. Am J Transplant. 2006;6:2535–42.
2. KDIGO. Clinical practice guideline for the care of kidney transplant recipients. Am J Transplant. 2009;9(Suppl 3):S1–S157.
3. Chandrakantan A, Ratanapanichkich P, Said M, Barker CV, Julian BA. Recurrent IgA nephropathy after renal transplantation despite immunosuppressive regimens with mycophenolate mofetil. Nephrol Dial Transplant. 2005;20:1214–21.
4. Briganti EM, Russ GR, McNeil JJ, Atkins RC, Chadban SJ. Risk of renal allograft loss from recurrent glomerulonephritis. N Engl J Med. 2002;347:103–9.
5. Berger J, Hinglais N. Intercapillary deposits of IgA-IgG. J Urol Nephrol. 1968; 74:694–5.
6. Xie Y, Nishi S, Ueno M, Imai N, Sakatsume M, Narita I, Suzuki Y, et al. The efficacy of tonsillectomy on long-term renal survival in patients with IgA nephropathy. Kidney Int. 2003;63:1861–7.
7. Xie Y, Chen X, Nishi S, Narita I, Gejyo F. Relationship between tonsils and IgA nephropathy as well as indication of tonsillectomy. Kidney Int. 2004;65: 1135–44.
8. Nishi S, Xie Y, Ueno M, Imai N, Suzuki Y, Iguchi S, Fukase S, et al. A clinicopathological study on the long-term efficacy of tonsillectomy in patients with IgA nephropathy. Acta Otolaryngol Suppl. 2004;555:49–53.
9. Abe K, Miyazaki M, Shioshita K, Harada T, Koji T, Kohno S. Clinical and immunohistochemical study of immunoglobulin A nephropathy (IgAN) before and after tonsillectomy. Acta Otolaryngol Suppl. 2004;555:20–4.
10. Solez K, Colvin RB, Racusen LC, Haas M, Sis B, Mengel M, Halloran PF, et al. Banff 07 classification of renal allograft pathology: updates and future direction. Am J Transplant. 2008;8:753–60.

11. Roberts IS, Coook HT, Troyanov S, Alpers CE, Amore A, Barratt J, Berthoux F, et al. Development of the Oxford Classification of IgA nephropathy: pathology definitions, correlations and reproducibility. Kidney Int. 2009;76:546–56.

12. Cattran DC, Coppo R, Cook HT, Feehally J, Roberts IS, Troyanov S, Alpers CE, et al. The Oxford classification of IgA nephropathy. Part 1: rationale, clinicopathological correlations, and proposal for classification. Kidney Int. 2009;76:534–42.

13. Hotta O, Miyazaki M, Furuta T, Tomioka S, Chiba S, Horigome I, Abe K, et al. Tonsillectomy and steroid pulse therapy significantly impact on clinical remission in patients with IgA nephropathy. Am J Kidney Dis. 2001;38:736–42.

14. Kennoli T, Ishida H, Yamaguchi Y, Tanabe K. Proteinuria-reducing effects of tonsillectomy alone in IgA nephropathy recurring after kidney transplantation. Transplantation. 2009;88:935–41.

15. Ushigome H, Suzuki T, Fujiki M, Nobori S, Sakamoto S, Okamoto M, Urasaki K, et al. Efficacy of tonsillectomy for patients with recurrence of IgA nephropathy after kidney transplantation. Clin Transplant. 2009;23:17–22.

16. Koshino K, Ushigome H, Sakai K, Suzuki T, Nobori S, Okajima H, Masuzawa N, et al. Outcome of tonsillectomy for recurrent IgA nephropathy after kidney transplantation. Clin Transplant. 2013;27:22–8.

17. Iseki K, Ikemiya Y, Iseki C, Takishita S. Proteinuria and the risk of developing end-stage renal disease. Kidney Int. 2003;63:1468–74.

18. Ohya M, Otani H, Minami Y, Yamanaka S, Mima T, Negi S, Yukawa S, et al. Tonsillectomy with steroid pulse therapy has more effect on the relapse rate than steroid pulse monotherapy in IgA nephropathy patients. Clin Nephro. 2013;80(1):47–52.

19. Hotta O. Use of corticosteroids, other immunosuppressive therapies, and tonsillectomy in the treatment of IgA nephropathy. Semin Nephrol. 2004; 24:244–55.

20. Hotta K, Fukasawa Y, Akimoto M, Tanabe T, Sasaki H, Fukuzawa N, Seki T, et al. Tonsillectomy ameliorates histological damage of recurrent immunoglobulin A nephropathy after kidney transplantation. Nephrology. 2013;18:808–12.

21. Eitner F, Floege J. Glomerular disease: The Oxford classification-predicting progression of IgAN. Nat Rev Nephrol. 2009;5:557–9.

22. Hotta O, Furuta T, Chiba S, Tomioka S, Taguma Y. Regression of IgA nephropathy: a repeat biopsy study. Am J Kidney Dis. 2002;39:493–502.

23. Pham PTT, Pham PCT. The impact of mycophenolate mofetil versus azathioprine as adjunctive therapy to cyclosporine on the rates of renal allograft loss due to glomerular disease recurrence. Nephrol Dial Transplant. 2012;27:2965–71.

17

Significance of new membrane formation in peritoneal biopsies of peritoneal dialysis patients: a case–control study

Kazuho Honda[1*], Chieko Hamada[2], Kunio Kawanishi[3], Masaaki Nakayama[4], Masanobu Miyazaki[5], Yasuhiko Ito[6] and on behalf of the Peritoneal Pathology Study Committee of Japanese Society of Peritoneal Dialysis (JSPD)[7]

Abstract

Background: Newly formed membrane (NFM) on the peritoneal membrane proper is a unique pathological hallmark of encapsulating peritoneal sclerosis (EPS), but its definition and diagnostic significance have not been well described. This study investigated the pathological features of NFM in EPS and prevalence of NFM in peritoneal biopsy at catheter removal.

Methods: This multicenter retrospective, observational study was conducted by the Japanese Society of Peritoneal Dialysis and enrolled ten patients with and 52 without EPS at peritoneal biopsy during enterolysis surgery or catheter removal. All patients were treated using conventional, acidic peritoneal dialysis (PD) solutions. Thirty of the 52 non-EPS patients perform peritoneal lavage once daily after completing PD to prevent the development of EPS and 22 discontinued PD without lavage. NFM was defined as additional membrane structure on the peritoneum that is properly characterized by exudative or fibrous matrices and fibroblast-like cells. Immunostaining of fibrin and podoplanin was performed for the evaluation of NFM.

Results: NFM was confirmed histologically in eight of the ten patients with EPS. It was also detected in 13 of the 30 patients (43.3%) in the post-PD lavage group and in one of the 22 patients (4.5%) in the non-lavage group. The NFM histology showed various stages of EPS pathology, from early exudative changes with fibrin deposition (stage I; $n = 5$), progressing to proliferative and fibrosing changes with podoplanin-positive fibroblast-like cells (stage II; $n = 9$), and finally resulting in adhesive and fibrous scar formation (stage III; $n = 8$). Immunostaining of fibrin and podoplanin was helpful for evaluating the stage of the NFM.

Conclusions: NFM contributes the encapsulation of intestines and is a pathological hallmark of EPS, but can be detected microscopically in patients without EPS, especially those with peritoneal lavage after PD. New membrane formation starts insidiously in peritoneal membrane damaged by PD treatment, but does not necessarily lead to the development of EPS.

Keywords: Encapsulating peritoneal sclerosis, Simple peritoneal fibrosis, Encapsulating membrane, Newly formed membrane, Fibrin, Podoplanin, Peritoneal permeability

* Correspondence: kzhonda@med.showa-u.ac.jp
[1]Department of Anatomy, Showa University School of Medicine, 1-5-8 Hatanodai, Shinagawa-ku, Tokyo 142-8555, Japan
Full list of author information is available at the end of the article

Background

Encapsulating peritoneal sclerosis (EPS) is a rare but serious complication of peritoneal dialysis (PD) [1–4]. The diagnosis of EPS is based on clinical signs of obstructive ileus and pathological evidence of encapsulation of entire abdominal organs (cocoon formation) [5]. Histological evaluation of peritoneal tissues in EPS revealed that fibrin deposition, increased fibrosis, inflammatory cell infiltration, and angiogenesis were characteristic of EPS [6–9]; however, they were nonspecific inflammatory findings, and none were pathognomonic for the diagnosis of EPS. Macroscopic findings of abdominal organs suggested a newly formed encapsulating membrane, mainly in the visceral peritoneum, was unique to EPS [10]. Histologically, the structure of encapsulating membrane was described as organized fibrosing tissue formed on the peritoneal membrane proper with swollen fibroblast-like cells immunohistochemically positive for podoplanin [11, 12]. These observations suggested that a definite pathological diagnosis of EPS requires macroscopic and/or histological confirmation of an encapsulating membrane. However, we have occasionally observed a newly formed membrane (NFM) similar to the encapsulating membrane of EPS in peritoneal biopsy specimens obtained from non-EPS patients with peritoneal lavage after PD withdrawal. Peritoneal lavage is frequently performed in Japan, especially in long-term PD patients, to prevent the development of EPS. It is believed to prevent EPS by elimination of exudates that lead to the formation of encapsulating membranes [13, 14].

The purpose of this study was to investigate the pathological features of encapsulating membranes as a diagnostic criterion of EPS and to evaluate the prevalence and significance of NFMs in peritoneal biopsies obtained at catheter removal. We also sought to identify the factors associated with new membrane formation, focusing on the extent of simple peritoneal sclerosis induced by PD and the effects of peritoneal lavage. We found that encapsulating membranes were diagnostic for EPS but that NFMs were frequently observed microscopically in biopsies of patients with peritoneal lavage after PD discontinuation but did not develop EPS. The presence of microscopic NFMs in peritoneal biopsies at catheter removal indicated increased peritoneal permeability and exudation but did not predict the subsequent development of EPS.

Methods

Patients

The Peritoneal Biopsy Program in Japan was conducted from 1994 to 2006. A total of 1928 peritoneal biopsy samples were collected from 227 medical institutes. Of these, 569 were excluded because of uncertain clinical information. Of the remaining 1359 samples, 230 were obtained at the initiation of PD and 1129 were obtained

after PD of 66.4 ± 44.4 months duration. Patients with peritonitis within 1 month before PD withdrawal ($n = 360$) were excluded, and 79 of the remaining 769 samples were from patients with medical records indicating that they had been diagnosed with EPS or suspected EPS. We confirmed the diagnosis of EPS based on the Japanese guidelines for EPS [5] and International Society for Peritoneal Dialysis statement [15]. Clinical signs and symptoms of gastrointestinal obstruction were an essential diagnostic criterion of EPS. Image findings suggesting peritoneal membrane thickening or encapsulation of abdominal organs, bowel obstruction, or cocoon formation were supportive findings for the diagnosis. To ensure the diagnosis of EPS, only peritoneal biopsy samples obtained at enterolysis surgery were selected for inclusion of the EPS group ($n = 10$, five men and five women; PD duration of 124.5 ± 34.2 months). Consequently, most biopsy samples of the EPS patients were obtained from the adhering visceral peritoneum.

We selected 52 non-EPS patients with a PD duration of more than 60 months as matched-duration controls for the EPS group. The non-EPS patients were divided into two groups by the performance of peritoneal lavage treatment after PD withdrawal. The peritoneal lavage group included 30 patients, 19 men and 11 women, 58.5 ± 9.5 years of age, a PD duration of 98.4 ± 33.7 months, and a lavage duration of 12.8 ± 5.1 months. The non-EPS patients without peritoneal lavage included 22 patients, 13 men and nine women, 44.1 ± 17.5 years of age, and PD duration of 91.4 ± 30.3 months. All biopsy samples of non-EPS patients were taken at catheter removal from the parietal peritoneum. No patient in the non-EPS groups, either with or without lavage, had clinical signs and symptoms of EPS. The reasons for PD discontinuation in the lavage group were ultrafiltration failure ($n = 7$), under-dialysis ($n = 1$), cerebral infarction ($n = 1$), EPS prevention ($n = 2$), and unknown ($n = 19$). Peritoneal lavage was usually performed once a day by exchange of PD solution with low glucose concentration ($n = 25$) or icodextrin ($n = 5$) solution for several months to years. The mean duration of peritoneal lavage was 12.8 ± 5.1 months. The clinical status of the non-lavage group varied, including patients who stopped PD because of ultrafiltration failure ($n = 6$), transplantation ($n = 4$), under-dialysis ($n = 1$), catheter-related problems ($n = 3$), malignancy ($n = 2$), and unknown ($n = 1$). Other patients were biopsied at catheter exchange ($n = 4$) or on exploratory laparotomy for the evaluation of peritoneal condition ($n = 1$). All patients in the EPS and non-EPS groups were treated using conventional acidic PD solutions. The study design was approved by the ethics committee of Juntendo Medical University (No. 370, May 2009). Written informed consent was obtained from all study subjects.

Histopathological analysis

Peritoneal biopsy specimens were cut from the parietal peritoneum using a scalpel or peeled from the encapsulated visceral peritoneum and processed by routine histological procedures as previously described [16]. The adequacy of specimens for histological evaluation was determined in terms of size, site, and direction of the samples as described in the previous report [16]. All specimens included in the study were regarded as adequate for the evaluation of the peritoneal thickness, vasculopathy at post-capillary venules (PCVs), and presence or absence of NFM and its histological features. Two pathologists (KH and KK) reviewed the samples together to arrive at a consensus evaluation. The extent of fibrosis and vascular sclerosis was evaluated as previously described [16]. In brief, to evaluate peritoneal fibrosis, we calculated average thickness (µm) at five random points within the submesothelial compact zone (SMC) between the basal border of the surface mesothelial cells and upper border of the peritoneal adipose tissue. To evaluate vascular sclerosis, average ratio of lumen to vessel diameter was calculated at three to five randomly selected PCVs with external diameters ranging 25–50 µm. NFMs were defined as formation of an additional membrane structure on the surface of the peritoneal membrane proper and comprised of fibrin exudation, collagenous fibrotic tissue, fibroblast-like cells, and capillary vessels. NFMs differ from peritoneal membrane proper, with simple peritoneal fibrosis and do not contain dense bundle of collagen, fascia, fat, or small arteries and veins that are seen in peritoneal tissue. The histological staging of NFMs included an early exudative phase with fibrin deposition and podoplanin-positive fibroblast-like cells (stage I), a proliferative and fibrosing phase with podoplanin-positive fibroblast-like cells but without fibrin deposition (stage II), and an adhesive and fibrous scarring phase without fibrin deposition or podoplanin-positive fibroblast-like cells (stage III). Immunostaining of fibrin and podoplanin was helpful for evaluating the stage of NFMs (Fig. 2j).

Immunohistochemistry

Mouse monoclonal anti-fibrin (MAB1901, Chemicon International) and human anti-podoplanin (#11-003, AngioBio, Del Mar, CA, USA) were used as primary antibodies. The Envision+ System (Dako Cytomation) was used for detection of antibody binding and was visualized using diaminobenzidine tetrahydrochloride (0.02%). Cell nuclei were counterstained with hematoxylin.

Statistical analysis

Data were reported as means ± standard deviation. Differences were assessed for significance by χ^2 tests, Student's t tests, Mann–Whitney U test, or Kruskal–Wallis test, depending on whether the variables were categorical or continuous. Correlation coefficients were assessed for significance using the F test. In all analyses, $p < 0.05$ was considered significant.

Results

Clinical and histological data of the ten EPS-developed cases

The clinical and histological findings of each patient in the EPS group are shown in Table 1. The average PD duration was 124.5 ± 34.2 months. The biopsy samples were obtained during enterolysis surgery, which was performed at 23.6 ± 19.2 months after PD discontinuation to dissect intestinal adhesions. Peritoneal lavage was performed in three patients (no. 1, 3, and 4) for several months (7, 15, and 2 months, respectively) before enterolysis surgery to prevent or reduce abdominal adhesions. NFMs were identified microscopically in eight patients (80%) and macroscopically during surgery in two

Table 1 Clinical and pathological characteristics of the EPS patients ($n = 10$)

Patient no.	Age	Sex	PD duration (m)	Post-PD duration (m)	Peritoneal lavage (m)	NFM (stage)	SMC (µm)	L/V ratio
1	55	F	79	15	7	I	389.2	0.352
2	57	M	166	74	–	III	283	0.166
3	68	F	80	26	15	I	622	0.196
4	56	F	144	11	2	I	1269.6	0.186
5	57	M	116	16	–	I	614.4	0.234
6	60	M	151	35	–	n.d.	259.4	0.9
7	56	F	165	18	–	II	389	0.192
8	60	F	142	18	–	II	985.6	0.382
9	52	M	84	9	–	n.d.	247	0.442
10	46	M	118	14	–	I	1302.8	0.263
	56.7 ± 5.7	M5 F5	124.5 ± 34.2	23.6 ± 19.2	3/10 (30%) 8.0 ± 6.6	8/10 (80%) [5/2/1]	636.2 ± 409.4	0.33 ± 0.22

Mean ± sd

NFM newly formed membrane, *SMC* submesothelial compact zone, *L/V* lumen/vessel diameter, *n.d.* not detected

patients (20%). In these two patients (no. 6 and 9), NFMs were not confirmed in the biopsy specimens. Histologically, most NFMs were stage I ($n = 5$), followed by stage II ($n = 2$), and stage III ($n = 1$), showing a predominance of early exudative stages in the encapsulating membrane formation. The stage III NFM was obtained from patient 2, who had the longest PD duration (166 months) and the longest post-PD duration (74 months). The extent of PD-related peritoneal sclerosis was evaluated by the thickness of the SMC and the lumen/vessel diameter ratio (L/V ratio) of the PCVs in the peritoneal membrane proper that was attached to the NFM in the biopsy specimens. The increased thickness of the SMC (636.2 ± 409.4 μm) and the decreased L/V ratio (0.33 ± 0.22) suggested a tendency of advanced peritoneal sclerosis in the EPS patients.

Pathology of NFMs in EPS patients

Figure 1 shows an NFM in an EPS patient (no. 4) obtained during enterolysis surgery. Microscopically, the NFM was identified as a fibrotic structure on the visceral peritoneum proper of the intestine (Fig. 1a). The thickness of the NFM was approximately 200–500 μm and characterized by interlacing homogenous fibrous bundles with fibroblast-like cells (Fig. 1b). Fibrin deposition was observed on the membrane surface by Masson trichrome staining (Fig. 1b) and confirmed by immunohistochemical staining (Fig. 1c).

Podoplanin was strongly positive on the cellular membranes of intercalating fibroblast-like cells and the inner surface of vessel-like clefts in the NFM (Fig. 1d).

Histological staging of NFMs

Histological observation revealed several stages of NFMs (Fig. 2), an early exudative phase (stage I), fibrosing phase (stage II), and late scarring phase (stage III). In the early exudative phase (stage I), fibrin was deposited, as detected by Masson trichrome staining (Fig. 2a) and confirmed by fibrin immunostaining (Fig. 2b). Podoplanin-positive fibroblasts were abundantly distributed in the NFM (Fig. 2c). In the fibrosing phase (stage II), fibrous matrices were dominant, with many collagen fibers and sparsely distributed fibroblast-like cells (Fig. 2d). In this stage, no fibrin deposition was detected immunohistochemically (Fig. 2e), whereas podoplanin was weakly positive in the fibroblast-like cells (Fig. 2f). In the scarring phase (stage III), the NFM was characterized by loose fibrous matrices covering the peritoneal surface and sometimes forming peritoneal adhesions with few cellular components (Fig. 2g). Neither fibrin (Fig. 2h) nor podoplanin (Fig. 2i) was detected in this phase. NFM stage was determined by Masson trichrome staining of fibrin and podoplanin or by immunohistochemistry (Fig. 2j). Other histological findings such as hemorrhage, inflammatory cell infiltration, and capillary proliferation were preferentially observed in

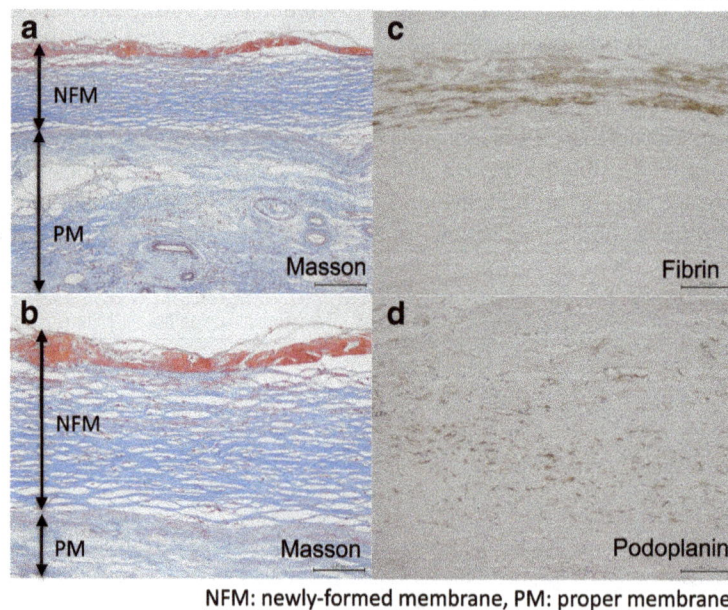

NFM: newly-formed membrane, PM: proper membrane

Fig. 1 Histological findings of an NFM in a representative EPS patient. An NFM is a fibrous membrane-like structure attached to the surface of the visceral peritoneum proper (PM). **a** The NFM is located on the visceral peritoneal membrane and has the histological appearance of simple peritoneal sclerosis with severe fibrosis and obstructive vasculopathy (Masson stain, ×100, and bar = 200 μm). **b** The NFM is characterized by surface fibrin deposition and an interlacing of homogenous fibrous bundles with fibroblast-like cells (Masson stain, ×200, and bar = 100 μm). **c** Fibrin is deposited on the surface of the NFM and confirmed by immunohistochemical fibrin staining (IHC for fibrin, ×200, and bar = 100 μm). **d** Podoplanin is strongly positive on the cell membranes of intercalating fibroblast-like cells in the NFM (IHC for podoplanin, ×200, and bar = 100 μm)

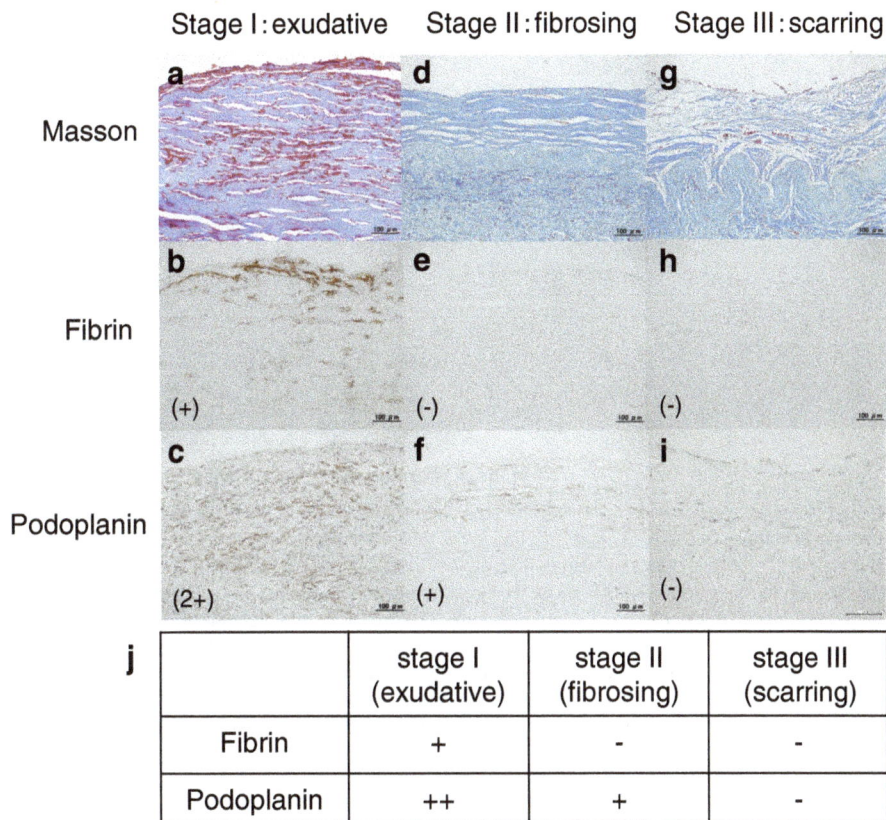

Fig. 2 Histological staging of NFMs. Histological observation revealed several stages of NFM. In the early exudative phase (stage I), fibrin deposition is apparent, as indicated by the bright red color in Masson trichrome staining (**a**) and confirmed by fibrin immunostaining (**b**). Podoplanin-positive fibroblasts are abundantly distributed in the encapsulating membrane (**c**). In the fibrotic phase (stage II), fibrosis is dominant, with many collagen fibers and sparsely distributed fibroblasts (**d**). In this stage, no fibrin deposition is detected immunohistochemically (**e**), whereas podoplanin is weakly positive in the fibroblast-like cells (**f**). In the scarring phase (stage III), the NFM is characterized by loose fibrous matrices covering the peritoneal surface, occasionally forming peritoneal adhesions with scant cellular components. Mesothelial cell coverage is observed on some areas of the peritoneal surface (**g**). Both fibrin (**h**) and podoplanin (**i**) were no longer detected in this phase. NFM staging was determined by the detection of fibrin and podoplanin by Masson trichrome staining or immunohistochemistry (**j**). All figures are ×200 and bars = 100 μm

the earlier stages (stages I and II). The mesothelial lining of the peritoneal surface was occasionally seen in later stages (stages II and III), but usually not in stage I.

NFMs were observed in non-EPS patients

NFMs were frequently observed in EPS patients and considered necessary for a diagnosis of EPS. However, NFMs were also identified microscopically in peritoneal samples of non-EPS patients, especially those with peritoneal lavage after PD discontinuation (Fig. 3). The NFM was usually identified histologically as a thin membrane on the peritoneal membrane proper and distinguished from the peritoneum proper by the presence of exudative features, swollen fibroblast-like cells, and absence of the expected vascular structure of arteries and veins present in the peritoneum proper (Fig. 3a, c, e). The detection of a layer of elastic fibers by Masson trichrome staining was helpful to distinguish the peritoneum proper from the new membrane because elastic

fibers occur in the submesothelial zone of the peritoneal membrane but not in the NFM (Fig. 1a). Podoplanin immunostaining was also helpful to confirm the NFM because its expression in fibroblast-like cells was a characteristic finding in the NFM (Fig. 3b, d).

Comparison of clinical and histological findings in EPS and non-EPS with or without peritoneal lavage

All patients in the three groups were treated with conventional acidic PD solutions (Table 2). The non-EPS patients without lavage were younger (44.1 ± 17.5 years of age) than both the EPS patients (56.7 ± 5.7 years old) and the non-EPS patients with lavage (58.5 ± 9.5 years old). The PD duration was longer in the EPS patients (124.5 ± 34.2 months) than in both the non-EPS patients with lavage (94.8 ± 33.7 months) and in those without lavage (91.4 ± 30.3 months). Peritoneal lavage was performed in three of the EPS patients to prevent peritoneal adhesions before peritoneal dissecting surgery.

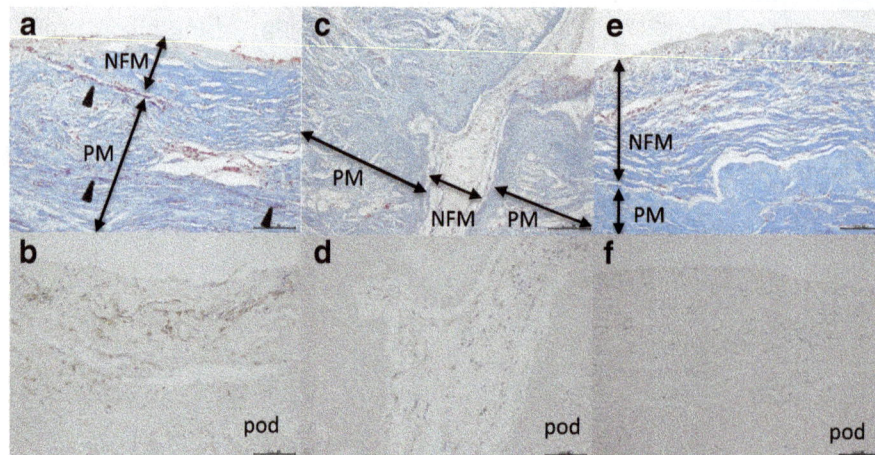

NFM: newly-formed membrane, PM: proper membrane

Fig. 3 Histological findings of NFMs in non-EPS patients. NFMs were observed microscopically in the peritoneal biopsies of non-EPS patients with peritoneal lavage treatment after completing PD. NFMs were attached to the peritoneal membrane proper and distinguished from the peritoneal membrane (PM) by the presence of exudative or fibrous features (**a**, **c**, **e**). The presence of an elastic fiber layer detected by elastic-Masson trichrome staining was helpful to distinguish the NFM from the PM because the elastic fiber layer was located in the upper part of PM but not in the NFM (**a**). Podoplanin immunostaining was helpful to identify the NFM and determine its histological stage. Podoplanin expression in fibroblast-like cells is characteristic of the NFM (**b**, **d**). Negative podoplanin expression in fibroblast-like cells indicates stage III NFM (scarring phase) (**e**, **f**). Absence of the original vascular structure including artery and vein complexes is another index of NFM (**a**, **c**, **e**). NFMs in non-EPS patients shifted to later histological stages: stage II (seven cases) and stage III (seven cases), compared with NFMs in EPS patients: stage I (five cases), stage II (two cases), and stage III (one case). **a** Elastic-Masson staining, ×200. **c**, **e** Masson staining, ×200. **b**, **d**, **f** IHC for podoplanin, ×200, bar = 100 μm

The category data of peritoneal equilibration test (PET) was available in 30 of non-EPS patients (16 with lavage and 14 without lavage), suggesting no difference between patients with and without peritoneal lavage.

Histological evaluation of the background peritoneum revealed that the average thickness of the SMC in EPS patients (636.2 ± 409.4 μm) and in the non-EPS patients with lavage (603.8 ± 386.6 μm) was greater than in non-EPS patients without lavage (336.0 ± 116.3 μm). It also

Table 2 Clinical and pathological characteristics of EPS patients (n = 10), non-EPS patients with lavage (n = 30), and non-EPS patients without lavage (n = 22)

	EPS patients (n = 10)	Non-EPS patients with lavage (n = 30)	Non-EPS patients without lavage (n = 22)	p value
Age	56.7 ± 5.7‡	58.5 ± 9.5*	44.1 ± 17.5*‡	<0.0041* <0.011‡ <0.0001 (KW)
Gender	M5/F5	M19/F11	M13/F9	NS (X2 test)
PD duration (m)	124.5 ± 34.2*‡	94.8 ± 33.7*	91.4 ± 30.3‡	<0.031* <0.021‡ <0.0001 (KW)
Lavage (%)	3/10 (30%)	30/30 (100%)	0/22 (0%)	ND
PET category: H/HA/LA/L	ND	4/7/4/1	4/5/5/0	NS (X2 test)
Average thickness of SMC (μm)	636.2 ± 409.4‡	603.8 ± 386.6*	336.0 ± 116.3*‡	<0.0031* <0.05‡ 0.063 (KW)
Average L/V ratio	0.33 ± 0.22‡	0.39 ± 0.20*	0.53 ± 0.24*‡	<0.028* <0.031‡ 0.048 (KW)
Prevalence of NFM	8/10 (80%)	13/30 (43.3%)	1/22(4.5%)	<0.0001 (X2 test)
Stage of NFMs (I/II/III)	5/2/1	0/6/7	0/1/0	ND

Mean ± sd

PET peritoneal equilibration test, H high, HA high average, LA low average, L low, SMC submesothelial compact zone, L/V lumen/vessel diameter, NFM newly formed membrane, NS not significant, ND not done, KW Kruskal–Wallis

revealed that the average L/V in EPS patients (0.33 ± 0.22) was smaller than that of the non-EPS patients without lavage (0.53 ± 0.24). The average L/V in the non-EPS patients with lavage (0.39 ± 0.20) was also smaller than that of the non-EPS patients without lavage. The decreased occurrence of peritoneal sclerosis in non-EPS patients without lavage might be explained by either treatment selection bias associated with peritoneal lavage after PD discontinuation or the younger age of that group. The frequency of NFM detection was significantly higher in EPS patients (8/10, 80%) than that in non-EPS patients with lavage (13/30, 43.3%) and those without lavage (1/22, 4.5%). The histological stages of NFM were predominantly earlier in EPS patients: stage I in five cases (62.5%), stage II in two cases (25%), and stage III in one case (12.5%), and shifted to later stages in non-EPS patients: stage II and stage III in seven cases each (50%) (Table 2). The comparison of the clinical and pathological characteristics of EPS patients (n = 10) and non-EPS patients (n = 52) was shown in Additional file 1: Table S1. The correlations between peritoneal sclerosis and PD duration in the three groups were represented in Additional file 1: Figure S1.

Clinical and histological significance of new membrane formation in peritoneal biopsy tissue

To investigate the clinical and histological significance of new membrane formation, we compared the biopsy data of cases with NFM (n = 13) and those without NFM (n = 17) in non-EPS patients with peritoneal lavage (Table 3). There were no significant differences of age, gender, PD duration, or post-PD duration (i.e., lavage duration) in the two groups. The PET category tended to be in high (H) and high average (HA) in the patients with NFM, whereas shifted to be in low average (LA) and low (L) in those

without NFM, but the difference did not reach significance. Histologically, the average SMC thickness and L/V ratio were not significantly different in the two groups; the L/V ratio in patients with NFM was lower than that in patients without new membranes (0.33 ± 0.12 vs. 0.43 ± 0.24, p = 0.16) but the difference did not reach significance. The clinical and histological relevance of histological staging of NFMs in EPS patients (n = 8) and in all patients with NFMs in the three groups (n = 22) was shown in Additional file 1: Tables S2 and S3, respectively.

Discussion
Definition of NFM and its histological features

Encapsulation in EPS is caused by an NFM on the peritoneal membrane proper, which can be distinguished by careful macroscopic and microscopic observation. Surgeon can usually identify the NFM by peeling it away from the intestinal serosa during enterolysis surgery. Laparoscopic observation can also confirm the NFM by its unique cocoon-like appearance over the gastroenteric organs. The histological appearance of NFMs resembles to that of fibrotic regions of simple peritoneal sclerosis; however, the NFM can be distinguished by the absence of large vessels, nerves, and adipose tissue that are usually observed in the peritoneum proper.

Various histological features and the stages of NFMs are suggestive of the initiation and progression of EPS. At early stages, NFMs are primarily composed of exudative fibrin, suggesting that the exudation of plasma containing fibrin/fibrinogen and other blood coagulation factors is required for encapsulating membrane formation [17]. The cocoon-like encapsulating membrane recognized macroscopically during the enterolysis surgery is usually characterized histologically by exudative fibrin and its organization and consistent with NFM in stage I. Increased permeability of the peritoneal membrane, a very common complication of long-term PD [18–20], may be an important background factor for the pathogenesis of EPS. Increased peritoneal vascularity is thought to be associated with the peritoneal hyperpermeability observed in the previous histological studies of PD peritoneum [21–23]. Recently, Tawada et al. reported that damage to vascular endothelium, represented by hyalinizing vasculopathy of the peritoneal membrane, was predictive of the development of EPS and suggested that peritoneal hyperpermeability could result from vascular endothelial injury [24]. Morelle et al. demonstrated that an early, relatively large reduction in osmotic conductance (sodium sieving) during PD was an independent predictor of EPS and that such functional disorders were associated with the extent of peritoneal fibrosis, but not with vasculopathy [25]. Although the precise mechanism of peritoneal hyperpermeability in long-term PD patients is still controversial, disturbance of peritoneal membrane transport across the peritoneal microvasculature has a significant role in the pathogenesis of EPS.

Table 3 Clinical and histological significance of new membrane formation in peritoneal biopsies obtained at catheter removal in non-EPS patients with lavage (n = 30)

	Non-EPS patients with NFM (n = 13)	Non-EPS patients without NFM (n = 17)	p value
Age	58.2 ± 11.1	58.7 ± 9.2	NS
Gender	M9/F4	M10/F7	NS
PD duration (m)	91.9 ± 18.8	97.6 ± 37.5	NS
Post-PD duration (m)	12.6 ± 5.2	12.9 ± 5.4	NS
PET category: H/HA/LA/L	4/3/1/0	0/4/3/1	NS (0.16)
Average thickness of SMC (μm)	560.8 ± 315.5	636.1 ± 475.3	NS
Average L/V ratio	0.33 ± 0.12	0.43 ± 0.24	NS (0.16)
Stage of NFM (I/II/III)	0/6/7	0/0/0	ND

Mean ± sd

PET peritoneal equilibration test, *H* high, *HA* high average, *LA* low average, *L* low, *SMC* submesothelial compact zone, *L/V* lumen/vessel diameter, *NFM* newly formed membrane, *NS* not significant, *ND* not done

This study also identified differences in the histological stages of NFM in different clinical situations. Early stages of NFM were frequently observed in EPS patients who experienced enterolysis surgery. On the other hand, later stages of NFM were seen in non-EPS patients with peritoneal lavage after completing PD. This difference could be associated with temporal phase of inflammatory process, showing active peritoneal injury in EPS patients with enterolysis surgery and chronic subsiding peritoneal damage in non-EPS patients with peritoneal lavage for several months after completion of PD. Therefore, the fresh fibrin deposition in histological stage I may be a possible diagnostic criterion for EPS in acute/active phase and it may disappear in chronic/subsiding phase. The predominance of early stages in EPS patients might be associated with a bias of biopsy sampling from visceral peritoneum. There may be some pathophysiological differences between visceral and parietal peritoneum, although they have not been fully established so far. Yaginuma et al. demonstrated increased lymphatic vessels in visceral peritoneum rather than parietal peritoneum [26], and this difference might be related to the susceptibility of encapsulating membrane formation in visceral peritoneum via increased exudation. The histological stage may also indicate the consequences of NFMs, that is progression to encapsulation and adhesion or scar formation without the development of EPS.

Significance of podoplanin expression in new membranes

This study confirmed the utility of podoplanin staining in the pathological diagnosis and staging of EPS. Braun et al. first reported that the presence podoplanin-positive fibroblast-like cells was a good marker of EPS [11, 12]. Podoplanin was first described as a molecule expressed on glomerular podocytes [27] and was later was found to be a useful marker of lymphatic endothelial [28] and mesothelial cells [29]. Recent investigations revealed that podoplanin is a transmembranous glycoprotein whose ligand is C-type lectin receptor-2 (CLEC-2) on platelets and inflammatory cells [30]. This protein is involved in cell motility, migration, and proliferation during development, in the immune system, and in cancer [31]. Because EPS develops in association with increased accumulation of serum and high concentrations of fibrin [17, 32], secretion of cytokines and growth factors [26, 33–35] may activate the transformation of peritoneal mesenchymal cells into swollen fibroblast-like cells that highly express podoplanin on their cell membranes. Podoplanin-positive fibroblast-like cells in the peritoneum of EPS patients may be activated by platelets and inflammatory cells expressing podoplanin-ligand, CLEC-2 [30], and by the surrounding extracellular matrix containing hyaluronic acid [31]. Thus, podoplanin expression may be associated with the disease activity or the histological stage of EPS.

NFMs were detected in non-EPS patients

To evaluate the diagnostic specificity of the NFM in EPS, we investigated the prevalence of NFM in the peritoneal biopsy specimens obtained from EPS patients at enterolysis surgery and in non-EPS patients at catheter removal. NFMs were detected in most of the EPS patients (8/10 cases, 80%), and although biopsies were not efficient for the detection of NFM in the other two patients, NFMs encapsulating the intestines had been macroscopically confirmed during enterolysis surgery. Therefore, it is reasonable to conclude that the detection of NFM, either macroscopically or microscopically, is required for a pathological diagnosis of EPS. On the other hand, NFMs were also detected microscopically in non-EPS patients (14/52 cases, 26.9%) suggesting that microscopic NFMs could not predict the development of EPS and was not a sufficient condition for the diagnosis of EPS. A similar result has been previously reported in a study by Sherif et al. comparing the peritoneal pathology of EPS and non-EPS patients, in which NFMs were observed in 6/23 non-EPS patients (26.1%) [8]. In an evaluation of new membrane formation in peritoneal biopsies at catheter removal, Tawada et al. also observed the presence of NFMs in non-EPS patients and found increased histological scores of NFMs in EPS patients, but the difference in comparison with non-EPS patients did not reach significance [24]. Because new membrane formation is a result of increased exudation on the peritoneal surface, the detection of NFM suggests the increased permeability of the peritoneal vessels. The increased incidence of NFMs in the peritoneal lavage group suggested that new membrane formation occurred primarily during the period of lavage after completion of PD. Nevertheless, the detection of NFMs did not predict the subsequent development of EPS in this study, indicating that microscopically detected NFMs probably regressed and did not progress to encapsulation of abdominal organs.

Role of peritoneal sclerosis in new membrane formation

We also evaluated pathological differences of the background peritoneum in EPS patients and non-EPS patients. The results indicated a tendency for an advanced grade of peritoneal vasculopathy in the EPS patients. These observations support previous observations that prolonged PD duration was the most important risk factor for EPS [18, 36–38] and that histological damage of the peritoneum is closely associated with high peritoneal transport, which is another risk factor for EPS [19, 20]. Increased microvascular density of the background peritoneum proper is thought to be associated with hyperpermeability of the peritoneal membrane and to promote EPS development [21–23]. However, we observed no significant difference of microvascular density in the peritoneum proper in EPS patients and non-EPS patients (data not shown). Further investigation is required to elucidate the functional and morphological relationships of microvascular density and peritoneal hyperpermeability in the pathogenesis of EPS.

Vascular density may not necessarily be associated with increased peritoneal permeability and subsequent formation of encapsulating membranes. The nonphysiological state of the vascular barrier, an endothelial layer of the peritoneal capillary, may be associated with impaired peritoneal barrier function observed with long-term PD treatment [39–41]. Functional deterioration of peritoneal microvascular permeability induced by PD, rather than morphological damages, might be associated with the onset of EPS and should be considered for understanding the pathogenesis of EPS.

Effect of neutral, low glucose degradation product (GDP) dialysate on peritoneal sclerosis, and EPS

Since biocompatible PD solutions with neutral pH and low GDP have become available, the incidence and extent of PD-induced peritoneal deterioration, characterized as simple peritoneal sclerosis, has decreased [42–44]. As simple peritoneal sclerosis is the most important risk factor for EPS, the incidence of EPS is expected to decrease. A recent report has shown a decrease in EPS incidence (1.0%) in Japan [45]. This tendency suggests that the use of biocompatible PD solution is the most effective, and indispensable, strategy for the prevention of EPS. The merits of biocompatible PD solutions are probably attributable to its low GDP concentration, which is the component with the highest toxicity for cellular and extracellular matrix components such as collagen fibers [46]. Peritoneal permeability is primarily determined by the capillary endothelium [41]. Preservation of the physiological integrity of peritoneal tissue contributes to vascular integrity and prevents increased permeability of the peritoneal membrane, a key factor in encapsulating membrane formation.

Limitations of the present study

Some limitations must be considered when interpreting the study results. First, this was a multicenter retrospective observational study, and not all the patients with PD withdrawal were included, thus there must be a selection bias in each cohort. Second, the clinical information was limited, and many factors like the daily ultrafiltration volume, the peritoneal equilibration test, the amount of glucose exposure, and the method of peritoneal lavage could not be evaluated. Third, the number of patients in each group limited the power of the statistical comparisons. Fourth, the long-term follow-up was not available to determine the clinical outcome, such as the development of EPS. Fifth, the method of peritoneal biopsy was not standardized, so the quality and quantity of the biopsy samples were not always adequate for histological evaluation. Sixth, there was a sampling bias of biopsy materials, which were taken from visceral peritoneum in most of the EPS patients (8/10) and from parietal in all of the non-EPS patients ($n = 52$). It might have some

influences on the staging of NFMs and predominance of stage I in the EPS patients. The above limitations may be associated with some inconclusive results. Nevertheless, the study reports important evidence of the appearance of NFM in peritoneal biopsy samples from both EPS patients and non-EPS patients.

Conclusions

The pathological diagnosis of EPS requires confirmation of NFM, either macroscopically or microscopically, which is a strong pathological hallmark of EPS. However, NFMs were detected microscopically in non-EPS patients, especially those with peritoneal lavage after completion of PD discontinuation. New membrane formation, which is believed to be an early pathological phenomenon of EPS, reflects increased exudation from peritoneal vasculature, associated with the initiation of, but does not always predict, the development of EPS.

Additional file

Additional file 1: Table S1. Clinical and pathological characteristics of EPS patients ($n = 10$) and non-EPS patients ($n = 52$). To identify the factors associated with the development of EPS, we compared the demographic and clinical characteristics EPS patients ($n = 10$) and non-EPS patients ($n = 52$) but could not find any differences except the prevalence of microscopic NFM; more frequent in EPS patients than in non-EPS patients (80% vs. 36.9%, $p < 0.0026$). **Table S2.** Clinical and histological relevance of histological staging of NFMs in EPS patients ($n = 8$). To evaluate the clinical and histological relevance of histological grading of NFM in the eight EPS patients with NFM, we compared the clinical and histological findings in the three groups stratified by NFM stage. No significant associations were found between the histological stages of NFM and the clinical and histological findings. **Table S3.** Clinical and histological relevance of histological staging in 22 patients with NFMs; EPS ($n = 8$) and non-EPS ($n = 14$) patients. To evaluate the clinical and histological relevance of histological grading of NFM, we compared the clinical and histological findings in the 22 patients with NFM in the three groups stratified by NFM stage. No significant associations were found between the histological stages of NFM and the clinical and histological findings. **Figure S1.** Degree of peritoneal sclerosis in the background peritoneum in EPS patients and non-EPS patients with or without peritoneal lavage. The SMC thickness and L/V ratio are plotted against PD duration. In EPS patients, there was no significant correlation of peritoneal sclerosis (SMC thickness and L/V ratio) and PD duration (1-a, -4-d). On the other hand, a weak correlation was observed between peritoneal sclerosis and PD duration in non-EPS patients (1-b, c, e, and f). The correlation seemed to be evident in non-EPS patients without lavage. SMC: submesothelial compact zone, L/V: lumen/vessel ratio, PD: peritoneal dialysis, M: month.

Abbreviations

EPS: Encapsulating peritoneal sclerosis; L/V ratio: Lumen/vessel ratio; NFM: Newly formed membrane; PCV: Post-capillary venule; PD: Peritoneal dialysis; SMC: Submesothelial compact zone

Acknowledgements

The authors would like to express their special thanks to Dr. Hiroshi Hirano for his significant contribution to the Peritoneal Biopsy Program in Japan. The authors also thank all the clinical physicians who participated in this program. The authors would like to thank Enago (www.enago.com) for the English language review.

Funding

The Peritoneal Biopsy Program in Japan conducted from 1994 to 2006 was financially supported by Baxter Japan Co. Ltd. The funder had no role in this study design, data collection and analysis, decision to publish, or preparation of the manuscript.

Authors' contributions

KH and KK performed the histological examination of peritoneal biopsy tissue and analyzed and interpreted the clinical and histological data. CH and MN analyzed and interpreted the clinical and histological data. MM and YI contributed to interpretation of the data and writing of the manuscript. JSPD organized the Peritoneal Pathology Study Committee and supported the activity. All authors read and approved the final manuscript.

Competing interests

The authors, except YI, declare that they have no competing interests regarding this article. YI is a professor in endowed chair supported by Baxter Japan Co. Ltd.

Author details

[1]Department of Anatomy, Showa University School of Medicine, 1-5-8 Hatanodai, Shinagawa-ku, Tokyo 142-8555, Japan. [2]Division of Nephrology, Juntendo Medical University Faculty of Medicine, 2-1-1 Hongo, Bunkyo-ku, Tokyo 113-8421, Japan. [3]Department of Surgical Pathology, Tokyo Women's Medical University, 8-1 Kawada-cho, Shinjuku-ku, Tokyo 162-8666, Japan. [4]Research Division of Chronic Kidney Disease and Dialysis Treatment, Tohoku University Hospital, 1-1 Seiryo-cho, Aoba-ku, Sendai-shi, Miyagi 980-0872, Japan. [5]Miyazaki Clinic, 3-12 Shiratori-cho, Nagasaki-shi, Nagasaki 852-8042, Japan. [6]Department of Nephrology and Renal Replacement Therapy, Nagoya University Graduate School of Medicine, 65 Tsurumai-cho, Showa-ku, Nagoya 466-8550, Japan. [7]Japanese Society of Peritoneal Dialysis (JSPD), 1-39 Kitasakoichiban-cho, Tokushima-shi, Tokushima 770-0011, Japan.

References

1.   Gandhi VC, Humayun HM, Ing TS, Daugirdas JT, Jablokow VR, Iwatsuki S, Geis WP, Hano JE. Sclerotic thickening of the peritoneal membrane in maintenance peritoneal dialysis patients. Arch Intern Med. 1980;140:1201–3.
2.   Dobbie JW. Pathogenesis of peritoneal fibrosing syndromes (sclerosing peritonitis) in peritoneal dialysis. Perit Dial Int. 1992;12:14–27.
3.   Nomoto Y, Kawaguchi Y, Kubo H, Hirano H, Sakai S, Kurokawa K. Sclerosing encapsulating peritonitis in patients undergoing continuous ambulatory peritoneal dialysis: a report of the Japanese Sclerosing Encapsulating Peritonitis Study Group. Am J Kidney Dis. 1996;28:420–7.
4.   Kawaguchi Y, Kawanishi H, Mujais S, Topley N, Oreopoulos DG. Encapsulating peritoneal sclerosis: definition, etiology, diagnosis, and treatment. International Society for Peritoneal Dialysis Ad Hoc Committee on Ultrafiltration Management in Peritoneal Dialysis. Perit Dial Int. 2000;20 (Suppl 4):S43–55.
5.   Kawaguchi Y, Saito A, Kawanishi H, Nakayama M, Miyazaki M, Nakamoto H, Tranaeus A. Recommendations on the management of encapsulating peritoneal sclerosis in Japan, 2005: diagnosis, predictive markers, treatment, and preventive measures. Perit Dial Int. 2005;25 (Suppl 4):S83–95.
6.   Honda K, Oda H. Pathology of encapsulating peritoneal sclerosis. Perit Dial Int. 2005;25 (Suppl 4):S19–29.
7.   Honda K, Nitta K, Horita S, Tsukada M, Itabashi M, Nihei H, Akiba T, Oda H. Histologic criteria for diagnosing encapsulating peritoneal sclerosis in continuous ambulatory peritoneal dialysis patients. Adv Perit Dial. 2003;19: 169–75.
8.   Sherif AM, Yoshida H, Maruyama Y, Yamamoto H, Yokoyama K, Hosoya T, Kawakami M, Nakayama M. Comparison between the pathology of encapsulating sclerosis and simple sclerosis of the peritoneal membrane in chronic peritoneal dialysis. Ther Apher Dial. 2008;12:33–41.
9.   Braun N, Fritz P, Ulmer C, Latus J, Kimmel M, Biegger D, Ott G, Reimold F, Thon KP, Dippon J, Segerer S, Alscher MD. Histological criteria for encapsulating peritoneal sclerosis—a standardized approach. PLoS ONE. 2012;7:e48647.
10. Latus J, Ulmer C, Fritz P, Rettenmaier B, Biegger D, Lang T, Ott G, Kimmel M, Steurer W, Alscher MD, Segerer S, Braun N. Phenotypes of encapsulating peritoneal sclerosis—macroscopic appearance, histologic findings, and outcome. Perit Dial Int. 2013;33:495–502.
11. Braun N, Alscher DM, Fritz P, Edenhofer I, Kimmel M, Gaspert A, Reimold F, Bode-Lesniewska B, Ziegler U, Biegger D, Wüthrich RP, Segerer S. Podoplanin-positive cells are a hallmark of encapsulating peritoneal sclerosis. Nephrol Dial Transplant. 2011;26:1033–41.
12. Braun N, Alscher MD, Fritz P, Latus J, Edenhofer I, Reimold F, Alper SL, Kimmel M, Biegger D, Lindenmeyer M, Cohen CD, Wüthrich RP, Segerer S. The spectrum of podoplanin expression in encapsulating peritoneal sclerosis. PLoS ONE. 2012;7:e53382.
13. Yamamoto T, Nagasue K, Okuno S, Yamakawa T. The role of peritoneal lavage and the prognostic significance of mesothelial cell area in preventing encapsulating peritoneal sclerosis. Perit Dial Int. 2010;30:343–52.
14. Ubara Y, Tagami T, Hara S. Successful peritoneal lavage therapy for prevention of encapsulating peritoneal sclerosis: a case report. Ther Apher Dial. 2011;15:211–3.
15. Brown EA, Van Biesen W, Finkelstein FO, Hurst H, Johnson DW, Kawanishi H, Pecoits-Filho R, Woodrow G, ISPD Working Party. Length of time on peritoneal dialysis and encapsulating peritoneal sclerosis: position paper for ISPD. Perit Dial Int. 2009;29:595–600.
16. Honda K, Hamada C, Nakayama M, Miyazaki M, Sherif AM, Harada T, Hirano H, Peritoneal Biopsy Study Group of the Japanese Society for Peritoneal Dialysis. Impact of uremia, diabetes, and peritoneal dialysis itself on the pathogenesis of peritoneal sclerosis: a quantitative study of peritoneal membrane morphology. Clin J Am Soc Nephrol. 2008;3:720–8.
17. Dobbie JW, Jasani MK. Role of imbalance of intracavity fibrin formation and removal in the pathogenesis of peritoneal lesions in CAPD. Perit Dial Int. 1997;17:121–4.
18. Yamamoto R, Otsuka Y, Nakayama M, Maruyama Y, Katoh N, Ikeda M, Yamamoto H, Yokoyama K, Kawaguchi Y, Matsushima M. Risk factors for encapsulating peritoneal sclerosis in patients who have experienced peritoneal dialysis treatment. Clin Exp Nephrol. 2005;9:148–52.
19. Habib AM, Preston E, Davenport A. Risk factors for developing encapsulating peritoneal sclerosis in the icodextrin era of peritoneal dialysis prescription. Nephrol Dial Transplant. 2010;25:1633–8.
20. Lambie ML, John B, Mushahar L, Huckvale C, Davies SJ. The peritoneal osmotic conductance is low well before the diagnosis of encapsulating peritoneal sclerosis is made. Kidney Int. 2010;78:611–8.
21. Mateijsen MA, van der Wal AC, Hendriks PM, Zweers MM, Mulder J, Struijk DG, Krediet RT. Vascular and interstitial changes in the peritoneum of CAPD patients with peritoneal sclerosis. Perit Dial Int. 1999;19:517–25.
22. Numata M, Nakayama M, Nimura S, Kawakami M, Lindholm B, Kawaguchi Y. Association between an increased surface area of peritoneal microvessels and a high peritoneal solute transport rate. Perit Dial Int. 2003;23:116–22.
23. Sherif AM, Nakayama M, Maruyama Y, Yoshida H, Yamamoto H, Yokoyama K, Kawakami M. Quantitative assessment of the peritoneal vessel density and vasculopathy in CAPD patients. Nephrol Dial Transplant. 2006;21:1675–81.
24. Tawada M, Ito Y, Hamada C, Honda K, Mizuno M, Suzuki Y, Sakata F, Terabayashi T, Matsukawa Y, Maruyama S, Imai E, Matsuo S, Takei Y. Vascular endothelial cell injury is an important factor in the development of encapsulating peritoneal sclerosis in long-term peritoneal dialysis patients. PLoS ONE. 2016;11:e0154644.
25. Morelle J, Sow A, Hautem N, Bouzin C, Crott R, Devuyst O, Goffin E. Interstitial fibrosis restricts osmotic water transport in encapsulating peritoneal sclerosis. J Am Soc Nephrol. 2015;26:2521–33.

26. Yaginuma T, Yamamoto I, Yamamoto H, Mitome J, Tanno Y, Yokoyama K, Hayashi T, Kobayashi T, Watanabe M, Yamaguchi Y, Hosoya T. Increased lymphatic vessels in patients with encapsulating peritoneal sclerosis. Perit Dial Int. 2012;32:617–27.

27. Breiteneder-Geleff S, Matsui K, Soleiman A, Meraner P, Poczewski H, Kalt R, Schaffner G, Kerjaschki D. Podoplanin, novel 43-kd membrane protein of glomerular epithelial cells, is down-regulated in puromycin nephrosis. Am J Pathol. 1997;151:1141–52.

28. Wetterwald A, Hoffstetter W, Cecchini MG, Lanske B, Wagner C, Fleisch H, Atkinson M. Characterization and cloning of the E11 antigen, a marker expressed by rat osteoblasts and osteocytes. Bone. 1996;18:125–32.

29. Kimura N, Kimura I. Podoplanin as a marker for mesothelioma. Pathol Int. 2005;55:83–6.

30. Suzuki-Inoue K, Kato Y, Inoue O, Kaneko MK, Mishima K, Yatomi Y, Yamazaki Y, Narimatsu H, Ozaki Y. Involvement of the snake toxin receptor CLEC-2, in podoplanin-mediated platelet activation, by cancer cells. J Biol Chem. 2007; 282:25993–6001.

31. Astarita JL, Acton SE, Turley SJ. Podoplanin: emerging functions in development, the immune system, and cancer. Front Immunol. 2012;3:283.

32. Fang CC, Huang JW, Shyu RS, Yen CJ, Shiao CH, Chiang CK, Hu RH, Tsai TJ. Fibrin-Induced epithelial-to-mesenchymal transition of peritoneal mesothelial cells as a mechanism of peritoneal fibrosis: effects of pentoxifylline. PLoS ONE. 2012;7:e44765.

33. Patel P, West-Mays J, Kolb M, Rodrigues JC, Hoff CM, Margetts PJ. Platelet derived growth factor B and epithelial mesenchymal transition of peritoneal mesothelial cells. Matrix Biol. 2010;29:97–106.

34. Pérez-Lozano ML, Sandoval P, Rynne-Vidal A, Aguilera A, Jiménez-Heffernan JA, Albar-Vizcaíno P, Majano PL, Sánchez-Tomero JA, Selgas R, López-Cabrera M. Functional relevance of the switch of VEGF receptors/co-receptors during peritoneal dialysis-induced mesothelial to mesenchymal transition. PLoS ONE. 2013;8:e60776.

35. Kinashi H, Ito Y, Mizuno M, Suzuki Y, Terabayashi T, Nagura F, Hattori R, Matsukawa Y, Mizuno T, Noda Y, Nishimura H, Nishio R, Maruyama S, Imai E, Matsuo S, Takei Y. TGF-β1 promotes lymphangiogenesis during peritoneal fibrosis. J Am Soc Nephrol. 2013;24:1627–42.

36. Kawanishi H, Kawaguchi Y, Fukui H, Hara S, Imada A, Kubo H, et al. Encapsulating peritoneal sclerosis in Japan: a prospective, controlled, multicenter study. Am J Kidney Dis. 2004;44:729–37.

37. Brown MC, Simpson K, Kerssens JJ, Mactier RA, Scottish Renal Registry. Encapsulating peritoneal sclerosis in the new millennium: a national cohort study. Clin J Am Soc Nephrol. 2009;4:1222–9.

38. Johnson DW, Cho Y, Livingston BE, Hawley CM, McDonald SP, Brown FG, Rosman JB, Bannister KM, Wiggins KJ. Encapsulating peritoneal sclerosis: incidence, predictors, and outcomes. Kidney Int. 2010;77:904–12.

39. Davies SJ. Peritoneal solute transport—we know it is important, but what is it? Nephrol Dial Transplant. 2000;15:1120–3.

40. Flessner MF. Endothelial glycocalyx and the peritoneal barrier. Perit Dial Int. 2008;28:6–12.

41. Rippe B, Davies S. Permeability of peritoneal and glomerular capillaries: what are the differences according to pore theory? Perit Dial Int. 2011;31:249–58.

42. Ayuzawa N, Ishibashi Y, Takazawa Y, Kume H, Fujita T. Peritoneal morphology after long-term peritoneal dialysis with biocompatible fluid: recent clinical practice in Japan. Perit Dial Int. 2012;32:159–67.

43. Kawanishi K, Honda K, Tsukada M, Oda H, Nitta K. Neutral solution low in glucose degradation products is associated with less peritoneal fibrosis and vascular sclerosis in patients receiving peritoneal dialysis. Perit Dial Int. 2013; 33:242–51.

44. Hamada C, Honda K, Kawanishi K, Nakamoto H, Ito Y, Sakurada T, Tanno Y, Mizumasa T, Miyazaki M, Moriishi M, Nakayama M. Morphological characteristics in peritoneum in patients with neutral peritoneal dialysis solution. J Artif Organs. 2015;18:243–50.

45. Nakayama M, Miyazaki M, Honda K, Kasai K, Tomo T, Nakamoto H, Kawanishi H. Encapsulating peritoneal sclerosis in the era of a multi-disciplinary approach based on biocompatible solutions: the NEXT-PD study. Perit Dial Int. 2014;34:766–74.

46. Cho Y, Johnson DW, Badve SV, Craig JC, Strippoli GF, Wiggins KJ. The impact of neutral-pH peritoneal dialysates with reduced glucose degradation products on clinical outcomes in peritoneal dialysis patients. Kidney Int. 2013;84:969–79.

18

Is hemodialysis itself a risk factor for dementia? An analysis of nationwide registry data of patients on maintenance hemodialysis

Shigeru Nakai[1]*[iD], Kenji Wakai[2], Eiichiro Kanda[3], Kazunori Kawaguchi[1], Kazuyoshi Sakai[1] and Nobuya Kitaguchi[1]

Abstract

Background: Chronic kidney disease is a major risk factor for dementia, but the influence of hemodialysis itself on the development of dementia remains unclear. We previously reported that non-diabetic patients on maintenance hemodialysis have preserved cognitive function; hemodialysis removes blood amyloid β (Aβ), which is a major cause of Alzheimer's disease in the brain; and the number of Aβ deposits in the postmortem brains of hemodialysis patients was significantly less compared to that in age-matched controls not undergoing hemodialysis. We aimed to evaluate the influence of hemodialysis on the development of dementia.

Methods: We accessed the Japanese Society for Dialysis Therapy Renal Data Registry between December 31, 2009, and December 31, 2010. Dementia was identified in 120,101 patients undergoing maintenance hemodialysis. The association between hemodialysis duration and dementia risk was analyzed using logistic regression analysis.

Results: There was a significant decrease in the dementia risk with an increase in the hemodialysis duration, with odds ratios (95% confidence intervals) of 0.78 (0.74–0.82) and 0.88 (0.78–0.99) for every 10 years in non-diabetic and diabetic patients, respectively. However, in diabetic patients, the correlation between hemodialysis duration and dementia risk was not consistent.

Conclusion: A longer hemodialysis duration was correlated with a lower dementia risk, but the correlation between hemodialysis duration and dementia risk in diabetic patients was much weaker and vaguer than that in non-diabetic patients. This finding does not appear to contradict greatly the assumption that the reduction in dementia risk with a prolonged hemodialysis duration in non-diabetic patients was caused not only by the survivor effect but also by hemodialysis itself.

Keywords: Dementia, Dialysis, Epidemiology, Hemodialysis duration, Amyloid β

Background

Chronic kidney disease (CKD) is a major risk factor for dementia [1, 2]. Fukunishi et al. [3] reported that the annual incidence rate of dementia among elderly patients was 7.4 times higher in those on hemodialysis than in those from the general population. Lin et al. [4] showed that there is no significant difference in dementia risk between patients undergoing hemodialysis and those undergoing peritoneal dialysis. However, the influence of long-term hemodialysis itself on the development of dementia remains unclear.

Alzheimer's disease (AD) is a major cause of dementia [5], and the accumulation of amyloid β (Aβ) protein in the brain in this condition was thought to cause cognitive impairment [6]. Moreover, the metabolic degradation of Aβ and its clearance from the brain are impaired in patients with AD [7]. If Aβ clearance from the brain can be increased, it is considered that AD could be prevented or even treated. To this end, treatment with antibodies

* Correspondence: s-nakai@fujita-hu.ac.jp
[1]Faculty of Clinical Engineering Technology, Fujita Health University School of Health Sciences, Dengakugakubo 1-98, Kutsukake-cho, Toyoake, Aichi 470-1192, Japan
Full list of author information is available at the end of the article

against Aβ has been shown to result in cognitive improvement and reduced Aβ burden in the brain among patients with AD [8]. Furthermore, in a current human clinical trial, patients with AD are being treated with peripheral administration of albumin, which is an Aβ-binding substance, and this phase 2 trial already has reported improved cognitive function in patients with AD [9]. Kato et al. [10] showed that hemodialysis removes Aβ, and Kitaguchi et al. [11] showed that cognitive function was maintained or improved in most patients undergoing maintenance non-diabetic hemodialysis over a period of 18 to 36 months. Sakai et al. [12] reported that the deposition of Aβ in postmortem brain tissue was decreased significantly in patients who had undergone hemodialysis compared to that in age-matched patients who had not undergone hemodialysis. Reusche et al. [13] reported similar results. These reports suggest that hemodialysis itself may prevent development of AD through removal of Aβ from the blood.

The Japanese Society for Dialysis Therapy (JSDT) has been conducting epidemiologic studies in dialysis facilities throughout Japan since 1968. Since 1983, more than 700,000 patients have been registered in an electronic database, including those who have died (JSDT Renal Data Registry [JRDR]) [14]. The influence of hemodialysis therapy itself on the development of dementia is unclear. Therefore, we evaluated the influence of hemodialysis therapy itself on the development of dementia using data from the JRDR.

Methods
Database search
The JSDT has been conducting annual surveys at dialysis facilities in Japan since 1968, and since 1983, all patients undergoing dialysis at the target facilities have been registered in the JRDR for monitoring [14]. The present study used the JRDR.

Subjects
Data from 282,010 patients undergoing chronic hemodialysis therapy at the end of 2009 were extracted from the JRDR (JRDR09002 dataset). At first, we selected the target patients based on their status at the end of 2009. To ensure uniformity of treatment conditions of the target patients, we excluded patients who underwent treatments other than hemodialysis. Cerebrovascular disease (CVD) is known to be a major risk factor for the development of dementia [5], but the type of dementia expected to be responsive to the preventive effects of hemodialysis is AD [10, 11]. Therefore, we excluded patients with preexisting brain infarction or brain hemorrhage. Furthermore, to analyze the dementia incidence, we excluded patients with preexisting dementia and those with missing data at the

end of 2009. A total of 149,534 patients were included in the baseline dataset. Next, based on the data obtained at the end of 2010, we excluded patients who had died, were lost to follow-up, and had an unclear history of dementia. To avoid the influence of dementia caused by CVD, we excluded those with newly developed brain infarction or hemorrhage and those without information regarding these conditions. Finally, 120,101 patients were included in the analysis.

Diabetic patients are regarded as a high-risk group for AD and vascular dementia (VaD) [15]. Therefore, we speculated that the effect of blood Aβ removal by hemodialysis might be weakened by diabetes with strong risk of dementia, particularly AD. Further, some parts of dementia among diabetic patients are reported as independent diseases because dementia developed in these patients has unique pathologic conditions [16]. Thus, we analyzed not only the whole target patient group but also patients without (non-diabetic group, $n = 80,207$) and with (diabetic group, $n = 39,894$) diabetes separately.

The baseline characteristics of these patients are summarized in Tables 1 and 2. The selection process for the target patients is summarized in Fig. 1.

Dementia survey
The presence or absence of concomitant dementia, brain infarction, and brain hemorrhage was investigated through surveys conducted in 2009 and 2010 [14, 17]. The questions and possible answers are shown in Table 3.

A note stating, "A patient's primary doctor should answer this question" was added. When assessing the dementia risk, patients designated as "with dementia (requiring no care)" and "with dementia (requiring care)" at the end of 2010, but not in 2009, were recorded as patients with newly developed dementia.

Covariates
Among the items included in the 2009 and 2010 surveys, the following were used as covariates in a logistic regression analysis: Kt/V for urea calculated with a single pool model (Kt/V) [18]; body mass index (BMI), predialysis serum albumin level (albumin level), predialysis serum C-reactive protein level (CRP level), and predialysis whole blood hemoglobin level (hemoglobin level); history of myocardial infarction, limb amputation, or hip fracture; activities of daily living (ADLs); and place of residence. The response options for the questions regarding history of brain infarction, brain hemorrhage, myocardial infarction, limb amputation, and hip fracture were "Yes" and "No." The response options for the items on ADLs and place of residence are presented in the footnotes of Tables 1 and 2.

Table 1 Baseline characteristics of non-diabetic patients

	Hemodialysis duration (year)														Total	(%)
	0~1	(%)	2~4	(%)	5~9	(%)	10~14	(%)	15~19	(%)	20~24	(%)	25~	(%)		
Total	14,787	(100.0)	17,293	(100.0)	19,984	(100.0)	12,479	(100.0)	7452	(100.0)	4138	(100.0)	4074	(100.0)	80,207	(100.0)
Sex Male	9106	(61.6)	10,515	(60.8)	11,814	(59.1)	7144	(57.2)	4169	(55.9)	2275	(55.0)	2251	(55.3)	47,274	(58.9)
Female	5681	(38.4)	6778	(39.2)	8170	(40.9)	5335	(42.8)	3283	(44.1)	1863	(45.0)	1823	(44.7)	32,933	(41.1)
Age (years old) 15–64	5980	(40.4)	7584	(43.9)	10,258	(51.3)	7245	(58.1)	4654	(62.5)	2635	(63.7)	2732	(67.1)	41,088	(51.2)
65–74	4066	(27.5)	4900	(28.3)	5612	(28.1)	3499	(28.0)	2092	(28.1)	1196	(28.9)	1133	(27.8)	22,498	(28.0)
<75	4741	(32.1)	4809	(27.8)	4114	(20.6)	1735	(13.9)	706	(9.5)	307	(7.4)	209	(5.1)	16,621	(20.7)
With history of myocardial infarction	630	(4.3)	780	(4.5)	767	(3.8)	467	(3.7)	314	(4.2)	187	(4.5)	190	(4.7)	3335	(4.2)
With history of limb amputation	101	(0.7)	101	(0.6)	137	(0.7)	100	(0.8)	44	(0.6)	33	(0.8)	48	(1.2)	564	(0.7)
With history of hip fracture	181	(1.2)	279	(1.6)	310	(1.6)	175	(1.4)	104	(1.4)	89	(2.2)	190	(4.7)	1328	(1.7)
ADL No symptoms[†]	8122	(54.9)	10,072	(58.2)	12,140	(60.7)	7742	(62.0)	4553	(61.1)	2282	(55.1)	1733	(42.5)	46,644	(58.2)
Moderate symptoms[‡]	4512	(30.5)	5153	(29.8)	5896	(29.5)	3641	(29.2)	2269	(30.4)	1414	(34.2)	1518	(37.3)	24,403	(30.4)
≥50% sitting up[§]	1333	(9.0)	1307	(7.6)	1174	(5.9)	704	(5.6)	370	(5.0)	257	(6.2)	466	(11.4)	5611	(7.0)
≥50% in bed[#]	496	(3.4)	429	(2.5)	416	(2.1)	176	(1.4)	125	(1.7)	96	(2.3)	206	(5.1)	1944	(2.4)
Whole day in bed[¶]	154	(1.0)	100	(0.6)	115	(0.6)	58	(0.5)	42	(0.6)	32	(0.8)	87	(2.1)	588	(0.7)
Place of residence Homes[¶¶]	13,836	(93.6)	16,614	(96.1)	19,359	(96.9)	12,138	(97.3)	7250	(97.3)	4022	(97.2)	3838	(94.2)	77,057	(96.1)
Care facilities[^]	164	(1.1)	203	(1.2)	162	(0.8)	76	(0.6)	38	(0.5)	16	(0.4)	27	(0.7)	686	(0.9)
Hospitals[‡‡]	694	(4.7)	335	(1.9)	316	(1.6)	170	(1.4)	106	(1.4)	62	(1.5)	163	(4.0)	1846	(2.3)
With dementia at the end of 2010	669	(4.5)	681	(3.9)	599	(3.0)	285	(2.3)	108	(1.4)	58	(1.4)	39	(1.0)	2439	(3.0)
Age (years old)*	66.2	±14.0	65.1	±13.8	63.0	±13.4	61.2	±12.5	60.2	±11.4	60.4	±10.1	60.8	±8.5	63.3	±13.1
Kt/V*	1.25	±0.3	1.39	±0.3	1.46	±0.3	1.52	±0.3	1.54	±0.3	1.56	±0.3	1.57	±0.3	1.43	±0.3
Body mass index (kg/m^2)*	21.4	±3.4	21.5	±3.4	21.3	±3.3	20.8	±3.0	20.4	±2.9	20.2	±2.7	19.8	±2.7	21.0	±3.2
Serum albumin level (g/dl)*	3.70	±0.4	3.77	±0.4	3.79	±0.4	3.80	±0.4	3.80	±0.4	3.77	±0.4	3.71	±0.4	3.77	±0.4
Serum CRP level (mg/dl)*	0.46	±1.6	0.38	±1.2	0.36	±1.2	0.36	±1.3	0.39	±1.3	0.38	±1.4	0.47	±1.4	0.39	±1.3
Hemoglobin level (g/dl)*	10.5	±1.3	10.6	±1.2	10.6	±1.2	10.7	±1.2	10.7	±1.2	10.7	±1.2	10.6	±1.3	10.6	±1.2

ADLs activities of daily living, *CRP* C-reactive protein

*Data are presented as mean ± standard deviation

[†] No symptoms (the patient can perform social activities without symptoms and behave without restrictions)

[‡] Moderate symptoms (the patient has mild symptoms and has trouble with physical work, but can walk and do light and sedentary work, such as light domestic and clerical work)

[§] ≥50% sitting up (the patient can walk and take care of him/herself, but sometimes requires care. The patient can sit up at least half of the day, but cannot do light work)

[#] ≥50% in bed (the patient can take care of him/herself to some extent, but often requires care and is in bed at least half of the day)

[¶] Whole day in bed (the patient cannot take care of him/herself and requires constant care. The patient must be in bed all day)

[¶¶] Patients' own home

[^] Care facilities (e.g., homes with care services; nursing homes, such as private nursing homes without national aid and nursing homes for families with financial difficulties; group homes; vocational centers; or relief facilities)

[‡‡] Hospitals (e.g., health service facilities for the elderly; beds for general patients, patients at chronic stage, patients requiring rehabilitation, and patients with mental illness and infectious diseases, such as tuberculosis)

Table 2 Baseline characteristics of diabetic patients

		Hemodialysis duration (year)													
		0~1	(%)	2~4	(%)	5~9	(%)	10~14	(%)	15~19	(%)	20~24	(%)	25~	(%)	Total	(%)
Total		12,756	(100.0)	13,342	(100.0)	10,273	(100.0)	2785	(100.0)	605	(100.0)	98	(100.0)	35	(100.0)	39,894	(100.0)
Sex	Male	8949	(70.2)	9215	(69.1)	6819	(66.4)	1767	(63.4)	369	(61.0)	61	(62.2)	18	(51.4)	27,198	(68.2)
	Female	3807	(29.8)	4127	(30.9)	3454	(33.6)	1018	(36.6)	236	(39.0)	37	(37.8)	17	(48.6)	12,696	(31.8)
Age (years old)	15~64	6378	(50.0)	6495	(48.7)	5040	(49.1)	1415	(50.8)	276	(45.6)	57	(58.2)	23	(65.7)	19,684	(49.3)
	65~74	3940	(30.9)	4434	(33.2)	3518	(34.2)	970	(34.8)	234	(38.7)	28	(28.6)	8	(22.9)	13,132	(32.9)
	<75	2438	(19.1)	2413	(18.1)	1715	(16.7)	400	(14.4)	95	(15.7)	13	(13.3)	4	(11.4)	7078	(17.7)
With history of myocardial infarction		913	(7.2)	1154	(8.6)	896	(8.7)	241	(8.7)	57	(9.4)	12	(12.2)	2	(5.7)	3275	(8.2)
With history of limb amputation		383	(3.0)	571	(4.3)	638	(6.2)	220	(7.9)	66	(10.9)	8	(8.2)	5	(14.3)	1891	(4.7)
With history of hip fracture		201	(1.6)	250	(1.9)	251	(2.4)	65	(2.3)	21	(3.5)	4	(4.1)	1	(2.9)	793	(2.0)
ADL	No symptoms[†]	6419	(50.3)	6685	(50.1)	4942	(48.1)	1277	(45.9)	234	(38.7)	43	(43.9)	9	(25.7)	19,609	(49.2)
	Moderate symptoms[‡]	4121	(32.3)	4323	(32.4)	3323	(32.3)	906	(32.5)	193	(31.9)	28	(28.6)	12	(34.3)	12,906	(32.4)
	≥50% sitting up[§]	1425	(11.2)	1401	(10.5)	1244	(12.1)	375	(13.5)	100	(16.5)	20	(20.4)	8	(22.9)	4573	(11.5)
	≥50% in bed[#]	471	(3.7)	562	(4.2)	496	(4.8)	151	(5.4)	51	(8.4)	3	(3.1)	2	(5.7)	1736	(4.4)
	Whole day in bed[¶]	155	(1.2)	184	(1.4)	133	(1.3)	51	(1.8)	16	(2.6)	3	(3.1)	2	(5.7)	544	(1.4)
Place of residence	Homes[¶]	11,912	(93.4)	12,656	(94.9)	9769	(95.1)	2617	(94.0)	557	(92.1)	93	(94.9)	29	(82.9)	37,633	(94.3)
	Care facilities[^]	136	(1.1)	141	(1.1)	107	(1.0)	29	(1.0)	9	(1.5)	1	(1.0)	0	(0.0)	423	(1.1)
	Hospitals[‡]	619	(4.9)	438	(3.3)	324	(3.2)	125	(4.5)	33	(5.5)	3	(3.1)	5	(14.3)	1547	(3.9)
With dementia at the end of 2010		512	(4.0)	578	(4.3)	375	(3.7)	97	(3.5)	24	(4.0)	4	(4.1)	2	(5.7)	1592	(4.0)
Age (years old)*		64.0	±11.5	64.2	±11.1	64.4	±10.5	63.9	±10.0	64.5	±9.9	62.9	±9.8	60.5	±10.5	64.2	±11.0
Kt/V*		1.18	±0.3	1.32	±0.3	1.38	±0.2	1.45	±0.3	1.49	±0.3	1.49	±0.3	1.52	±0.2	1.30	±0.3
Body mass index (kg/m²)*		22.5	±3.5	22.7	±3.6	22.4	±3.5	21.7	±3.3	20.7	±3.3	20.6	±3.4	19.8	±3.1	22.4	±3.5
Serum albumin level (g/dl)*		3.66	±0.4	3.77	±0.4	3.77	±0.3	3.74	±0.4	3.69	±0.4	3.73	±0.3	3.63	±0.4	3.73	±0.4
Serum CRP level (mg/dl)*		0.45	±1.5	0.39	±1.3	0.43	±1.5	0.53	±2.0	0.47	±1.4	0.39	±0.9	1.02	±2.3	0.43	±1.5
Hemoglobin level (g/dl)*		10.5	±1.3	10.6	±1.2	10.6	±1.2	10.6	±1.3	10.6	±1.3	10.6	±1.4	10.6	±1.4	10.6	±1.3

ADLs activities of daily living, *CRP* C-reactive protein

*Data are presented as mean ± standard deviation

[†]No symptoms (the patient can perform social activities without symptoms and behave without restrictions)

[‡]Moderate symptoms (the patient has mild symptoms and has trouble with physical work, but can walk and do light and sedentary work, such as light domestic and clerical work)

[§]≥50% sitting up (the patient can walk and take care of him/herself, but sometimes requires care. The patient can sit up at least half of the day, but cannot do light work)

[#]≥50% in bed (The patient can take care of him/herself to some extent, but often requires care and is in bed at least half of the day)

[¶]Whole day in bed (The patient cannot take care of him/herself and requires constant care. The patient must be in bed all day)

[¶]Patients' own home

[^]Care facilities (e.g., homes with care services; nursing homes, such as private nursing homes without national aid and nursing homes for families with financial difficulties; group homes; vocational centers; relief facilities)

[‡]Hospitals (e.g., health service facilities for the elderly; beds for general patients, patients at chronic stage, patients requiring rehabilitation, and patients with mental illness and infectious diseases, such as tuberculosis)

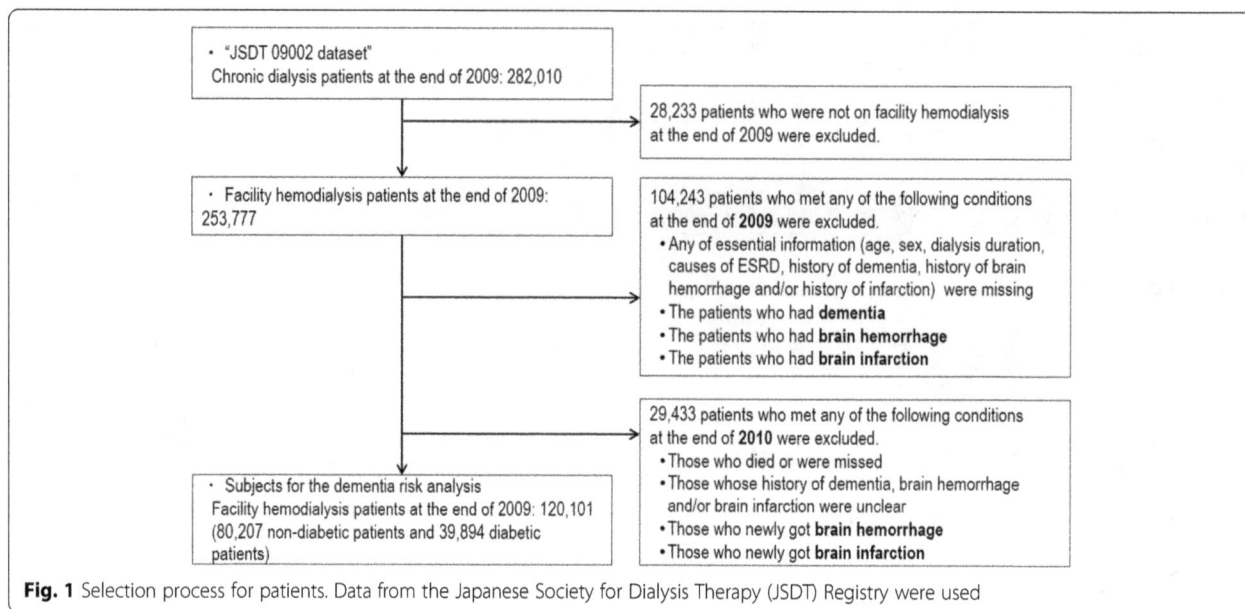

Fig. 1 Selection process for patients. Data from the Japanese Society for Dialysis Therapy (JSDT) Registry were used

Statistical analysis

All analyses were performed using the Statistical Analysis System, version 9.4 (SAS Institute, Inc., Cary, NC, USA). The incidence rate of dementia from the end of 2009 to the end of 2010 was calculated using the following formula: incidence rate of dementia (cases/1000 person-years) = the number of patients with newly developed dementia during the observation period (cases)/the total person-years of the target patients during the observation period (person-years) × 1000.

The time of dementia onset was not recorded in this survey. Therefore, the length of follow-up for patients who suffered dementia during 2010 was assumed to be 0.5 years when the incidence rate of dementia was calculated.

Because of the lack of data on the time of dementia onset, for the analyses of dementia risk, logistic regression models were constructed. All P values were two sided. In all models, the hemodialysis duration at

Table 3 The questions and answer options in the dementia survey

• Questions

   Please indicate the presence or absence of dementia in the patient.

   Please provide as much information as you can about the conditions of the patient during dialysis treatment or consultation.

   (Note that the primary doctor should provide the answer.)

• Answer options

   Without dementia

   Without dementia (requiring no care)

   Without dementia (requiring care)

   Unspecified

the end of 2009 was used as the independent variable and the prevalence of dementia at the end of 2010 was used as the dependent variable. In these analyses, age-adjusted and multifactor models were used.

The age and hemodialysis duration values used in this report were calculated as of the end of 2009. As age is the most independent risk factor of dementia, the age-adjusted model included only age and hemodialysis duration as independent variables. The multifactor model included baseline factors from the age-adjusted model plus additional clinical covariates (i.e., sex; comorbidity of diabetes; Kt/V; BMI; albumin level; CRP level; hemoglobin level, history of myocardial infarction, limb amputation, or hip fracture; ADLs; and place of residence). Age, hemodialysis duration, Kt/V, BMI, albumin level, CRP level, and hemoglobin level were incorporated as continuous variables, whereas the other factors were incorporated as stratified categorical variables (Tables 1 and 2). A missing value of each covariate was treated as "a missing value group" and was analyzed.

In the multifactor model analysis, we analyzed not only the whole target patients but also non-diabetic and diabetic patients separately, to compare the tendency of dementia risk of these two patient groups. In these separated analyses, we incorporated hemodialysis duration as a stratified variable into the analytic model to confirm the dementia risk trend associated with elongation of hemodialysis duration. The hemodialysis duration was stratified into the following intervals: 0 to 1, 2 to 4, 5 to 9, 10 to 14, 15 to 19, 20 to 24, and ≥ 25 years. Because patients initiated on hemodialysis within 2 years frequently have significant residual renal function, we considered hemodialysis duration of < 2 years as a separate category. The mean value of age, which is the most independent risk factor, was quite similar between the hemodialysis duration groups (Tables 1 and 2).

Finally, to evaluate how the exclusion of patients by the end of 2010 affected the results (Fig. 1, $n = 29,433$), we conducted the following sensitivity analyses. We analyzed the dementia risk under the assumptions that none of the excluded patients suffered dementia (negative analysis) and that all excluded patients suffered dementia (positive analysis). These analyses were conducted on the non-diabetic and diabetic patients separately, using the multifactor model.

Results

Diabetes and dementia risk

The overall dementia incidence was higher in diabetic than in non-diabetic patients (35.5 cases/1000 person-years; 95% confidence interval [CI], 33.8–37.3 vs. 30.9 cases/1000 person-years, 95% CI, 29.7–32.1; Table 4). In the multifactor model analysis, the diabetic patients did not have significant risk of dementia compared with non-diabetic patients. (Table 5).

Covariates and dementia risk

The associations between the covariates and dementia risk, which were obtained from the whole patient analysis using the multifactor model, are shown in Table 5. Female sex, elder age, and higher CRP level were associated with higher dementia risk. The dementia risk was higher in those with than in those without a history of hip fracture, whereas the risk was lower in those with than in those without a history of amputation. Predictably, reduced ADLs and residence at a hospital or care facility were associated with dementia.

Hemodialysis duration and dementia risk

As shown in Table 4, there was a decrease in the dementia incidence with an increase in hemodialysis duration in non-diabetic patients, but there was no such association in diabetic patients.

When we analyzed the whole target patient group, which included those without and with diabetes simultaneously, longer hemodialysis duration was associated significantly with lower dementia risk in the age-adjusted and multifactor model analyses (Fig. 2a).

On the other hand, when we analyzed patients without and with diabetes separately, the analytic results were different. In non-diabetic patients, longer hemodialysis duration was associated significantly with lower dementia risk in the age-adjusted and multifactor model analyses, similar to the whole patient group analyses (Fig. 2b). However, in diabetic patients, we found no significant association between hemodialysis duration and dementia risk in the age-adjusted model analysis. The multifactor model analysis showed a significant correlation between hemodialysis duration and dementia risk, but the correlation was much weaker than that found in non-diabetic patients (Fig. 2c).

Figure 3 shows the results of the analyses in which hemodialysis duration was treated as a stratified but not as a continuous variable. These analyses were done using a multifactor model. Non-diabetic patients had a consistent decrease in dementia risk with an increase in hemodialysis duration from the shortest to the longest duration strata (Fig. 3a). However, in contrast, diabetic patients had only a vague association between hemodialysis duration and dementia risk. The association between hemodialysis duration and dementia risk was not consistent along with the elongation of hemodialysis duration (Fig. 3b). At less than 5 years of hemodialysis

Table 4 Dementia incidence according to hemodialysis duration

Hemodialysis duration (year)	Non-diabetic patients					Diabetic patients				
	Number of patients	Person-years	Number of patients who developed dementia	Incidence rates of dementia (cases/1000 person-year)	(95% CI)	Number of patients	Person-years	Number of patients who developed dementia	Incidence rates of dementia (cases/1000 person-year)	(95% CI)
0–1	14,787	14,452.5	669	46.3	(42.9 – 49.9)	12,756	12,500.0	512	35.8	(32.9 – 39.1)
2–4	17,293	16,952.5	681	40.2	(37.3 – 43.3)	13,342	13,053.0	578	39.1	(36.1 – 42.4)
5–9	19,984	19,684.5	599	30.4	(28.1 – 33.0)	10,273	10,085.5	375	32.2	(29.1 – 35.6)
10–14	12,479	12,336.5	285	23.1	(20.6 – 25.9)	2785	2736.5	97	30.1	(24.7 – 36.8)
15–19	7452	7398.0	108	14.6	(12.1 – 17.6)	605	593.0	24	34.5	(23.1 – 51.4)
20–24	4138	4109.0	58	14.1	(10.9 – 18.3)	98	96.0	4	34.9	(13.1 – 93.1)
25–	4074	4054.5	39	9.6	(7.0 – 13.2)	35	34.0	2	50.6	(12.7 – 202.5)
Total	80,207	78,987.5	2439	30.9	(29.7 – 32.1)	39,894	39,098.0	1592	35.5	(33.8 – 37.3)

Incidence rate of dementia (cases/1000 person-years) = the number of patients with newly developed dementia during the observation period (cases)/the total person-years of the target patients during the observation period (person-years) × 1000. The length of follow-up for patients with dementia was assumed to be 0.5 years

CI confidence interval

Table 5 ORs of dementia with covariates

Covariates	Number of patients	Incident number*	OR for development of dementia	(95% CI)	p value
Age					
For every 10 years old	120,101	4031	1.05	(1.02 – 1.07)	0.0003
Sex					
Male	74,472	2112	1.00	Reference	
Female	45,629	1919	1.14	(1.08 – 1.21)	0.0001
Comorbidity of diabetes					
Without diabetes	80,207	2439	1.00	Reference	
With diabetes	39,894	1592	1.00	(0.94 – 1.07)	0.9
Kt/V					
For every 0.1 increase	112,533	3690	1.00	(0.99 – 1.01)	0.5
No information available	7568	341	1.00	(0.83 – 1.19)	1.0
Body mass index					
For every 1 kg/m² increase	105,234	3390	0.99	(0.98 – 1.00)	0.2
No information available	14,867	641	1.01	(0.81 – 1.25)	1.0
Serum albumin level					
For every 1.0 g/dl increase	116,318	3923	0.96	(0.89 – 1.04)	0.3
No information available	3783	108	0.76	(0.55 – 1.06)	0.1
CRP level					
For every 1.0 mg/dl increase	58,498	2276	1.02	(1.00 – 1.04)	0.03
No information available	61,603	1755	0.94	(0.88 – 1.02)	0.1

Covariates	Number of patients	Incident number*	OR for development of dementia	(95% CI)	p value
History of myocardial infarction					
No	113,283	3762	1.00	Reference	
Yes	6610	265	1.02	(0.91 – 1.14)	0.7
No information available	208	4	0.61	(0.30 – 1.25)	0.2
History of limb amputation					
No	117,449	3911	1.00	Reference	
Yes	2455	111	0.66	(0.56 – 0.77)	0.0001
No information available	197	9	1.03	(0.53 – 2.00)	0.9
History of hip fracture					
No	117,467	3789	1.00	Reference	
Yes	2121	219	2.38	(2.10 – 2.71)	0.0001
No information available	513	23	1.26	(0.82 – 1.93)	0.3
Activities of daily living					
No symptoms†	66,253	1009	1.00	Reference	
Moderate symptoms‡	37,309	1159	1.13	(1.05 – 1.22)	0.001
≥ 50% sitting up§	10,184	1050	4.49	(4.14 – 4.88)	0.0001
≥ 50% in bed#	3680	548	9.60	(8.69 – 10.6)	0.0001
Whole day in bed¶	1132	224	21.70	(18.7 – 25.2)	0.0001
No information available	1543	41	0.95	(0.66 – 1.37)	0.8
Place of residence					

Table 5 ORs of dementia with covariates (*Continued*)

Covariates	Number of patients	Incident number*	OR for development of dementia	(95% CI)	p value	Covariates	Number of patients	Incident number*	OR for development of dementia	(95% CI)	p value
Hemoglobin level						Homes§¶	114,690	3286	1.00	Reference	
For every 1.0 g/dl increase	118,829	3967	0.99	(0.97 ~ 1.01)	0.5	Care facilities^	1109	191	10.95	(9.53 ~ 12.6)	0.0001
No information available	1272	64	1.18	(0.84 ~ 1.65)	0.3	Hospitals‡	3393	526	5.32	(4.86 ~ 5.84)	0.0001
						No information available	909	28	1.15	(0.73 ~ 1.82)	0.5

The associations between the covariates and dementia risk, which were obtained from the whole patient group analysis using a multifactor model, are shown

ADLs activities of daily living, *CI* confidence interval, *CRP* C-reactive protein, *OR* odds ratio

*Number of patients with dementia

†No symptoms (the patient can perform social activities without symptoms and behave without restrictions)

‡Moderate symptoms (the patient has mild symptoms and has trouble with physical work, but can walk and do light and sedentary work, such as light domestic and clerical work)

§≥ 50% sitting up (the patient can walk and take care of him/herself, but sometimes requires care. The patient can sit up at least half of the day, but cannot do light work)

∥≥ 50% in bed (the patient can take care of him/herself to some extent, but often requires care and is in bed at least half of the day)

¶Whole day in bed (the patient cannot take care of him/herself and requires constant care. The patient must be in bed all day)

§Patients' own home

^Care facilities (e.g., homes with care services; nursing homes, such as private nursing homes without national aid and nursing homes for families with financial difficulties; group homes; vocational centers; or relief facilities)

‡Hospitals (e.g., health service facilities for the elderly; beds for general patients, patients at chronic stage, patients requiring rehabilitation, and patients with mental illness and infectious diseases, such as tuberculosis)

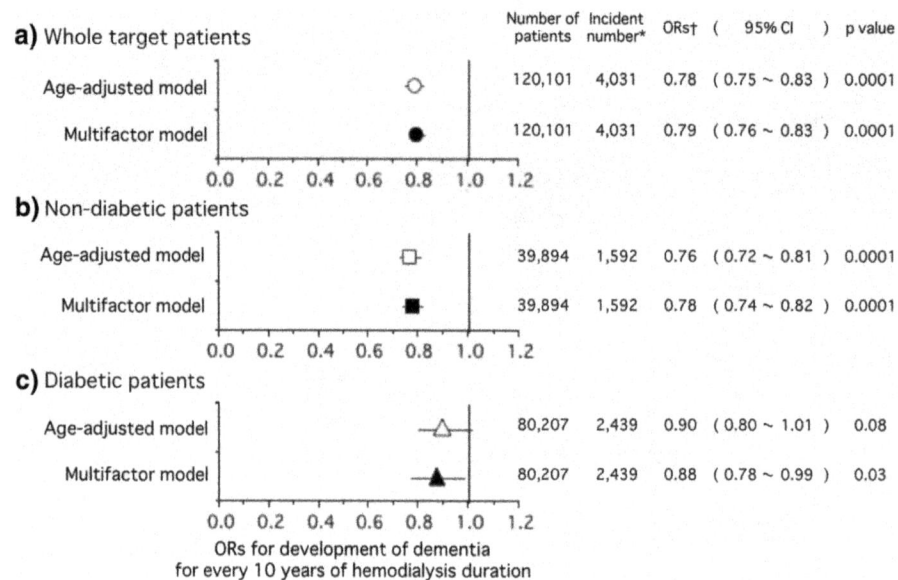

Fig. 2 Dementia risk for hemodialysis duration. The dementia risk for hemodialysis duration was analyzed for each different patient group using the age-adjusted or multifactor model. The age-adjusted model included only age and hemodialysis duration as independent variables. The multifactor model included baseline factors from the age-adjusted model plus additional clinical covariates (i.e., sex, comorbidity of diabetes, Kt/V, BMI, albumin level, CRP level, hemoglobin level, history of myocardial infarction, limb amputation, or hip fracture, ADLs, and place of residence). The duration of hemodialysis was treated as a continuous variable. Please note that the X axis is a linear plot. **a** The target patients of the analysis were the whole target patients. **b** The target patients of the analysis were only the non-diabetic patients. **c** The target patients of the analysis were only the diabetic patients. Asterisk indicates the number of patients who suffered dementia. Dagger indicates ORs for development of dementia for every 10 years of hemodialysis duration. ADLs activities of daily living, BMI body mass index, CI confidence interval, CRP C-reactive protein, OR odds ratio

duration, the dementia risk seemed to increase along with the elongation of the hemodialysis duration, but, on the contrary, from five to 19 years, it seemed to decrease. At over 20 years of hemodialysis duration, the dementia risk seemed to increase again along with elongation of the duration.

Figure 4 shows the result of sensitivity analysis. In the negative and positive analyses in the non-diabetic patients, the dementia risk decreased with increasing hemodialysis duration (Fig. 4a). However, in the positive analysis of diabetic patients, the risk of dementia tended to increase with prolongation of hemodialysis duration (Fig. 4b).

Discussion

Our study showed that the dementia risk in non-diabetic patients decreased with prolongation of hemodialysis duration. However, we must consider the survivor effect when analyzing the relationship between hemodialysis duration and dementia incidence.

The survivor effect is a bias caused by a prolonged period of observation for incidence in the target cohort. As the observation period increases, more patients with risk factors will drop out from the target cohort upon reaching the designated endpoints. As a result, the incidence rate tends to decrease with an increase in the observation period. In our study, hemodialysis duration also was the exposure period, with hemodialysis as a risk factor. Therefore, we must consider the survivor effect of hemodialysis duration in this study.

On the other hand, CKD is a reported risk factor of dementia [1, 2]. If we consider hemodialysis duration as the exposure period and consider CKD as a risk factor, a longer hemodialysis duration may be expected to increase dementia risk. However, in our study, the dementia risk in non-diabetic patients decreased as the hemodialysis duration increased. This result may suggest that the risk-reducing power of the survivor effect overcame the risk-enhancing power of CKD in non-diabetic patients throughout the entire hemodialysis period. However, we could not necessarily identify a clear relationship between dialysis duration and dementia risk in diabetic patients.

In general, the survivor effect appears to be stronger when more patients drop out from the target cohort as they reach the designated endpoints. For example, the dementia risk was significantly lower in patients with a history of limb amputation (odds ratio [OR], 0.66 [95% CI, 0.56–0.77]; the OR compares patients "with limb amputation history" to those "without limb amputation history"; Table 5). Moreover, previous research has shown that the survival rate was low in hemodialysis

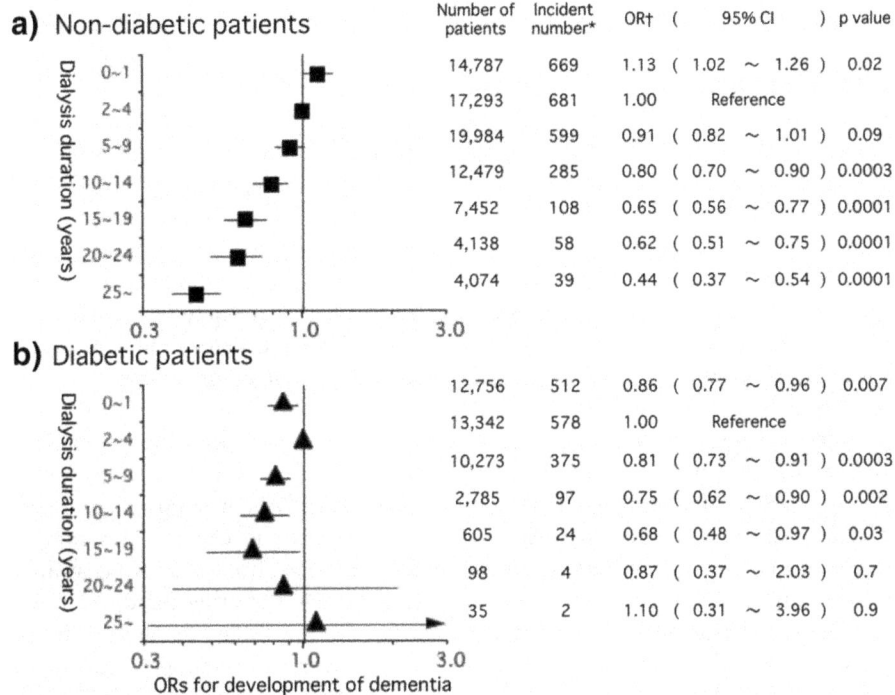

Fig. 3 Dementia risk for hemodialysis duration as a stratified variable. The dementia risk for hemodialysis duration was analyzed as a stratified variable using the multifactor model. The multifactor model included the following factors as independent variables: hemodialysis duration, age, sex, comorbidity of diabetes, Kt/V, BMI, albumin level, CRP level, hemoglobin level, history of myocardial infarction, limb amputation, or hip fracture, ADLs, and place of residence. Please note that the X axis is a log-linear plot. **a** The target patients of the analysis were only the non-diabetic patients. **b** The target patients of the analysis were only the diabetic patients. Asterisk indicates the number of patients who suffered dementia. Dagger indicates ORs for development of dementia. ADLs activities of daily living, BMI body mass index, CI confidence interval, CRP C-reactive protein, OR odds ratio

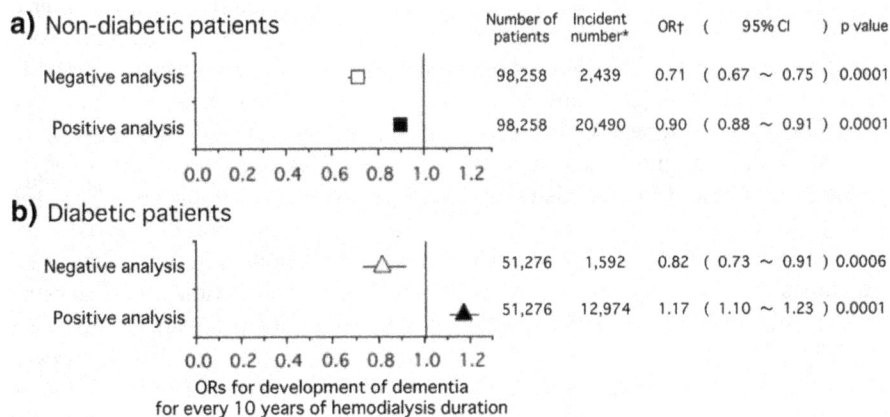

Fig. 4 Sensitivity analyses for the excluded patients' influence evaluation. The sensitivity analyses were conducted to evaluate how the exclusion of patients affected the results. We analyzed the dementia risk under the assumptions that none of the excluded patients had dementia (negative analysis) and that all the excluded patients had dementia (positive analysis). These analyses were conducted using the multifactor model, which included the following factors as independent variables; hemodialysis duration, age, sex, comorbidity of diabetes, Kt/V, BMI, albumin level, CRP level, hemoglobin level, history of myocardial infarction, limb amputation, or hip fracture, ADLs, and place of residence. Please note that the X axis is a linear plot. **a** The target patients of the analysis were only the non-diabetic patients. **b** The target patients of the analysis were only the diabetic patients. Asterisk indicates the number of patients with dementia. Dagger indicates ORs for development of dementia for every 10 years of hemodialysis duration. ADLs activities of daily living, BMI body mass index, CI confidence interval, CRP C-reactive protein, OR odds ratio

patients with a history of limb amputation [19]. This also is confirmed in our mortality risk analysis (Additional file 1: Table S1). The mortality risk increased significantly when hemodialysis duration increased in non-diabetic and diabetic (Additional file 1: Table S2). However, the relationship between mortality risk and hemodialysis duration was much stronger in the diabetic patients than in non-diabetic patients. Based on these findings, we may be able to assume that the survivor effect was stronger in diabetic patients than in non-diabetic patients. However, the relationship between dementia risk and hemodialysis duration in diabetic patients was much weaker or vaguer than that in non-diabetic patients (Figs. 2 and 3). Therefore, we might be able to consider that the reduction in dementia risk with prolonged hemodialysis duration in non-diabetic patients was caused not only by the survivor effect but also by some other factors, such as hemodialysis itself.

AD is a major cause of dementia [5], in which accumulation of Aβ in the brain results in cognitive impairment [6]. Moreover, in these patients, the metabolic degradation of Aβ and its clearance from the brain are impaired [7]. If Aβ clearance from the brain can be increased, AD might be prevented or even treated. It has been shown that hemodialysis removes Aβ [10] and that the cognitive function of non-diabetic patients was maintained or improved among those undergoing maintenance hemodialysis over a period of 18 to 36 months [11]. Additionally, Aβ deposition was significantly weaker in the postmortem brains of patients who had undergone hemodialysis than in age-matched controls who had not undergone hemodialysis [12], and this finding is comparable to the finding in the study by Reusche et al. [13]. Although Lin et al. [4] showed that there is no significant difference in dementia risk between patients undergoing hemodialysis and those undergoing peritoneal dialysis, Jin et al. [20] showed that Aβ removal from the blood by peritoneal dialysis also reduces Aβ in the brain interstitial fluid. These reports suggest that hemodialysis might reduce the dementia risk through removal of Aβ from the blood of patients.

It is known that hemodialysis patients have a high morbidity risk of cerebrovascular events [21], and CVD is a major risk factor for VaD. We excluded patients with a clear history of CVD (Fig. 1). Therefore, we may assume that most cases in our analysis had a type of dementia other than VaD. In the study by Sekita et al. [22] on dementia in the general population in Japan, approximately 46% of individuals had AD and 30% had VaD. If we apply this finding to our study in which patients with CVD were excluded, we might be able to assume that approximately two thirds of our patients with dementia had AD. However, we may have to consider the possibility that patients suffered VaD without

presenting with clear symptoms of CVD, and it is known that patients with CKD tend to experience VaD rather than AD [23]. Therefore, we may have to consider that the patients with dementia among our target patients still include many with VaD. However, it is reported that the vascular lesion of patients with CKD also is a risk for AD [24]. Furthermore, it has been reported that many patients with cerebrovascular dementia have concomitant AD [5]; thus, we believe that hemodialysis may suppress the development of dementia in this patient group to some extent.

In this survey, despite the notification that the primary physician should determine the presence or absence of dementia, no standard criteria were specified and there was no information on dementia severity. We cannot exclude the possibility that this ambiguity of dementia diagnosis influenced the analytic results. Patients with long hemodialysis duration might be well known by their own physicians in charge. This situation might make it easier for the physicians to be aware of their patients' dementia. On the other hand, the physicians might tend to answer "without dementia" from force of habit. However, even if we suppose the possibility of "negative diagnosis bias" of long-term dialysis patients, we cannot explain the reason why the risk suppression effect of hemodialysis duration in diabetic patients is weaker than that of non-diabetic patients.

On assessing patients in this study, we found no apparent relationship between hemodialysis duration and age (Tables 1 and 2). Moreover, the influence of age was adjusted using the logistic regression analysis. Therefore, it is difficult to consider that a deviation in age with a prolonged hemodialysis duration affected the analytical results.

The discontinuation of dialysis after dementia onset by a substantial number of patients could exacerbate the survivor effect. However, among the 8367 patients excluded from our analytical cohort due to death during 2010, only 33 (0.4%) died due to discontinuation of dialysis. Thus, discontinuation of dialysis does not appear to contribute substantially to the survivor effect.

Considering the aforementioned findings, the assumption that hemodialysis itself may prevent development of AD in non-diabetic patients does not appear to have a major conflict with our results. Our results may not show clearly the dementia-preventing effect of hemodialysis therapy. However, if we can interpret this result as "the first finding," showing the dementia-preventing effect of hemodialysis therapy based on the real clinical data obtained from a large cohort of patients, this result may have important implications in the prevention of dementia. Therefore, we reported this result in this study.

Although hemodialysis is considered to be preventive against the incidence of dementia, it does not imply that the incidence of dementia in the hemodialysis patients is absolutely lower than that in the general population. The incidence of dementia in the > 65-year-old target patients was 50.0 and 59.0 cases/1000 person-years among those without and with diabetes, respectively (Additional file 1: Table S3). On the other hand, it is reported that the incidence of dementia in the > 65-year-old Japanese general population was 30.5–35.6 cases/1000 person-years [25]. This finding suggests that the absolute value of the incidence of dementia in hemodialysis patients is still higher than that in the general population. This may suggest that the dementia risk-reducing effect of hemodialysis did not overcome the risk caused by CKD itself, which every hemodialysis patient faced.

Because it is known that renal failure patients without hemodialysis have a 2.86 times higher risk of cognitive impairment than healthy subjects [2], we consider that the high dementia risk of hemodialysis patients may not have resulted from hemodialysis therapy but from their renal failure. There may be some patients who had dementia or cognitive impairment prior to dialysis initiation. Therefore, in this study, we evaluated the relationship between dementia risk and the patients' hemodialysis duration.

In the present analysis, we found no significant risk of dementia related to Kt/V (Table 5). Kt/V is considered to be the dialysis efficiency indicator of the small substance because the target substance of Kt/V is urea and its molecular weight is only 60 Da. On the other hand, the molecular weight of Aβ, which is considered to be related to the occurrence of AD, is 4 kDa and is much heavier than urea. Recently, Kawaguchi et al. [26] reported that dialyzers remove Aβ from the blood, not by the dialysis phenomenon but by adsorption during hemodialysis therapy [26]. Kato et al. [10] also reported that the reduction rate of blood Aβ concentration of a 4-h hemodialysis session is approximately 34.9 to 53.0%. Based on these reports, we may be able to assume that the reduction rate of Aβ in our target patients was similar to that reported by Kato et al. [10]. These findings suggest that our result of Kt/V having no dementia risk does not necessarily conflict with our hypothesis that the hemodialysis prevents development of AD through removing Aβ.

Regarding removal of large molecular weight substances from the blood, the hemodiafiltration therapy, which uses dialysis and the filtration phenomenon, generally is considered to have a higher efficiency than hemodialysis. However, because the main mechanism of removing Aβ from blood is not dialysis but the adsorption phenomenon of the dialyzer membrane, we may be able to consider that the choice of blood purification method, such as hemodialysis or hemodiafiltration,

may not make much difference in the dementia preventive effect.

Diabetes is a known risk factor for dementia [15]. Hanyu et al. [16] recently mentioned that dementia in diabetic patients should be regarded as an independent disease (i.e., diabetes-related dementia) because it results from pathologic conditions related to diabetes. Following their concept, we separated the target patients based on their comorbidity of diabetes in our study. A unique disease entity causing dementia also may explain the weak or absent association between hemodialysis duration and dementia risk in diabetic patients. In our analysis, the multifactor model showed no significant dementia risk in diabetic patients compared with non-diabetic patients (Table 5). When we tentatively analyzed the dementia risk for the comorbidity of diabetes using a simple analytic model that contains only age and hemodialysis duration as covariates other than comorbidity of diabetes, we showed that diabetic patients had a significant OR for dementia of 1.13 (95% CI, 1.07–1.20, $P = 0.0001$; Additional file 1: Table S4). We considered that this finding may show that the influence of the comorbidity of diabetes was confounded by other covariates in the multifactor model analysis.

We conducted a sensitivity analysis to evaluate how the exclusion of patients by the end of 2010 affected the results. In the negative and positive analyses of non-diabetic patients, the dementia risk decreased with increasing hemodialysis duration (Fig. 4a). This result suggested that the exclusion of patients by the end of 2010 did not affect the relationship between dementia risk and hemodialysis duration among the non-diabetic patients. Although the negative analysis of diabetic patients showed that the dementia risk decreased with prolongation of hemodialysis duration, the positive analysis of diabetic patients showed to the contrary that the risk of dementia increased with prolongation of hemodialysis duration (Fig. 4b). This result showed that the dementia risk possibly may increase along with prolongation of hemodialysis duration in diabetic patients. But the diabetic patients may also have a weak negative relationship between the dementia risk and their hemodialysis duration because the multifactor model analysis of the diabetic patients showed a weak but significant negative relationship between the dementia risk and hemodialysis duration (Fig. 2c).

Our analysis showed that advancing age, female sex, a high CRP level, history of hip fracture, low ADLs, and admission to facilities or hospitals were significant risk factors for dementia (Table 5). These risk factors have been reported as significant for dementia in previous studies [27–30]. Anemia has been reported to be a risk factor for cognitive impairment [31]. However, our analysis did not show a significant association between hemoglobin level and dementia risk. We considered that the effects of hemoglobin on dementia probably were confounded by other covariates (Additional file 1: Table S5).

Our study had several limitations. First, the diagnostic criteria for dementia were not specified clearly, and the assessment of dementia was based on a simple query to the respondents at each facility. Despite the notification that the primary physician should determine the presence or absence of dementia, no standard criteria were specified and there was no information on dementia severity. Second, the database used did not include many factors, including hypertension, hyperlipidemia, low socioeconomic status, and low education status, which have been reported to affect dementia risk in patients with CKD [32]. Third, we could not completely exclude survivor bias despite our efforts to mitigate the effect by incorporating many covariates in the regression model. To resolve these problems in the future, extensive cohort studies should be performed among patients undergoing hemodialysis and care should be taken to collect detailed information related to the onset of AD.

Conclusion

A longer hemodialysis duration was correlated with a lower dementia risk in non-diabetic patients, but not in diabetic patients. This finding does not appear to contradict greatly the assumption that the reduction in dementia risk with a prolonged hemodialysis duration in non-diabetic patients was caused not only by the survivor effect but also by hemodialysis itself.

Abbreviations
AD: Alzheimer's disease; ADLs: Activities of daily living; Aβ: Amyloid β; BMI: Body mass index; CI: Confidence interval; CKD: Chronic kidney disease; CRP: C-reactive protein; CVD: Cerebrovascular disease; ESRD: End-stage renal disease; JRDR: Japanese Society for Dialysis Therapy Renal Data Registry; JSDT: Japanese Society for Dialysis Therapy; OR: Odds ratio; VaD: Vascular dementia

Acknowledgements
We are grateful to Dr. Takayuki Hamano, Dr. Takeshi Hasegawa, Dr. Shoichi Maruyama, and Dr. Takahiro Shinzato, for their advice and encouragement. We also appreciate Ms. Shinobu Hattori for her kind English editing.

Funding
The authors did not receive any funding for this study.

Authors' contributions
SN, KW, and NK devised the study design. SN and EK analyzed the data. KS assisted with the pathophysiologic assessment. KK assisted with the etiologic assessment. SN wrote the original draft, prepared the tables and figures, and searched the literature. All authors interpreted the data and reviewed the manuscript. All authors read and approved the final manuscript.

Authors' information
S.N. and E.K. are present members of Committee of Renal Data Registry of JSDT, and K.W. was a previous member of this committee.

Competing interests
The authors declare that they have no competing interests.

Author details
[1]Faculty of Clinical Engineering Technology, Fujita Health University School of Health Sciences, Dengakugakubo 1-98, Kutsukake-cho, Toyoake, Aichi 470-1192, Japan. [2]Department of Preventive Medicine, Nagoya University Graduate School of Medicine, Tsurumai-cho 65, Showa-ku, Nagoya, Aichi 466-8550, Japan. [3]Department of Nephrology, Tokyo Kyosai Hospital, Nakameguro 2-3-8, Meguro-ku, Tokyo 153-8934, Japan.

References
1. Yaffe K, Ackerson L, Kurella Tamura M, Le Blanc P, Kusek JW, Sehgal AR, et al. Chronic kidney disease and cognitive function in older adults: findings from the chronic renal insufficiency cohort cognitive study. J Am Geriatr Soc. 2010;58:338–45.
2. Kurella M, Chertow GM, Fried LF, Cummings SR, Harris T, Simonsick E, et al. Chronic kidney disease and cognitive impairment in the elderly: the health, aging, and body composition study. J Am Soc Nephrol. 2005;16:2127–33.
3. Fukunishi I, Kitaoka T, Shirai T, Kino K, Kanematsu E, Sato Y. Psychiatric disorders among patients undergoing hemodialysis therapy. Nephron. 2002;91:344–7.
4. Lin YT, Wu PH, Kuo MC, Chen CS, Chiu YW, Yang YH, et al. Comparison of dementia risk between end stage renal disease patients with hemodialysis and peritoneal dialysis—a population based study. Sci Rep. 2015;5:8224. https://doi.org/10.1038/srep08224.
5. World Health Organization and Alzheimer's disease international. Dementia: a public health priority. http://www.who.int/mental_health/publications/dementia_report_2012/en/. Accessed 5 Nov 2017.
6. Selkoe DJ. Alzheimer's disease: genes, proteins, and therapy. Physiol Rev. 2001;81:741–66.
7. Mawuenyega KG, Sigurdson W, Ovod V, Munsell L, Kasten T, Morris JC, et al. Decreased clearance of CNS beta-amyloid in Alzheimer's disease. Science. 2010;330:1774.
8. Hock C, Konietzko U, Streffer JR, Tracy J, Signorell A, Müller-Tillmanns B, et al. Antibodies against beta-amyloid slow cognitive decline in Alzheimer's disease. Neuron. 2003;38:547–54.
9. Boada M, Ramos-Fernández E, Guivernau B, Muñoz FJ, Costa M, Ortiz AM, et al. Treatment of Alzheimer disease using combination therapy with plasma exchange and haemapheresis with albumin and intravenous immunoglobulin: rationale and treatment approach of the AMBAR (Alzheimer management by albumin replacement) study. Neurologia. 2016;31:473–81.
10. Kato M, Kawaguchi K, Nakai S, Murakami K, Hori H, Ohashi A, et al. Potential therapeutic system for Alzheimer's disease: removal of blood Aβs by hemodialyzers and its effect on the cognitive functions of renal-failure patients. J Neural Transm. 2012;12:1533–44.
11. Kitaguchi N, Hasegawa M, Ito S, Kawaguchi K, Hiki Y, Nakai S, et al. A prospective study on blood Aβ levels and the cognitive function of patients with hemodialysis: a potential therapeutic strategy for AD. J Neural Transm. 2015;122:1593–607.
12. Sakai K, Senda T, Hata R, Kuroda M, Hasegawa M, Kato M, et al. Patients that have undergone hemodialysis exhibit lower amyloid deposition in the brain: evidence supporting a therapeutic strategy for ad by removal of blood amyloid. J Alzheimers Dis. 2016;51:997–1002.
13. Reusche E, Koch V, Lindner B, Harrison AP, Friedrich HJ. Alzheimer morphology is not increased in dialysis-associated encephalopathy and long-term hemodialysis. Acta Neuropathol. 2001;101:211–6.
14. Nakai S, Iseki K, Itami N, Ogata S, Kazama JJ, Kimata N, et al. An overview of regular dialysis treatment in Japan (as of 31 December 2010). Ther Apher Dial. 2012;16:483–521.

Is hemodialysis itself a risk factor for dementia? An analysis of nationwide registry data of patients...

171

15. Kopf D, Frölich L. Risk of incident Alzheimer's disease in diabetic patients: a systematic review of prospective trials. J Alzheimers Dis. 2009;16:677–85.

16. Hanyu H, Hirose D, Fukasawa R, Hatanaka H, Namioka N, Sakurai H. Guidelines for the clinical diagnosis of diabetes mellitus-related dementia. J Am Geriatr Soc. 2015;63:1721–3.

17. Nakai S, Iseki K, Itami N, Ogata S, Kazama JJ, Kimata N, et al. Overview of regular dialysis treatment in Japan (as of 31 December 2009). Ther Apher Dial. 2012;16:11–53.

18. Shinzato T, Nakai S, Fujita Y, Takai I, Morita H, Nakane K, et al. Determination of Kt/V and protein catabolic rate using pre- and postdialysis blood urea nitrogen concentrations. Nephron. 1994;67:280–90.

19. Constantinescu MI, Constantinescu DP, Chiş B, Andercou A, Mironiuc IA. Influence of risk factors and comorbidities on the successful therapy and survival of patients with critical limb ischemia. Clujul Med. 2013;86:57–64.

20. Jin WS, Shen LL, Bu XL, Zhang WW, Chen SH, Huang ZL, et al. Peritoneal dialysis reduces amyloid-beta plasma levels in humans and attenuates Alzheimer-associated phenotypes in an APP/PS1 mouse model. Acta Neuropathol. 2017;134:207–20.

21. Fu J, Huang J, Lei M, Luo Z, Zhong X, Huang Y, et al. Prevalence and impact on stroke in patients receiving maintenance hemodialysis versus peritoneal dialysis: a prospective observational study. PLoS One. 2015;10:e0140887.

22. Sekita A, Ninomiya T, Tanizaki Y, Hata J, Yonemoto K, Arima H, et al. Trends in prevalence of Alzheimer's disease and vascular dementia in a Japanese community: the Hisayama study. Acta Psychiatr Scand. 2010;122:319–25.

23. Naganuma T, Takemoto Y. New aspects of cerebrovascular diseases in dialysis patients. Contrib Nephrol. 2015;185:138–46.

24. Hardy JA, Mann DM, Wester P, Winblad B. An integrative hypothesis concerning the pathogenesis and progression of Alzheimer's disease. Neurobiol Aging. 1986;7:489–502.

25. Kishimoto H, Ohara T, Hata J, Ninomiya T, Yoshida D, Mukai N, et al. The long-term association between physical activity and risk of dementia in the community: the Hisayama study. Eur J Epidemiol. 2016;31:267–74.

26. Kawaguchi K, Saigusa A, Yamada S, Gotoh T, Nakai S, Hiki Y, et al. Toward the treatment for Alzheimer's disease: adsorption is primary mechanism of removing amyloid β protein with hollow-fiber dialyzers of the suitable materials, polysulfone and polymethyl methacrylate. J Artif Organs. 2016;19:149–58.

27. Moser VA, Pike CJ. Obesity and sex interact in the regulation of Alzheimer's disease. Neurosci Biobehav Rev. 2016;67:102–18.

28. Monastero R, Palmer K, Qiu C, Winblad B, Fratiglioni L. Heterogeneity in risk factors for cognitive impairment, no dementia: population-based longitudinal study from the Kungsholmen project. Am J Geriatr Psychiatry. 2007;15:60–9.

29. Lilamand M, Cesari M, del Campo N, Cantet C, Soto M, Ousset PJ, et al. Brain amyloid deposition is associated with lower instrumental activities of daily living abilities in older adults. Results from the MAPT study. J Gerontol A Biol Sci Med Sci. 2016;71:391–7.

30. Guerra C, Hua M, Wunsch H. Risk of a diagnosis of dementia for elderly medicare beneficiaries after intensive care. Anesthesiology. 2015;123:1105–12.

31. Grimm G, Stockenhuber F, Schneeweiss B, Madl C, Zeitlhofer J, Schneider B. Improvement of brain function in hemodialysis patients treated with erythropoietin. Kidney Int. 1990;38:480–6.

32. Kurella Tamura M, Yaffe K. Dementia and cognitive impairment in ESRD: diagnostic and therapeutic strategies. Kidney Int. 2011;79:14–22.

19

Positive association of residual kidney function with hemoglobin level in patients on peritoneal dialysis independent of endogenous erythropoietin concentration

Kazuhiko Tsuruya[1,2*†], Kumiko Torisu[2†], Hisako Yoshida[1,3], Shunsuke Yamada[2], Shigeru Tanaka[2], Akihiro Tsuchimoto[2], Masahiro Eriguchi[2], Kiichiro Fujisaki[2], Kosuke Masutani[2] and Takanari Kitazono[2]

Abstract

Background: How residual kidney function (RKF) functions in the prevention of anemia in peritoneal dialysis (PD) patients is unclear. In this study, we investigated the association between RKF and hemoglobin (Hb) level.

Methods: We performed a cross-sectional analysis of the association between RKF, defined as the mean renal creatinine and urea clearance (rCUC), and the Hb level in 50 PD patients registered retrospectively. The independent variable was mean rCUC as continuous or categorical variable by tertile, and the dependent variable was Hb level as continuous or dichotomous variable using Hb cutoff of 10 g/dL. We conducted a multivariable regression analysis and calculated the c-statistic for Hb level < 10 g/dL using a receiver operating characteristic curve.

Results: In multivariable regression analysis, mean rCUC was significantly associated with Hb level independent of dose of erythropoiesis-stimulating agent (ESA) and endogenous erythropoietin (eEPO) concentration. Multivariable adjusted least square means of the Hb level were higher with increase in the mean rCUC tertile. The c-statistic (95% confidential interval) for a Hb level < 10 g/dL was significantly greater in the model with mean rCUC than without [0.931 (0.789–0.980) vs. 0.856 (0.697–0.939), $P = 0.044$].

Conclusion: A decline in RKF is associated with anemia in PD patients independent of ESA dose and eEPO concentration.

Keywords: Anemia, Creatinine clearance, Erythropoietin, Hemoglobin, Kt/V, Residual kidney function

Background

The introduction of erythropoiesis-stimulating agent (ESA) to clinical settings for renal anemia has allowed the easy management of anemia in patients with chronic kidney disease (CKD). Anemia control is considered important for the prediction of mortality and increase in quality of life in CKD patients. However, recent studies have demonstrated that a large dose of ESA results in a high mortality rate and high incidence of cardiovascular events such as stroke in hemodialysis (HD) patients [1] and those with non-dialysis-dependent CKD [2–4].

The importance of residual kidney function (RKF) in the survival of chronic dialysis patients, especially peritoneal dialysis (PD) patients, was recently reported [5–7]. The "Cardiovascular and Metabolic Clinical Practice Guidelines for Peritoneal Dialysis Patients" by the International Society for Peritoneal Dialysis in 2015 also emphasize the importance of RKF in cardiovascular disease and mortality, recommending that PD patients undergo monitoring of RKF at least once every 6 months [8].

* Correspondence: tsuruya@intmed2.med.kyushu-u.ac.jp
†Equal contributors
[1]Department of Integrated Therapy for Chronic Kidney Disease, Graduate School of Medical Sciences, Kyushu University, 3-1-1 Maidashi, Higashi-ku, Fukuoka 812-8582, Japan
[2]Department of Medicine and Clinical Science, Graduate School of Medical Sciences, Kyushu University, Fukuoka, Japan
Full list of author information is available at the end of the article

Wang and Lai [5] also stressed the importance of RKF in anemia management. Lopez-Menchero et al. [9] reported that in addition to ESA use and iron levels, RKF also correlated significantly with hemoglobin (Hb) levels in PD patients. A recent report by Penne et al. [10] showed a strong relation between RKF and improved anemia control in HD patients. However, how RKF functions and how the endogenous erythropoietin (eEPO) concentration is involved in the prevention of anemia in CKD patients is unclear.

This study investigated the association between RKF and Hb levels from the perspective of the mechanism by measuring eEPO concentrations in PD patients.

Methods

Study participants

The study population comprised 50 patients aged > 18 years who were treated with PD at our hospital between May 2006 and March 2011 and had been followed for at least 6 months. Patients, who did not have any bone marrow disease or cirrhosis of the liver, were registered retrospectively. This study is a subanalysis of our multicenter cohort study (Fukuoka Peritoneal Dialysis Database Study), which was conducted in accordance with the Declaration of Helsinki, was approved by the Institutional Review Boards of Kyushu University Hospital (no. 26-223), and was registered at the University Hospital Medical Information Network (UMIN000018902).

Data collection

Blood, 24-h urine, and peritoneal dialysate samples were collected from PD patients at least every 6 months to evaluate their dialysis and peritoneal status as well as medical condition [11]. Demographic, clinical, and prescription data at each 6-monthly examination were also recorded based on the guidelines [12]. Venous blood was collected at a regular outpatient clinic visit after fasting, and part of the blood sample was centrifuged at $3000 \times g$ at 4 °C for 15 min and stored at − 80 °C until analysis, except for those used for standard biochemical analyses.

Calculation of Hb levels and ESA dose

Hb levels were assessed based on mean values during the last 3 months of the observation period. Darbepoetin alfa was administered as the ESA in all 50 patients to achieve and maintain a Hb level of approximately 11 g/dL according to the guidelines for anemia in CKD [13, 14]. The ESA dose was evaluated based on the weekly dose calculated from the total dose during the last 3 months of the observation period.

Measurements of RKF, dialysis adequacy, and peritoneal membrane solute transport

RKF and dialysis adequacy, which were measured every 6 months in each patient, were calculated as the weekly urea clearance (Kt/V) and creatinine clearance (Ccr) from 24-h urinary and dialysate clearance, by direct measurement of urea in the urine and each dialysate exchange. The volume of urea distribution in a patient, which is the patient's total body water (TBW), was calculated according to the equations of Hume and Weyers—men: TBW (L) = 0.297 body weight (kg) + 0.195 body height (cm) – 14.013; women: TBW (L) = 0.184 body weight (kg) + 0345 body height (cm) – 35.27 [15]. RKF was defined as the mean renal creatinine and urea clearance (rCUC). Peritoneal membrane solute transport was assessed by the peritoneal equilibration test. A standard 4-h dwell period was used (first exchange of the day), with a 2.27% glucose concentration 2-L volume exchange. The patients used their usual overnight dialysis regimes, and both the overnight and the test drainage volumes were measured. The dialysate-to-plasma ratio of creatinine at the completion of the 4-h dwell period (D/Pcr) was used as the estimate of low molecular weight solute transport.

Measurement of serum eEPO concentration

Serum eEPO concentration was measured by a chemiluminescent enzyme immunoassay (SRL Inc., Fukuoka, Japan).

Statistical analysis

Results are expressed as the mean ± standard deviation, median (interquartile range [IQR]), or number (percentage) as appropriate. The trend among mean rCUC groups was assessed using Cochran-Armitage test for the categorical variables and Jonckheere-Terpstra test for continuous variables. The primary outcome variable was the mean Hb level during the last 3 months of the observation period. Both univariable and multivariable linear regression analyses were conducted to assess the associations between the Hb level and the variables. Variables showing a P value of < 0.05 in the univariable analysis were included in addition to cardiothoracic ratio (CTR), ESA dose, and log-transformed eEPO concentration in the multivariable analyses. To investigate whether the accuracy of predicting Hb levels improved after addition of the mean rCUC into a basic model (model 1) including the potential risk factors that were significantly associated with Hb levels in the univariable analysis in addition to CTR, ESA dose, and eEPO concentration, we calculated the c-statistic for Hb levels < 10 g/dL using a receiver operating characteristic curve. For two-tailed tests, $P < 0.05$ was considered significant in all analyses. All statistical analyses were conducted using JMP 11.2 software (SAS Institute, Tokyo, Japan) and RStudio Version 0.99.896.

Results

The characteristics and laboratory data of the 50 patients according to the tertiles of mean rCUC are

Table 1 Clinical characteristics according to tertiles of mean rCUC

	Total (N = 50)	T1 (mean rCUC < 11.7 L/week/1.73m^2), n = 17	T2 (mean rCUC 11.8–29.8 L/week/1.73m^2), n = 17	T3 (mean rCUC ≥ 29.9 L/week/1.73m^2), n = 16	P for trend
Male sex, n (%)	37 (74.0)	12 (70.6)	11 (64.7)	14 (87.5)	0.277
Age, years	54 ± 14	53 ± 14	55 ± 15	55 ± 15	0.499
Dialysis duration, months	20.2 ± 11.6	23.4 ± 12.3	18.1 ± 9.7	18.8 ± 12.5	0.213
Original disease					
DN, n (%)	16 (32.0)	7 (41.2)	6 (35.3)	3 (18.8)	0.167
Non-DN, n (%)	34 (68.0)	10 (58.8)	11 (64.7)	13 (81.2)	
Blood pressure, mmHg					
Systolic	139 ± 14	141 ± 11	137 ± 18	139 ± 13	0.845
Diastolic	81 ± 11	82 ± 9	78 ± 16	82 ± 7	0.581
Daily alcohol consumption, n (%)	20 (40.0)	5 (29.4)	8 (47.1)	7 (43.8)	0.394
Current smoker, n (%)	9 (18.0)	3 (17.7)	2 (11.8)	4 (25.0)	0.593
Past histories of CVD, n (%)	8 (16.0)	2 (11.8)	4 (23.5)	2 (12.5)	0.939
History of peritonitis, n (%)	8 (16.0)	1 (5.9)	3 (17.7)	4 (25.0)	0.133
Body mass index, kg/m^2	22.9 ± 2.9	22.4 ± 2.4	22.1 ± 2.7	24.2 ± 3.2	0.124
CTR, %	48.2 ± 5.4	49.8 ± 4.7	48.3 ± 4.6	46.6 ± 6.7	0.075
Dialysis modality					
APD, n (%)	22 (44.0)	11 (64.7)	8 (47.1)	9 (56.3)	0.614
CAPD, n (%)	28 (56.0)	6 (35.3)	9 (52.9)	7 (43.7)	
Use of icodextrin, n (%)	41 (82.0)	16 (94.1)	13 (76.5)	12 (75.0)	0.150
Use of HG dialysate, n (%)	17 (34.0)	11 (64.7)	4 (23.5)	2 (12.5)	0.002
Dose of ESA, μg/week	34 ± 18	37 ± 16	32 ± 16	31 ± 23	0.206
Total Kt/V, /week	1.71 ± 0.34	1.66 ± 0.42	1.61 ± 0.31	1.87 ± 0.23	0.011
Renal Kt/V, /week	0.46 ± 0.37	0.10 ± 0.11	0.42 ± 0.18	0.88 ± 0.27	< 0.001
Peritoneal Kt/V, /week	1.25 ± 0.38	1.56 ± 0.41	1.19 ± 0.21	0.99 ± 0.22	< 0.001
Renal Ccr, L/week, /week	29.2 ± 26.9	5.1 ± 4.9	27.4 ± 8.9	56.8 ± 27.8	< 0.001
Urine volume, L/day	0.80 ± 0.64	0.22 ± 0.24	0.76 ± 0.38	1.44 ± 0.55	< 0.001
Mean rCUC, L/week/1.73m^2	22.7 ± 19.4	4.2 ± 4.2	20.5 ± 6.2	44.5 ± 16.5	< 0.001
D/Pcr	0.73 ± 0.16	0.76 ± 0.16	0.72 ± 0.17	0.70 ± 0.16	0.328
Prescriptions, n (%)					
RAS inhibitors	48 (96.0)	17 (100.0)	15 (88.2)	16 (100)	0.972
Calcium channel blockers	37 (74.0)	15 (88.2)	10 (58.8)	12 (75.0)	0.370
β blockers	23 (46.0)	11 (64.7)	6 (35.3)	6 (37.5)	0.113
Calcium-containing PBs	44 (88.0)	13 (76.5)	16 (94.1)	15 (93.8)	0.123
Non-calcium containing PBs	29 (58.0)	14 (82.4)	6 (35.3)	9 (56.3)	0.119
Iron preparations	11 (22.5)	7 (41.2)	2 (11.8)	2 (13.3)	0.054
Vitamin D	27 (54.0)	9 (52.9)	7 (41.2)	11 (68.8)	0.375
Cinacalcet hydrochloride	4 (8.0)	1 (5.9)	1 (5.9)	2 (12.5)	0.488

Values are expressed as mean ± standard deviation or number (percentage) as appropriate

Abbreviations: *APD* automated peritoneal dialysis, *CAPD* continuous ambulatory peritoneal dialysis, *Ccr* creatinine clearance, *CTR* cardiothoracic ratio, *CVD* cardiovascular disease, *DN* diabetic nephropathy, *D/Pcr* dialysate-to-plasma creatinine ratio, *ESA* erythropoiesis-stimulating agent, *HG* high-glucose (2.5%), *Kt/V* urea clearance, *PBs* phosphate binders, *RAS* renin-angiotensin system, *rCUC* renal creatinine and urea clearance

shown in Tables 1 and 2, respectively. Total Kt/V, renal Kt/V, renal Ccr, urine volume, sodium, and chloride were significantly higher with greater mean rCUC, while the prevalence of diabetic nephropathy (DN) and high-glucose dialysate users, peritoneal Kt/V, serum creatinine, brain natriuretic peptide (BNP), and β_2-microglobulin (BMG) were lower with greater mean rCUC.

Positive association of residual kidney function with hemoglobin level in patients on peritoneal...

175

Table 2 Laboratory data according to tertiles of mean rCUC

	Total (N = 50)	T1 (mean rCUC < 11.7 L/week/1.73m²), n = 17	T2 (mean rCUC 11.8–29.8 L/week/1.73m²), n = 17	T3 (mean rCUC ≥ 29.9 L/week/1.73m²), n = 16	P for trend
Total protein, g/dL	6.4 ± 0.7	6.5 ± 0.6	6.2 ± 0.6	6.4 ± 0.7	0.539
Albumin, g/dL	3.5 ± 0.4	3.5 ± 0.4	3.4 ± 0.5	3.6 ± 0.4	0.270
Blood urea nitrogen, mg/dL	65 ± 13	63 ± 10	68 ± 17	67 ± 12	0.460
Creatinine, mg/dL	11.5 ± 3.0	13.1 ± 3.1	11.1 ± 2.3	10.1 ± 3.0	0.003
Uric acid, mg/dL	6.8 ± 1.1	6.7 ± 1.2	6.7 ± 1.0	6.9 ± 1.1	0.341
Sodium, mEq/L	136 ± 4	134 ± 3	137 ± 3	139 ± 2	< 0.001
Potassium, mEq/L	4.4 ± 0.6	4.4 ± 0.7	4.2 ± 0.6	4.7 ± 0.5	0.306
Chloride, mEq/L	98 ± 5	94 ± 3	98 ± 4	102 ± 4	< 0.001
Calcium, mg/dL	9.5 ± 0.4	9.5 ± 0.4	9.5 ± 0.5	9.5 ± 0.4	0.643
Phosphate, mg/dL	5.4 ± 1.2	5.4 ± 1.7	5.3 ± 0.7	5.4 ± 1.2	0.894
Glucose, mg/dL	108 ± 31	112 ± 35	105 ± 26	107 ± 34	0.408
Total cholesterol, mg/dL	182 ± 44	168 ± 33	195 ± 58	183 ± 37	0.355
Triglyceride, mg/dL	126 ± 73	126 ± 84	114 ± 53	138 ± 82	0.569
LDL-C, mg/dL	96 ± 27	85 ± 22	105 ± 26	100 ± 30	0.176
HDL-C, mg/dL	52 ± 18	53 ± 14	53 ± 22	52 ± 16	0.794
Hb, g/dL	10.2 ± 1.1	9.8 ± 1.0	10.0 ± 1.2	10.9 ± 0.7	< 0.001
C-reactive protein, mg/dL	0.08 (0.03–0.13)	0.07 (0.04–0.15)	0.08 (0.03–0.22)	0.06 (0.03–0.11)	0.631
Serum iron, μg/dL	87 ± 26	84 ± 26	87 ± 31	88 ± 22	0.735
TIBC, μg/dL	283 ± 34	301 ± 34	268 ± 37	281 ± 22	0.074
TSAT, %	30.7 ± 9.3	28.2 ± 8.8	32.2 ± 10.3	31.7 ± 8.7	0.213
Ferritin, ng/mL	130 (80–220)	108 (73–205)	216 (89–306)	113 (59–177)	0.643
Whole PTH, pg/mL	94 (55–151)	89 (55–128)	92 (37–173)	97 (52–163)	0.801
BNP, pg/mL	86 (37–298)	222 (67–468)	101 (34–433)	47 (20–116)	0.023
eEPO, U/mL	16.0 (13.6–25.1)	22.1 (13.9–24.9)	17.7 (13.9–24.3)	18.6 (14.0–23.7)	0.618
BMG, mg/L	23.2 (18.1–28.8)	28.6 (26.6–37.3)	22.8 (19.9–29.6)	17.6 (14.6–18.9)	< 0.001
HbA1c, %	5.4 ± 0.7	5.3 ± 0.8	5.5 ± 0.7	5.5 ± 0.8	0.128

Values are expressed as mean ± standard deviation or median (interquartile range) as appropriate

Abbreviations: *BMG* β$_2$-microglobulin, *BNP* brain natriuretic peptide, *eEPO* endogenous erythropoietin, *Hb* hemoglobin, *HbA1c* hemoglobin A1c, *HDL-C* high-density lipoprotein cholesterol, *LDL-C* low-density lipoprotein cholesterol, *PTH* parathyroid hormone, *rCUC* renal creatinine and urea clearance, *TIBC* total iron binding capacity, *TSAT* transferrin saturation

The mean Hb levels were higher with greater mean rCUC (Table 2). This trend remained statistically significant [least square mean ± standard error: 9.7 ± 0.2, 10.2 ± 0.2, and 10.8 ± 0.2 in T1, T2, and T3, respectively; P for trend = 0.002] even after adjustment for model 1 (dialysis duration, current smoking habit, dose of ESA, log-transformed ferritin, log-transformed BNP, log-transformed eEPO, total Kt/V, and CTR) by analysis of covariance (Fig. 1).

Univariable regression analysis revealed that dialysis duration, current smoker, total Kt/V, renal Kt/V, renal Ccr, mean rCUC, and urine volume were positively associated and that log-transformed ferritin and log-transformed BNP were negatively associated with Hb levels. In the multivariable regression analysis, containing model 1 plus mean rCUC, dialysis duration and mean rCUC remained

significant (Table 3). We did not enter renal Kt/V, renal Ccr, and urine volume in the multivariable model because of their multicollinearity with mean rCUC (r = 0.919, 0.980, and − 0.756) in the multivariable analysis.

To evaluate the impact of the mean rCUC on the accuracy of assessment, we compared the discriminatory abilities between model 1 (dialysis duration, current smoking habit, dose of ESA, log-transformed ferritin, log-transformed BNP, log-transformed eEPO, total Kt/V, and CTR) and the following models: model 1 plus mean rCUC, urine volume, renal Kt/V, renal Ccr, or log-transformed BMG. The c-statistic (95% confidential interval) for a Hb level < 10 g/dL was significantly greater in model 1 plus mean rCUC than model 1 [0.931 (0.789–0.980) vs. 0.856 (0.697–0.939), P = 0.044]. However, no significant increases in the c-statistic (95% confidential

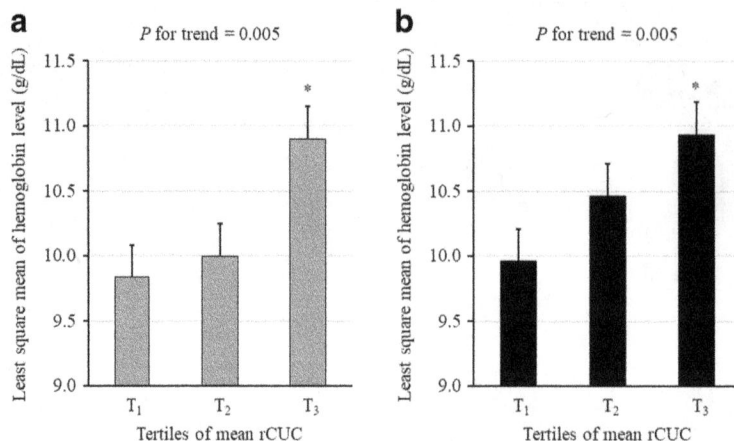

Fig. 1 Hb level according to the tertiles of mean rCUC. Least square means of Hb level according to the tertiles of mean rCUC in the univariable model (**a**) and the multivariable-adjusted regression model (**b**). A linear regression model was used to compare the least square mean among the tertile groups. *$P < 0.01$ vs. T1. Abbreviations: *Hb* hemoglobin, *rCUC* renal creatinine and urea clearance, *T* tertile

interval) were found in model 1 plus urine volume [0.906 (0.776–0.964), $P = 0.192$], renal Kt/V [0.924 (0.767–0.978), $P = 0.061$], renal Ccr [0.929 (0.795–0.978), $P = 0.058$], or log-transformed BMG [0.880 (0.738–0.950), $P = 0.491$] compared with model 1.

Discussion

The present study suggests that RKF represents an important correlate of Hb level in PD patients and that this correlation is independent of ESA dose and eEPO concentration. Therefore, the findings suggest that hematopoiesis-inhibiting uremic toxins, which are mainly removed by RKF, but not by PD, are a major cause of anemia in PD patients.

Ifudu et al. [16] reported an independent positive correlation between dialysis dose and hematocrit level when investigating the contribution of hematocrit in 135 HD patients receiving ESA. A comparison of 20 patients whose dialysis dose was increased with 20 patients with similar baseline characteristics whose dialysis dose was unaltered showed that the hematocrit level was significantly increased in the former group after 6 weeks, but remained unchanged in the latter group, demonstrating the importance of dialysis dose on anemia management. In a retrospective study by Matsuo et al. [17], in which 53 patients on PD monotherapy were moved to a combined regimen of HD + PD following a diagnosis of underdialysis and/or overhydration with declining RKF, a significant increase in Hb levels (from 8.2 to 10.7 g/dL) was found without an increase in ESA dose. The present study of PD monotherapy, however, found no evidence to suggest a significant correlation between dialysis dose (peritoneal Kt/V) and Hb level. We consider that this was because of the superior solute clearance of HD compared with PD. Evenepoel et al. [18] reported that high-flux HD delivered significantly higher clearance of all retention

solutes, especially BMG and p-cresol compared with peritoneal dialysis, although renal clearances, conversely, were significantly higher in patients in PD.

A significant association of total Kt/V, calculated by the addition of renal Kt/V to peritoneal Kt/V, with Hb level, was observed in the univariable regression analysis. However, the significant association was diminished in the multivariable regression analysis (Table 3). Furthermore, no association was found between peritoneal Kt/V and Hb level. According to these findings, maintaining RKF, but not an increase in dialysis dose, is important for the control of Hb levels in PD patients. Taken together, these findings show that standard PD is insufficient to eliminate factors influencing anemia, suggesting the presence of a hematopoiesis-inhibiting substance that is typically removed and eliminated by RKF, but not by PD.

The mechanism of the association between RKF and Hb remains to be elucidated. In the present study, log-transformed BMG was closely correlated with mean rCUC ($r = -0.736$, $P < 0.001$), suggesting the possibility of this factor as an important cause of low RKF-associated anemia. However, a significant association was not observed in the univariable regression analysis (Table 3) and also in the multivariable regression analysis when log-transformed BMG was entered instead of mean rCUC (Additional file 1: Table S1).

However, Pawlak et al. [19] described the contribution of quinolinic acid in the development of anemia in CKD patients. Quinolinic acid is an intermediate of the metabolic pathway responsible for the conversion of tryptophan into nicotinic acid and is an N-methyl-D-aspartate (NMDA) receptor agonist with putative neuroexcitatory and neurotoxic properties [20]. Another candidate for the potential contributing factor of anemia is indoxyl sulfate, a representative uremic toxin. Chiang et al. [21]

Table 3 Univariable and multivariable regression analysis for Hb levels

	Univariable		Multivariable		
	β-coefficient	P	β-coefficient	Standardized β	P
Male sex	− 0.223	0.534			
Age, years	0.005	0.658			
Primary disease of kidney disease, DN	− 0.383	0.254			
Dialysis duration, months	*0.038*	*0.004*	*0.033*	*0.346*	*0.008*
Body mass index, kg/m²	− 0.020	0.713			
Systolic blood pressure, mmHg	− 0.014	0.199			
Diastolic blood pressure, mmHg	0.007	0.605			
Daily alcohol consumption	0.405	0.204			
Current smoker	*0.927*	*0.020*	0.240	0.170	0.211
Past histories of CVD	0.553	0.194			
History of peritonitis	− 0.134	0.756			
CTR, %	− 0.032	0.277	0.037	0.181	0.280
Dose of ESA, µg/week	− 0.002	0.823	0.001	0.010	0.943
Dialysis modality, APD	− 0.078	0.805			
Use of icodextrin	0.319	0.435			
Use of HG dialysate	0.258	0.437			
Total Kt/V, /week	*1.038*	*0.021*	0.330	0.104	0.425
Renal Kt/V, /week	*1.400*	*< 0.001*			
Peritoneal Kt/V, /week	− 0.501	0.232			
Renal Ccr, L/week, /week/1.73m²	*0.017*	*0.003*			
Mean rCUC, L/week	*0.024*	*0.002*	*0.018*	*0.321*	*0.045*
Urine volume, L/day	*0.630*	*0.009*			
D/Pcr	− 0.881	0.371			
Total protein, g/dL	0.322	0.183			
Albumin, g/dL	0.517	0.150			
Blood urea nitrogen, mg/dL	− 0.020	0.103			
Creatinine, mg/dL	− 0.092	0.077			
Uric acid, mg/dL	0.123	0.393			
Sodium, mEq/L	0.048	0.272			
Potassium, mEq/L	0.082	0.752			
Chloride, mEq/L	0.055	0.109			
Calcium, mg/dL	0.098	0.802			
Phosphate, mg/dL	− 0.136	0.291			
Glucose, mg/dL	0.001	0.835			
Total cholesterol, mg/dL	− 0.0001	0.969			
Triglyceride, mg/dL	0.003	0.209			
LDL-C, mg/dL	0.005	0.390			
HDL-C, mg/dL	− 0.010	0.283			
Ln C-reactive protein, mg/dL	− 0.123	0.329			
Serum iron, µg/dL	− 0.004	0.539			
TIBC, µg/dL	− 0.005	0.252			
TSAT, %	− 0.004	0.813			

Table 3 Univariable and multivariable regression analysis for Hb levels *(Continued)*

Ln ferritin, ng/dL	*− 0.569*	*0.009*	− 0.276	− 0.177	0.221
Ln whole PTH, pg/mL	− 0.018	0.924			
Ln BNP, pg/mL	*− 0.216*	*0.021*	− 0.146	− 0.220	0.233
Ln eEPO, U/mL	− 0.042	0.897	− 0.046	− 0.021	0.884
Ln BMG, mg/L	− 0.545	0.200			
HbA1c, %	0.098	0.649			
Use of RAS inhibitors	1.248	0.116			
Use of calcium channel blockers	− 0.431	0.227			
Use of β blockers	− 0.153	0.629			
Use of calcium-containing PBs	− 0.135	0.780			
Use of non-calcium-containing PBs	− 0.145	0.650			
Use of iron preparations	0.044	0.908			
Use of vitamin D	− 0.108	0.733			
Use of cinacalcet hydrochloride	0.175	0.764			

Variables with a *P* value of < 0.05 in the univariable analysis were included in addition to CTR, ESA dose, and log-transformed eEPO in the multivariable analyses. Renal Kt/V, renal Ccr, and urine volume were excluded from multivariable analysis because of their multicollinearity with mean rCUC. The values written in Italic letter show significant association with Hb levels. A *P* value of < 0.05 was considered statistically significant

Abbreviations: *APD* automated peritoneal dialysis, *BMG* β₂-microglobulin, *BNP* brain natriuretic peptide, *CTR* cardiothoracic ratio, *Ccr* creatinine clearance, *DN* diabetic nephropathy, *D/Pcr* dialysate-to-plasma creatinine ratio, *eEPO* endogenous erythropoietin, *ESA* erythropoiesis-stimulating agent, *Hb* hemoglobin, *HbA1c* hemoglobin A1c, *HDL-C* high-density lipoprotein cholesterol, *HG* high-glucose (2.5%), *Kt/V* urea clearance, *LDL-C* low-density lipoprotein cholesterol, *Ln* log-transformed, *PBs* phosphate binders, *PTH* parathyroid hormone, *RAS* renin-angiotensin system, *rCUC* renal creatinine and urea clearance, *TIBC* total iron binding capacity, *TSAT* transferrin saturation

demonstrated that indoxyl sulfate treatment suppressed EPO mRNA expression and decreased the nuclear accumulation of hypoxia-inducible factor-α proteins and hypoxia-responsive element-luciferase activity following hypoxia. This suggested a potential connection between a uremic toxin and the desensitization of the oxygen-sensing mechanism in EPO-producing cells, which may explain anemia in CKD patients. However, these mechanisms are mediated by decreased eEPO production and do not explain the lack of a relationship between eEPO concentration and Hb levels observed in the present study.

More recently, two observational reports on anemia in PD patients have been published [22, 23]. Huang et al. [22] reported that serum indoxyl sulfate was negatively correlated with Hb level in 90 non-anuric PD patients but did not show the association of Kt/V and Hb levels. Meanwhile, Ryta et al. [23] reported the association of total Kt/V with Hb levels both in 2180 prevalent and 88 incident PD patients. However, this report unfortunately did not show the association of renal Kt/V and Hb level. The findings of the two reports are slightly different from the present study but support our speculation that accumulation of uremic toxins may be involved in anemia in PD patients.

While several studies have reported the role of iron metabolism, renin-angiotensin system inhibitors, BMG levels, serum albumin levels, parathyroid hormone, C-reactive protein, and other factors in anemia management

[24–26], we did not find any correlations of these factors in the present study.

Distribution of original disease was different among three tertiles; that is, prevalence of DN increased with a decrease in mean rCUC, although not significant. To date, there have been a few reports on the association between Hb levels and diabetes, in which diabetic patients were reported to require less ESA than non-diabetic patients [27], whereas no association was reported between diabetes and anemia [28]. In our study, no significant association was observed between DN and Hb levels in the univariable analysis, and the association between mean rCUC and Hb level was robust even when the variable "diabetic nephropathy" was added to the multivariable model. Thus, we consider that this bias would not affect this association.

This study had some limitations. It had a cross-sectional design, which limited the interpretation of the results with respect to cause and effect. Another limitation is the small number of subjects included in our study. Moreover, we could not identify the uremic toxin that might inhibit erythropoiesis or shorten the red blood cell life span. Nevertheless, there are some strengths in this study that eEPO concentration was measured and the involvement of eEPO concentration was examined in the association between RKF and Hb level. To the best of our knowledge, this study is the first report which focused on these associations.

Conclusion

The findings in the present study demonstrated that a decline in RKF is associated with a low Hb level independent of ESA dose and eEPO concentration. This suggests the existence of a uremic toxin as an inducer of anemia, which is probably eliminated mainly by RKF, but not by PD. Further research is needed to clarify the specific mechanism responsible for anemia in PD patients.

Acknowledgements
We thank the investigators and the doctors who participated in the present study. We thank Edanz Editing (http://www.edanzediting.co.jp/) for carefully reading and preparing our manuscript.

Funding
None to declare.

Authors' contributions
KaT and KuT contributed to the research idea and study design. KaT, KuT, HY, SY, ST, AT, ME, KF, and KM carried out the data acquisition. KuT and HY participated in the data cleaning. KaT and KuT interpreted the data. KaT and HY participated in the statistical analysis. TK carried out the supervision. Each author contributed important intellectual content during manuscript drafting or revision and accepts accountability for the overall work by ensuring that questions pertaining to the accuracy or integrity of any portion of the work are appropriately investigated and resolved. KaT takes responsibility that this study has been reported honestly, accurately, and transparently; that no important aspects of the study have been omitted; and that any discrepancies from the study as planned have been explained. All authors read and approved the final manuscript.

Competing interests
The authors declare that they have no competing interests.

Author details
[1]Department of Integrated Therapy for Chronic Kidney Disease, Graduate School of Medical Sciences, Kyushu University, 3-1-1 Maidashi, Higashi-ku, Fukuoka 812-8582, Japan. [2]Department of Medicine and Clinical Science, Graduate School of Medical Sciences, Kyushu University, Fukuoka, Japan. [3]Clinical Research Center, Saga University Hospital, Saga, Japan.

References
1. Besarab A, Bolton WK, Browne JK, Egrie JC, Nissenson AR, Okamoto DM, et al. The effects of normal as compared with low hematocrit values in patients with cardiac disease who are receiving hemodialysis and epoetin. N Engl J Med. 1998;339:584–90.
2. Drueke TB, Locatelli F, Clyne N, Eckardt KU, Macdougall IC, Tsakiris D, et al. Normalization of hemoglobin level in patients with chronic kidney disease and anemia. N Engl J Med. 2006;355:2071–84.
3. Singh AK, Szczech L, Tang KL, Barnhart H, Sapp S, Wolfson M, et al. Correction of anemia with epoetin alfa in chronic kidney disease. N Engl J Med. 2006;355:2085–98.
4. Pfeffer MA, Burdmann EA, Chen CY, Cooper ME, de Zeeuw D, Eckardt KU, et al. A trial of darbepoetin alfa in type 2 diabetes and chronic kidney disease. N Engl J Med. 2009;361:2019–32.
5. Wang AY, Lai KN. The importance of residual renal function in dialysis patients. Kidney Int. 2006;69:1726–32.

6. Marron B, Remon C, Perez-Fontan M, Quiros P, Ortiz A. Benefits of preserving residual renal function in peritoneal dialysis. Kidney Int Suppl. 2008;108:S42–51.
7. Perl J, Bargman JM. The importance of residual kidney function for patients on dialysis: a critical review. Am J Kidney Dis. 2009;53:1068–81.
8. Wang AY, Brimble KS, Brunier G, Holt SG, Jha V, Johnson DW, et al. ISPD cardiovascular and metabolic guidelines in adult peritoneal dialysis patients part I—assessment and management of various cardiovascular risk factors. Perit Dial Int. 2015;35:379–87.
9. Lopez-Menchero R, Miguel A, Garcia-Ramon R, Perez-Contreras J, Girbes V. Importance of residual renal function in continuous ambulatory peritoneal dialysis: its influence on different parameters of renal replacement treatment. Nephron. 1999;83:219–25.
10. Penne EL, van der Weerd NC, Grooteman MP, Mazairac AH, van den Dorpel MA, Nube MJ, et al. Role of residual renal function in phosphate control and anemia management in chronic hemodialysis patients. Clin J Am Soc Nephrol. 2011;6:281–9.
11. Yamada S, Tsuruya K, Taniguchi M, Yoshida H, Tokumoto M, Hasegawa S, et al. Relationship between residual renal function and serum fibroblast growth factor 23 in patients on peritoneal dialysis. Ther Apher Dial. 2014;18:383–90.
12. Working Group Committee for Preparation of Guidelines for Peritoneal Dialysis, Japanese Society for Dialysis Therapy. 2009 Japanese Society for Dialysis Therapy guidelines for peritoneal dialysis. Ther Apher Dial. 2010;14:489–504.
13. KDOQI, National Kidney Foundation. KDOQI clinical practice guidelines and clinical practice recommendations for anemia in chronic kidney disease. Am J Kidney Dis. 2006;47:S11–145.
14. Tsubakihara Y, Nishi S, Akiba T, Hirakata H, Iseki K, Kubota M, et al. 2008 Japanese Society for Dialysis Therapy: guidelines for renal anemia in chronic kidney disease. Ther Apher Dial. 2010;14:240–75.
15. Hume R, Weyers E. Relationship between total body water and surface area in normal and obese subjects. J Clin Pathol. 1971;24:234–8.
16. Ifudu O, Feldman J, Friedman EA. The intensity of hemodialysis and the response to erythropoietin in patients with end-stage renal disease. N Engl J Med. 1996;334:420–5.
17. Matsuo N, Yokoyama K, Maruyama Y, Ueda Y, Yoshida H, Tanno Y, et al. Clinical impact of a combined therapy of peritoneal dialysis and hemodialysis. Clin Nephrol. 2010;74:209–16.
18. Evenepoel P, Bammens B, Verbeke K, Vanrenterghem Y. Superior dialytic clearance of beta(2)-microglobulin and p-cresol by high-flux hemodialysis as compared to peritoneal dialysis. Kidney Int. 2006;70:794–9.
19. Pawlak D, Koda M, Pawlak S, Wolczynski S, Buczko W. Contribution of quinolinic acid in the development of anemia in renal insufficiency. Am J Physiol Renal Physiol. 2003;284:F693–700.
20. Schwarcz R, Whetsell WO Jr, Mangano RM. Quinolinic acid: an endogenous metabolite that produces axon-sparing lesions in rat brain. Science. 1983;219:316–8.
21. Chiang CK, Tanaka T, Inagi R, Fujita T, Nangaku M. Indoxyl sulfate, a representative uremic toxin, suppresses erythropoietin production in a HIF-dependent manner. Lab Investig. 2011;91:1564–71.
22. Huang JY, Hsu CW, Yang CW, Hung CC, Huang WH. Role of anuria in the relationship between indoxyl sulfate and anemia in peritoneal dialysis patients. Ther Clin Risk Manag. 2016;12:1797–803.
23. Ryta A, Chmielewski M, Debska-Slizien A, Jagodzinski P, Sikorska-Wisniewska M, Lichodziejewska-Niemierko M. Impact of gender and dialysis adequacy on anaemia in peritoneal dialysis. Int Urol Nephrol. 2017;49:903-8.
24. Tonelli M, Blake PG, Muirhead N. Predictors of erythropoietin responsiveness in chronic hemodialysis patients. ASAIO J. 2001;47:82–5.
25. Nakamoto H, Kanno Y, Okada H, Suzuki H. Erythropoietin resistance in patients on continuous ambulatory peritoneal dialysis. Adv Perit Dial. 2004;20:111–6.
26. Pajek J, Bucar-Pajek M, Grego K, Gucek A, Bevc S, Ekart R, et al. Epoetin responsiveness in peritoneal dialysis patients: a multi-center Slovenian study. Ther Apher Dial. 2005;9:228–32.
27. Mitwalli A, Alsuwaida A, Wakeel JA, Usama S, Zainalddain N, Al Ghonaim M, et al. Do diabetic dialysis patients require more or less of erythropoietin? Ann Saudi Med. 2013;33:457–63.
28. Oliveira MC, Ammirati AL, Andreolli MC, Nadalleto MA, Barros CB, Canziani ME. Anemia in patients undergoing ambulatory peritoneal dialysis: prevalence and associated factors. J Bras Nefrol. 2016;38:76–81.

20

Cardiovascular disease, mortality, and magnesium in chronic kidney disease: growing interest in magnesium-related interventions

Ryota Ikee

Abstract

Magnesium (Mg) is an essential element that plays pivotal roles in a number of biological processes in the human body. Hypomagnesemia is involved in the pathophysiology of hypertension, vascular calcification, and metabolic derangements including diabetes mellitus and dyslipidemia, which are all risk factors for cardiovascular disease, the leading cause of mortality and morbidity in patients with chronic kidney disease (CKD). Hypomagnesemia is also associated with the development and progression of CKD. As CKD advances, renal Mg excretion decreases and hypermagnesemia emerges in end-stage renal disease (ESRD). In addition, dialysates with high Mg concentrations, which were used in the early era of dialysis therapy, increased the risk of hypermagnesemia, and thus, the dialysate Mg composition has since been reduced. Accordingly, dialysis patients in the modern era commonly have normomagnesemia or even hypomagnesemia. The relationships between hypomagnesemia and cardiovascular disease and mortality have been increasingly reported in observational studies in CKD/ESRD. However, these relationships may be attenuated by a patient's race or region. Although dialysates with higher Mg concentrations or Mg-containing phosphate binders appear to be promising in this setting, only a few interventional studies have examined the effects of Mg supplementation on cardiovascular lesions. Furthermore, the effects of Mg supplementation on mortality have not yet been investigated as a primary end-point in randomized controlled trials. Further studies are required in order to establish the efficacy and safety of Mg in CKD patients.

Keywords: Magnesium, Chronic kidney disease, Dialysis, Cardiovascular disease, Vascular calcification, Mortality, Dialysate composition, Phosphate binder

Background

Magnesium (Mg), the fourth most abundant cation in the human body, is a co-factor in more than 300 enzyme systems that regulate a number of biological processes, such as protein synthesis, muscle and nerve transmission, neuromuscular conduction, and signal transduction. It is also involved in the cardiovascular system via the regulation of vascular tone, heart rhythm, endothelial function, and platelet-activated thrombosis [1–5]. An insufficient Mg intake and hypomagnesemia are associated with inflammation, oxidative stress, and metabolic derangements, such as diabetes mellitus (DM) and dyslipidemia [5–8], all

of which contribute to the development of cardiovascular disease. It is well known that cardiovascular mortality is 10–30-fold higher in dialysis patients than in the general population [9]. Recent clinical studies reported the negative impact of hypomagnesemia in patients with chronic kidney disease (CKD). The potentially protective role of Mg in this population has been attracting increasing attention. We herein review clinical studies that examined the effects of serum Mg levels on cardiovascular disease and mortality and discuss Mg-related interventions in CKD patients.

Mg and the kidney

The human body stores approximately 25 g of Mg: 66% of this is in bone, 33% in intracellular spaces,

Correspondence: ryota.ikee@gmail.com
Department of Nephrology and Dialysis, H. N. Medic Kitahiroshima, 5-6-1
Kyoeicho, Kitahiroshima, Hokkaido 061-1113, Japan

and 1% in extracellular spaces [5, 10]. Serum Mg levels in healthy subjects are maintained within a narrow range primarily by the balance between intestinal absorption and renal excretion. In the kidney, most Mg filtered by the glomeruli is immediately reabsorbed and only 3–5% is excreted in the urine [5]. Reabsorption occurs in the ascending limb of Henle's loop mainly via paracellular transport, and transcellular transport in the distal convoluted segment contributes to maintaining the regulation of Mg. Renal tubular reabsorption of Mg is increased by extracellular volume contraction, hypomagnesemia, and high parathyroid hormone (PTH) levels [10].

Several observational studies identified hypomagnesemia as a predictor of a decline in renal function [11–14]. Tin et al. evaluated the risk of renal function loss in association with serum Mg levels in 13,226 patients during a median follow-up period of 21 years [13]. In a multivariate analysis adjusted for demographics, baseline renal function, nutrition markers, and comorbidities, patients with low serum Mg levels ≤ 1.70 mg/dL (0.70 mmol/L) showed a 58% higher hazard ratio (HR) for incident CKD and a 139% higher HR for end-stage renal disease (ESRD) than those with the highest quartile of serum Mg levels (2.19–2.80 mg/dL [0.90–1.15 mmol/L]). Sakaguchi et al. demonstrated a significant interaction between serum Mg and P levels on CKD progression [14]. Among 311 non-diabetic CKD patients, those in the lower Mg and higher P group were at a 2.07-fold risk for incident ESRD compared with those in the higher Mg and higher P group. The mechanisms contributing to the relationship between hypomagnesemia and renal function loss have not yet been elucidated in detail, but endothelial dysfunction, inflammation, vascular calcification, DM, insulin resistance, hyperaldosteronism, and pro-thrombotic effects may be involved [13, 15]. Lower dietary Mg intake may also induce renal function loss [16].

Glomerular filtration of Mg decreases as CKD progresses, whereas tubular reabsorption of Mg is impaired due to tubulointerstitial injury, thus causing an increase in fractional Mg excretion [17, 18]. However, the quantitative excretion of Mg tends to decrease regardless of the compensatory increase in fractional Mg excretion if glomerular filtration rate (GFR) falls to < 30 mL/min/1.73 m^2 [19], particularly < 10–15 mL/min/1.73 m^2 [20, 21]. Overt hypermagnesemia emerges when GFR falls to < 10 mL/min/1.73 m^2 [20]. Previous studies reported an inverse correlation between renal function and serum Mg levels in non-diabetic CKD [11, 22]. However, this correlation was not observed in diabetic CKD [11, 22], which would be attributable to an insulin-induced increase in renal Mg excretion leading to hypomagnesemia in diabetic patients [5, 23].

Mg and dialysis therapy

Dialysate Mg concentrations are one of the main factors influencing the Mg balance and serum Mg levels in dialysis patients. Mg easily crosses the hemodialyzer membrane and peritoneal membrane, and the amount of Mg elimination depends on its concentration gradient between serum and dialysate. A small amount of Mg is also removed by ultrafiltration. Actually, hypertonic dialysate use has been associated with hypomagnesemia in patients treated with peritoneal dialysis (PD) [24]. Dialysate Mg concentrations have changed over time. Until the 1980s, hemodialysis (HD) dialysate with a Mg concentration of 0.75 mmol/L was commonly used, while that with a lower concentration of 0.5 mmol/L is now widely used. In PD, dialysate Mg concentrations have changed from 0.75 to 0.25 mmol/L. These changes may be attributable to concerns regarding the suggestion by some studies of the adverse influence of hypermagnesemia on renal osteodystrophy [25], uremic pruritus [26], and visceral calcification [27] and the introduction of Mg-containing phosphate binders. Serum Mg levels in dialysis patients have been decreased by the changes of dialysate Mg concentrations, and hypomagnesemia rather than hypermagnesemia is now becoming an issue of interest due to its potent harmful influence. Hypomagnesemia is more common in PD patients than in HD patients because of lower dialysate Mg concentrations as well as the continuous nature of PD therapy.

Dietary Mg intake is another factor that influences serum Mg levels [28]. Dietary Mg is mainly absorbed in the small intestine. The active form of vitamin D has been shown to stimulate intestinal Mg absorption [5], which may partly explain depressed Mg absorption reported in CKD patients with a deficiency in active vitamin D [29]. Schmulen et al. previously showed that the administration of vitamin D receptor activators enhanced intestinal Mg absorption in CKD patients [30]. Mg-rich foods include green vegetables, peas, beans, nuts, seeds, and some fish [28], which are often restricted to avoid hyperkalemia and hyperphosphatemia. Therefore, dietary Mg intake may be insufficient, particularly in dialysis patients, as described by Luis et al. [31]. Serum Mg levels may be used as nutritional markers in dialysis patients because they correlate with serum albumin levels [24, 32–36], body mass index [24, 32], normalized protein catabolic rate [32, 34, 36], muscle mass [32] and strength [37], and subjective global assessment scores [32]. Of interest, the use of a low Mg PD dialysate induced a decrease in serum albumin levels [38].

In order to treat the complications that occur during long-term CKD, a number of drugs, such as diuretics, antibiotics, chemotherapeutic agents, β-blockers, and proton-pump inhibitors, are often used and may induce hypomagnesemia [5].

Observational studies on hypomagnesemia, cardiovascular disease, and mortality

In CKD patients, cardiovascular calcification begins during the pre-dialysis period and relentlessly progresses after the induction of dialysis therapy [39, 40]. In addition to hypertension, inflammation, an increase in serum Ca/P levels, the high prevalence of DM and warfarin use, and chronic micro-inflammation [41], hypomagnesemia may accelerate the progression of vascular calcification. Recently, the mechanisms of inhibition of vascular calcification by Mg have been widely investigated in experimental studies. Currently, there are two leading hypotheses [42]. First, Mg may bind P and delay Ca-P crystal growth in the circulation, thereby passively interfere with Ca-P deposition in the vessel wall. Elevated serum Mg interferes with amorphous Ca-P maturation into hydroxyapatite [43]. Calciprotein particle (CPP) is a recent issue of interest. Ca and P combine with fetuin-A to form amorphous Ca-P containing primary CPPs. Primary CPP is considered to inhibit crystal growth and aggregation [44], but it undergo spontaneous maturation and develop crystalline structures to form secondary CPP. Aghagolzadeh et al. have recently reported that secondary CPP has a potential to induce vascular calcification [45]. In addition, CPP maturation time (T_{50}) has been reported as an independent predictor of mortality in HD patients [46] and renal transplant recipients [47]. It is notable that Mg suppresses CPP maturation [48]. Second, Mg may regulate transdifferentiation of vascular smooth muscle cells (VSMC) toward an osteogenic phenotype by active cellular modulation of factors associated with calcification. It has been reported that Mg suppresses expression of osteogenic transcription factors (bone morphogenetic protein [BMP]-2, runt-related transcription factor 2, Msh homeobox 2, SRY-box 9), bone proteins, and genes associated with matrix mineralization (osteocalcin, alkaline phosphatase) [42]. In addition, Mg prevents the loss of calcification inhibitors (BMP-7, matrix Gla protein, osteopontin) that protect against osteogenic conversion [42]. Montes de Oca et al. reported that Mg inhibited Wnt/β-catenin signaling pathway and reversed osteogenic transformation of VSMC [49]. Mg transport through the cell membrane mediated by transient receptor potential melastatin 7 (TRPM7) is important in VSMC calcification [49–51]. Previous studies have suggested that P uptake through phosphate transporter-1 (Pit-1) is also essential in calcification [52]. Sonou et al. reported that Mg supplementation decreased Pit-1 protein expression in aortic rings incubated in high-phosphate medium [51].

PTH has been suggested to be involved in vascular calcification [53, 54]. Serum Mg levels showed an independent inverse relationship with intact PTH levels in pre-dialysis ESRD patients [55] and dialysis patients [56, 57]. Interventional studies showed that dialysate Mg concentration and Mg-containing phosphate binders affected intact PTH levels [58, 59]. Mg suppresses PTH secretion via the activation of Ca sensing receptor, although Mg is 2- to 3-fold less potent than Ca. Suppression of PTH secretion induced by Mg supplementation may have a favorable effect on vascular calcification to some extent.

Changes in serum Mg levels during HD sessions may acutely influence cardiovascular hemodynamics and electrophysiological functioning. Kyriazis et al. investigated the influence of intradialytic changes in serum Mg levels on blood pressure [60]. Decreased serum Mg levels induced by a low Mg dialysate enhanced susceptibility to intradialytic hypotension, possibly because of impaired cardiac contractility. Limited information is currently available on the effects of Mg on arrhythmia, but Alabd et al. reported that the post-dialysis QTc interval duration inversely correlated with a decrease in serum Mg levels during the HD session [61].

Table 1 shows observational studies that examined the relationship between serum Mg levels and cardiovascular calcification/atherosclerosis in CKD/ESRD patients [32, 62–68]. Most of these studies indicated an association between hypomagnesemia and cardiovascular lesions. Sakaguchi et al. performed a cross-sectional study to evaluate coronary artery calcification using multidetector-row computed tomography in 109 pre-dialysis CKD patients with DM [67]. A multivariate analysis showed that serum Mg levels were inversely associated with the density of coronary artery calcification, after adjustments for demographics, renal function, and indices related to nutrition, inflammation, and mineral and bone disorders. This relationship was more pronounced in patients with serum phosphate levels ≥ 3.4 mg/dL (1.40 mmol/L). Liu et al. reported an independent relationship between hypomagnesemia and carotid intima-media thickness (IMT) in 98 HD patients [32].

The relationship between serum Mg levels and mortality in CKD patients is shown in Table 2 [12, 33–35, 69–72]. Van Laecke et al. found that adjusted HR for all-cause mortality decreased by 7% with a 0.1-mg/dL (0.04 mmol/L) increase in serum Mg levels in non-dialysis CKD patients [12]. In the study by Cai et al. which included 253 incident PD patients, all-cause and cardiovascular mortalities were significantly lower in the high-serum-Mg group than in the low-Mg group [35]. Yang et al. examined 10,692 incident PD patients in the USA and found a significant association between hypomagnesemia and hospitalization [72]. However, hypomagnesemia was not an independent predictor of all-cause death after adjustments for laboratory variables. In HD patients, Ishimura et al. were the first to report an independent relationship between hypomagnesemia and all-cause mortality [73]. This study included 515 patients, and the mortality risk

Table 1 Observational studies examining the relationship between serum Mg levels and cardiovascular calcification/atherosclerosis

Authors (year)	Subjects	Study design	Dialysate Mg (mmol/L)	Outcome	Adverse effects of hypomagnesemia
Meema et al. (1987) [62]	44, PD	Prospective follow-up for an average of 27 months	0.75	Progression and regression of artery calcification evaluated by plain X-ray	Yes
Tzanakis et al. (1997) [63]	56, HD	Cross-sectional analysis	0.81	Mitral annular calcification detected by echocardiography	Yes
Tamashiro et al. (2001) [64]	24, HD	Prospective follow-up for an average of 17 months	0.5	Changes in coronary artery calcification scores evaluated by CT	No
Tzanakis et al. (2004) [65]	93, HD	Cross-sectional analysis	0.48	Carotid intima-media thickness evaluated by ultrasound	Yes
Ishimura et al. (2007) [66]	390, HD, non-DM	Cross-sectional analysis	0.5	Arterial calcification of the hands detected by plain X-ray	Yes
Liu et al. (2013) [32]	98, HD	Cross-sectional analysis	0.5	Carotid intima-media thickness evaluated by ultrasound	Yes
Sakaguchi et al. (2016) [67]	109, pre-dialysis CKD, DM	Cross-sectional analysis	–	Density of coronary artery calcification evaluated by CT using Agatston scores	Yes
Molnar et al. (2017) [68]	80, PD	Cross-sectional analysis	0.25	Abdominal aortic calcification scores on lateral lumbar spine X-ray	Yes

Abbreviations: *CKD* chronic kidney disease, *CT* computed tomography, *DM* diabetes mellitus, *HD* hemodialysis, *PD* peritoneal dialysis

decreased by 52% with a 1-mg/dL increase in serum Mg levels. Recently, similar findings have been increasingly reported in large-scale studies [33, 34, 69–71]. Sakaguchi et al. examined this relationship using the Japanese National Registry data [69]. Although the follow-up period was limited to 1 year, the lowest Mg sextile group (serum Mg levels < 2.3 mg/dL [0.95 mmol/L]) showed the highest all-cause and non-cardiovascular mortality risks, whereas the second highest Mg sextile (2.8–3.1 mg/dL [1.15–1.28 mmol/L]) showed the lowest mortality risk. It was notable that the second highest all-cause mortality risk and highest cardiovascular mortality risk were found in the highest Mg sextile (≥ 3.1 mg/dL [1.28 mmol/L]). Consistent with these findings, a restricted cubic spline analysis showed that the shape of the fully adjusted relationship between serum Mg levels and all-cause mortality was J shaped. Kurita et al. also employed a restricted cubic spline analysis in 2165 Japanese patients and found a similar curve for the relationship between serum Mg levels and all-cause mortality [70]. In Europe, de Roji van Zuijdewijn et al. demonstrated that lower serum Mg levels were associated with a high risk of all-cause and cardiovascular death as well as sudden death [71]. In these three studies [69–71], the relationship between hypomagnesemia and the mortality risk remained significant after the full adjustments. However, the findings from the USA [33, 34] were different. In Lacson's study [33], a linear decline was observed in the risk of all-cause death adjusted for case-mix variables (see Table 2) from the lowest to the highest serum Mg category, with the best survival in the category with the highest serum Mg levels (> 3.04 mg/dL [1.25 mmol/L]). However, the relationship between hypomagnesemia and mortality was not significant after additional adjustments for laboratory variables. Similarly, Li et

al. reported that time-varying serum Mg levels did not predict the death in incident HD patients after adjustment for laboratory variables [34].

Thus, a relationship exists between hypomagnesemia and mortality, even after full adjustment for laboratory variables in patients from Asia and Europe [35, 69–71], but not in those from the USA [33, 34, 72]. Based on these results, it seems that patient's race or region may be involved in susceptibility to the harmful effects of hypomagnesemia. There may be another opinion that in the studies from the USA with the short dialysis duration (Table 2), the prognostic impact of hypomagnesemia might be confounded or diluted by residual renal function. Residual renal function is considered to be beneficial for the prognosis and has a negative impact on Mg balance even in HD patients. The median of HD duration in Lacson's study [33] was comparable to that in de Roji van Zuijdewijn's study [71]. Both Cai's [35] and Yang's study [72] included incident PD patients. However, hypomagnesemia was an independent predictor of mortality only in Cai's (from China) and de Roji van Zuijdewijn's study (from Europe).

Mg-related interventions in CKD/ESRD patients

There are two methods to increase serum Mg levels: increasing dialysate Mg concentrations and Mg supplementation. However, evidence from interventional studies to prove the favorable effects of Mg on cardiovascular disease and mortality is limited, which is not in proportion to the increasing interest in Mg. These interventions should be employed with careful monitoring of serum Mg levels to avoid hypermagnesemia.

Table 2 Observational studies examining the relationship between serum Mg levels and mortality

Authors (year)	Subjects	Dialysis duration	Dialysate Mg (mmol/L)	Follow-up period	Adjusted HR	Adjustments
Pre-dialysis CKD						
Van Laecke et al. (2013) [12]	1650	–	–	Median 5.1 years	All-cause mortality 0.930 per 0.1-mg/dL increase in serum Mg levels. All-cause mortality 1.613 in the low Mg group (< 1.8 mg/dL) vs. the high Mg group (> 2.2 mg/dL)	Age, sex, DM, hypertension, obesity, smoking, eGFR, diuretics, RAAS blockade, UA, Na, K, P, CRP
Dialysis						
Sakaguchi et al. (2014) [69]	142,555, HD	Median 7 years	0.5	1 year	All-cause mortality 1.28, cardiovascular mortality 1.24, non-cardiovascular mortality 1.32 in the lowest Mg sextile (< 2.3 mg/dL) vs. the second highest sextile (≥ 2.8, < 3.1 mg/dL)	Age, sex, HD duration, weekly HD time, BMI, DM, CVD, parathyroidectomy, hip fracture, BUN, albumin, ALP, hemoglobin, Ca, P, CRP, iPTH, VDRAs, PBs, cinacalcet
Kurita et al. (2015) [70]	2165, HD	Median 8.3 years	0.5	3 years	All-cause mortality 1.734 in the lowest Mg quintile (≤ 2.3 mg/dL) vs. the middle quintile (> 2.5, ≤ 2.7 mg/dL). All-cause mortality 1.649 in the second lowest quintile (> 2.3, ≤ 2.5 mg/dL) vs. the middle quintile	Age, sex, HD duration, Kt/V, primary renal disease, BMI, CVD, lung disease, liver disease, malignancy, parathyroidectomy, albumin, hemoglobin, K, Ca, P, CRP, iPTH, serum iron, ferritin
de Roji van Zuijdewijn et al. (2015) [71]	HD 184, HDF 181	Median 1.8 years	0.5	Mean 3.1 years	All-cause mortality 0.88, cardiovascular mortality 0.73, sudden death 0.78 per 0.1-mmol/L (0.24 mg/dL) increase in serum Mg levels	Age, sex, HD duration, weekly HD time, dialysis modality (HD/HDF), residual renal function, BMI, BP, DM, CVD, albumin, Ca, P, iPTH
Lacson et al. (2015) [33]	27,544, HD	Median 2.5 years	Various	1 year	All-cause mortality 0.89 in the highest Mg group (≥ 1.25 mmol/L) vs. the reference group (≥ 0.80, < 0.95 mmol/L) (not significant)	Case mix: age, sex, race/ethnicity, HD duration, vascular access type, BSA. Laboratory: Kt/V, DM, albumin, hemoglobin, Ca, P, iPTH
Li et al. (2015) [34]	9359, HD	Incident patients	Not mentioned	Mean 19 months	No relationship between time-varying serum Mg levels and all-cause mortality after all adjustments	Age, sex, race/ethnicity, Kt/V, BMI, DM, hypertension, dyslipidemia, CVD, lung disease, liver disease, cancer, BUN, albumin, ALP, hemoglobin, K, Ca, P, iPTH, ferritin, nPCR
Cai et al. (2016) [35]	253, PD	Incident patients	0.25	Median 29 months	All-cause mortality 0.075 in the normomagnesemia group (≥ 1.7 mg/dL) vs. the hypomagnesemia group (< 1.7 mg/dL). Cardiovascular mortality 0.003 in the normomagnesemia group vs. the hypomagnesemia group	Age, sex, BMI, DM, BP, urine output, net UF, weekly Ccr, residual renal function, albumin, total cholesterol, triglycerides, hemoglobin, Na, Ca, P, iPTH, calcium carbonate, VDRAs
Yang et al. (2016) [72]	10,692, PD	Incident patients	Not mentioned	Median 13 months	Hospitalization risk 1.09 in the lowest Mg quintile (< 1.8 mg/dL) vs. the middle quintile (≥ 2.0, < 2.2 mg/dL). All-cause mortality 0.97 in the lowest Mg quintile vs. the middle quintile (not significant)	Age, sex, race/ethnicity, primary insurance, primary renal disease, total weekly Kt/V, residual renal function, 4-h D/P Cr ratio, DM, hypertension, CVD, albumin, hemoglobin, K, Ca, P, bicarbonate, iPTH, ferritin, iron saturation

Abbreviations: 4-h D/P Cr ratio 4-h dialysate to plasma creatinine ratio from the peritoneal equilibration test, *ALP* alkaline phosphatase, *BMI* body mass index, *BP* blood pressure, *BUN* blood urea nitrogen, *BSA* body surface area, *Ccr* creatinine clearance, *CKD* chronic kidney disease, *CRP* C-reactive protein, *CVD* cardiovascular disease, *DM* diabetes mellitus, *eGFR* estimated glomerular filtration rate, *HD* hemodialysis, *HDF* hemodiafiltration, *HR* hazard ratio, *iPTH* intact parathyroid hormone, *nPCR* normalized protein catabolic rate, *PBs* phosphate binders, *PD* peritoneal dialysis, *RAAS* renin-angiotensin-aldosterone system, *UA* uric acid, *UF* ultrafiltration, *VDRAs* vitamin D receptor agonists

Dialysates with higher Mg concentrations

Dialysates with higher Mg concentrations are feasible and effective for increasing serum Mg levels. In Nilsson's study including 22 HD patients who had been treated with 0.75 mmol/L-Mg dialysate, 12 were assigned to 0.2 mmol/L dialysate and 10 continued to use 0.75 mmol/L dialysate [58]. Four months later, the former patients showed a significant decrease in serum Mg levels from 2.71 ± 0.55 mg/dL (1.11 ± 0.23 mmol/L) to 2.26 ± 0.54 mg/dL (0.93 ± 0.22 mmol/L, $P < 0.01$), whereas the latter did not. Similar findings have been also reported in PD by Ejaz et al. [38]. None of the 33 patients had hypomagnesemia (defined as < 1.52 mg/dL [0.625 mmol/L]) with the use of 0.75 mmol/L-Mg dialysate. After the change to 0.25 mmol/L Mg-dialysate, 21 patients (63.6%) developed hypomagnesemia. This change also resulted in lower serum albumin levels in those with than in those without hypomagnesemia (2.5 ± 0.12 g/dL vs. 3.2 ± 0.12 g/dL, $P < 0.01$). Regardless of these findings, the effects of dialysates with higher Mg concentrations on cardiovascular disease and mortality have not yet been examined. Dialysate Mg-related clinical trials are of interest and need to be conducted in the future.

Mg-containing phosphate binders

It is important to control hyperphosphatemia, which leads to cardiovascular calcification and increased morbidity and mortality in CKD patients [74]. Mg is contained in some phosphate binders and its affinity for P is weaker than that of Al and Ca. Since the mid-1980s, magnesium hydroxide was used to replace Al-containing phosphate binders but caused diarrhea and mild hyperkalemia [75]. Magnesium carbonate effectively controlled serum P levels with less adverse effects [75]. However, Mg-containing phosphate binders have not been widely used because of concerns regarding hypermagnesemia. In 2010, a randomized controlled trial (RCT), the CALMAG study, which compared the efficacy of calcium acetate/magnesium carbonate and sevelamer hydrochloride in HD patients, was reported [59]. At week 25, mean reductions in serum P from baseline in the calcium acetate/magnesium carbonate group and sevelamer group were similar. Serum Mg levels in the former group significantly increased from baseline (0.73 ± 0.56 mg/dL [0.30 ± 0.23 mmol/L]), whereas a slight increase was observed in the latter group (0.10 ± 0.36 mg/ dL [0.04 ± 0.15 mmol/L]). Gastrointestinal adverse events occurred more frequently in the sevelamer group (23.6 vs. 13.6%). The authors concluded that magnesium carbonate was a tolerable and effective agent in the treatment of hyperphosphatemia.

A few interventional studies have examined the effects of Mg-containing phosphate binders on cardiovascular lesions, as shown in Table 3 [76, 77]. Furthermore, their effects on mortality currently remain unknown. Tzanakis et al. randomly assigned 59 HD patients to calcium acetate or calcium acetate/magnesium carbonate for 12 months [77]. At the end of the study, the number of patients with improved carotid IMT was significantly higher in the Mg-containing phosphate binder group than in the Ca-containing binder group ($P = 0.04$). Turgut et al. also showed the beneficial effects of Mg supplementation [76]. However, these findings appeared to be inconclusive because of the relatively small sample size as well as the accuracy and reproducibility of the evaluation methods.

In a sub-analysis of the aforementioned Japanese National Registry data [69], Sakaguchi et al. reported that the mortality risk of HD patients with hyperphosphatemia was attenuated with increases in serum Mg levels [78]. If large-scale RCTs successfully show the benefits of Mg-containing phosphate binders for cardiovascular disease and mortality, these drugs may be widely used in the control of hyperphosphatemia.

Mg-containing laxatives

The prevalence of constipation requiring laxative therapy is high in ESRD patients [79, 80]. Mg-containing laxatives may be used to concurrently treat constipation and hypomagnesemia. However, these drugs should be used carefully. Serum Mg levels were increased to approximately 10 mg/dL (4.11 mmol/L) by magnesium oxide administered at 3 g/day in dialysis patients, resulting in muscle paresis or impaired consciousness [81, 82]. Toprak et al. conducted a RCT including 128 prediabetic patients with hypomagnesemia (< 1.8 mg/dL [0.74 mmol/L] in males and < 1.9 mg/dL [0.78 mmol/L] in females) and mild to moderate CKD (estimated GFR 30–60 mL/min/1.73 m^2) [83]. Patients were assigned to magnesium oxide or placebo for 3 months. Magnesium oxide was administered at 613.2 mg/day and serum Mg levels increased from 1.70 ± 0.13 mg/dL (0.70 ± 0.05 mmol/L) to 1.91 ± 0.22 mg/dL (0.79 ± 0.09 mmol/ L). At the end of this study, insulin resistance, glycemic control, and uric acid levels were better in the former than in the latter patient group. These improvements in metabolic indices were accompanied by an increase in not only serum Mg, but also albumin levels.

Table 3 Interventional studies examining effects of Mg-containing phosphate binders on cardiovascular calcification/atherosclerosis

Authors (year)	Subjects	Study design	Outcome	Serum Mg levels in the Mg group (mg/dL)	Benefits of Mg supplementation
Turgut et al. (2008) [76]	47, HD	RCT with assignment to magnesium citrate or calcium acetate for 2 months	Changes in carotid intima-media thickness evaluated by ultrasound	Pre: 2.50 ± 0.36 Post: 2.69 ± 0.39	Yes
Tzanakis et al. (2014) [77]	72, HD	RCT with assignment to calcium acetate or calcium acetate/magnesium carbonate for 12 months	Changes in arterial calcification of the femur, pelvis, hands, and abdomen evaluated by plain X-ray using vascular calcification scores	Pre: 2.59 ± 0.29 Post: 2.83 ± 0.38	Yes

Abbreviations: HD hemodialysis, RCT randomized controlled trial

Sevelamer

Sevelamer is a Ca-free, Mg-free, non-absorbable anion exchange resin that is used to control hyperphosphatemia. There are two salts of sevelamer: sevelamer hydrochloride and sevelamer carbonate. This drug has been reported to increase serum Mg levels. Mitsopoulos et al. found that the mean serum Mg levels significantly increased from 2.75 mg/dL (1.13 mmol/L) to 2.90 mg/dL (1.19 mmol/L) during an 8-week treatment with sevelamer [84]. Chertow et al. also reported a significant increase in serum Mg levels induced by sevelamer [85]. In addition, two cross-sectional studies showed an independent relationship between sevelamer and higher serum Mg levels [36, 86]. It seems plausible to speculate that this effect of sevelamer depends on its adsorptive action on some substances other than P. Free fatty acids in the intestinal lumen may combine with Mg to form non-absorbable soaps. Therefore, Mitsopoulos et al. speculated that sevelamer binds biliary salts, thereby increasing the quantity of free Mg available for intestinal absorption [84]. On the other hand, Nagano et al. reported the contribution of magnesium stearate, which is included as a pharmaceutical excipient in phosphate binders, to increases in serum Mg levels [87].

Sevelamer has been reported to exert favorable effects on inflammation, oxidative stress, glucose metabolism, lipid profiles, and cardiovascular disease [88, 89], similar to Mg supplementation. Although the precise mechanisms responsible for these effects of sevelamer have not yet been elucidated, the increases in serum Mg levels induced by the drug itself may be included in these mechanisms.

Conclusions

In the clinical practice of dialysis therapy, concerns need to shift from hypermagnesemia to hypomagnesemia. Dialysis patients, particularly those treated with PD, are exposed to the risk of hypomagnesemia because of the use of dialysates with low Mg concentrations as well as decreased intake/absorption and the adverse effects of some drugs. Observational studies have almost consistently indicated that hypomagnesemia is associated with cardiovascular disease and mortality in CKD. However, this relationship may depend on a patient's race or region. Dialysates with higher Mg concentrations and some drugs including phosphate binders are useful for increasing serum Mg levels, but few interventional studies have examined the benefits of the correction of hypomagnesemia. Further studies are required in order to establish the efficacy of Mg supplementation in CKD patients. In addition, it is important to establish the harmless upper limit of serum Mg levels.

Abbreviations

BMP: Bone morphogenetic protein; CKD: Chronic kidney disease; CPP: Calciprotein particle; DM: Diabetes mellitus; ESRD: End-stage renal disease; GFR: Glomerular filtration rate; HD: Hemodialysis; HR: Hazard ratio; IMT: Intima-media thickness; PD: Peritoneal dialysis; PTH: Parathyroid hormone; RCT: Randomized controlled trial; VSMC: Vascular smooth muscle cell

Acknowledgements

Not applicable

Funding

Not applicable

Competing interests

The author declares no competing interest.

References

1. Altura BM, Altura BT. New perspectives on the role of magnesium in the pathophysiology of the cardiovascular system. I Clinical aspects Magnesium. 1985;4:226–44.
2. Shechter M, Merz CN, Paul-Labrador M, Meisel SR, Rude RK, Molloy MD, et al. Oral magnesium supplementation inhibits platelet-dependent thrombosis in patients with coronary artery disease. Am J Cardiol. 1999;84: 152–6.
3. Shechter M, Sharir M, Labrador MJ, Forrester I, Silver R, Bairey Merz CN. Oral magnesium therapy improves endothelial function in patients with coronary artery disease. Circulation. 2000;102:2353–8.
4. Chen X, Mak IT. Mg supplementation protects against ritonavir-mediated endothelial oxidative stress and hepatic eNOS downregulation. Free Radic Biol Med. 2014;69:77–85.
5. Grober U, Schmidt J, Kisters K. Magnesium in prevention and therapy. Nutrients. 2015;7:8199–226.
6. Guerrero-Romero F, Rodriguez-Moran M. Low serum magnesium levels and metabolic syndrome. Acta Diabetol. 2002;39:209–13.
7. Song Y, Ridker PM, Manson JE, Cook NR, Buring JE, Liu S. Magnesium intake, C-reactive protein, and the prevalence of metabolic syndrome in middle-aged and older U.S. women. Diabetes Care. 2005;28:1438–44.
8. Evangelopoulos AA, Vallianou NG, Panagiotakos DB, Georgiou A, Zacharias GA, Alevra AN, et al. An inverse relationship between cumulating components of the metabolic syndrome and serum magnesium levels. Nutr Res. 2008;28:659–63.
9. Sarnak MJ, Levey AS, Schoolwerth AC, Coresh J, Culleton B, Hamm LL, et al. Kidney disease as a risk factor for development of cardiovascular disease: a statement from the American Heart Association Councils on Kidney in Cardiovascular Disease, High Blood Pressure Research, Clinical Cardiology, and Epidemiology and Prevention. Circulation. 2003;108:2154–69.
10. Kanbay M, Goldsmith D, Uyar ME, Turgut F, Covic A. Magnesium in chronic kidney disease: challenges and opportunities. Blood Purif. 2010;29:280–92.
11. Sakaguchi Y, Shoji T, Hayashi T, Suzuki A, Shimizu M, Mitsumoto K, et al. Hypomagnesemia in type 2 diabetic nephropathy: a novel predictor of end-stage renal disease. Diabetes Care. 2012;35:1591–7.
12. Van Laecke S, Nagler EV, Verbeke F, Van Biesen W, Vanholder R. Hypomagnesemia and the risk of death and GFR decline in chronic kidney disease. Am J Med. 2013;126:825–31.

13. Tin A, Grams ME, Maruthur NM, Astor BC, Couper D, Mosley TH, et al. Results from the Atherosclerosis Risk in Communities study suggest that low serum magnesium is associated with incident kidney disease. Kidney Int. 2015;87:820–7.

14. Sakaguchi Y, Iwatani H, Hamano T, Tomida K, Kawabata H, Kusunoki Y, et al. Magnesium modifies the association between serum phosphate and the risk of progression to end-stage kidney disease in patients with non-diabetic chronic kidney disease. Kidney Int. 2015;88:833–42.

15. Dousdampanis P, Trigka K, Fourtounas C. Hypomagnesemia, chronic kidney disease and cardiovascular mortality: pronounced association but unproven causation. Hemodial Int. 2014;18:730–9.

16. Rebholz CM, Tin A, Liu Y, Kuczmarski MF, Evans MK, Zonderman AB, et al. Dietary magnesium and kidney function decline: the healthy aging in neighborhoods of diversity across the life span study. Am J Nephrol. 2016; 44:381–7.

17. Futrakul P, Yenrudi S, Futrakul N, Sensirivatana R, Kingwatanakul P, Jungthirapanich J, et al. Tubular function and tubulointerstitial disease. Am J Kidney Dis. 1999;33:886–91.

18. Noiri C, Shimizu T, Takayanagi K, Tayama Y, Iwashita T, Okazaki S, et al. Clinical significance of fractional magnesium excretion (FEMg) as a predictor of interstitial nephropathy and its correlation with conventional parameters. Clin Exp Nephrol. 2015;19:1071–8.

19. Mordes JP, Wacker WE. Excess magnesium. Pharmacol Rev. 1977;29:273–300.

20. Coburn JW, Popovtzer MM, Massry SG, Kleeman CR. The physicochemical state and renal handling of divalent ions in chronic renal failure. Arch Intern Med. 1969;124:302–11.

21. Massry SG. Magnesium homeostasis in patients with renal failure. Contrib Nephrol. 1984;38:175–84.

22. Dewitte K, Dhondt A, Giri M, Stockl D, Rottiers R, Lameire N, et al. Differences in serum ionized and total magnesium values during chronic renal failure between nondiabetic and diabetic patients: a cross-sectional study. Diabetes Care. 2004;27:2503–5.

23. Djurhuus MS, Skott P, Hother-Nielson O, Klitgaard NA, Beck-Nielsen H. Insulin increases renal magnesium excretion: a possible cause of magnesium depletion in hyperinsulinaemic states. Diabet Med. 1995;12: 664–9.

24. Ye H, Zhang X, Guo Q, Huang N, Mao H, Yu X, et al. Prevalence and factors associated with hypomagnesemia in Southern Chinese continuous ambulatory peritoneal dialysis patients. Perit Dial Int. 2013;33:450–4.

25. Gonella M, Ballanti P, Della Rocca C, Calabrese G, Pratesi G, Vagelli G, et al. Improved bone morphology by normalizing serum magnesium in chronically hemodialyzed patients. Miner Electrolyte Metab. 1988;14:240–5.

26. Graf H, Kovarik J, Stummvoll HK, Wolf A. Disappearance of uraemic pruritus after lowering dialysate magnesium concentration. Br Med J. 1979;2:1478–9.

27. Contiguglia SR, Alfrey AC, Miller NL, Runnells DE, Le Geros RZ. Nature of soft tissue calcification in uremia. Kidney Int. 1973;4:229–35.

28. Wyskida K, Witkowicz J, Chudek J, Więcek A. Daily magnesium intake and hypermagnesemia in hemodialysis patients with chronic kidney disease. J Ren Nutr. 2012;22:19–26.

29. Brannan PG, Vergne-Marini P, Pak CY, Hull AR, Fordtran JS. Magnesium absorption in the human small intestine. Results in normal subjects, patients with chronic renal disease, and patients with absorptive hypercalciuria. J Clin Invest. 1976;57:1412–8.

30. Schmulen AC, Lerman M, Pak CY, Zerwekh J, Morawski S, Fordtran JS, et al. Effect of 1,25-(OH)₂D₃ on jejunal absorption of magnesium in patients with chronic renal disease. Am J Phys. 1980;238:G349–52.

31. Luis D, Zlatkis K, Comenge B, Garcia Z, Navarro JF, Lorenzo V, et al. Dietary quality and adherence to dietary recommendations in patients undergoing hemodialysis. J Ren Nutr. 2016;26:190–5.

32. Liu F, Zhang X, Qi H, Wang J, Wang M, Zhang Y, et al. Correlation of serum magnesium with cardiovascular risk factors in maintenance hemodialysis patients-a cross-sectional study. Magnes Res. 2013;26:100–8.

33. Lacson E Jr, Wang W, Ma L, Passlick-Deetjen J. Serum magnesium and mortality in hemodialysis patients in the United States: a cohort study. Am J Kidney Dis. 2015;66:1056–66.

34. Li L, Streja E, Rhee CM, Mehrotra R, Soohoo M, Brunelli SM, et al. Hypomagnesemia and mortality in incident hemodialysis patients. Am J Kidney Dis. 2015;66:1047–55.

35. Cai K, Luo Q, Dai Z, Zhu B, Fei J, Xue C, et al. Hypomagnesemia is associated with increased mortality among peritoneal dialysis patients. PLoS One. 2016;1:e0152488.

36. Ikee R, Toyoyama T, Endo T, Tsunoda M, Hashimoto N. Impact of sevelamer hydrochloride on serum magnesium concentrations in hemodialysis patients. Magnes Res. 2016;29:184–90.

37. Okazaki H, Ishimura E, Okuno S, Norimine K, Yamakawa K, Yamakawa T, et al. Significant positive relationship between serum magnesium and muscle quality in maintenance hemodialysis patients. Magnes Res. 2013;26:182–7.

38. Ejaz AA, McShane AP, Gandhi VC, Leehey DJ, Ing TS. Hypomagnesemia in continuous ambulatory peritoneal dialysis patients dialyzed with a low-magnesium peritoneal dialysis solution. Perit Dial Int. 1995;15:61–4.

39. Shroff RC, McNair R, Figg N, Skepper JN, Schurgers L, Gupta A, et al. Dialysis accelerates medial vascular calcification in part by triggering smooth muscle cell apoptosis. Circulation. 2008;118:1748–57.

40. Temmar M, Liabeuf S, Renard C, Czernichow S, Esper NE, Shahapuni I, et al. Pulse wave velocity and vascular calcification at different stages of chronic kidney disease. J Hypertens. 2010;28:163–9.

41. Ohtake T, Kobayashi S. Impact of vascular calcification on cardiovascular mortality in hemodialysis patients: clinical significance, mechanisms and possible strategies for treatment. Renal Replacement Therapy. 2017;3:13.

42. ter Braake AD, Shanahan CM, de Baaij JH. Magnesium counteracts vascular calcification: passive interference or active modulation? Arterioscler Thromb Vasc Biol. 2017;37:1431–45.

43. Apfelbaum F, Mayer I, Rey C, Lebugle A. Magnesium in maturing synthetic apatite: a Fourier transform infrared analysis. J Cryst Growth. 1994;144:304–10.

44. Heiss A, DuChesne A, Denecke B, Grotzinger J, Yamamoto K, Renne T, et al. Structural basis of calcification inhibition by α 2-HS glycoprotein/fetuin-A. Formation of colloidal calciprotein particles. J Biol Chem. 2003; 278:13333–41.

45. Aghagolzadeh P, Bachtler M, Bijarnia R, Jackson C, Smith ER, Odermatt A, et al. Calcification of vascular smooth muscle cells is induced by secondary calciprotein particles and enhanced by tumor necrosis factor-α. Atherosclerosis. 2016;251:404–14.

46. Pasch A, Block GA, Bachtler M, Smith ER, Jahnen-Dechent W, Arampatzis S, et al. Blood calcification propensity, cardiovascular events, and survival in patients receiving hemodialysis in the EVOLVE trial. Clin J Am Soc Nephrol. 2017;12:315–22.

47. Keyzer CA, de Borst MH, van den Berg E, Jahnen-Dechent W, Arampatzis S, Farese S, et al. Calcification propensity and survival among renal transplant recipients. J Am Soc Nephrol. 2016;27:239–48.

48. Pasch A, Farese S, Graber S, Wald J, Richtering W, Floege J, et al. Nanoparticle-based test measures overall propensity for calcification in serum. J Am Soc Nephrol. 2012;23:1744–52.

49. Montes de Oca A, Guerrero F, Martinez-Moreno JM, Madueno JA, Herencia C, Peralta A, et al. Magnesium inhibits Wnt/β-catenin activity and reverses the osteogenic transformation of vascular smooth muscle cells. PLoS One. 2014;9:e89525.

50. Montezano AC, Zimmerman D, Yusuf H, Burger D, Chignalia AZ, Wadhera V, et al. Vascular smooth muscle cell differentiation to an osteogenic phenotype involves TRPM7 modulation by magnesium. Hypertension. 2010; 56:453–62.

51. Sonou T, Ohya M, Yashiro M, Masumoto A, Nakashima Y, Ito T, et al. Magnesium prevents phosphate-induced vascular calcification via TRPM7 and Pit-1 in an aortic tissue culture model. Hypertens Res. 2017;40:562–7.

52. Mune S, Shibata M, Hatamura I, Saji F, Okada T, Maeda Y, et al. Mechanism of phosphate-induced calcification in rat aortic tissue culture: possible involvement of Pit-1 and apoptosis. Clin Exp Nephrol. 2009;13:571–7.

53. Coen G, Manni M, Mantella D, Pierantozzi A, Balducci A, Condo S, et al. Are PTH serum levels predictive of coronary calcifications in haemodialysis patients? Nephrol Dial Transplant. 2007;22:3262–7.

54. Neves KR, Graciolli FG, dos Reis LM, Graciolli RG, Neves CL, Magalhaes AO, et al. Vascular calcification: contribution of parathyroid hormone in renal failure. Kidney Int. 2007;71:1262–70.

55. Ohya M, Negi S, Sakaguchi T, Koiwa F, Ando R, Komatsu Y, et al. Significance of serum magnesium as an independent correlative factor on the parathyroid hormone level in uremic patients. J Clin Endocrinol Metab. 2014;99:3873–8.

56. Navarro JF, Mora C, Macia M, Garcia J. Serum magnesium concentration is an independent predictor of parathyroid hormone levels in peritoneal dialysis patients. Perit Dial Int. 1999;19:455–61.

57. Gohda T, Shou I, Fukui M, Funabiki K, Horikoshi S, Shirato I, et al. Parathyroid hormone gene polymorphism and secondary hyperparathyroidism in hemodialysis patients. Am J Kidney Dis. 2002;39:1255–60.

58. Nilsson P, Johansson SG, Danielson BG. Magnesium studies in hemodialysis patients before and after treatment with low dialysate magnesium. Nephron. 1984;37:25–9.

59. de Francisco AL, Leidig M, Covic AC, Ketteler M, Benedyk-Lorens E, Mircescu GM, et al. Evaluation of calcium acetate/magnesium carbonate as a phosphate binder compared with sevelamer hydrochloride in haemodialysis patients: a controlled randomized study (CALMAG study) assessing efficacy and tolerability. Nephrol Dial Transplant. 2010;25:3707–17.

60. Kyriazis J, Kalogeropoulou K, Bilirakis L, Smirnioudis N, Pikounis V, Stamatiadis D, et al. Dialysate magnesium level and blood pressure. Kidney Int. 2004;66:1221–31.

61. Alabd MA, El-Hammady W, Shawky A, Nammas W, El-Tayeb M. QT interval and QT dispersion in patients undergoing hemodialysis: revisiting the old theory. Nephron Extra. 2011;1:1–8.

62. Meema HE, Oreopoulos DG, Rapoport A. Serum magnesium level and arterial calcification in end-stage renal disease. Kidney Int. 1987;32:388–94.

63. Tzanakis I, Pras A, Kounali D, Mamali V, Kartsonakis V, Mayopoulou-Symvoulidou D, et al. Mitral annular calcifications in haemodialysis patients: a possible protective role of magnesium. Nephrol Dial Transplant. 1997;12: 2036–7.

64. Tamashiro M, Iseki K, Sunagawa O, Inoue T, Higa S, Afuso H, et al. Significant association between the progression of coronary artery calcification and dyslipidemia in patients on chronic hemodialysis. Am J Kidney Dis. 2001;38: 64–9.

65. Tzanakis I, Virvidakis K, Tsomi A, Mantakas E, Girousis N, Karefyllakis N, et al. Intra- and extracellular magnesium levels and atheromatosis in haemodialysis patients. Magnes Res. 2004;17:102–8.

66. Ishimura E, Okuno S, Kitatani K, Tsuchida T, Yamakawa T, Shioi A, et al. Significant association between the presence of peripheral vascular calcification and lower serum magnesium in hemodialysis patients. Clin Nephrol. 2007;68:222–7.

67. Sakaguchi Y, Hamano T, Nakano C, Obi Y, Matsui I, Kusunoki Y, et al. Association between density of coronary artery calcification and serum magnesium levels among patients with chronic kidney disease. PLoS One. 2016;11:e0163673.

68. Molnar AO, Biyani M, Hammond I, Harmon JP, Lavoie S, McCormick B, et al. Lower serum magnesium is associated with vascular calcification in peritoneal dialysis patients: a cross sectional study. BMC Nephrol. 2017;18:129.

69. Sakaguchi Y, Fujii N, Shoji T, Hayashi T, Rakugi H, Isaka Y. Hypomagnesemia is a significant predictor of cardiovascular and non-cardiovascular mortality in patients undergoing hemodialysis. Kidney Int. 2014;85:174–81.

70. Kurita N, Akizawa T, Fukagawa M, Onishi Y, Kurokawa K, Fukuhara S. Contribution of dysregulated serum magnesium to mortality in hemodialysis patients with secondary hyperparathyroidism: a 3-year cohort study. Clin Kidney J. 2015;8:744–52.

71. de Roij van Zuijdewijn CL, Grooteman MP, Bots ML, Blankestijn PJ, Steppan S, Buchel J, et al. Serum magnesium and sudden death in European hemodialysis patients. PLoS One. 2015;10:e0143104.

72. Yang X, Soohoo M, Streja E, Rivara MB, Obi Y, Adams SV, et al. Serum magnesium levels and hospitalization and mortality in incident peritoneal dialysis patients: a cohort study. Am J Kidney Dis. 2016;68:619–27.

73. Ishimura E, Okuno S, Yamakawa T, Inaba M, Nishizawa Y. Serum magnesium concentration is a significant predictor of mortality in maintenance hemodialysis patients. Magnes Res. 2007;20:237–44.

74. Covic A, Kothawala P, Bernal M, Robbins S, Chalian A, Goldsmith D. Systematic review of the evidence underlying the association between mineral metabolism disturbances and risk of all-cause mortality, cardiovascular mortality and cardiovascular events in chronic kidney disease. Nephrol Dial Transplant. 2009;24:1506–23.

75. Spiegel DM. The role of magnesium binders in chronic kidney disease. Semin Dial. 2007;20:333–6.

76. Turgut F, Kanbay M, Metin MR, Uz E, Akcay A, Covic A. Magnesium supplementation helps to improve carotid intima media thickness in patients on hemodialysis. Int Urol Nephrol. 2008;40:1075–82.

77. Tzanakis IP, Stamataki EE, Papadaki AN, Giannakis N, Damianakis NE, Oreopoulos DG. Magnesium retards the progress of the arterial calcifications in hemodialysis patients: a pilot study. Int Urol Nephrol. 2014;46:2199–205.

78. Sakaguchi Y, Fujii N, Shoji T, Hayashi T, Rakugi H, Iseki K, et al. Magnesium modifies the cardiovascular mortality risk associated with hyperphosphatemia in patients undergoing hemodialysis: a cohort study. PLoS One. 2014;9:e116273.

79. Sutton D, Dumbleton S, Allaway C. Can increased dietary fibre reduce laxative requirement in peritoneal dialysis patients? J Ren Care. 2007;33: 174–8.

80. Ikee R, Toyoyama T, Endo T, Tsunoda M, Hashimoto N. Clinical factors associated with constipation in hemodialysis patients. Int Urol Nephrol. 2016;48:1741–2.

81. Matsuo H, Nakamura K, Nishida A, Kubo K, Nakagawa R, Sumida Y. A case of hypermagnesemia accompanied by hypercalcemia induced by a magnesium laxative in a hemodialysis patient. Nephron. 1995;71:477–8.

82. Jung GJ, Gil HW, Yang JO, Lee EY, Hong SY. Severe hypermagnesemia causing quadriparesis in a CAPD patient. Perit Dial Int. 2008;28:206.

83. Toprak O, Kurt H, Sari Y, Sarkis C, Us H, Kirik A. Magnesium replacement improves the metabolic profile in obese and pre-diabetic patients with mild-to-moderate chronic kidney disease: a 3-month, randomised, double-blind, placebo-controlled study. Kidney Blood Press Res. 2017;42: 33–42.

84. Mitsopoulos E, Griveas I, Zanos S, Anagnostopoulos K, Giannakou A, Pavlitou A, et al. Increase in serum magnesium level in haemodialysis patients receiving sevelamer hydrochloride. Int Urol Nephrol. 2005;37:321–8.

85. Chertow GM, Burke SK, Dillon MA, Slatopolsky E. Long-term effects of sevelamer hydrochloride on the calcium × phosphate product and lipid profile of haemodialysis patients. Nephrol Dial Transplant. 1999;14:2907–14.

86. Rosa-Diez G, Negri AL, Crucelegui MS, Philippi R, Perez-Teysseyre H, Sarabia-Reyes C, et al. Sevelamer carbonate reduces the risk of hypomagnesemia in hemodialysis-requiring end-stage renal disease patients. Clin Kidney J. 2016; 9:481–5.

87. Nagano N, Ito K, Honda M, Sunaga S, Tagahara A, Nohara T, et al. The magnesium included as a pharmaceutical excipient in phosphate binders might affect the serum magnesium levels of dialysis patients. J Jpn Soc Dial Ther. 2016;49:571–80. (in Japanese)

88. Ikee R, Tsunoda M, Sasaki N, Sato N, Hashimoto N. Emerging effects of sevelamer in chronic kidney disease. Kidney Blood Press Res. 2013;37:24–32.

89. Ikee R, Hashimoto N. Glucose-lowering effect of sevelamer hydrochloride in hemodialysis patients. Ther Apher Dial. 2015;19:412–3.

21

Lower Hb at the initiation of dialysis does not adversely affect 1-year mortality rate

Shinya Kawamoto[*], Yu Kaneko, Hideo Misawa, Katsuhiro Nagahori, Atsushi Kitazawa, Atsunori Yoshino and Tetsuro Takeda

Abstract

Background: The management of renal anemia in the pre-dialysis period has been remarkably improved by long-acting erythropoiesis-stimulating agents (ESA). However, many incident dialysis patients cannot achieve target hemoglobin (Hb) levels (> 10 g/dL) and sometimes require blood transfusions. Anemia at the time of dialysis initiation is reportedly correlated with cardiomegaly and early cardiovascular events. Here, we investigated whether this V-shaped depression in Hb level at dialysis initiation adversely affects short-term prognosis.

Methods: The medical charts of 166 patients who underwent initial dialysis were retrospectively reviewed for Hb level, ESA treatment status, dry weight (DW), cardiothoracic rate (CTR), and brain natriuretic peptide (BNP) level at dialysis initiation and 1 year later. Patients were subdivided into three groups according to the tertile of Hb levels. The risk of mortality within 1 year after initiation was analyzed using multivariable-adjusted Cox proportional hazard model.

Result: Mean Hb level at initiation was 8.6 ± 1.3 g/dL despite the administration of sufficient ESA. After initiation, Hb levels rapidly increased and the Hb time course showed a V-shape with the bottom at initiation. Hb level, CTR, and log BNP showed a significant negative correlation. The Hb level and CTR 1 year after initiation did not correlate with Hb levels at initiation. Lower Hb levels at initiation as a V-shaped depression do not adversely affect 1-year mortality rate by multivariable-adjusted Cox proportional hazard model.

Conclusion: Hb level around dialysis initiation showed a V-shaped depression despite ESA use. Our findings suggest that the V-shaped Hb depression at initiation does not affect short-term prognosis.

Keywords: CTR, ESA, Hemodialysis initiation, Short-term prognosis, V-shaped Hb depression

Background

Before the advent of erythropoiesis-stimulating agents (ESA), renal anemia arose as an almost obligatory complication of chronic kidney failure requiring blood transfusions and early dialysis initiation for patients with end-stage kidney disease (ESKD). With ESA use, the management of renal anemia in the pre-dialysis period has been dramatically improved, reducing blood transfusion rates and postponing dialysis initiation by symptomatically relieving anemia and creating a renal protective effect. However, it has been reported that hemoglobin (Hb) decreases to 8.4 g/dL during the initial dialysis phase

despite recombinant human erythropoietin (rHuEPO) treatment [1].

This study aimed to evaluate the influence of Hb depression at dialysis initiation on short-term prognosis. Our principal goal was to investigate if a V-shaped Hb depression at initiation has any effect on short-term prognosis.

Methods

Patients

We retrospectively reviewed the charts of inpatients who underwent initial dialysis between January 2012 and May 2015 at Dokkyo Medical University Saitama Medical Center (Koshigaya, Saitama, Japan). After initiation, all patients were treated in an ordinary outpatient clinic according to Japanese guidelines.

* Correspondence: kwmt@dokkyomed.ac.jp
Department of Nephrology, Dokkyo Medical University Saitama Medical Center, 2-1-50 Minami-Koshigaya, Koshigaya, Saitama 343-8555, Japan

This was an observational study and approved by the Dokkyo Medical University Saitama Medical Center Ethics Committee (2017/1716). Observations and inspections were conducted according to the items and methods below, and the collected data were used in the study.

Basic patient information included date of initiation, age, sex, primary disease, main reason for dialysis initiation, body weight, and blood pressure at initiation. Laboratory values including levels of Hb, blood urea nitrogen (BUN), creatinine (Cr), potassium (K), calcium (Ca), phosphorus (P), albumin, Fe, ferritin, and C-reactive protein; estimated glomerular filtration rate (eGFR); total iron binding capacity (TIBC); and transferrin saturation (TSAT) were collected from 6 months prior to 1 year after initiation. Data on B-type natriuretic peptide (BNP) level were collected at initiation, while data on cardiothoracic rate (CTR) were collected at initiation and 1 year after initiation.

State of ESA administration included ESA drug name and dosage. Erythropoietin resistance index (ERI) (IU/kg/week/g/100 mL) = weekly ESA dose (unit as Epo conversion rate)/(Hb [g/dL] × body weight [kg]). Considering the use of different ESA, the dose conversion ratio was rHuEpo to darbepoetin to epoetin beta pegol of 1:200:240 [2, 3]. The usual ESA treatment interval is once a month, although some patients received it biweekly.

A total of 166 incident patients were followed up for 1 year; of them, 12 died (7.2%), 6 were lost to follow-up, 4 underwent transplantation, and 144 remained on dialysis (Fig. 1).

Patients were subdivided into three groups according to the tertile of Hb levels and compared Hb levels and CTR at 1 year after initiation.

The risk of mortality within 1 year after initiation was analyzed using multivariable-adjusted Cox proportional hazard model.

Statistical analyses

Statistical analysis was performed using SPSS version 23 (SPSS Inc., Chicago, IL, USA). All results are expressed as mean ± SD. To measure intergroup differences, paired t tests, the Kruskal-Wallis test, and Fisher's exact test were used as appropriate. The risk of mortality was analyzed using multivariable-adjusted Cox proportional hazard model. The correlation between the two groups was determined using Pearson's correlation coefficient. Values of $P < 0.05$ were considered statistically significant.

Results

Patient characteristics

This study comprised 166 patients who started undergoing dialysis between January 2012 and May 2015. Men accounted for 67% of the subjects, and the mean age was 61.5 ± 14.3 years. The patient characteristics are shown in Table 1. The ESKD was caused by diabetic nephropathy (89 cases, 49%), nephrosclerosis (41 cases, 25%), chronic glomerulonephritis (13 cases, 8%), and polycystic kidney (PKD) (4 cases, 2.4%). The primary reasons for dialysis initiation included uremia (57 cases, 34%), uremia with edema (47 cases, 28%), congestion or dyspnea (33 cases, 20%), and edema (15 cases, 9%). The mean blood pressure was $147 \pm 21/76 \pm 16$ mmHg. The mean body weight was 62.6 ± 15.7 kg. Of the total patients, dialysis was initiated in 125 (75.3%) using arteriovenous fistulae (AVF) and in 41 (24.7%) using a catheter. The mean Hb was 8.56 ± 1.3 g/dL. The mean Fe was 61 ± 31 /dL, TIBC was 212 ± 44 μg/dL, and ferritin was 305 ± 315 ng/dL. The mean BUN was 103 ± 33 mg/dL; Cr was 11.1 ± 4.3 mg/dL. The mean eGFR was 4.5 ± 1.8 mL/min/1.73 m^2. The mean K was 4.7 ± 1.0 mEq/L. The mean corrected Ca was 8.5 ± 1.1 mg/dL, and P was 7.6 ± 2.1 mg/dL. The mean intact parathyroid hormone was 186 ± 107 pg/mL. The mean BNP was 954 ± 2136 ng/mL (4~18,258). The mean CTR was 54.8 ± 6.0%.

A total of 129 patients (78%) were treated with long-acting ESA (epoetin beta pegol in 89 and darbepoetin in 40). The mean ESA dosage was 4871 ± 3259 U/week (Epo conversion rate: Hb [g/dL] × body weight [kg]). The mean ERI was 9.95 ± 7.35 IU/kg/week/g/100. Forty-six patients (28%) were treated with an oral iron supplement.

The Hb distribution at initiation was normal. At initiation, the associations between Hb level and both CTR

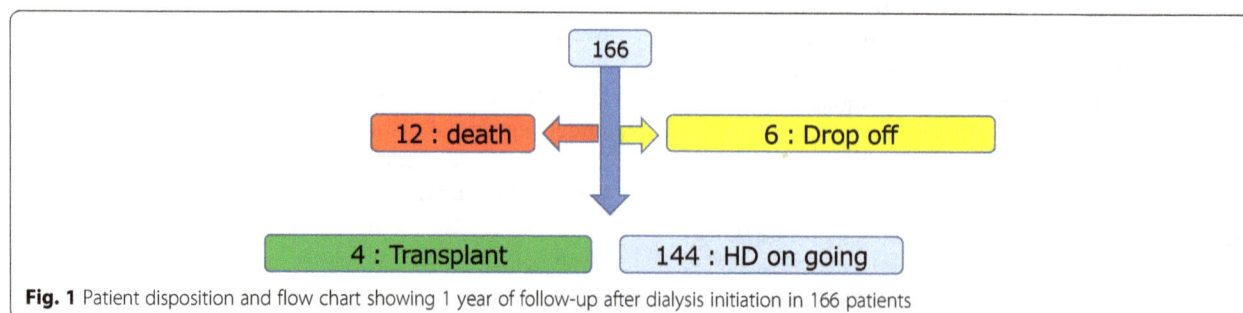

Fig. 1 Patient disposition and flow chart showing 1 year of follow-up after dialysis initiation in 166 patients

Table 1 Patient characteristics at initiation of HD ($n = 166$)

Clinical findings	
Age (years)	61.5 ± 14.3(30~89)
Gender (male/female)	110/56
Systolic/diastolic blood pressure (mmHg)	147 ± 21/76 ± 16
BW (kg; mean ± SD)	62.6 ± 15.7
Method of HD initiation (AVF/catheter)	125/41
Primary disease of ESKD	
Diabetic nephropathy	87 (49%)
Chronic glomerulonephritis	13 (8%)
Nephrosclerosis	41 (25%)
Polycystic kidney disease	4 (2.4%)
Others	21 (12.7%)
Laboratory findings	
Hb (g/dL)	8.56 ± 1.3
Fe/TIBC (µg/dL)	61 ± 31/212 ± 44
Ferritin (ng/dL)	305 ± 315
Serum albumin (g/dL)	3.0 ± 0.6
BUN/creatinine (mg/dL)	103 ± 33/11.1 ± 4.3
eGFR (mL/m/1.73m²)	4.5 ± 1.8
K (mEq/L)	4.7 ± 1.0
Ca/P (mg/dL)	8.5 ± 1.1/7.6 ± 2.1
Intact PTH(pg/mL)	186 ± 107
B-type natriuretic peptide (BNP) (ng/mL)	954 ± 2136 (4~18258)
Cardiothoracic rate (CTR) (%)	54.8 ± 6.0
ESA treatment	129 (78%) epoetin beta pegol:89 darbepoetin:40
ESA dosage (U/week; converted in Epo dosage)	4871 ± 3259
Erythropoietin resistance index(U/week/Hb (g/dL) × BW (kg))	9.95 ± 7.36
Fe treatment	46 (28%)

and log BNP were significantly negative ($R = -0.175$, $P = 0.025$; $R = -0.29$, $P < 0.01$) (Fig. 2).

The time course of Hb levels and percentages of ESA usage in 105 patients obserbed from 6 months prior to initiation are shown in Fig. 3. At 6 months prior to initiation, the Hb level was 9.7 ± 1.2 g/dL with 62% of patients treated with ESA. Although the ESA usage rate gradually increased up to nearly 100% toward the initiation, the Hb level gradually decreased to 9.3 ± 1.2 g/dL at 1 month prior to initiation and then dramatically dropped to 8.6 ± 1.3 g/dL at initiation. After initiation, Hb level rapidly increased to > 10 g/dL and a V-shaped curve was seen at the bottom at the time of initiation.

We compared the Hb level, CTR, ESA dose, and ERI between the time of initiation and 1 year later in 144 patients (Fig. 4). Hb level at 1 year after initiation showed a significant increase compared with the level at initiation (10.6 ± 1.0 vs 8.6 ± 1.3 g/dL, $P < 0.001$). CTR showed a significant decrease compared with that at initiation (49.3 ± 5.0 vs 54.8 ± 6.0%, $P < 0.001$). ESA dose at 1 year after initiation showed an insignificant decrease compared with that at initiation. (4232 ± 3044 vs 4872 ± 3259 U/week, $P = 0.068$). ERI showed a significant decrease compared with that at initiation (7.74 ± 6.92 vs 9.95 ± 7.35, $P < 0.001$) (Fig. 4).

The patient characteristics of three groups according to the tertile of Hb levels at initiation are shown in Table 2. There was a significant difference only in Hb and CTR at initiation between the three groups. The mean Hb level at initiation and 1 year after among three groups and the association between the Hb levels at initiation and 1 year later are shown in Fig. 5. There were no differences in Hb level among the three groups at 1 year after initiation. Thus, there was no significant correlation between Hb levels at initiation and 1 year later.

Changes in CTR at 1 year after initiation among the three groups are shown in Fig. 6. CTR showed significant differences at initiation but no significant differences at 1 year after initiation among the three groups.

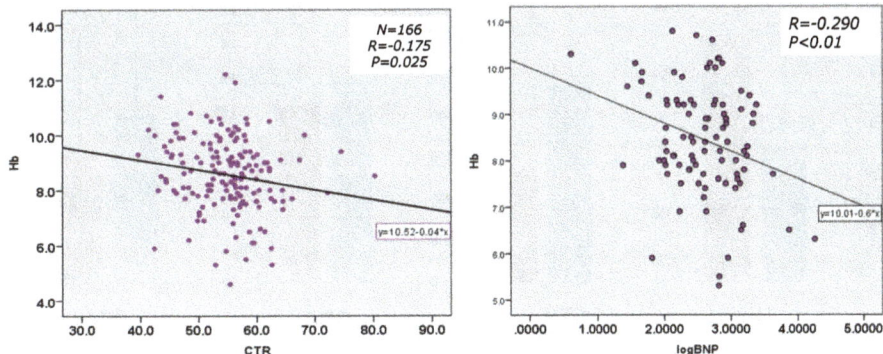

Fig. 2 Association between hemoglobin (Hb) level and cardiothoracic rate (CTR), log brain natriuretic protein (BNP) at dialysis initiation. At initiation, both association between Hb level, CTR, and log BNP had a significant negative correlation

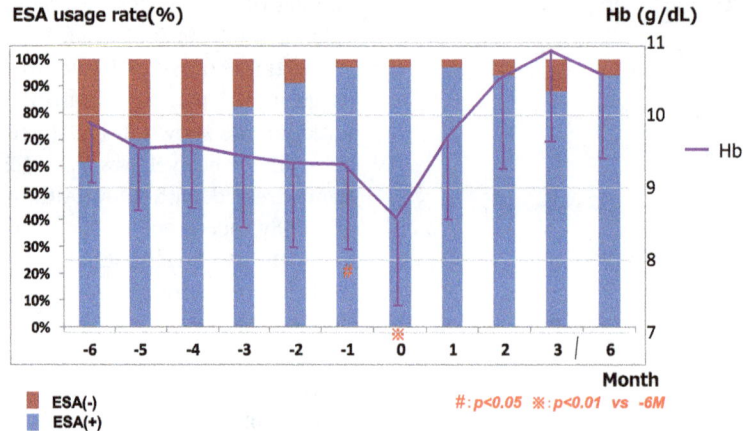

Fig. 3 Time course of hemoglobin (Hb) and erythropoiesis-stimulating agent (ESA) usage rate between 6 months before and after dialysis initiation. Despite the ESA usage rate gradually increasing to nearly 100% as initiation approached, the Hb level gradually decreased until 1 month prior to initiation and then dramatically decreased to 8.6 g/dL at initiation. After initiation, Hb level rapidly increased to > 10 g/dL and exhibited a V-shaped curve with the bottom at the time of initiation

Twelve patients were dead. Three deaths in higher and middle tertile group and 6 in lower tertile group. The cause of death was pneumonia in three patients, cardiovascular event including sudden death in three patients, and cerebral infarction, gastrointestinal bleeding, colon cancer, subdural hemorrhage, hyperkalemia, and myelodysplastic syndrome (MDS) in each one. The results of multivariate Cox proportional hazard model indicated that eGFR at initiation was the only significant risk factor for mortality within 1 year after dialysis initiation (hazard ratio 1.419, $P = 0.006$) (Table 3).

Discussion
Nevertheless, the Hb level gradually decreased at 1 month prior to initiation and then dramatically decreased at initiation despite the administration of the long acting ESA. ERI also increased as patients approached the initiation of dialysis. Kawahara reported that the monthly Hb decreased gradually during 6-month period before initiation of dialysis, whereas ESA dose and ERI increased as patients approached the initiation of dialysis [4]. Our data showed a tendency similar to that reported by Kawahara. It could be thought that the point at which a maximum ERI was reached would be the ideal timing for the initiation.

Regarding the V-shaped depression of Hb at dialysis initiation, it was previously not observed after use of long-acting ESA in a limited number of cases [5]. Kataoka reported that this depression was observed even after use of long-acting ESA in 72 incident dialysis patients [6]. The difference in this study was thought to be due to both number of patients and initiation timing.

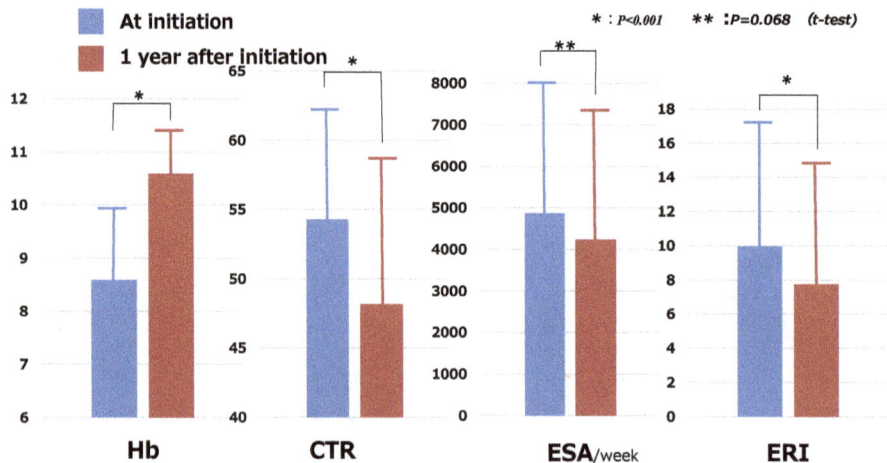

Fig. 4 Changes in hemoglobin (Hb), cardiothoracic rate (CTR), erythropoiesis-stimulating agent (ESA) dosage, and erythropoietin resistance index (ERI) from initiation to 1 year after initiation Hb at 1 year after initiation showed a significant increase, and CTR and ERI showed a significant decrease compared with initiation. ESA dose at 1 year after initiation showed an insignificant decrease compared with the initiation

Table 2 Patient characteristics of three cohorts ($n = 166$)

Variables	Hb $\leqq$ 8	8 < Hb $\leqq$ 9.2	9.2 < Hb (g/dL)	P value
	60	57	49	
Clinical findings				
Age (years)	60.6 ± 16.1	62.3 ± 12.4	61.7 ± 14.2	0.11
Gender (male/female)	39/21	35/22	36/13	0.40
DM/non DM	26/34	33/24	28/21	0.22
CVD history (+/−)	18/42	7/50	12/37	0.064
Method of HD initiation (AVF/catheter)	41/19	49/8	35/14	0.057
Laboratory findings				
Hb (g/dL) at initiation	7.23 ± 0.84	8.69 ± 0.37	10.05 ± 0.63	0.00
Hb (g/dL) at 6 months prior to initiation	9.48 ± 1.50	9.81 ± 1.07	9.84 ± 1.02	0.62
Hb (g/dL) at 1 year after initiation	10.45 ± 1.04	10.61 ± 0.98	10.76 ± 0.90	0.66
Creatinine (mg/dL)	11.6 ± 4.6	11.5 ± 4.7	10.1 ± 3.4	0.196
eGFR (mL/m/1.73m^2)	4.4 ± 1.8	4.2 ± 1.6	5.0 ± 2.4	0.196
Cardiothoracic rate (CTR) at initiation (%)	56.3 ± 5.9	55.0 ± 5.0	52.8 ± 6.8	0.007
CTR at 1 year after initiation (%)	48.5 ± 5.2	50.7 ± 5.1	48.6 ± 4.5	0.057
Log BNP (ng/mL)	2.7 ± 0.6	2.7 ± 0.4	2.3 ± 0.6	0.069
Treatment				
ESA dosage (U/week; converted in Epo dosage)	4760 ± 3223	5231 ± 2803	4580 ± 3796	0.439
Erythropoietin resistance index (ERI)	11.1 ± 8.4	10.1 ± 6.0	8.4 ± 7.4	0.21

Our result supported Kataoka's observation of V-shaped depression at initiation even after long-acting ESA use. Since almost all patients in our study underwent dialysis initiation with serious symptoms such as uremia, edema, and dyspnea at a mean Cr level of 11.1 mg/dL, the timing of dialysis initiation was relatively late, so anemia was considered to be progressing.

In our cohort, the average Hb was 8.6 ± 1.3 g/dL with a peak at 8.0–8.9 g/dL and showed a normal distribution. Asakawa et al. demonstrated the same tendency in 2249 Japanese initiation patients with a normally distributed mean Hb level of 8.7 ± 1.6 g/dL with a peak at 8.0–8.9 g/dL [7] and a negative relationship between Hb and CTR [8]. Koibuchi et al.

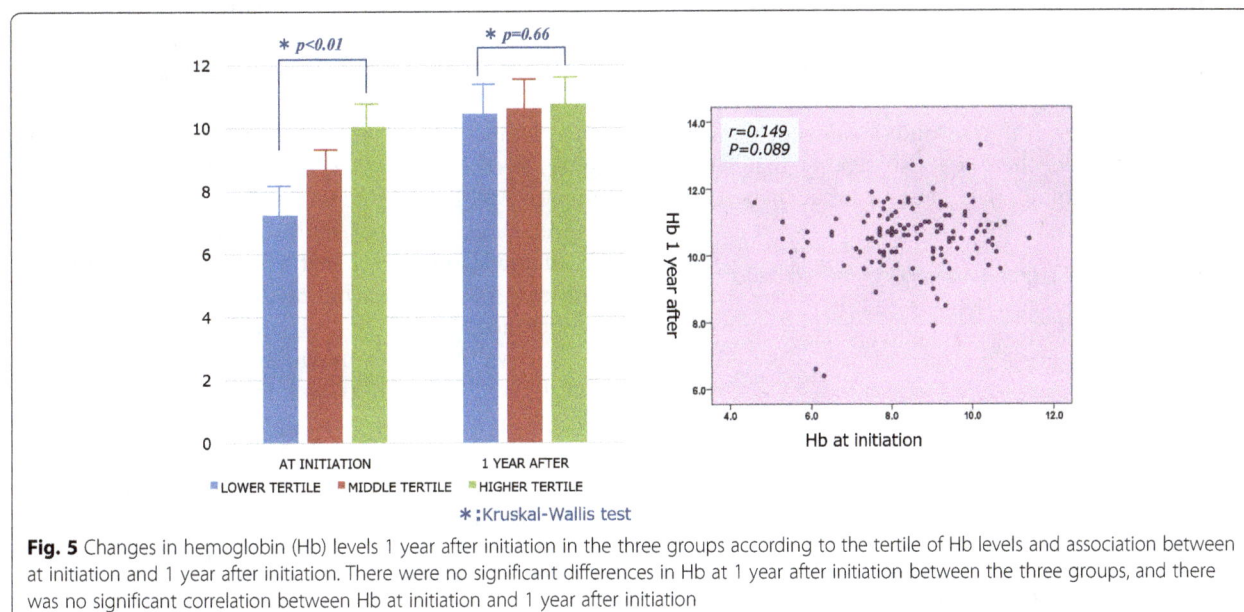

Fig. 5 Changes in hemoglobin (Hb) levels 1 year after initiation in the three groups according to the tertile of Hb levels and association between at initiation and 1 year after initiation. There were no significant differences in Hb at 1 year after initiation between the three groups, and there was no significant correlation between Hb at initiation and 1 year after initiation

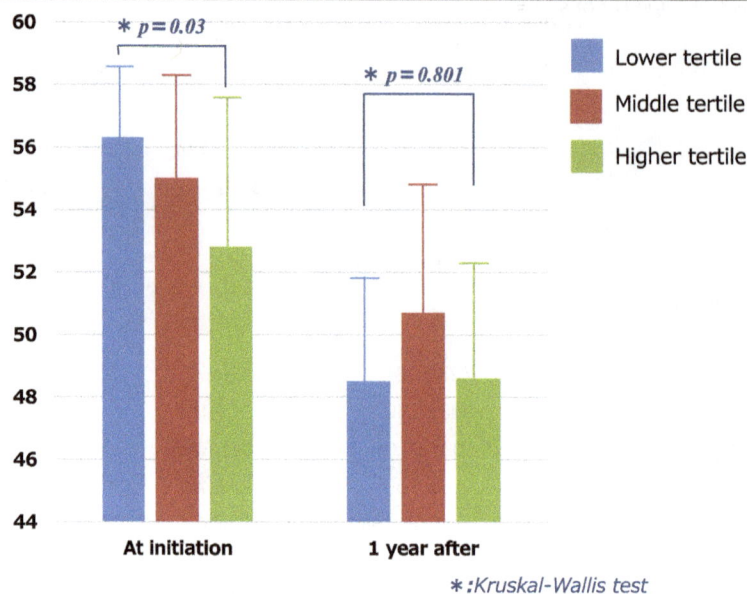

Fig. 6 Changes in cardiothoracic rate (CTR) from dialysis initiation to 1 year after initiation in the three groups according to the tertile of Hb levels. Though there was a significant difference in CTR among the three groups at initiation, this significant difference could not be observed at 1 year after

also reported the same correlation between them [9]. In our patients, there was a significant negative relationship between Hb and CTR at initiation. Moreover, the negative relationship between Hb and log BNP was also observed in our patients. Negative correlations of Hb with CTR and BNP are considered to be associated with fluid volume status. With progression of renal failure, the progression of renal anemia and over fluid volume status is presented. In addition, at the time of initiation, it also exhibits dilutable Hb reduction due to over fluid volume status. Regarding the relationship between anemia and cardiovascular parameters, a negative correlation has been noted between anemia and cardiac hypertrophy [10]. Moreover, correlations exit between the LVMI coefficient and both the survival rate and incidence of cardiac events. Meanwhile, there are also reports that low Hb levels during hemodialysis cause cardiac hypertrophy

[11]. Accordingly, a persistent lower Hb of dialysis patients could be a high-risk factor for cardiovascular events. However, this V-shaped depression of Hb was corrected promptly after initiation and a shift to a stable state of dialysis was achieved within a few months. Although a lower level of Hb at initiation presents a higher CTR or BNP level, which is considered high-risk factors of cardiovascular events [12], CTR at 1 year after initiation showed a significant decrease in relation to Hb levels and the fluid volume reduction induced by dialysis.

Death was considered much more likely in the early stage after initiation, and the mortality rate immediately post-hemodialysis has been noted to be high even by global standards [13, 14]. Regarding the mortality within 1 year after initiation, it seems to be higher in the lower Hb tertile group in six cases, compared with the middle tertile and higher tertile, in three cases each, but multivariate Cox proportional hazard model indicated that Hb at initiation was not significant risk factor. One of the reasons for the lack of differences by Hb level would be the very good 1-year survival rate after initiation as over 90% in Japan recently, and our cohort size may not have been big enough to recognize as a significant difference. We think that one reason for this good survival rate in Japan is that almost all of the incident dialysis patients were admitted to the hospital for initiation in this dangerous period. And after discharge from the hospital at initiation, the very low mortality rate in Japan during the stable dialysis period was proven by

Table 3 Multivariate regression analysis of risk factors for mortality within 1 year after dialysis initiation

Variables	β	S.E	Hazard ratio	95% CI	P value
Age	0.015	0.027	1.016	0.964–1.070	0.562
Gender (male (1))	0.514	0.814	1.671	0.339–8.243	0.528
Hb	−0.150	0.254	0.860	0.523–1.415	0.554
ERI	−0.013	0.038	0.987	0.916–1.063	0.554
eGFR	−0.350	0.126	1.419	1.108–1.817	0.006
CTR	0.001	0.055	1.001	0.898–1.115	0.991
sBP	−0.022	0.018	0.978	0.944–1.013	0.978

Dialysis Outcomes and Practice Patterns Study (DOPPS) [11].

A statistical analysis from Japan [15] indicated a 10% mortality rate in the first year for 35,864 incident dialysis patients in 2014, most commonly caused by infection, followed by heart failure, malignancy, cerebrovascular disease, and myocardial infarction. The high probability of attribution to cardiovascular disease is well known, reaching 25%. In this study, 12 patients died. Our results are consistent with the annual dialysis data report from the Japanese Society for Dialysis Therapy (JSDT).

In the 1-year follow-up survey of 29,716 patients among 36,173 Japanese incident patients in 2007, a comparison of mortality by cohorts regarding as Hb level at initiation showed no significant differences in cohorts in Hb level from 7 to 11 g/dL [16].

Yamagata et al. investigated the ideal timing for dialysis initiation to determine whether eGFR was associated with better mortality after initiation in 9695 incident dialysis patients in 2007 based on these data and reported a lowest 1-year odds ratio (OR) of mortality in patients with an eGFR of 4–6 mL/min/1.73 m^2, but the OR was identical among groups with an eGFR of 2–8 mL/min/1.73 m^2. The average Hb of patients with an eGFR of 4–6 mL/min/1.73 m^2 was 8.4 g/dL, while that of those with an eGFR of 2–8 mL/min/1.73 m^2 was equivalent to 8.0–8.6 g/dL [17].

These data were investigated in incident patients in 2007 when long-acting ESA could not be used. At the present time, long-acting ESA can be used, the anemia management around the initiation phase is improved, and Hb level at initiation is increasing [18]. The mortality rate 1 year after initiation showed some improvement compared with that in 2007 as 10.3% in 2014 vs 12.6% in 2007. The average age in our cohort was a little bit younger than that reported in the annual dialysis data report from the JSDT, and this is the one reason for our low mortality (7.2% in 2015).

Watanabe et al. recently reported that the 1-year survival rate was 95.36% in the rHuEPO and 90.36% in the non-treatment group despite the mean Hb at initiation being 8.35 g/dL in the rHuEPO and 8.25 g/dL in the non-treatment group [19].

In Japan, patients with a low Hb that could indicate a risk of cardiovascular events could safely initiate dialysis because the majority of initiation patients are hospitalized during high-risk period.

Finally, from an economical view for initiation patients, ESA costs before initiation require a corresponding self-burden vs almost no self-burden after initiation in Japan. It is economically beneficial for initiation patients when short-term Hb depression before initiation quickly catches up with ESA treatment after initiation

without self-burden, and no difference is noted in short-term prognosis.

Study limitation

Our study has several limitations. First, this was a retrospective study, there were constraints regarding the number of the subjects and the length of the observation period. Our subject's age was younger than the JSDT statistics; it had become sticking to the initiation point where the symptom appears. Second, comparison of the three cohorts examined important factors for survival rates such as age and diabetes and did not show any significant difference, but other comorbidities could not be considered. Third, cardiac function at initiation was not evaluated by UCG but only with CTR and BNP in our study.

Conclusion

In the dialysis initiation period, incident patients showed severe renal anemia that was resistant even to long-acting ESA as well as a high CTR and elevated BNP, both of which were considered high-risk factors of cardiovascular events. This was corrected promptly by dialysis initiation and a short-term V-shaped depression of Hb level had no effects on short-term prognosis including cardiovascular events under current ordinary hemodialysis treatment in Japan.

Acknowledgements
Not applicable

Funding
This study was not supported by any fundings.

Authors' contributions
SK designed and promoted the study. YK, HM, KN, AK, and AY participated in data collection. TT conceived of the study and participated in its design and coordination and helped draft the manuscript. All authors read and approved the final manuscript.

Competing interests
All authors declare that they have no competing interests.

References

1. Akisawa T, Saito A, Gejyo F, et al. Impacts of recombinant human erythropoietin treatment during predialysis periods on the progression of chronic kidney disease in a large-scale cohort study (Co-JET study). Ther Apher Dial. 2014;18:140–8.

2. Bonafont X, Bock A, Carter D, Brunkhorst R, Carrera F, Iskedjian M, et al. A meta-analysis of the relative doses of erythropoiesis-stimulating agents in patients undergoing dialysis. Nephrol Dial Transplant Plus. 2009;2:347–35.

3. Vega A, Abad S, Verdalles U, et al. Dose equivalence between continuous erythropoietin receptor activator (CERA), darbepoiet and epoetin in patients with advanced chronic kidney disease. Hippokratia Med J. 2014;18:315–8.

4. Kawahara K, Minakuchi J, Yokota N, Suekane H, Tsuchida K, Kawashima S. Treatment of renal anemia with erythropoiesis-stimulating agents in predialysis chronic kidney disease patients: haemoglobin profile during the 6 months before initiation of dialysis. Nephrology. 2015;20(Suppl. 4):29–32.

5. Yoshiya K, Tsukuda M, Hara A, Anpuku T. The efficacy of continuous erythropoietin receptor activator (C.E.R.A) in renal anemia during dialysis initiation. Japanese J Clin Dial. 2013;29(9):115–7. (Japanese)

6. Kataoka H, Tsuchiya K, Naganuma T, Okazaki M, Komatsu M, Kimura T, Shiohira S, Kawaguchi H, Nitta K. Relationship between anaemia management at haemodialysis initiation and patient prognosis. Nephrology. 2015;20:14–21.

7. Asakawa T, Komatsu Y, Ando R, Joki N, Tanaka Y, Iwasaki M, Hase H, Ikeda M, Inaguma D, Sakaguchi T, Shinoda T, Koiwa F, Negi S, Yamaka T, Shigematsu T. Effect of long-acting erythropoiesis-stimulating agents on hemoglobin levels at the initiation of dialysis. Renal Replace Ther. 2016;2:12.

8. Asakawa T, Joki N, Tanaka Y, Hayashi T, Hase H, Komatsu Y, Ando R, Ikeda M, Inaguma D, Sakaguchi T, Shinoda T, Koiwa F, Negi S, Yamaka T, Shigematsu T. Association between the hemoglobin level and cardiothoracic ratio in patients on incident dialysis. Cardiorenal Med. 2014;4:189–200.

9. Koibuchi K, Miyagi M, Arai T, Aoki T, Aikawa A, Sakai K. Comparing the efficacy of continuous erythropoietin receptor activator and darbepoetin alfa treatments in Japanese patients with chronic kidney disease during the predialysis period: a propensity-matched analysis. Nephrology. 2015; 20(Suppl. 4):22–8.

10. London GM, Marchais SJ, Guerin AP, Fabiani F, Metivier F. Cardiovascular function in hemodialysis patients. Adv Nephrol. 1991;20:249–73.

11. Zoccali C, Benedetto FA, Mallamaci F, et al. Left ventricular mass monitoring I the follow-up of dialysis patients: prognostic value of left ventricular hypertrophy progression. Kidney Int. 2004;65:1492–8.

12. Koch M, Trapp R, Kohnle M, Aker S, Haastert B, Rump LC. B-type natriuretic peptide and severe heart failure at baseline predict overall mortality in incident dialysis patients. Clin Nephrol. 2010;73(1):21–9.

13. Robinson BM, Zhang J, Morgenstern H, Bradbury BD, Ng LJ, McCullough KP, Gillespie BW, Hakim R, Rayner H, Fort J, Akizawa T, Tentori F, Pisoni RL. Worldwide, mortality risk is high soon after initiation of hemodialysis. Kidney Int. 2014;85(1):158–65.

14. Eckardt KU, Gillespie IA, Kronenberg F, Richards S, Stenvinkel P, Anker SD, Wheeler DC, de Francisco AL, Marcelli D, Froissart M, Floege J, ARO Steering Committee. High cardiovascular event rates occur within the first weeks of starting hemodialysis. Kidney Int. 2015;88(5):1117–25.

15. Masakane I, Taniguchi M, Nakai S, et al. Annual dialysis data report 2015, JSDT registry J. Jpn Soc Dial Ther. 2017;50(1):1–62.

16. The committee of Renal Data Registry of the Japanese Society for Dialysis. Therapy analysis on factors influencing the mortality of dialysis initiation patients in 2007 an overview of regular dialysis treatment in Japan (as 31 December 2007). Tokyo: Japanese Society of Dialysis therapy; 2008. p. 54–78.

17. Yamagata K, Nakai S, Masakane I, Hanafusa N, Iseki K, Tsubakihara Y. The committee of renal data ideal timing and predialysis nephrology care duration for dialysis initiation: from analysis of Japanese dialysis initiation survey. Ther Apher Dial. 2012;16(1):54–62.

18. Asakawa T, Komatsu Y, Ando R, et al. Effect of long-acting erythropoiesis stimulating agents on hemoglobin levels at the initiation of dialysis. Renal Replace Ther. 2016;2:12P.

19. Watanabe Y, Akizawa T, Saito T, et al. Effect of predialysis recombinant human erythropoietin on early survival after hemodialysis initiation in patients with chronic kidney disease: Co-JET study. Ther Apher Dial. 2016; 20(6):598–607.

Biocompatibility and small protein permeability of hydrophilic-coated membrane dialyzer (NV) in hemodialysis patients

Hirotoshi Kodama[1]* (iD), Akira Tsuji[2], Akihiro Fujinoki[1], Koujirou Ooshima[2], Kaori Ishizeki[2] and Tatsuo Inoue[1]

Abstract

Background: We evaluated the biocompatibility and small protein permeability of a newly developed hydrophilic-coated membrane dialyzer (NV) compared with conventional polysulfone dialyzer (APS) for hemodialysis (HD) therapy.

Methods: In a prospective crossover study, 11 maintenance HD patients (7 males; mean age 67.0 ± 10.2 years) received HD three times a week for 4 weeks with the NV membrane and then for another 4 weeks with the APS membrane. We evaluated the variation in several parameters including white blood cell (WBC) count and fibrinogen as indexes for biocompatibility. The plasma and dialysate concentrations of β_2-microglobulin (β_2-M), α_1-microglobulin (α_1-M), and albumin were measured at baseline and after 4 h of each study treatment in order to assess the removal of small proteins.

Results: Reductions in the WBC count were seen with APS compared with NV at 60 min (NV 5.65 ± 1.60, APS $5.17 \pm 1.65 \times 10^3/\mu L$, $p < 0.05$) and 240 min (NV 5.28 ± 1.38, APS $4.63 \pm 1.2 \times 10^3/\mu L$, $p < 0.005$) after the start of HD. With NV, we found significantly greater rates of variation of β_2-M (NV 45.5 ± 1.2, APS $40.1 \pm 1.2\%$, $p < 0.0001$), α_1-M (NV 41.2 ± 9.9, APS $34.2 \pm 18.5\%$, $p < 0.05$), and albumin (NV 31.6 ± 7.8, APS $18.1 \pm 6.5\%$, $p < 0.0001$) during HD than with APS. However, there were no significant differences in the removal of β_2-M between the two dialyzers.

Conclusions: The clinical characteristics of NV may reveal an improved biocompatibility and a comparable efficiency in small protein removal as compared to those of APS.

Keywords: Hemodialysis, Polysulfone, Hydrophilic-coated membrane, Biocompatibility, Small protein permeability

Background

Biocompatibility and middle molecule clearance of hemodialysis (HD) membranes affect the survival, morbidity, and quality of life of uremic patients undergoing maintenance HD therapy. In particular, malnutrition [1] and dialysis-related amyloidosis due to the reference middle molecule β_2-microglobulin (β_2-M) [2] are the major long-term complications. A polysulfone (PS) dialyzer is the mainstay of HD treatment because of its high performance. However, TORAYLIGHT® NV dialyzer (NV; Toray Industries, Inc., Tokyo, Japan) is expected to have different characteristics from the conventional PS due to its newly developed hydrophilic-coated membrane [3]. We therefore designed this prospective, crossover study to evaluate the biocompatibility and low-molecular-weight protein permeability (small protein permeability) of NV compared with a conventional PS (APS; ASAHIKASEI Industries, Inc., Tokyo, Japan).

---

* Correspondence: hiro25@jcom.zaq.ne.jp
[1]Division of Blood Purification Center, Kamifukuoka General Hospital, 931 Fukuoka, Fujimino, Saitama 356-0011, Japan
Full list of author information is available at the end of the article

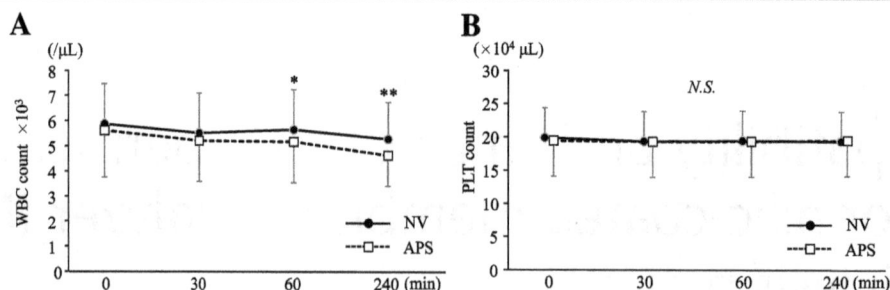

Fig 1 a WBC count and **b** PLT count. **a** Reduction in the white blood cell count were seen with the APS compared with the NV in 60 min (*$p < 0.05$) and 240 min (**$p < 0.005$) after the start of HD. **b** There were no significant differences between NV and APS

Methods

Eleven maintenance HD patients (7 males; mean age 67.0 ± 10.2 years) on regular thrice-weekly HD treatment for 4 h were enrolled in the study after they had given their written informed consent. The underlying renal diseases were diabetes mellitus ($N = 3$), glomerulonephritis ($N = 2$), and unknown ($N = 6$). The mean duration of dialysis treatment was 48.6 ± 45.0 (range 15 to 258) months. All of the patients underwent 12 consecutive HD treatments with NV-13U (1.3 m^2) and then switched with APS-13SA (1.3 m^2) as a control after a 2-week wash-out period.

Laboratory measurements

The platelet (PLT) count, white blood cell (WBC) count, and hematocrit (Hct) were measured at the beginning of dialysis and after 30, 60, and 240 min. To adjust for differences in the cell counts at the beginning of dialysis, we calculated the change ratio at each point using the following formula (1):

Change ratio X min $= 100 + 100 \times \{($Cell count $\times$ min$)/$
$\qquad\qquad\qquad\qquad\qquad\qquad$ (Cell count 0 min$)-1\}$

Cell count 0 min : Cell count at the beginning of dialysis

Cell count X min : Cell count after X minutes from the
$\qquad\qquad\qquad\qquad\qquad$ beginning of dialysis

$\qquad\qquad\qquad\qquad\qquad\qquad\qquad\qquad\qquad$ (1)

We measured the urea nitrogen, serum creatinine, inorganic phosphorus, single-pool Kt/V [4], and hemoglobin levels; the removal rate of β_2-M; and the rate of variation of β_2-M, α_1-microglobulin (α_1-M), and albumin. We also measured the levels of platelet factor-4 (PF-4), β-thromboglobulin (β-TG), fibrinogen/fibrin degradation products (FDP), D-dimer, and fibrinogen (FIB).

Dialysate samples were collected at the final two dialysis sessions at a speed of 1.0 L/h using a fixed-quantity pump from the dialysate discharge line for 0–60, 60–180, and 180–240 min after the start of HD. On the assumption that each value measured before dialysis was 100%, the results were evaluated for variability.

This study was conducted in accordance with the guidelines of the Declaration of Helsinki and approved by the ethics committees of Kamifukuoka General Hospital and National Defense Medical College Hospital.

Statistical analyses

The continuous values of variables are expressed as the mean $\pm$ standard deviation or as the median (25th, 75th percentile). The comparative p values for continuous variables were calculated by an analysis of variance (ANOVA). All of the statistical analyses were carried out using the JMP Pro Version 11.2.0 software program (SAS Institute, Cary, NC, USA), setting the significance level at a p value of less than 0.05.

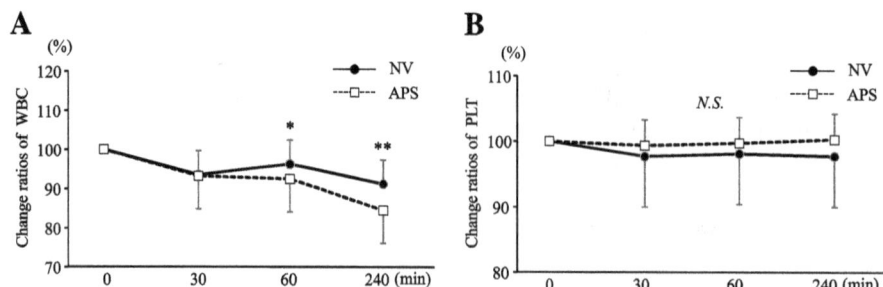

Fig 2 Change ratios of **a** WBC and **b** PLT. **a** The change ratios of the white blood cell count were significantly smaller with the NV than with the APS after 60 min (*$p < 0.01$) and 240 min (**$p < 0.05$). **b** There were no significant differences between NV and APS

Table 1 Clinical parameters of Hct, PF-4, β-TG, FDP, D-dimer, and change ratio of FIB

		0 (min)	30 (min)	60 (min)	240 (min)
Hct (%)	NV	32.2 ± 2.4	31.4 ± 2.7	32.1 ± 2.6	34.9 ± 3.3
	APS	32.0 ± 2.4	30.9 ± 2.3	31.5 ± 2.3	34.4 ± 2.8
PF-4 (ng/mL)	NV	7.45 ± 7.09	29.2 ± 13.5	16.9 ± 8.1	12.3 ± 7.4
	APS	6.77 ± 3.69	32.3 ± 21.5	17.3 ± 6.9	12.1 ± 5.8
β-TG (ng/mL)	NV	146 ± 41	128 ± 42	118 ± 36	104 ± 39
	APS	135 ± 33	125 ± 40	119 ± 36	101 ± 30
FDP (μg/mL)	NV	2.0(2.0, 2.0)	2.0(2.0, 2.0)	2.0(2.0, 2.0)	2.0(2.0, 3.0)
	APS	2.0(2.0, 2.0)	2.0(2.0, 2.0)	2.0(2.0, 3.0)	2.0(2.0, 2.0)
D-dimer (μg/mL)	NV	0.4(0.2, 0.5)	0.3(0.2, 0.5)	0.3(0.2, 0.5)	0.4(0.2, 0.5)
	APS	0.4(0.4, 0.5)	0.3(0.2, 0.5)	0.3(0.2, 0.5)	0.3(0.2, 0.5)
Change ratio of FIB (%)	NV	–	98.6 ± 2.8	102 ± 3	117 ± 8
	APS	–	97.8 ± 3.3	101 ± 4	116 ± 11

FDP and D-dimer are expressed as medians with 25th–75th percentiles

Hct hematocrit, *PF-4* platelet factor-4, *β-TG* thromboglobulin, *FDP* fibrinogen/fibrin degradation products, *FIB* fibrinogen

Results

Biocompatibility

Reductions in the WBC count were seen with APS compared with NV at 60 min (NV $5.65 ± 1.60$, APS $5.17 ± 1.65 \times 10^3/\mu L$, $p < 0.05$) and 240 min (NV $5.28 ± 1.38$, APS $4.63 ± 1.20 \times 10^3/\mu L$, $p < 0.005$) after the start of HD (Fig. 1). The PLT count was not markedly different between the two dialyzers. The change ratios of the WBC count were significantly smaller with NV than with APS after 60 min (NV $96.3 ± 2.3$, APS $92.5 ± 7.5\%$, $p < 0.01$) and 240 min (NV $91.3 ± 2.3$, APS $84.6 ± 11.3\%$, $p < 0.05$) (Fig. 2).

No significant differences were seen in the levels of Hct, PF-4, β-TG, FDP, or D-dimer or in the change ratio of FIB between NV and APS (Table 1). There were also no significant differences in the urea nitrogen, creatinine, inorganic phosphorus, single-pool Kt/V, or hemoglobin values between the two dialyzers (Table 2).

Small protein permeability

The intradialytic removal of α_1-M was greater with NV than with APS in the first hour (NV $15.7 ± 4.0$, APS $10.7 ± 3.0$ mg, $p < 0.001$) and last hour (NV $6.47 ± 2.35$, APS $3.23 ± 0.74$ mg, $p < 0.001$) as well as over the total HD session (NV $32.0 ± 11.3$, APS $17.7 ± 6.3$ mg, $p < 0.0001$)

Table 2 Clinical parameters

	NV	APS	p
Urea nitrogen (mg/dL)	61.1 ± 13.8	62.1 ± 11.7	N.S.
Creatinine (mg/dL)	9.98 ± 2.39	9.87 ± 2.23	N.S.
Phosphorus (mg/dL)	4.84 ± 1.31	4.95 ± 1.25	N.S.
Single-poor Kt/V	1.55 ± 0.22	1.63 ± 0.21	N.S.
Hemoglobin (g/dL)	10.5 ± 0.9	10.3 ± 0.7	N.S.

N.S. not significant

(Fig. 3). In addition, the removal of albumin was greater with NV than with APS in the first hour (NV $340 ± 125$, APS $198 ± 59$ mg, $p < 0.001$) and last hour (NV $109 ± 46$, APS $32.0 ± 3.8$ mg, $p < 0.001$) as well as over the total HD session (NV $693 ± 283$, APS $249 ± 90$ mg, $p < 0.001$) (Fig. 4). There were no significant differences in the removal of β_2-M between the two dialyzers (Fig. 5). However, the rates of variation during HD were greater with NV than with APS for β_2-M (NV $45.5 ± 1.2$, APS $40.1 ± 1.2\%$, $p < 0.001$), α_1-M (NV $41.2 ± 9.9$, APS $34.2 ± 18.5\%$, $p < 0.05$), and albumin (NV $31.6 ± 7.8$, APS $18.1 ± 6.5\%$, $p < 0.001$).

Discussion

The PS membrane has shown a very good biocompatibility due to its superior removal performance for small-molecule proteins such as β_2-M, high clearance of small-molecule solutes such as urea and creatinine [5], and low rate of complications such as leukopenia or disorders associated with the complement system [6]. Therefore, the PS membrane is widely used for HD treatment in Japan [7]. The NV membrane was developed as an alternative to PS. With NV, the mobility of water adjacent to the membrane surface is enhanced using a new hydrophilic polymer to reform the membrane surface. NV has antithrombotic activity and less platelet and leukocyte activation than PS, as well as the ability to sufficiently remove small solutes and low-molecular-weight proteins [3]. Further, NV induces less interleukin-6 activity, which may reduce the risk of erythropoiesis-stimulating agent hyporesponsiveness [8]. In this study, we evaluated the biocompatibility and protein permeability of NV compared with those of APS as a conventional PS.

The variation of several parameters such as the WBC, PLT, Hct and levels of PF-4, β-TG, FDP, D-dimer, and

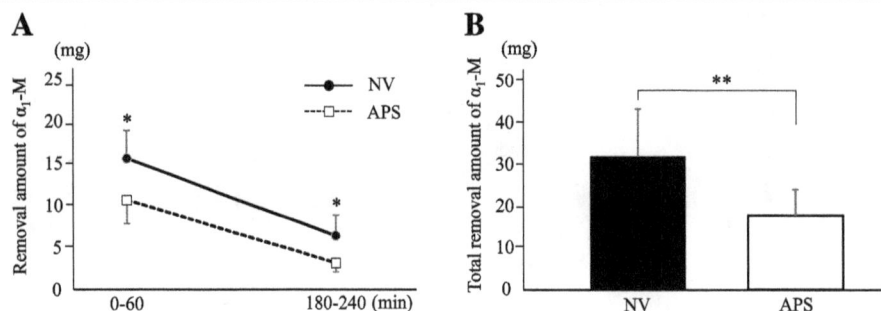

Fig 3 a Removal amount of α_1-M and **b** total removal amounts of α_1-M. Compared to APS. $*p < 0.001$ and $**p < 0.0001$ by paired t test. α_1-M α_1-microglobulin

FIB were compared to evaluate the biocompatibility of NV. PF4 and β-TG are substances contained within platelet α-granules, and changes in platelet PF4 or β-TG levels are useful indicators of platelet degranulation and activation during dialysis [9]. However, there were no significant changes observed in the coagulation factor values with either dialyzer. Although acute leukopenia is known to occur in all patients during the first 30 min of HD treatment [10], our study showed no reduction in the WBC during dialysis with either dialyzer. The platelet count usually decreases 5 to 15% at 15 to 30 min from the start of HD and recovers to the normal level by the end of the dialysis session [9, 11]. Oshihara [3] reported that the numbers of platelets adhering to the membrane surface were lower with NV than with the conventional PS (CX) membrane. In our results, the variations in the platelet counts with both membranes were stable, suggesting that both may prevent HD-associated thrombocytopenia.

It is known that WBC adhesion occurs with protein adsorption, and FIB adsorption promotes PLT adhesion on the dialysis membrane surface by blood exposure in HD treatment [12]. Platelet-derived microparticles are released from activated platelets during HD [13]. Although the biocompatibility of PS is generally regarded to be good, there are some reports that the PS dialyzer caused PLT depletion [14, 15]. On the other hand, the NV membrane has been reported that it not only inhibits the adhesion of blood components such as PLT and FIB but also acts as a highly biocompatible membrane to reduce blood cell stimulation because it is developed as a new hydrophilic polymer membrane [3]. With NV, the reduction rate of the WBC count was inhibited to a greater degree than with APS. However, the change ratio of FIB showed no significant difference between NV and APS. These results suggest that NV improves the biocompatibility compared with APS.

Dialysis-related amyloidosis is a major complication with long-term HD treatment and greatly affects patients' quality of life. The removal of β_2-M is therefore important to avoid this complication. However, there have been no reports of the small protein permeability of NV. We therefore designed this prospective crossover study to evaluate whether or not NV offers any advantages over APS. We found that the intradialytic removal of α_1-M and albumin but not β_2-M was significantly greater with NV than with APS. The rates of variation in the β_2-M and α_1-M levels during HD with NV were higher than with APS, but the differences were small. These results suggest that the removal performance of β_2-M with NV and APS should be almost equivalent.

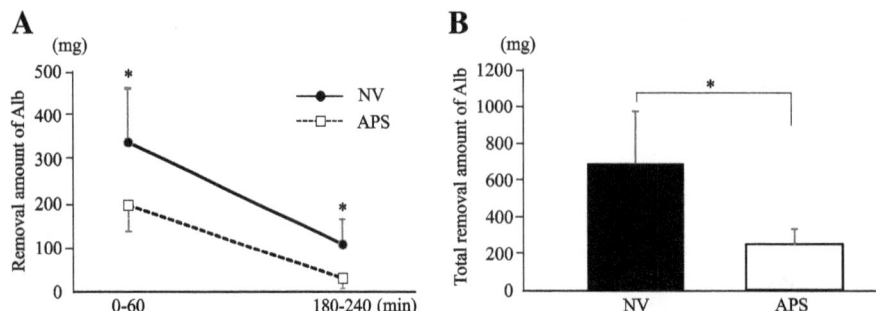

Fig 4 a Removal amount of Alb and **b** total removal amounts of Alb. Compared to APS. $*p < 0.0001$ by paired t test. *Alb* albumin

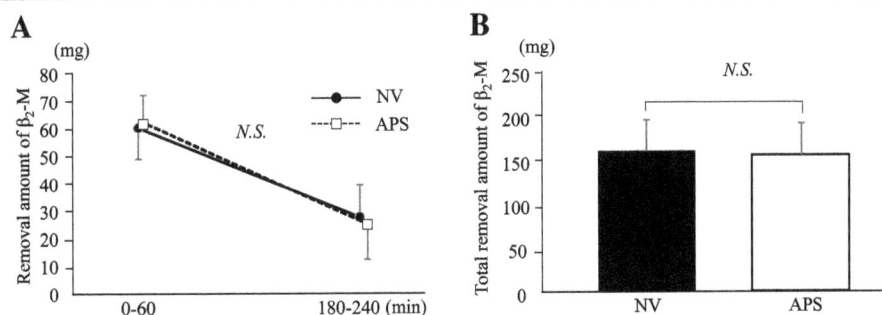

Fig 5 a Removal amount of β_2-M and **b** total removal amounts of β_2-M. There were no significant differences between NV and APS. β_2-M β_2-microglobulin

In addition, since the decrease in the serum albumin may cause low muscle mass [16], malnutrition [17], and mortality risk [18], it is important to select dialyzers with consideration of the laboratory data. NV removed significantly greater albumin than APS. Therefore, we should be cautious when using the NV membrane in elderly or malnourished patients, although the amount of albumin removed was less than 1 g (NV 693 ± 283, APS 249 ± 90 mg) in either dialyzer.

Because this was a short-term, prospective, crossover study involving only a few cases, large-scale and long-term future trials are necessary to corroborate our findings.

Conclusions

We designed this crossover study of the NV and APS membranes to evaluate the biocompatibility and small protein removal ability. The clinical characteristics of NV may reveal an improved biocompatibility and a comparable efficiency in small protein removal as compared to APS.

Abbreviations

Alb: Albumin; FDP: Fibrinogen/fibrin degradation products; FIB: Fibrinogen; Hct: Hematocrit; HD: Hemodialysis; PF-4: Platelet factor-4; PLT: Platelet; PS: Polysulfone; WBC: White blood cell; α_1-M: α_1-Microglobulin; β_2-M: β_2-Microglobulin; β-TG: β-Thromboglobulin

Acknowledgements

The authors thank all the staff members working at the Division of Blood Purification Center, Kamifukuoka General Hospital and Department of Blood Purification Therapy, National Defense Medical College Hospital.

Funding

This study has received research funds from the Foundation for Promotion of Defense Medicine.

Authors' contributions

HK designed the study, collected the clinical data, analyzed the data, and wrote the manuscript. AT designed the study and wrote the manuscript. AF collected the clinical data. KI, KO, and TI participated in its design and coordination. All authors read and approved the final manuscript.

Competing interests

The authors declare that they have no competing interests.

Author details

[1]Division of Blood Purification Center, Kamifukuoka General Hospital, 931 Fukuoka, Fujimino, Saitama 356-0011, Japan. [2]Department of Blood Purification, National Defense Medical College Hospital, 3-2 Namiki, Tokorozawa, Saitama 359-8513, Japan.

References

1. Kalantar-Zadeh K, Kopple JD, Block G, Humphreys MH. A malnutrition-inflammation score is correlated with morbidity and mortality in maintenance hemodialysis patients. Am J Kidney Dis. 2001;38:1251–63.
2. Gejyo F, Yamada T, Odani S, Nakagawa Y, Arakawa M, Kunitomo T, et al. A new form of amyloid protein associated with chronic hemodialysis was identified as beta 2-microgulobulin. Biophys Res Commun. 1985;129:701–6.
3. Oshihara W, Ueno Y, Fujieda H. A new polysulfone membrane dialyzer, NV, with low-founding and antithrombotic properties. Contrib Nephrol. 2017;189:222–9.
4. Shinzato T, Nakai S, Fujita Y, Takai I, Morita E, Nakane K, Maeda K. Determination of Kt/V and protein catabolic rate using pre- and postdialysis blood urea nitrogen concentrations. Nephron. 1994;67:280–90.
5. Fukuda M, Miyazaki M, Uezumi S, Yoshida M. Design and assessment of the new APS dialyzer (APS-SA series). J Artifs Organs. 2006;9:192–8.
6. Yamashita S, Mochizuki A, Nakazaki T, Seita Y, Sawamoto J, Endo F, et al. A new blood compatible and permselective hollow fiber membrane for hemodialysis. ASAIO J. 1996;42(6):1019–26.
7. Nakai S, Suzuki K, Masakane I, et al. Overview of regular dialysis treatment in Japan (as of 31 December 2009). Ther Apher Dial. 2010;14:505–40.
8. Kakuta T, Komaba H, Takagi N, Takahashi Y, Suzuki K, et al. A prospective multicenter randomized controlled study on interleukin-6 removal and induction by a new hemodialyzer with improved biocompatibility in hemodialysis patients: a pilot study. Ther Apher Dial. 2016;20(6):569–78.
9. Daugirdas JT, Bernardo AA. Hemodialysis effect on platelet count and function and hemodialysis-associated thrombocytoperia. Kidney Int. 2012;82:147–57.
10. Kaplow LS, Goffinet JA. Profound neutropenia during the early phase of hemodialysis. JAMA. 1968;203:1135–7.
11. Amato M, Salvadori M, Bergesio F, Messeri A, Filimberti E, Morfini M. Aspects of biocompatibility of two different dialysis membranes: cuprophane and polysulfone. Int J Artif Organs. 1988;11:175–80.
12. Reginald G. Mason, Hanson Y.K. chuang, S. Fazal Mohammad. Extracorporeal thrombogenesis: mechanisms and prevention. replacement of renal function by dialysis. 1983: 186-200.
13. Daniel L, Fakhouri F, Joly D, et al. Increase of circulating neutrophil and platelet microparticles during acute vasculitis and hemodialysis. Kidney Int. 2006;69:1416–23.
14. Kobari E, Terawaki H, Takahashi Y, et al. Dialyzer-related thrombocytopenia due to a polysulfone membrane. Intern Med. 2016;55:965–8.

15. Deprada L, Lee J, Gillespie A, Benjamin J. Thrombocytopenia associated with one type of polysulfone hemodialysis membrane: a report of 5 cases. Am J Kidney Dis. 2013;61:131–3.

16. Yasui S, Shirai Y, Tanimura M, Matsuura S, Saito Y, Miyata K. Prevalence of protein-energy wasting (PEW) and evaluation of diagnostic criteria in Japanese maintenance hemodialysis patients. Asia Pac J Clin Nutr. 2016;25(2):292–9.

17. Pifer TB, McCullough K, Port FK, Goodkin DA, Maroni BJ, Held PJ, et al. Mortality risk in hemodialysis patients and changes in nutritional indicators: DOPPS. Kidney Int. 2002;62:2338–245.

18. Dwyer JT, Larive B, Leung J, Rocco MV, Greene T, Burrowes J, et al. Are nutritional status indicators associated with mortality in hemodialysis (HEMO) study? Kidney Int. 2005;68:1766–76.

23

Asymptomatic peripheral artery disease and mortality in patients on hemodialysis

Manae Harada[1], Ryota Matsuzawa[2], Naoyoshi Aoyama[3], Kaoru Uemura[4], Yoriko Horiguchi[4], Junko Yoneyama[4], Keika Hoshi[5], Kei Yoneki[1], Takaaki Watanabe[1,4], Takahiro Shimoda[1,4], Yasuo Takeuchi[6], Shokichi Naito[6], Atsushi Yoshida[4] and Atsuhiko Matsunaga[1*]

Abstract

Background: Asymptomatic peripheral artery disease (PAD) increases the risk of mortality in non-hemodialysis patients. However, the association between asymptomatic PAD and mortality rate remains unclear in patients on hemodialysis.

Methods: This retrospective cohort study aimed to assess the prognostic significance of asymptomatic PAD in a population of 310 hemodialysis patients. Patients with an ankle–brachial index of < 1.00, or > 1.40 with a toe–brachial index of < 0.70, were diagnosed as having PAD. The San Diego Claudication Questionnaire was used to characterize leg symptoms in patients with PAD, and asymptomatic PAD was defined as the absence of symptoms in the legs or buttocks while walking. The mortality risk of asymptomatic PAD was assessed using the Cox proportional hazard model.

Results: The rate of PAD was 28.1%. Among 87 patients, those with PAD, 66.7% were asymptomatic. Fifty-eight patients died during a mean follow-up of 38.9 months. Multivariate analysis revealed hazard ratios of 1.963 (95% confidence interval (CI), 1.012 to 3.740; $P = 0.046$) and 3.237 (95% CI, 1.402 to 7.020; $P = 0.007$) in patients with asymptomatic PAD and symptomatic PAD, respectively, compared to patients without PAD. No significant difference was observed between patients with asymptomatic PAD and symptomatic PAD in terms of survival.

Conclusions: Hemodialysis patients with asymptomatic PAD have an elevated mortality risk compared to patients without PAD, with no significant difference compared to patients with symptomatic PAD.

Keywords: Ankle–brachial index, Hemodialysis, Leg symptoms, Mortality, Peripheral artery disease, Toe–brachial index

Background

Peripheral artery disease (PAD) is associated with an increased risk of all-cause and atherosclerotic mortality [1]. Leg symptoms are typical complaints of patients with PAD, and the severity of PAD is classified according to the degree of leg symptoms, such as the Fontaine and Rutherford classifications [2–5]. Although intermittent claudication and leg pain are well known and the most common symptoms of PAD, the majority of PAD patients are asymptomatic. In 2009, Diehm et al. [6] reported that the mortality risk among asymptomatic PAD patients did not differ significantly from that among symptomatic PAD patients in community-dwelling adults. However, few reports are available regarding

the usefulness of medical therapy for asymptomatic PAD to derive a meaningful conclusion. The current American Heart Association/American College of Cardiology guidelines [7] and Society for Vascular Surgery guidelines [8] do not strongly recommend treatment interventions for patients with asymptomatic PAD.

The risk of atherosclerosis is elevated regardless of the stage of chronic kidney disease, especially among patients undergoing hemodialysis (HD patients) [9]. PAD is an important manifestation of systemic atherosclerosis and is observed commonly in HD patients. The prevalence of PAD is markedly high in HD patients, although approximately 68.7% are asymptomatic [10]. One reason for the high proportion of asymptomatic PAD among HD patients is that habitual physical activity levels are reportedly low in these patients [11], and given that HD patients often have peripheral neuropathy due to a high prevalence of diabetes [12], their leg symptoms such as pain and numbness are masked.

* Correspondence: atsuhikonet@gmail.com
[1]Department of Rehabilitation Sciences, Kitasato University Graduate School of Medical Sciences, 1-15-1 Kitasato, Minami-ku, Sagamihara, Kanagawa 252-0373, Japan
Full list of author information is available at the end of the article

As a result, these patients have a similar risk of poor prognosis. Previous studies in HD patients reported a relationship between PAD and elevated mortality risk [13, 14]; however, no report has focused on the presence of leg symptoms. Moreover, the mortality risk associated with asymptomatic PAD remains unclear in HD patients. Accordingly, the present retrospective cohort study aimed to examine the mortality risk of asymptomatic PAD in HD patients.

Methods

This retrospective cohort study (registry number UMIN000020830) was reported in accordance with the STROBE guidelines (Additional file 1) [15].

Study design and patients

This study was a single-center, retrospective, and longitudinal cohort study. We conducted a retrospective analysis of patient data from another prospective study. The study was performed in accordance with the Declaration of Helsinki and the protocol was approved by the Kitasato University Allied Health Sciences Research Ethics Committee (approval no. 2012-020), and informed consent was obtained from all the patients.

We performed a retrospective cohort study of 390 patients undergoing maintenance HD at Sagami Junkanki Clinic (HD treatment organization certified by the Japanese Society for Dialysis Therapy) between May 2012 and May 2015. Inclusion criteria in this study were age > 20 years and provided informed consent for another prospective study. The exclusion criteria were patients with an ankle–brachial index (ABI) > 0.99 with lower extremity peripheral revascularization and amputation at baseline. Patients were analyzed from the date of first measurement of ABI until death or end of follow-up on Oct 2016. The date and cause of death for patients who died were obtained from their medical records. Patients who left the facilities or underwent kidney transplantation were censored. The date of death or censoring was recorded for the time-to-event analysis of all-cause mortality.

Among 390 patients undergoing HD between May 2012 and May 2015, 62 patients did not provide informed consent. Therefore, 328 patients followed up were included in this retrospective study. Additionally, we excluded 13 patients with missing data, and 5 patients with an ABI > 0.99 with lower extremity peripheral revascularization and amputation from this study. Thus, 310 HD patients were analyzed. Of these, 87 (28.1%) patients had PAD, including 58 (66.7%) with asymptomatic PAD (Fig. 1).

Baseline characteristics

Baseline characteristics of patients, including age, sex, body mass index, dialysis vintage (time since initiation of dialysis), cause of end-stage renal disease (ESRD), diabetes, comorbidities (e.g., coronary artery disease, cerebrovascular disease, and spinal stenosis), medications (e.g., angiotensin-converting enzyme inhibitors, angiotensin receptor blockers, calcium channel blockers, beta-blockers, lipid-lowering agents, antiplatelet agents, and anticoagulant agents), smoking status (ever or never), systolic blood pressure, diastolic blood pressure, pulse pressure, pulse rate, levels of serum albumin, creatinine, calcium, phosphorus, hemoglobin, hematocrit, high-density lipoprotein cholesterol (HDL-C), low-density lipoprotein cholesterol, and triglycerides, and geriatric nutritional risk index (GNRI) were obtained from medical records at the time of study entry. Blood data were measured immediately before the hemodialysis session. GNRI was calculated from the patient's serum albumin, body weight, and height as follows: GNRI = (14.89 × albumin) + (41.7 × (body weight/body weight at BMI of 22)) [16].

Diagnosis of PAD

PAD was diagnosed based on the ankle–brachial index (ABI) and toe–brachial index (TBI), which were obtained using a blood pressure pulse-wave inspection apparatus (Form3; Omron Colin, Tokyo, Japan) that allows for simultaneous measurement of arm (without dialysis access) and ankle or toe blood pressure. All patients were examined at rest in the supine position by clinical laboratory technologists using the same apparatus. ABI was calculated as the ratio of ankle systolic blood pressure to arm systolic blood pressure and TBI as the ratio of toe systolic blood pressure to arm systolic blood pressure. The lowest values of ankle and toe pressure were used for the calculations. ABI is generally used as a tool for detecting PAD, with a cutoff value of < 0.90 for detecting PAD in the general population [3]. However, since ABI values are high in HD patients and may be influenced by vascular calcification [17], an ABI cutoff of < 0.90 could result in underdiagnosing PAD in this patient population. Therefore, given that current guidelines specify a normal ABI range to be 1.00 to 1.40 and recommend follow-up for those with an ABI of > 1.4, with a TBI of < 0.7 indicating PAD [7], PAD was diagnosed in the present study using an ABI of < 1.00, or > 1.4 and a TBI of < 0.7, in HD patients.

Leg symptoms

A structured interview was conducted to assess leg symptoms in patients. Leg symptoms in patients with PAD were characterized using the San Diego Claudication Questionnaire [18, 19], which is derived from the Rose Claudication Questionnaire [20], and is used to classify symptoms as intermittent claudication, leg pain on exertion and rest, atypical exertional leg pain/carry on (i.e., exertional leg symptoms that do not begin at rest and do not stop the individual while walking), atypical exertional leg pain/stop exertional leg symptoms (i.e., exertional leg symptoms that do not begin at rest, prevent the individual from walking, and do not involve the calves or resolve

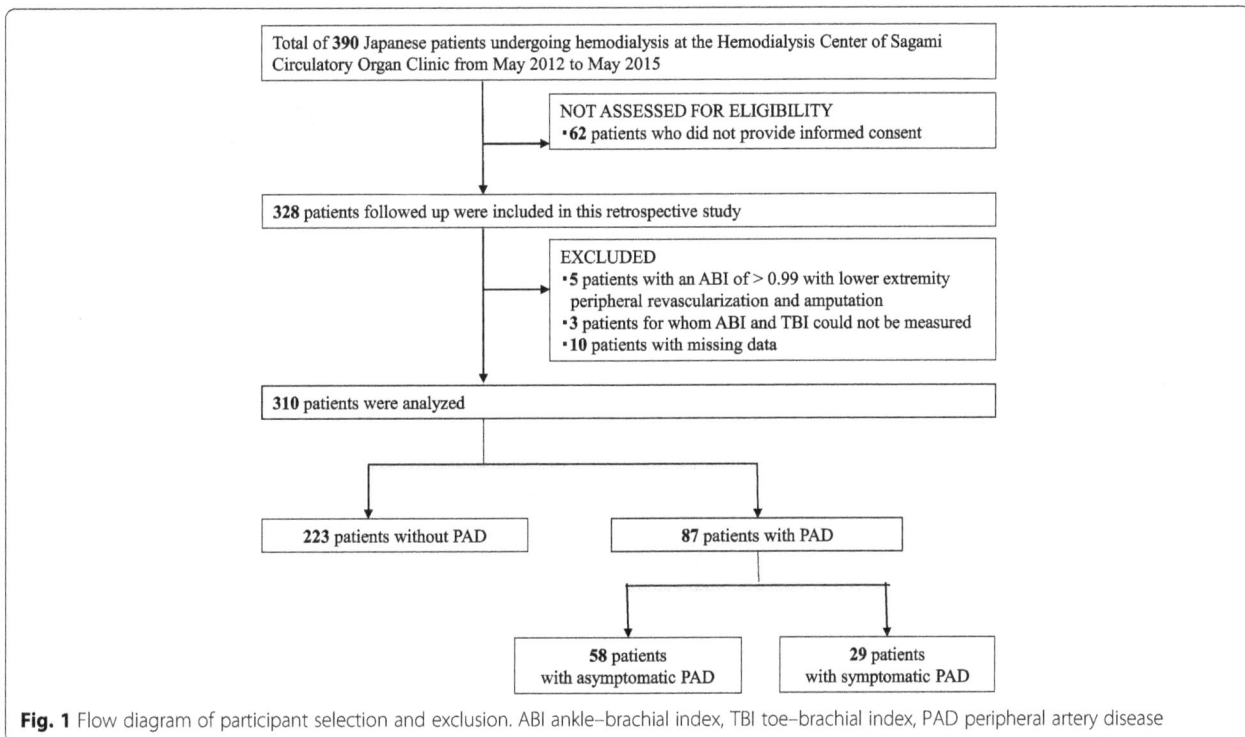

Fig. 1 Flow diagram of participant selection and exclusion. ABI ankle–brachial index, TBI toe–brachial index, PAD peripheral artery disease

within 10 min of rest), or the absence of clinical symptoms based on the response to the question, "Do you get pain in either the legs or buttocks while walking?" [21]. Symptomatic PAD was defined as PAD with exertional leg symptoms (i.e., intermittent claudication, leg pain on exertion and rest, and atypical exertional leg pain), while asymptomatic PAD was defined as PAD with no clinical symptoms [21].

Statistical analysis

The results of normally distributed continuous variables are expressed as the means ± standard deviation, and non-normally distributed variables are presented as the median (25th and 75th percentiles). Patients were divided into four groups according to PAD diagnosis and leg symptoms: non-PAD, total PAD (asymptomatic and symptomatic PAD), asymptomatic PAD, and symptomatic PAD groups. In addition, differences between non-PAD and total PAD groups and between asymptomatic PAD and symptomatic PAD groups at baseline were investigated exploratively with χ^2 tests, t tests, and Mann-Whitney U tests, respectively. The cumulative incidence of death was calculated in all groups using the Kaplan–Meier method, and comparisons were performed using the log-rank test.

Univariate and multivariate analyses were performed using Cox proportional hazards regression models to estimate the independent prognostic effect of PAD on survival after adjusting for confounders. Four separate models were used for comparisons: between non-PAD and total PAD groups (analysis included all patients), between non-PAD

and asymptomatic PAD groups (patients with symptomatic PAD were excluded), between non-PAD and symptomatic PAD groups (patients with asymptomatic PAD were excluded), and between asymptomatic PAD and symptomatic PAD groups (patients without PAD were excluded).

We initially considered the following variables as potential confounders: age, sex, body mass index, dialysis vintage, smoking status, cause of ESRD, diabetes, coronary artery disease, cerebrovascular disease, and levels of creatinine, albumin, hemoglobin, HDL-C, and GNRI. These variables were selected based on an a priori determined model and evaluation of patient characteristics associated with mortality. Multicollinearity was tested by investigating the variance inflation factor and tolerance in multiple linear regression analysis. Two levels of multivariate analyses were performed: model 1, with adjustment for demographic characteristics (age, sex, and body mass index); and model 2, an augmented version of model 1 with adjustment for age, cause of ESRD, cerebrovascular disease, creatinine, and GNRI. Unadjusted and adjusted hazard ratios for death with 95% confidence intervals (95% CIs) were obtained. Statistical analyses using the t tests, Mann-Whitney U tests, χ^2 tests, Kaplan–Meier method, and Cox proportional hazards regression models were performed using SPSS for Windows version 24.0 (IBM SPSS, Chicago, IL). In all analyses, $P < 0.05$ was considered statistically significant. The sample power was calculated with the number of patients in the asymptomatic PAD group, the hazard ratio for the non-PAD group compared to the asymptomatic PAD group, the median survival time in the non-PAD group, accrual time during which patients were recruited, additional follow-up time after the end of recruitment, and the ratio of non-PAD patients to asymptomatic PAD patients. The probability of type I error associated with the test of the null hypothesis was 0.05.

Results
Baseline characteristics
Table 1 summarizes the baseline characteristics of the study population comprising 183 (59.0%) men and 127 (41.0%) women. The median age was 66 (25th and 75th percentiles, 61, 74) years, median dialysis vintage was 5 (25th and 75th percentiles, 1, 13) years, and the most common cause of ESRD was diabetic nephropathy (34.5%) followed by glomerulonephritis (30.6%). Significant differences were observed between non-PAD and total PAD groups in age, cause of ESRD, prevalence of diabetes, coronary artery disease, cerebrovascular disease, spinal stenosis, use of beta-blockers, antiplatelet agents, and anticoagulant agents, smoking status, diastolic blood pressure, pulse pressure, ABI, TBI, and levels of creatinine, albumin, HDL-C, and triglycerides. A significant difference in dialysis vintage and ABI was observed between asymptomatic PAD and symptomatic PAD groups.

Kaplan–Meier estimate of patient survival
All patients were followed for up to 4 years. The follow-up period ranged from 2 to 48 months overall, with a median of 48.0 months for all groups, 48.0 months for the non-PAD group, 45.0 months for the total PAD group, 44.0 months for the asymptomatic PAD group, and 45.0 months for the symptomatic PAD group. Additional follow-up time after the end of recruitment was 17 months. In total, 58 patients died during the follow-up period due to the following causes: cardiovascular disease in 16, infection in 14, cancer in 7, cerebral vascular disease in 4, others in 7, and unknown in 10. Kaplan–Meier survival curves based on all-cause mortality for non-PAD and total PAD groups are shown in Fig. 2. The cumulative survival rate in the total PAD group was significantly lower than in the non-PAD group (log-rank $\chi^2 = 19.890$; $P < 0.001$). Kaplan–Meier survival curves based on all-cause mortality for non-PAD, total PAD, asymptomatic PAD, and symptomatic PAD groups are shown in Fig. 3. Cumulative survival rates were significantly lower in asymptomatic PAD and symptomatic PAD groups compared to the non-PAD group, but were not significant deference between

asymptomatic PAD and symptomatic PAD groups (log-rank $\chi^2 = 0.334$; $P = 0.564$).

Multivariate analysis of the effect of asymptomatic PAD on mortality
The results of univariate Cox proportional hazards analysis of covariates to predict all-cause mortality are shown in Table 2. Total PAD, asymptomatic PAD, and symptomatic PAD groups had crude hazard ratios of 3.040 (95% CI, 1.816 to 5.089; $P < 0.001$), 2.809 (95% CI, 1.559 to 5.059; $P = 0.001$), and 3.515 (95% CI, 1.755 to 7.041; $P < 0.001$), respectively, compared to the non-PAD group. The results of multivariate Cox proportional hazards analysis of covariates to predict all-cause mortality are shown in Table 3. We developed two multivariate models to adjust for demographic and clinical characteristics. There was no multicollinearity among independent variables. In model 1, after adjusting for the effects of demographic characteristics, total PAD, asymptomatic PAD, and symptomatic PAD groups had hazard ratios of 2.796 (95% CI, 1.654 to 4.730; $P < 0.001$), 2.323 (95% CI, 1.257 to 4.183; $P = 0.008$), and 4.159 (95% CI, 1.970 to 8.179; $P < 0.001$), respectively, compared to the non-PAD group. In model 2, after adjusting for age, cause of ESRD, cerebrovascular disease, creatinine and GNRI, total PAD, asymptomatic PAD, and symptomatic PAD groups had hazard ratios of 2.273 (95% CI, 1.262 to 4.110; $P = 0.006$), 1.963 (95% CI, 1.012 to 3.740; $P = 0.046$), and 3.237 (95% CI, 1.402 to 7.020; $P = 0.007$), respectively, compared to the non-PAD group. No significant difference was observed between asymptomatic PAD and symptomatic PAD groups in terms of survival. The sample size in this study was sufficient as reflected by the sample power of 0.950.

Discussion
We examined all-cause mortality in a population of patients undergoing HD ($n = 310$). In total, 58 (18.7%) patients died during the observation period of up to 4 years. The mortality rate was significantly higher in HD patients with PAD compared to those without PAD, but no significant difference was found between patients with symptomatic PAD and those with asymptomatic PAD. This is the first study to report on the association between asymptomatic PAD and mortality risk in patients undergoing HD. Therefore, we considered that HD patients with asymptomatic PAD should not be underestimated.

The prevalence of PAD is higher in HD patients than in the general population. According to the Dialysis Outcomes and Practice Patterns Study (DOPPS), a prospective cohort observational study of adult HD patients, PAD prevalence rates in the total study population, in the USA/Canada, in Europe, in Australia/New Zealand, and in Japan

Table 1 Patient characteristics

Characteristics	All patients (n = 310)	Non-PAD (n = 223)	PAD (n = 87)	P,* non-PAD vs. PAD	Asymptomatic PAD (n = 58)	Symptomatic PAD (n = 29)	P,† asymptomatic vs. symptomatic PAD
Age, years	66.0 (61.0, 74)	65.0 (60.0, 73.0)	69.0 (64.0, 75.5)	0.017	70.0 (65.0, 77.5)	66.0 (63.0, 73.0)	0.174
Male, %	183 (59.0%)	134 (60.1%)	49 (56.3%)	0.607	36 (62.1%)	13 (44.8%)	0.170
Body mass index, kg/m^2	20.7 (18.7, 23.0)	20.4 (18.7, 23.0)	21.0 (18.8, 22.8)	0.720	20.9 (18.4, 22.8)	21.3 (19.4, 22.8)	0.402
Time on hemodialysis, years	5 (1, 13)	5 (1, 14)	5 (2, 11)	0.675	4. (1, 8)	10 (4, 15)	0.019
Cause of ESRD, %				< 0.001			0.448
Glomerulonephritis	95 (30.6%)	78 (35.0%)	17 (19.5%)		12 (20.7%)	5 (17.2%)	
Diabetic nephropathy	107 (34.5%)	58 (26.0%)	49 (56.3%)		29 (50.0%)	20 (69.0%)	
Hypertension	28 (9.0%)	21 (9.4%)	7 (8.0%)		6 (10.3%)	1 (3.4%)	
Cystic disease	13 (4.2%)	11 (4.9%)	2 (2.3%)		1 (1.7%)	1 (3.4%)	
Other	43 (13.9%)	34 (15.2%)	9 (10.3%)		8 (13.8%)	1 (3.4%)	
Unknown	24 (7.7%)	21 (9.4%)	3 (3.4%)		2 (3.4%)	1 (3.4%)	
Comorbid conditions							
Diabetes, %	126 (40.6%)	76 (34.1%)	50 (57.5%)	0.001	30 (51.7%)	20 (69.0%)	0.260
Coronary artery disease, %	51 (16.5%)	24 (10.8%)	27 (31.0%)	< 0.001	15 (25.9%)	12 (41.4%)	0.150
Cerebrovascular disease, %	53 (17.1%)	32 (14.3%)	21 (24.1%)	0.045	15 (25.9%)	6 (20.7%)	0.791
Spinal stenosis, %	38 (12.3%)	17 (7.6%)	21 (24.1%)	< 0.001	10 (17.2%)	11 (37.9%)	0.061
Medication							
ACEI, %	23 (7.4%)	19 (8.5%)	4 (4.6%)	0.335	3 (5.2%)	1 (3.4%)	1.000
ARB, %	138 (44.5%)	104 (46.6%)	34 (39.1%)	0.254	27 (46.6%)	7 (24.1%)	0.062
CCB, %	136 (43.9%)	100 (42.9%)	36 (41.4%)	0.612	28 (48.3%)	8 (27.6%)	0.071
Beta-blockerv, %	85 (27.4%)	51 (22.9%)	34 (39.1%)	0.007	21 (36.2%)	13 (44.8%)	0.489
Lipid-lowering agent, %	50 (16.1%)	37 (16.6%)	13 (14.9%)	0.864	7 (12.1%)	6 (20.7%)	0.344
Antiplatelet agent, %	138 (44.5%)	81 (36.3%)	57 (65.5%)	< 0.001	36 (62.1%)	21 (72.4%)	0.473
Anticoagulant agent, %	13 (4.2%)	4 (1.8%)	9 (10.7%)	0.002	5 (8.6%)	4 (13.8%)	0.474
Smoking status (ever), %	182 (58.7%)	121 (54.3%)	61 (70.1%)	0.014	41 (70.7%)	20 (69.0%)	1.000
Systolic BP, mmHg	136.8 ± 25.3	136.8 ± 24.2	137 ± 27.9	0.930	137.9 ± 28.5	135.4 ± 27.1	0.303
Diastolic BP, mmHg	75.4 ± 13.5	77.2 ± 12.6	71.1 ± 14.6	0.001	72.4 ± 15.3	68.1 ± 12.7	0.162
Pulse pressure, mmHg	61.0 (49.0, 73.3)	58.0 (48.0, 71.0)	64.0 (53.0, 78.8)	0.006	63.0 (52.0, 78.0)	65.0 (56.0, 81.0)	0.459
Pulse rate	71.0 (64.5, 80.0)	70.0 (65.0, 80.8)	73.0 (64.0, 79.0)	0.708	72.0 (63.8, 78.3)	75.0 (66.0, 79.0)	0.447
Ankle–brachial index	1.12 (0.96, 1.19)	1.16 (1.10, 1.22)	0.82 (0.68, 0.92)	< 0.001	0.87 (0.79, 0.94)	0.73 (0.59, 0.82)	< 0.001
Toe–brachial index	0.75 ± 0.22	0.79 ± 0.20	0.58 ± 0.21	< 0.001	0.57 ± 0.16	0.66 ± 0.42	0.312
Creatinine, mEq/L	10.1 ± 2.6	10.4 ± 2.7	9.4 ± 2.4	0.002	9.2 ± 2.7	9.9 ± 1.6	0.214
Calcium, mg/dL	8.7 (8.4, 9.1)	8.8 (8.4, 9.1)	8.7 (8.4, 9.1)	0.342	8.7 (8.4, 9.0)	8.7 (8.4, 9.1)	0.787
Phosphorus, mg/dL	5.1 ± 1	5.1 ± 1	5 ± 1.1	0.809	5.1 ± 1.1	4.9 ± 1.1	0.593
Hemoglobin, g/dL	11.1 (10.5, 11.7)	11.1 (10.6, 11.7)	10.9 (10.5, 11.9)	0.702	10.9 (10.4, 11.9)	11.0 (10.5, 11.8)	0.665
Hematocrit, %	33.0 (31.3, 34.9)	33.0 (31.3, 34.8)	33.0 (31.2, 35.0)	0.942	33.0 (31.2, 35.1)	32.9 (31.1, 34.8)	0.928

Table 1 Patient characteristics *(Continued)*

Characteristics	All patients ($n = 310$)	Non-PAD ($n = 223$)	PAD ($n = 87$)	$P,$* non-PAD vs. PAD	Asymptomatic PAD ($n = 58$)	Symptomatic PAD ($n = 29$)	$P,$† asymptomatic vs. symptomatic PAD
Albumin, g/dL	3.7 (3.5, 3.9)	3.8 (3.5, 4.0)	3.7 (3.5, 3.9)	0.036	3.7 (3.5, 3.8)	3.7 (3.6, 3.9)	0.485
HDL-C, mg/dL	41.0 (32.0, 52.8)	43.0 (33.5, 55.0)	37.0 (30.0, 48.0)	< 0.001	37.0 (30.0, 45.8)	36.0 (30.0, 50.0)	0.939
LDL-C, mg/dL	86.0 (67.0, 105.0)	86.0 (66.50, 104.0)	87.0 (68.5, 107.0)	0.319	88.0 (71.0, 113.5)	86.0 (65.0, 100.0)	0.317
Triglycerides, mg/dL	111.5 (80.3, 173.8)	106.0 (75.5, 156.0)	126.0 (83.5, 189.0)	0.045	122.0 (82.3, 181.0)	132.0 (111.0, 211.0)	0.129
GNRI	94.0 (89.5, 98.3)	93.8 (90.1, 98.5)	95.1 (88.9, 97.6)	0.340	95.0 (87.1, 97.3)	95.3 (90.5, 98.3)	0.276

Values are expressed as means ± SD, *n* (%), or median (25th and 75th percentiles)

ESRD end-stage renal disease, *ACEI* angiotensin-converting enzyme inhibitor, *ARB* angiotensin receptor blocker, *BP* blood pressure, *CCB* calcium channel blocker, *HDL-C* high-density lipoprotein cholesterol, *LDL-C* low-density lipoprotein cholesterol, *GNRI* geriatric nutritional risk index, *PAD* peripheral artery disease

*Comparison between PAD and non-PAD groups (with *t*, Mann-Whitney *U*, or χ^2 tests)

†Comparison between symptomatic PAD and asymptomatic PAD groups (with *t*, Mann-Whitney *U*, or χ^2 tests)

were 25.3, 27.5–32.3, 17.5–38.0, 32.7, and 12.0%, respectively [13]. A large degree of variation in PAD prevalence was noted among 12 countries included in the DOPPS, with the highest rate of 38.0% in Belgium and lowest rate of 12.0% in Japan. DOPPS reports determined PAD by prior diagnosis of PAD, symptom, or surgical therapy for PAD. However, we provide prevalence of PAD by ABI and TBI. The prevalence of PAD in the present study was 28.1%, which is markedly higher than DOPPS reports. The diagnosis of PAD in HD patients is widely based on ABI; however, patients undergoing HD frequently show high ABI values due to medial artery calcification, despite limb ischemia [17]. TBI is a non-invasive and useful measure of PAD in patients with non-compressible arteries, which cause an artificial

elevation of ABI [7], and its use is recommended by current guidelines for diagnosing PAD [3, 7]. The cutoff value of ABI for detecting PAD has been reported to be < 1.06 in HD patients, with high sensitivity and specificity of 80.0 and 98.0%, respectively [17]. In addition, since current guidelines specify a normal ABI range of 1.00 to 1.40 [22], we used a cutoff ABI of 1.00, rather than 0.9, for detecting PAD. The frequency distribution of ABI < 1.0 in previous study targeting Japanese HD patients was 25.1% of patients in Japanese HD patients, which is nearly similar those reported in this study [14]. Thus, the high prevalence of PAD in the present study population could be due to the ABI cutoff (< 1.00) used, in addition to including TBI for diagnosis.

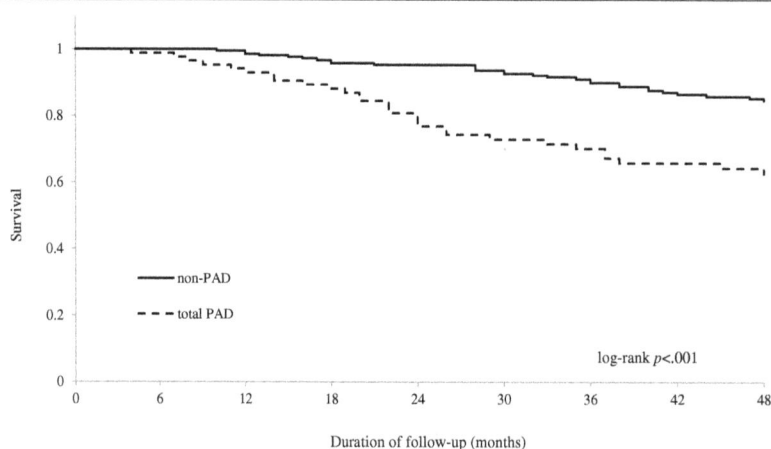

Fig. 2 Probabilities of overall survival in non-PAD and total PAD groups. Log-rank test for overall survival. *PAD* peripheral artery disease

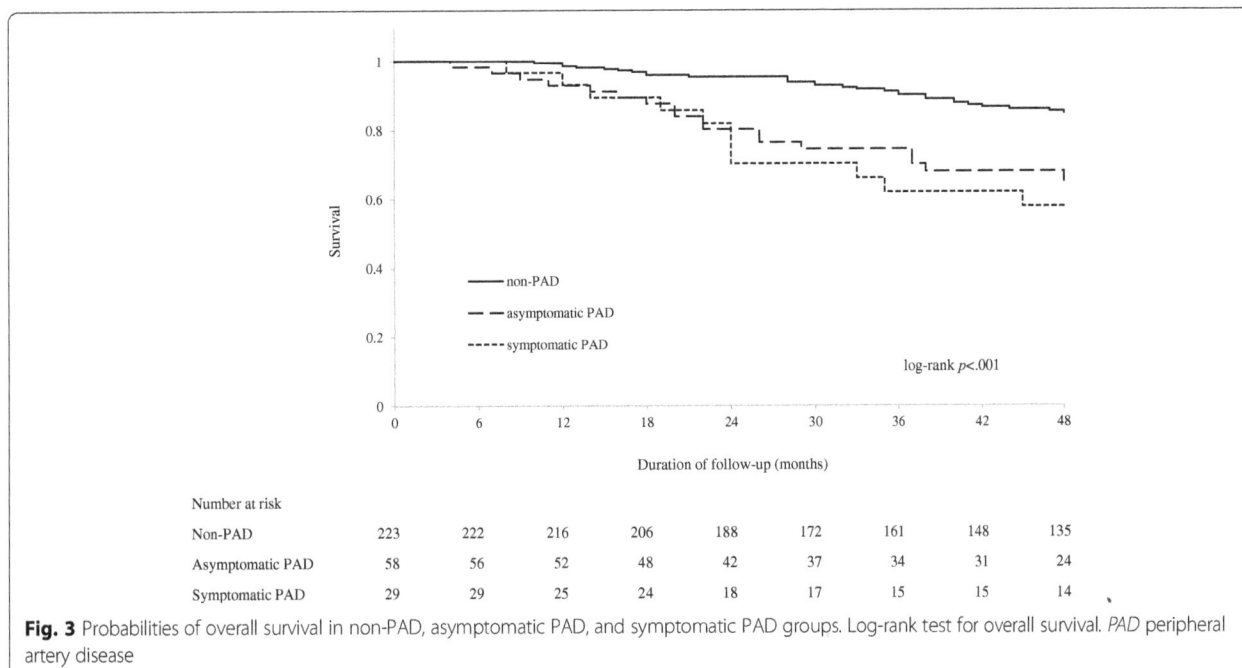

Fig. 3 Probabilities of overall survival in non-PAD, asymptomatic PAD, and symptomatic PAD groups. Log-rank test for overall survival. *PAD* peripheral artery disease

In the present study, HD patients with asymptomatic PAD had unfavorable prognoses compared with those without PAD. Previous studies showed that patients with asymptomatic PAD had significantly greater functional impairment and faster functional decline than those without PAD [18, 21, 23, 24]. Previously, we reported the prognostic significance of poor physical performance, including poor muscle strength and physical inactivity, on survival in a cohort of HD patients [25, 26]. Moreover, the first multicenter, randomized controlled trial conducted to examine the relative benefits of exercise training in patients with symptomatic PAD indicated that exercise training was associated with greater improvement of walking performance than primary aorto-iliac stent revascularization and optimal medical care [27]. Furthermore, exercise training has been shown to reduce atherosclerotic risk factors, including lipid disorders, insulin resistance, dysfunction of the cardiac autonomic system, and reduced maximal oxygen consumption, which also accelerate PAD progression [28–30]. However, it remains unclear whether exercise training interventions can improve or reverse the decline in physical performance among HD patients with asymptomatic PAD, although studies suggest that patients with PAD might benefit from adopting a more active lifestyle [8].

This study has several limitations. First, we conducted this study in Japan using a single-center, observational design, retrospective; and therefore, further multicenter studies are required for generalizability. Second, multivariate analysis was performed using Cox proportional hazards regression models to estimate the independent prognostic effect of asymptomatic PAD on mortality after adjusting for confounders. Differences in patient characteristics attributed to asymptomatic PAD in the present study were adjusted for only by observed factors. Therefore, additional information regarding characteristics that could potentially affect the prevalence of asymptomatic PAD in HD patients will be necessary. Thirdly, because of retrospective study and clinical problem, it was difficult to align the timing for performing ABI test. However, in previous study, Su HM et al. reported that the ABI remained constant before and after HD, or on the next dialysis-free day [31]. Additionally, Jimenez ZN et al. reported that they found no difference in ABI pre- and post-dialysis on the right or left side [32]. Finally, although we found that the mortality risk in patients with asymptomatic PAD was higher than that in patients without PAD, the underlying mechanisms remain unknown.

Conclusions

The prevalence of PAD is high in HD patients, and while most HD patients with PAD have no lower leg symptoms, these patients (i.e., asymptomatic PAD patients) have a significantly increased mortality risk compared to those without PAD. Moreover, the mortality risk of HD patients with asymptomatic PAD was no difference from patients with symptomatic PAD. These findings underscore the importance of screening and stratification of hemodialysis patients at risk of mortality as a part of routine care for HD patients regardless of whether or not patients present with leg symptoms. Additionally, further investigation

Table 2 Univariate cox proportional hazards regression analysis of mortality

Parameter	Univariate analysis		
	Hazard ratio (95% CI)		P value
PAD			
Non-PAD	Reference		
Total PAD (vs. non-PAD)	3.040	(1.816 to 5.089)	< 0.001
Asymptomatic PAD (vs. non-PAD)	2.809	(1.559 to 5.059)	0.001
Symptomatic PAD (vs. non-PAD)	3.515	(1.755 to 7.041)	< 0.001
Age, per 1 year	1.067	(1.040 to 1.095)	< 0.001
Male vs. female	1.637	(0.938 to 2.855)	0.083
Body mass index, per 1 kg/m^2	0.897	(0.824 to 0.977)	0.012
Dialysis vintage, per 1 year	1.009	(0.981 to 1.038)	0.541
Cause of ESRD			0.010
Glomerulonephritis	Reference		
Diabetic nephropathy	1.624	(0.767 to 3.440)	0.205
Hypertension	4.782	(2.066 to 11.069)	< 0.001
Cystic disease	1.642	(0.364 to 7.419)	0.519
Other	1.912	(0.792 to 4.614)	0.149
Unknown	2.794	(1.083 to 7.208)	0.034
Diabetes	1.033	(0.607 to 1.755)	0.906
Coronary artery disease	1.183	(0.598 to 2.337)	0.630
Cerebrovascular disease	2.040	(1.146 to 3.630)	0.015
Smoking status (ever vs. never)	1.305	(0.764 to 2.231)	0.329
Creatinine, per 1 mEq/L	0.842	(0.763 to 0.929)	0.001
Albumin, per 1 g/dL	0.138	(0.068 to 0.280)	< 0.001
Hemoglobin, per 1 g/dL	0.887	(0.679 to 1.159)	0.380
HDL-C, per 1 mg/dL	0.988	(0.968 to 1.008)	0.227
GNRI	0.220	(0.074 to 0.683)	0.009

Analyses were performed using cox proportional hazards regression (unadjusted for background factors on survival)
PAD peripheral artery disease, *ESRD* end-stage renal disease, *HDL-C* high-density lipoprotein cholesterol, *GNRI* geriatric nutritional risk index, *CI* confidence interval

Table 3 Multivariate cox proportional hazards regression analysis for mortality

Parameter	Hazard ratio (95% CI)		P value
Model 1[a]			
Non-PAD	Reference		
Total PAD (vs. non-PAD)	2.796	(1.654 to 4.730)	< 0.001
Asymptomatic PAD (vs. non-PAD)	2.323	(1.257 to 4.183)	0.008
Symptomatic PAD (vs. non-PAD)	4.159	(1.970 to 8.179)	< 0.001
Asymptomatic PAD vs. Symptomatic PAD	0.558	(0.264 to 1.234)	0.145
Model 2[b]			
Non-PAD	Reference		
Total PAD (vs. non-PAD)	2.273	(1.262 to 4.110)	0.006
Asymptomatic PAD (vs. non-PAD)	1.963	(1.012 to 3.740)	0.046
Symptomatic PAD (vs. non-PAD)	3.237	(1.402 to 7.020)	0.007
Asymptomatic PAD vs. Symptomatic PAD	0.606	(0.273 to 1.407)	0.236

Analyses were performed using cox proportional hazards regression
PAD peripheral artery disease, *CI* confidence interval
[a]Adjusted by age, sex, and body mass index
[b]Adjustment by age, cause of end-stage renal disease, cerebrovascular disease, creatinine, and geriatric nutritional risk index

is needed to establish treatment on asymptomatic and symptomatic PAD for HD patients.

Abbreviations
ABI: Ankle–brachial index; CI: Confidence interval; DOPPS: Dialysis Outcome and Patterns Study; ESRD: End-stage renal disease; GNRI: Geriatric nutritional risk index; HD: Hemodialysis; HDL-C: High-density lipoprotein cholesterol; PAD: Peripheral artery disease; SD: Standard deviation; TBI: Toe–brachial index

Acknowledgements
We thank all patients for their participation and commitment during the study. We also thank all investigators and contributors of our study.

Funding
This research was supported by a Kitasato University Research grant and JSPS KAKENHI grant number JP16K 16466.

Authors' contributions
MH, RM, NA, YH, and AM conceived the research idea and study design. MH, KU, JY, KY, TW, and TS were involved for the data acquisition. MH, RM, NA, and AM were responsible for the data analysis/interpretation and MH and KH were responsible for the statistical analysis, while NA, YT, SN, AY and AM were responsible for the supervision or mentorship. All authors read and approved the final manuscript.

Competing interests
The authors declare that they have no competing interests.

Author details
[1]Department of Rehabilitation Sciences, Kitasato University Graduate School of Medical Sciences, 1-15-1 Kitasato, Minami-ku, Sagamihara, Kanagawa 252-0373, Japan. [2]Department of Rehabilitation, Kitasato University Hospital, Sagamihara, Japan. [3]Department of General Medicine, Kitasato University School of Medicine, Sagamihara, Japan. [4]Sagami Junkanki Clinic, Sagamihara, Japan. [5]Department of Hygiene, Kitasato University School of Medicine, Sagamihara, Japan. [6]Division of Nephrology, Department of Internal Medicine, Kitasato University School of Medicine, Sagamihara, Japan.

References
1. Fowkes FG, Murray GD, Butcher I, Heald CL, Lee RJ, Chambless LE, et al. Ankle brachial index combined with Framingham Risk Score to predict cardiovascular events and mortality: a meta-analysis. JAMA. 2008;300(2):197–208.
2. Fontaine R, Kim M, Kieny R. Surgical treatment of peripheral circulation disorders. Helv Chir Acta. 1954;21(5-6):499–533.
3. Norgren L, Hiatt WR, Dormandy JA, Nehler MR, Harris KA, Fowkes FG, et al. Inter-Society Consensus for the Management of Peripheral Arterial Disease (TASC II). J Vasc Surg. 2007;45(Suppl S):S5–67.
4. Baker JD, Rutherford RB, Bernstein EF, Courbier R, Ernst CB, Kempczinski RF, et al. Suggested standards for reports dealing with cerebrovascular disease. Subcommittee on Reporting Standards for Cerebrovascular Disease, Ad Hoc Committee on Reporting Standards, Society for Vascular Surgery/North American Chapter, International Society for Cardiovascular Surgery. J Vasc Surg. 1988;8(6):721–9.
5. Rutherford RB, Baker JD, Ernst C, Johnston KW, Porter JM, Ahn S, et al. Recommended standards for reports dealing with lower extremity ischemia: revised version. J Vasc Surg. 1997;26(3):517–38.
6. Diehm C, Allenberg JR, Pittrow D, Mahn M, Tepohl G, Haberl RL, et al. Mortality and vascular morbidity in older adults with asymptomatic versus symptomatic peripheral artery disease. Circulation. 2009;120(21):2053–61.
7. Gerhard-Herman MD, Gornik HL, Barrett C, Barshes NR, Corriere MA, Drachman DE, et al. 2016 AHA/ACC Guideline on the Management of Patients With Lower Extremity Peripheral Artery Disease: a report of the American College of Cardiology/American Heart Association Task Force on Clinical Practice Guidelines. J Am Coll Cardiol. 2017;69(11):e71–e126.
8. Society for Vascular Surgery Lower Extremity Guidelines Writing Group, Conte MS, Pomposelli FB, Clair DG, Geraghty PJ, JF MK, et al. Society for vascular surgery practice guidelines for atherosclerotic occlusive disease of the lower extremities: management of asymptomatic disease and claudication. J Vasc Surg. 2015;61(Suppl):2S–41S.
9. Cheung AK, Sarnak MJ, Yan G, Dwyer JT, Heyka RJ, Rocco MV, et al. Atherosclerotic cardiovascular disease risks in chronic hemodialysis patients. Kidney Int. 2000;58(1):353–62.
10. Matsuzawa R, Aoyama N, Yoshida A. Clinical characteristics of patients on hemodialysis with peripheral arterial disease. Angiology. 2015;66(10):911–7.
11. Johansen KL, Chertow GM, Ng AV, Mulligan K, Carey S, Schoenfeld PY, et al. Physical activity levels in patients on hemodialysis and healthy sedentary controls. Kidney Int. 2000;57(6):2564–70.
12. Ndip A, Rutter MK, Vileikyte L, Vardhan A, Asari A, Jameel M, et al. Dialysis treatment is an independent risk factor for foot ulceration in patients with diabetes and stage 4 or 5 chronic kidney disease. Diabetes Care. 2010;33(8):1811–6.
13. Rajagopalan S, Dellegrottaglie S, Furniss AL, Gillespie BW, Satayathum S, Lameire N, et al. Peripheral arterial disease in patients with end-stage renal disease: observations from the Dialysis Outcomes and Practice Patterns Study (DOPPS). Circulation. 2006;114(18):1914–22.
14. Ono K, Tsuchida A, Kawai H, Matsuo H, Wakamatsu R, Maezawa A, et al. Ankle-brachial blood pressure index predicts all-cause and cardiovascular mortality in hemodialysis patients. J Am Soc Nephrol. 2003;14(6):1591–8.
15. von Elm E, Altman DG, Egger M, Pocock SJ, Gøtzsche PC, Vandenbroucke JP, et al. The Strengthening the Reporting of Observational Studies in Epidemiology (STROBE) statement: guidelines for reporting observational studies. PLoS Med. 2007;4(10):e296.
16. Bouillanne O, Morineau G, Dupont C, Coulombel I, Vincent JP, Nicolis I, et al. Geriatric nutritional risk index: a new index for evaluating at-risk elderly medical patients. Am J Clin Nutr. 2005;82(4):777–83.
17. Ohtake T, Oka M, Ikee R, Mochida Y, Ishioka K, Moriya H, et al. Impact of lower limbs' arterial calcification on the prevalence and severity of PAD in patients on hemodialysis. J Vasc Surg. 2011;53(3):676–83.
18. McDermott MM, Greenland P, Liu K, Guralnik JM, Criqui MH, Dolan NC, et al. Leg symptoms in peripheral arterial disease: associated clinical characteristics and functional impairment. JAMA. 2001;286(13):1599–606.
19. Criqui MH, Denenberg JO, Bird CE, Fronek A, Klauber MR, Langer RD. The correlation between symptoms and non-invasive test results in patients referred for peripheral arterial disease testing. Vasc Med. 1996;1(1):65–71.
20. Rose GA. The diagnosis of ischaemic heart pain and intermittent claudication in field surveys. Bull World Health Organ. 1962;27:645–58.
21. McDermott MM, Liu K, Greenland P, Guralnik JM, Criqui MH, Chan C, et al. Functional decline in peripheral arterial disease: associations with the ankle brachial index and leg symptoms. JAMA. 2004;292(4):453–61.
22. Rooke TW, Hirsch AT, Misra S, Sidawy AN, Beckman JA, Findeiss LK, et al. 2011 ACCF/AHA Focused Update of the Guideline for the Management of Patients With Peripheral Artery Disease (updating the 2005 guideline): a report of the American College of Cardiology Foundation/ American Heart Association Task Force on Practice Guidelines. J Am Coll Cardiol. 2011;58(19):2020–45.
23. McDermott MM, Ferrucci L, Liu K, Guralnik JM, Tian L, Liao Y, et al. Leg symptom categories and rates of mobility decline in peripheral arterial disease. J Am Geriatr Soc. 2010;58(7):1256–62.
24. McDermott MM, Guralnik JM, Ferrucci L, Tian L, Liu K, Liao Y, et al. Asymptomatic peripheral arterial disease is associated with more adverse lower extremity characteristics than intermittent claudication. Circulation. 2008;117(19):2484–91.
25. Matsuzawa R, Matsunaga A, Wang G, Kutsuna T, Ishii A, Abe Y, et al. Habitual physical activity measured by accelerometer and survival in maintenance hemodialysis patients. Clin J Am Soc Nephrol. 2012;7(12):2010–6.

26. Matsuzawa R, Matsunaga A, Wang G, Yamamoto S, Kutsuna T, Ishii A, et al. Relationship between lower extremity muscle strength and all-cause mortality in Japanese patients undergoing dialysis. Phys Ther. 2014;94(7):947–56.

27. Murphy TP, Cutlip DE, Regensteiner JG, Mohler ER, Cohen DJ, Reynolds MR, et al. Supervised exercise versus primary stenting for claudication resulting from aortoiliac peripheral artery disease: six-month outcomes from the claudication: exercise versus endoluminal revascularization (CLEVER) study. Circulation. 2012;125(1):130–9.

28. Matsuzawa R, Matsunaga A, Kutsuna T, Ishii A, Abe Y, Yoneki K, et al. Association of habitual physical activity measured by an accelerometer with high-density lipoprotein cholesterol levels in maintenance hemodialysis patients. ScientificWorldJournal. 2013;2013:780783.

29. Mustata S, Chan C, Lai V, Miller JA. Impact of an exercise program on arterial stiffness and insulin resistance in hemodialysis patients. J Am Soc Nephrol. 2004;15(10):2713–8.

30. Deligiannis A, Kouidi E, Tourkantonis A. Effects of physical training on heart rate variability in patients on hemodialysis. Am J Cardiol. 1999;84(2):197–202.

31. Su HM, Chang JM, Lin FH, Chen SC, Voon WC, Cheng KH, et al. Influence of different measurement time points on brachial-ankle pulse wave velocity and ankle-brachial index in hemodialysis patients. Hypertens Res. 2007;30(10):965–70.

32. Jimenez ZN, de Castro I, Pereira BJ, de Oliveira RB, Romao JE Jr, Elias RM, et al. When is the best moment to assess the ankle brachial index: pre- or post hemodialysis? Kidney Blood Press Res. 2012;35(4):242–6.

24

The geographical distribution of dialysis services

E. K. Tannor[1], Y. A. Awuku[2*], V. Boima[3] and S. Antwi[4]

Abstract

Background: Chronic kidney disease (CKD) is an important global health challenge with increasing burden worldwide. CKD and acute kidney injury (AKI) may require renal replacement therapy (RRT) at some stages of the disease. Ghana currently has no renal transplant program. Dialysis services still remain a mirage to many chronic kidney disease patients in Ghana due to cost and paucity of hemodialysis machines. This survey highlights the geographical distribution of dialysis services in Ghana.

Methods: A cross-sectional situational survey of dialysis centers in the ten regions of Ghana was conducted by interviewing doctors and other health care professionals in all health institutions. Information on dialysis services, staff status, and number of hemodialysis machines and presence of peritoneal dialysis services in both private and government facilities was obtained and mapped out.

Results: Fifteen dialysis centers with a total of 103 hemodialysis machines were identified with majority 59 (57.2%) in state-owned facilities. One half of regions in Ghana do not have any form of dialysis facilities. Majority 65 (63.1%) of hemodialysis machines are in the Greater Accra region. Private hemodialysis services are available only in Greater Accra and Ashanti regions. There is no chronic peritoneal dialysis in Ghana but limited acute peritoneal dialysis. Ghana currently has eight nephrologists found only in the three government teaching hospitals. Most dialysis units across the country are supported by non-nephrologists.

Conclusion: There are few hemodialysis centers in Ghana; the distribution of which is skewed to few regions across the country. There is a need to improve dialysis services and equitable distribution across the country.

Keywords: Hemodialysis, Peritoneal dialysis, Geographical distribution, Ghana

Background

Chronic kidney disease (CKD) is an important global health problem with increasing incidence and prevalence. Currently, the worldwide prevalence is 10–13% [1–3] and similar estimates of 13.9% have been reported in Africa in a recent meta-analysis [4]. The prevalence in Ghana is however not known. Chronic kidney disease inevitably progresses to end-stage renal disease (ESRD) which requires renal replacement therapy (RRT) in the form of hemodialysis, peritoneal dialysis, or renal transplantation as the main modalities of treatment. It has been shown consistently that renal transplantation is cost effective and improves patient survival and quality

of life as compared to peritoneal dialysis and hemodialysis [5–11].

Unfortunately, Ghana has no national renal transplantation program but has had limited renal transplantation services in the capital city Accra. This started in the Korle-bu Teaching Hospital, a 1600-bed teaching hospital [12] in 2008. Seventeen patients have since had renal transplants since its inception [13], but none has been done recently. A few well-to-do patients currently travel abroad for kidney transplantation services. Hemodialysis therefore remains the main form of renal replacement therapy in the country for patients with ESRD. Unfortunately, hemodialysis services are not widely available in Ghana. It was shown by Antwi [13] in 2015 that hemodialysis was mainly found in three teaching hospitals and three private institutions in Ghana and was inadequate to serve Ghana's population in the light

* Correspondence: ppawuku@gmail.com
[2]Department of Medicine and Therapeutics, School of Medical Sciences, University of Cape Coast, Cape Coast, Ghana
Full list of author information is available at the end of the article

of the increased burden of kidney diseases. Acute kidney injury is also reported in hospital admissions and may require renal replacement therapy in severe cases. Mortality rates of acute kidney injury in adults in Africa ranges from 13.5–43.5% [14] and may increase in settings where dialysis services are unavailable.

Peritoneal dialysis in adults with end-stage renal disease is non-existent in Ghana though the modality has been used for the management of acute kidney injury in children in some parts of the country [13].

Due to increased cost of hemodialysis, most patients after diagnoses are left to their fate when they cannot afford hemodialysis. The National Health Insurance Scheme (NHIS) does not cover patients with end-stage renal disease requiring hemodialysis. The high cost of renal replacement therapy is a deterrent in the management of end-stage renal disease as patients have to pay out of pocket for hemodialysis sessions in Ghana.

The cost of frequent laboratory investigations and the treatment for hypertension, anemia, and calcium and phosphate abnormalities will further increase the cost of treatment of end-stage renal disease. The tragedy for those who even start hemodialysis is that they impoverish their families and then eventually die very depressed with poor quality of life [15].

Furthermore, due to inadequate hemodialysis centers and machines, patients diagnosed with infections such as human immunodeficiency virus (HIV) and viral hepatitis B and C in some facilities are prevented from accessing the few hemodialysis machines available. This results in even fewer patients getting access to hemodialysis. Currently, the population of Ghana is about 27 million [16] and with the high prevalence rate of the causes of chronic kidney disease, there might be the need to increase the number and distribution of dialysis offered. The current number and geographical distribution of hemodialysis and peritoneal dialysis units remain unknown.

We set out to establish the number of hemodialysis machine in the various government and private facilities and to map out the regional distribution of renal replacement therapy in Ghana.

Methods

It was a cross-sectional situational survey of dialysis centers in all the ten regions of Ghana as at 31 December 2016. Information was sought by interviewing doctors and health care workers providing renal care in all health care facilities in all the regions in Ghana to ascertain the availability of dialysis services in both government and private facilities. The presence of peritoneal dialysis services, the availability of trained staff, specialist, and nephrologists were also documented. The number of patients on dialysis in the centers was also

documented. The distribution of facilities with hemodialysis centers across the country were mapped using Google Earth. For facilities not already mapped on Google maps, Google search was used to retrieve the physical address of the facility and this was used in estimating the location of the facility.

Ghana's administrative regions and population

Ghana is a country located in West Africa bounded by Burkina Faso on the north, Togo on the eastern border, Côte d'ivoire on the west, and the gulf of Guinea on the south. Ghana has a gross domestic product (GDP) of 37.54 billion US dollars and a GDP per capita of 1696.64 US dollars as at 2016 [17].

Ghana has a geographical surface area of 238,540 km and ten administrative regions. Greater Accra is the smallest region measuring 3245 km^2 and hosts the national capital Accra with a population of 4,010,054 [18]. The Northern region with its capital Tamale is the largest region in Ghana measuring 70,384 km^2 with a population of 2,479,461 followed by Brong Ahafo with a surface area of 39,557 km^2 in the middle belt of Ghana with a population of 2,310,983. Ashanti region also in the middle belt with capital Kumasi has a population of 4,780,380 and a surface area of 24,389 km^2 [18]. The other regions are the Western region, Central region, Brong Ahafo region, Upper East region, Upper West region, and the Volta region as shown in Fig. 1.

Results

As at December 2016, there were 15 centers offering in-center hemodialysis services in Ghana. This included 7 in the government-owned facilities and 8 in private-owned centers. There were 103 functioning hemodialysis machines in Ghana with 59 (57.3%) in the government-owned hospitals and 44 (42.7%) in private-owned health centers. The government-owned hospitals with hemodialysis machines were mainly the teaching hospitals in the Northern, Ashanti, Central, the Greater Accra, and the Volta regions.

This included 18 functioning machines in the Renal Unit of Korle-bu Teaching Hospital besides 10 machines in the National Cardiothoracic Unit within the Korle-bu Teaching Hospital. The cardiothoracic unit is a 32-bed facility established in the 1960s but was recommissioned in 1992 for the management of thoracic and cardiac cases surgically. It is one of the few functioning cardiothoracic centers in Africa. The National Cardiothoracic Centre receives referrals from other African countries such as Benin, Togo, Nigeria, Ivory Coast, Cameroon, Ethiopia, and Tanzania.

There are 8 functioning machines in the Police Hospital in Accra, 10 in the Cape Coast Teaching Hospital, 8 in the Komfo Anokye Teaching Hospital, 3

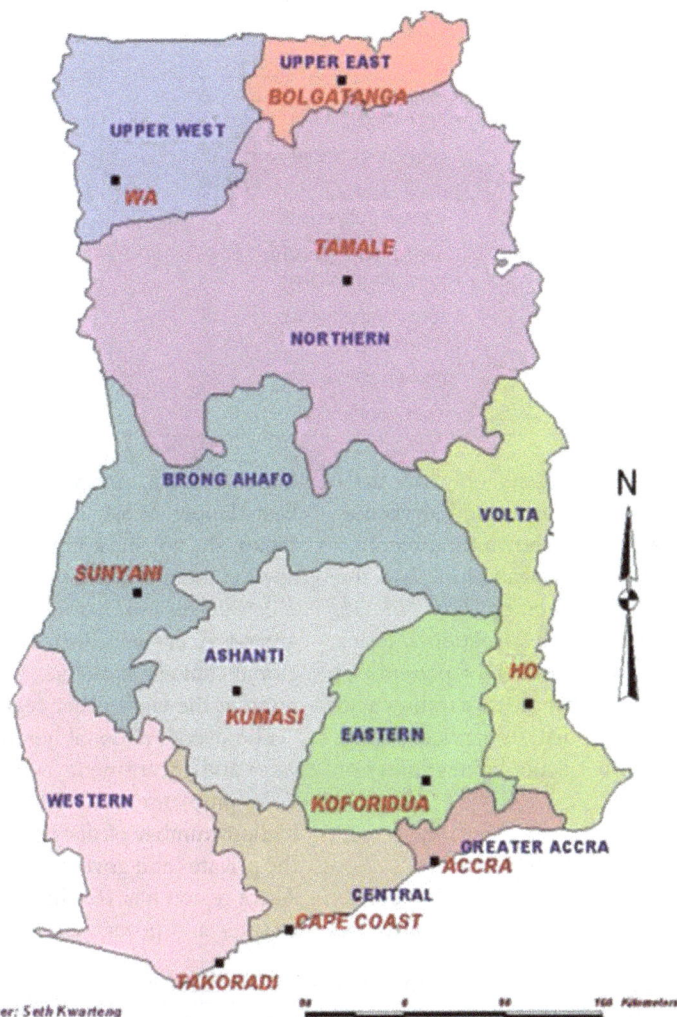

Fig. 1 The administrative regions of Ghana with regional capitals [18]. The regions and administrative capitals in Ghana [19, 20]

in the Tamale Teaching Hospital, and 2 in the Ho Regional Hospital in the Volta region as shown in Table 1. The Korle-bu Teaching Hospital has the greatest number of patients on dialysis in Ghana: 250 patients on hemodialysis as at December 2016. This was followed by the Cape Coast Teaching Hospital (68 patients) and the National cardiothoracic unit (65 patients). Komfo Anokye Teaching Hospital had the least number of patients on hemodialysis as shown in Table 1.

Chronic peritoneal dialysis was not available in any of the teaching hospital for the management of end-stage renal disease. Acute peritoneal dialysis was present in a large scale in Komfo Anokye Teaching Hospital for the management of acute kidney injury in pediatric population only. Acute peritoneal dialysis has recently been introduced in the Tamale Teaching Hospital, the Korle-bu Teaching Hospital and the Cape Coast Teaching Hospital on a small scale.

Some of the hemodialysis centers even in some teaching hospitals were not manned by trained nephrologists. The Cape Coast Teaching Hospital is manned by a consultant physician and two medical officers (specialist-in-training) and the Ho Regional Hospital is manned by a medical officer as shown in Table 1.

Private-owned dialysis centers in Ghana

Private-owned hemodialysis facilities were identified in only two out of the ten regions in Ghana. These facilities were found only in Accra and Kumasi, which are the regional capitals of the Greater Accra and Ashanti regions respectively. Six private facilities were identified in Accra and two in Kumasi in the Ashanti region within the study period. The private facilities in Accra include the Accra kidney clinic, the Trust Hospital, the Meridian Hospital, the Ghana Canada Hospital, Bengali Hospital, and the Labone dialysis clinic. It was found that most of the private-owned facilities were run by medical officers,

Table 1 Dialysis services within government-owned hospitals in Ghana

Government hospital	Number of functioning hemodialysis machines	Personnel in-charge of unit	Number of patients	Peritoneal dialysis availability
Korle-bu Teaching Hospital	18	4 nephrologists 4 nephrology trainees	250	No
Cardiothoracic unit	10	1 nephrology trainee	65	No
Komfo Anokye Teaching Hospital	8	3 nephrologists 2 specialist physicians	22	Yes for acute dialysis in children only
Tamale Teaching Hospital	3	1 nephrologist (Cuban) 1 specialist physician	45	Yes for acute dialysis in children only
Cape Coast Teaching Hospital	10	1 consultant physician 2 medical officers	68	Yes for acute dialysis both adult and children
Ho Teaching Hospital	2	1 medical officer	26	No
Police Hospital, Accra	8	1 medical officer	25	No

dialysis nurses, and some nephrologists only on part-time basis. The number of functioning hemodialysis machines identified in these facilities is shown in Table 2.

Among private-owned facilities, Bengali clinic had the highest number of patients on hemodialysis of 34, followed by Ghana Canada clinic with 24 patients. Peace and Love Hospital had the least number of patients of 10 on hemodialysis as at December 2016 as shown in Table 2. There were no peritoneal dialysis services in any of these private facilities for either acute kidney injury or chronic kidney disease.

Regional distribution of dialysis units in Ghana

As shown in Table 2, the distribution of government- and private-owned dialysis centers is skewed towards the Greater Accra, Ashanti, and Central regions. The Upper East, Upper West, Brong Ahafo, Eastern, and Western region do not have any form of renal replacement therapy for the management of renal diseases (Fig. 2).

Private-owned hemodialysis centers are only in the greater Accra and Ashanti regions. These are in the regional capitals alone, i.e., Accra and Kumasi. There were none in the eight other regions and as shown in Table 3.

The overall national hemodialysis machines in both private- and government-owned facilities per million population (pmp) are 4.20. The greater Accra region has the highest number of dialysis machines of 65 (63.1%) in both the private- and government-owned hospitals. The Greater Accra region has 16.2 hemodialysis machines pmp in both private- and government-owned facilities followed by the

Table 2 The regional distribution of dialysis services within private-owned facilities in Ghana

Region	Private facilities	Name of facility	Number of hemodialysis machines	Number of patients	Personnel in-charge of unit
Eastern	No	NA	NA	–	NA
Volta	No	NA	NA	–	NA
Greater Accra	Yes	Accra kidney clinic	7	23	1 nephrologist 1 medical officer
	Yes	Trust Hospital	4	20	1 medical officer
	Yes	Bengali clinic	5	34	1 nephrologist (locum) 1 medical officer
	Yes	Meridian clinic	5	12	1 renal nurse
	Yes	Ghana Canada Clinic	5	24	1 nephrologist (locum)
	Yes	Ababio clinic (Labone)	3	12	1 renal nurse
Central	No	NA	NA	–	NA
Western	No	NA	NA	–	NA
Brong Ahafo	No	NA	NA	–	NA
Ashanti	Yes	Peace and Love Hospital	5	10	1 senior medical officer
	Yes	Naghe Clinic	10	16	1 principal medical officer
Upper East	No	NA	NA	–	NA
Upper West	No	NA	NA	–	NA
Northern	No	NA	NA	–	NA

NA not available

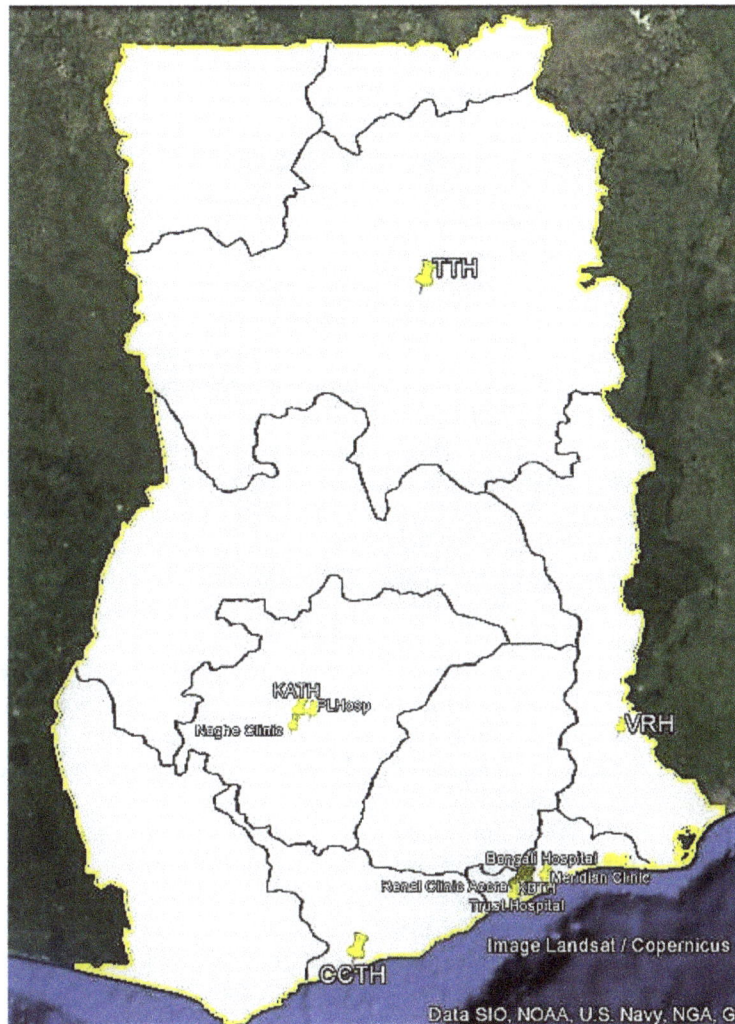

Fig. 2 The geographical distribution of the dialysis units in Ghana

Table 3 The regional distribution of hemodialysis machines per million population (pmp) in Ghana

Region	Public units (n)	Private units (n)	Total (n)	Total (%)	Population per region	Hemodialysis machines (pmp)
Eastern	0	0	0	0	2,633,154	0
Volta	2	0	2	1.9	2,118,525	0.94
Greater Accra	36	29	65	63.1	4,010,054	16.20
Central	10	0	10	9.7	2,201,863	4.54
Western	0	0	0	0	2,376,021	0
Brong Ahafo	0	0	0	0	2,310,938	0
Ashanti	8	15	23	22.3	4,780,380	4.81
Upper east	0	0	0	0	1,046,545	0
Upper West	0	0	0	0	702,110	0
Northern	3	0	3	2.9	2,479,461	1.21
Total	59	44	103		24,658,823	4.20

Ashanti region of 4.81 hemodialysis machines pmp and Central region of 4.54 as shown in Table 3.

Peritoneal dialysis in Ghana

Peritoneal dialysis as a modality for managing chronic dialysis is not practiced in Ghana currently. It is however available for the management of acute kidney injury in the Komfo Anokye Teaching Hospital, to a very less extent in the Korle-bu Teaching Hospital, Cape Coast Teaching Hospital, and Tamale Teaching Hospital.

Discussion

This study is an audit of hemodialysis services in Ghana showing the regional distribution of hemodialysis facilities and number of hemodialysis machines in Ghana. There have been some improvements in the dialysis facilities in Ghana since the study by Antwi in 2014 [13]. There are now more private hemodialysis facilities but not much improvement in numbers in the state-owned facilities. The use of peritoneal dialysis as a form of renal replacement therapy in the management of acute and chronic kidney diseases in Ghana is however still minimal. The unavailability of chronic peritoneal dialysis in many sub-Saharan Africa including Ghana has been attributed to the high cost of the peritoneal dialysis fluid making it comparable or even more expensive than in-center hemodialysis sessions [21]. In developed countries, the cost of providing peritoneal dialysis is less than the cost of hemodialysis due to economies of scale in the production of dialysate but this is not so in developing countries [22] such as Ghana. Measures to produce peritoneal dialysate locally and lowering of import duties on peritoneal dialysate and peritoneal dialysis catheters have been suggested as important in decreasing the cost of peritoneal dialysis. Training of surgeons and physicians on Tenckhoff catheter insertion may provide peritoneal dialysis valuable modality as a renal replacement therapy with comparable quality of life to hemodialysis [11].

Acute peritoneal dialysis is however practiced in many regional and district hospitals in Ghana using improvised techniques and self-constituted fluids to decrease cost [23]. This has proven very useful in children for the management of acute kidney injury in some teaching hospitals in the country. The cost of peritoneal fluid is still a challenge for chronic peritoneal dialysis.

All the hemodialysis facilities are concentrated in the capital cities of the Greater Accra region, Ashanti region, the Central region, and Volta region with most regions bereft of any form of renal replacement therapy for the management of acute and chronic kidney diseases.

The unavailability of kidney transplantation services in Ghana leaves a lot of end-stage renal disease patients on hemodialysis for longer duration. Most patients do not get kidney transplant though it has been shown to be the best modality for renal replacement therapy as compared to hemodialysis and peritoneal dialysis [5–10]. In Ghana, patients on hemodialysis have high mortality rate [24]. Our study reveals that hemodialysis machines per million population in Ghana is 4.20 much lower than other African countries such as Egypt, South Africa, and Nigeria [25]. The dialysis rates across Africa are less than 20 per million population as compared to a global prevalence of 223 pmp [26]. Ghana falls far below the 20 hemodialysis machines per million population. Most regions in Ghana do not have any form of renal replacement therapy and are therefore transferred to the few centers for management with varied outcomes.

There is the need to improve the number of dialysis machines per million population considering the perceived high prevalence of chronic kidney disease and acute kidney injury in Africa and Ghana as we work to establish a renal transplant services.

The regulation of the hemodialysis services to provide adequate dialysis, without the spread of infection with ultrapure water quality with the reverse osmosis (RO) system is imperative [27]. Unfortunately, dialysis service in Ghana is not officially regulated and regular checks for water quality are done at the discretion of the service providers. This needs to be addressed to provide quality dialysis services in all centers across the country to avoid cross infections among patients with end-stage renal disease and acute kidney injury.

Most hemodialysis facilities especially in the private-owned facilities are not managed by trained nephrologists or physicians but by medical officers and renal nurses. This is because Ghana has very few nephrologists of less than one per million population just as other African countries in sub-Saharan Africa [25]. These nephrologists are found only in the teaching hospitals in Accra and Kumasi. It was reported in an earlier study that Ghana had 0.1 nephrologists per million population as compared to 0.6 pmp in Nigeria, 0.5 pmp in Kenya, 4.5 pmp in Morocco, and 6.5 pmp in Egypt [21]. The total number of nephrologist have subsequently improved from 0.1pmp in 2010 to 0.26 pmp currently, but this is still inadequate for the population in Ghana. We do acknowledge the limitation of our study as data was obtained by interviewing staff or health care workers in each region. This is because there is no designated outfit responsible for registering dialysis facilities in Ghana.

The authors believe that kidney transplantation program should be established in the country. The country needs to educate the populace about prevention of kidney disease and sensitize the public about kidney donation. Chronic peritoneal dialysis should be introduced for the management of end-stage renal disease. Hemodialysis centers and machines per population should be increased in both private-owned and government-owned facilities. Since cost of dialysis is also an important limiting factor affecting accessibility of renal replacement, there is the need for governmental support for renal replacement therapy. There is the need for the various dialysis facilities in Ghana to be regulated to provide quality renal services to patients with renal diseases.

Conclusion

The distribution of renal dialysis services is skewed to a few cities and regions. There is an urgent need to establish more dialysis services equitably across the country to meet the need of the growing prevalence of chronic kidney disease and for the management of acute kidney injury in all the ten regions of Ghana.

Acknowledgements

We appreciate the effort and contribution of the doctors and other health workers across dialysis facilities in Ghana who contributed data towards this manuscript. We also acknowledge Mr. EvansXorseAmuzu for helping with the mapping out of the locations of all the facilities.

Funding

This study is self-funded by the authors.

Authors' contributions

All authors contributed equally to the study concept and design, acquisition of data, interpretation of data, and critical revision of the manuscript. All authors read and approved the final manuscript.

Competing interests

The authors declare that they have no competing interests.

Author details

[1]Department of Medicine and Renal Unit, Komfo Anokye Teaching Hospital, Kumasi, Ghana. [2]Department of Medicine and Therapeutics, School of Medical Sciences, University of Cape Coast, Cape Coast, Ghana. [3]Department of Medicine and Renal Unit, Korle-bu Teaching Hospital, Accra, Ghana. [4]Paediatric Nephrology Unit, Department of Child Health, Kwame Nkrumah University of Science and Technology/Komfo Anokye Teaching Hospital, Kumasi, Ghana.

References

1. Stenvinkel P. Chronic kidney disease: a public health priority and harbinger of premature cardiovascular disease. J Intern Med. 2010;268:456–67.
2. Coresh J, Selvin E, Stevens LA, Manzi J, Kusek JW, Eggers P, et al. Prevalence of chronic kidney disease in the United States. J Am Med Assoc. 2007; 298(17):2038–47.
3. Eknoyan G, Lameire N, Barsoum R, Eckardt KU, Levin A, Levin N, et al. The burden of kidney disease: improving global outcomes. Kidney Int. 2004;66(4):1310–4.
4. Stanifer JW, Jing B, Tolan S, Helmke N, Mukerjee R, Naicker S, et al. The epidemiology of chronic kidney disease in sub-Saharan Africa: a systematic review and meta-analysis. Lancet Glob Health. 2014;2(3):e174–81.
5. Valderrabano F, Jofre R, Lopez-Gomez JM. Quality of life in end-stage renal disease patients. Am J Kidney Dis. 2001;38(3):443–64.
6. Alvares J, Cesar CC, AcurcioFde A, Andrade EI, Cherchiglia ML. Quality of life of patients in renal replacement therapy in Brazil: comparison of treatment modalities. Qual Life Res. 2012;21(6):983–91.
7. Kovacs AZ, Molnar MZ, Szeifert L, Ambrus C, Molnar-Varga M, Szentkiralyi A, et al. Sleep disorders, depressive symptoms and health-related quality of life—a cross-sectional comparison between kidney transplant recipients and waitlisted patients on maintenance dialysis. Nephrol Dial Transplant. 2011;26(3):1058–65.
8. Purnell TS, Auguste P, Crews DC, Lamprea-Montealegre J, Olufade T, Greer R, et al. Comparison of life participation activities among adults treated by hemodialysis, peritoneal dialysis, and kidney transplantation: a systematic review. Am J Kidney Dis. 2013;62(5):953–73.
9. Czyzewski L, Sanko-Resmer J, Wyzgal J, Kurowski A. Assessment of health-related quality of life of patients after kidney transplantation in comparison with hemodialysis and peritoneal dialysis. Ann Transplant. 2014;19:576–85.
10. Liem YS, Bosch JL, Arends LR, Heijenbrok-Kal MH, Hunink MG. Quality of life assessed with the Medical Outcomes Study Short Form 36-Item Health Survey of patients on renal replacement therapy: a systematic review and meta-analysis. Value Health. 2007;10(5):390–7.
11. Tannor EK, et al. Quality of life in patients on chronic dialysis in South Africa: a comparative mixed methods study. BMC Nephrol. 2017;18(1):4.
12. Govindaraj R, Obuobi A, Enyimayew N, Antwi P, Ofosu-Amaah S. Hospital autonomy in Ghana: the experience of Korle Bu and Komfo Anokye Teaching hospitals. Boston: Data for Decision Making Project, Harvard School of Public Health; 1996.
13. Antwi S. State of renal replacement therapy services in Ghana. Blood Purif. 2015;39(1–3):137–40.
14. Adu D, Okyere P, Boima V, Matekole M, Osafo C. Community-acquired acute kidney injury in adults in Africa. Clin Nephrol. 2016;86(13):48.
15. Boima V, Ganu V, Adjei D et al. Psychological wellbeing and quality of life among chronic kidney disease patients in Ghana. Changing Trends Mental Health Care Res Ghana. 2015(3).
16. http://www.statsghana.gov.gh/pop_stats.html. Accessed 20 Feb 2017.
17. http://www.tradingeconomics.com/ghana/gdp. Accessed 2 Apr 2017.
18. Service GS. 2010 population and housing census: demographic, social, economic and housing characteristic report 2013.
19. https://en.wikipedia.org/wiki/List_of_Ghanaian_regions_by_area. Accessed 23 Dec 2016.
20. http://www.pub.iaea.org/MTCD/Publications/PDF/CNPP2012_CD/countryprofiles/Ghana/Ghana.htm2012. Accessed 2 Apr 2017.
21. Katz IJ, Gerntholtz T, Naicker S. Africa and nephrology: the forgotten continent. Nephron Clin Pract. 2010;117(4):320–7.
22. Karopadi AN, Mason G, Rettore E, Ronco C. Cost of peritoneal dialysis and haemodialysis across the world. Nephrol Dial Transplant. 2013:2553–69.
23. Antwi S. Peritoneal dialysis using improvised PD catheter and self-constituted dialysis solution. 2010.
24. Eghan BA, Amoako-Atta K, Kankam CA, Nsiah-Asare A. Survival pattern of hemodialysis patients in Kumasi, Ghana: a summary of forty patients initiated on hemodialysis at a new hemodialysis unit. Hemodial Int. 2009;13(4):467–71.
25. Naicker S, Eastwood JB, Plange-Rhule J, Tutt RC. Shortage of healthcare workers in sub-Saharan Africa: a nephrological perspective. Clin Nephrol. 2010;74:S129–33.
26. El Matri A. ESRD management in Africa during the last decade. Clin Nephrol. 2015;83(7 Suppl 1):11–3.
27. Laurence RA, Lapierre ST. Quality of hemodialysis water: a 7-year multicenter study. Am J Kidney Dis. 1995;25(5):738–50.

25

Fibroblast growth factor 23 and cardiovascular disease in patients with chronic kidney disease

Kosaku Nitta

Abstract

Chronic kidney disease (CKD) has been known to be associated with an increased risk of cardiovascular (CV) mortality and morbidity in Japan. Although traditional risk factors contribute to the development of CV disease in CKD patients, they cannot fully explain the unacceptably high incidence of CV mortality. Recently, non-traditional risk factors, including abnormal mineral metabolism, have been suggested to be involved in the increased risk of CV events. The medical treatment of CKD-mineral bone disorders (CKD-MBD) has been associated with encouraging, but inconsistent, improvement in CV disease complications and patient survival. A better understanding of the biomarkers and mechanisms involved in left ventricular hypertrophy (LVH) and vascular calcification might improve the diagnosis and treatment of the CV disease secondary to CKD-MBD, thus improving patient survival. Recent insights into fibroblast growth factor 23 (FGF23) and its co-receptor, Klotho, have led to marked advancements in the interpretation of data about CKD-MBD and CV damage.

Keywords: CKD-MBD, FGF23, Klotho, LVH, Arterial calcification

Background

Japan is one of the countries with the highest incidence of end-stage renal disease (ESRD) globally, and the number of Japanese patients with ESRD is continuously increasing [1]. Chronic kidney disease (CKD) is known to be associated with an increased risk for cardiovascular (CV) mortality and morbidity in Japan [2]. CV diseases account for 30–50% of all-cause mortality in CKD patients, especially dialysis patients worldwide [1, 3]. Although traditional risk factors contribute to the development of CV disease in CKD patients, they cannot fully explain the unacceptably high incidence of CV mortality in these patients. Hence, non-traditional risk factors, including abnormal mineral metabolism, are thought to be involved in the increased risk of CV events [4, 5].

There is growing interest in the issues surrounding CKD-mineral and bone disorder (CKD-MBD) [6]. CKD has been shown to be associated with bone and mineral disorder characterized by (i) laboratory abnormalities of calcium, phosphate, parathyroid hormone (PTH), and

vitamin D; (ii) evidence of bone disease; and (iii) vascular calcification. Vascular calcification is associated with adverse clinical outcomes, including ischemic CV events and subsequent vascular mortality [7]. The pathogenesis of vascular calcification in CKD is complex, and rather than being attributable to a simple process of calcium and phosphate precipitation, involves an active process where vascular smooth muscle cells (VSMCs) undergo apoptosis with release of matrix vesicles and are transformed into osteoblast-like cells [7].

The complex mechanisms by which aging leads to increased vascular calcification remain uncertain. However, there is no doubt that patients with ESRD are at high risk of and have a high prevalence of vascular calcification because of multiple risk factors that induce the phenotypic transformation of VSMCs into osteoblast-like cells capable of carrying out tissue mineralization [8]. Vascular calcification has been associated with numerous traditional CV risk factors, including advanced age, hypertension, diabetes, and dyslipidemia, as well as with non-traditional CV risk factors, including hyperphosphatemia, hyperparathyroidism, and excessive calcium intake [9]. There are two patterns of vascular calcification. One occurs in the

---

Correspondence: knitta@twmu.ac.jp
Department of Medicine, Kidney Center, Tokyo Women's Medical University, Tokyo, Japan

intimal layer and the other occurs in the medial layer of the vessel wall as in Mönckeberg's sclerosis, which is very common in ESRD patients. The hemodynamic consequences of vascular calcification include loss of arterial elasticity, an increase in pulse wave velocity, left ventricular hypertrophy, a decrease in coronary artery perfusion, and myocardial ischemia (Fig. 1).

Recent studies have shown that fibroblast growth factor 23 (FGF23), a bone-derived phosphatonin, and its co-receptor Klotho play an important role in the regulation of calcium and phosphate metabolism in CKD-MBD [10]. This review summarizes the pathophysiology involving the FGF23-Klotho axis, with particular focus on the recent advances elucidating its role in CV disease, which are characterized by left ventricular hypertrophy (LVH) and vascular calcification.

Mineral metabolism and vascular calcification

As earlier mentioned, numerous risk factors for vascular calcification have been reported. Traditional risk factors include advanced age, hypertension, diabetes, and dyslipidemia. Non-traditional risk factors in CKD include disorders of mineral metabolism, elevated serum PTH levels, excessive intake of calcium supplements, inflammation, malnutrition, and oxidative stress [11]. Patients with advanced CKD develop hyperphosphatemia secondary to impaired renal phosphate excretion. There is strong evidence that vascular calcification is closely associated with high serum calcium and phosphate levels. High serum phosphate levels can be considered a vascular toxin [12], and clinical studies have shown that patients with the poorest phosphate control experience the most rapid progression of vascular calcification [13].

Two different mechanisms of vascular calcification have been proposed to explain the relationship between calcium and phosphate disorders and vascular calcification. Experimental studies have demonstrated that calcium plays a role in the development of vascular calcification by stimulating mineralization of VSMCs under normal phosphate conditions [14]. When phosphate levels are elevated, this calcium-driven mineralization is accelerated synergistically and hyperphosphatemia may directly induce vascular injury, and it indirectly stimulates osteoblastic differentiation through a type III sodium-dependent phosphate co-transporter (PiT-1) [15]. New discoveries related to extracellular vesicles, microRNAs, and calci-protein particles (CPPs) further reveal the mechanisms involved in the initiation and progression of vascular calcification in CKD [16]. Thus, elevated intracellular phosphate concentration may directly stimulate VSMCs to transform into calcifying cells by activating genes associated with osteoblastic functions. These findings provide strong evidence that excess phosphate and calcium load is probably the most important pathogenic factor in vascular calcification.

Interaction between FGF23 and Klotho

FGF23 is a 32 kDa protein synthesized primarily in osteocytes, and the corresponding gene encodes a 251-amino-acid protein, including a 24-amino-acid signal peptide [17]. FGF23 circulates in two distinct forms, a single, intact, full-length active protein and a shorter, inactive protein. Intact-FGF23 activates FGF receptors (FGFRs) 1, 3, and 4 to elicit tissue-specific responses through the subsequent induction of two main pathways: (1) Klotho-dependent activation of the mitogen-activated protein kinase (MAPK) cascade, leading to extracellular

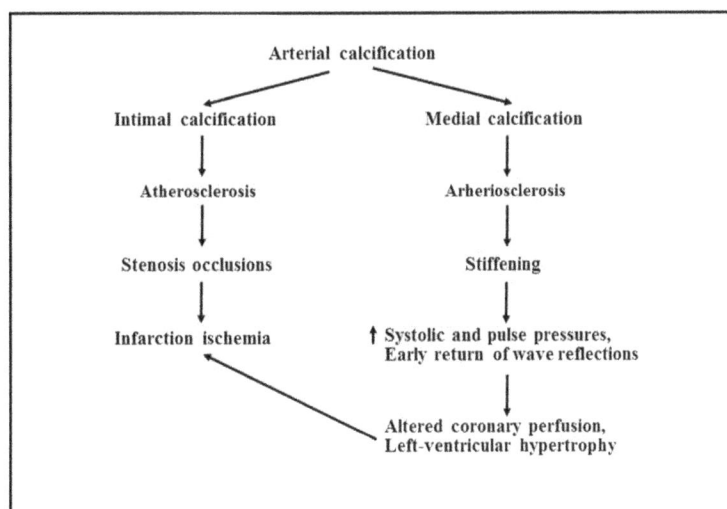

Fig. 1 Schematic representation of the clinical effects of arterial intimal and medial calcification. Cited from [7]

signal-regulated kinase (ERK) activation and Egr-1 expression, and (2) a Klotho-independent cascade, characterized by phosphoinositide-specific phospholipase C (PLC) γ-dependent activation of the calcineurin-nuclear factor of activated T-cells (NFAT) [18]. FGF23 appears to impair synthesis and accelerate degradation of 1, 25 (OH)$_2$D. Recombinant FGF23 also has a phosphaturic effect, which is attributable to reduced renal phosphate reabsorption. FGF23 downregulates the expression of both type IIa and type IIc sodium-phosphate cotransporters on the apical surface of renal proximal tubular epithelial cells in vivo [19].

The effects of FGF23 are influenced by Klotho, which is itself a 130-kDa transmembrane β-glucuronidase that catalyzes the hydrolysis of steroid β-glucuronides. Klotho was discovered by Kuro-o et al. in 1997 [20]. The *Klotho* gene is expressed in a limited number of tissues, mainly the kidneys, and mutations cause multiple aging-related disorders in nearly all organs and tissues. FGF23 exerts its biological effects through activation of FGFRs in a Klotho-dependent manner (Fig. 2), because a Klotho/FGFR complex binds to FGF23 with higher affinity than FGF-R or Klotho alone [21]. Thus, activation of FGF23 receptors requires not only circulating FGF23, but also the presence of Klotho as a specific promoter whose affinity dictates the selectivity towards its targets.

Because of the reduction in functioning nephrons during CKD progression, each nephron is required to excrete an increasing amount of phosphate to maintain normal serum phosphate levels. This can be attained by increasing serum FGF23 levels, which is an early sign of changes in phosphate metabolism during CKD progression. However,

because FGF23 is a counter-regulatory hormone for vitamin D, an increase in its levels is at the expense of vitamin D synthesis. Decreasing vitamin D in turn stimulates PTH secretion, leading to secondary hyperparathyroidism. In fact, decreases in serum 1, 25 (OH)$_2$D levels and increases in serum PTH levels are observed in patients with early-stage CKD with normophosphatemia. The fact that Klotho expression in the parathyroid gland is decreased in CKD patients may explain why elevated serum FGF23 levels fail to suppress PTH. The increase of FGF23 was associated with the decrease of 1, 25 (OH)$_2$D in CKD patients [22]. Moreover, the inhibition of FGF23 activity in the animal model of CKD increased serum 1, 25 (OH)$_2$D [23]. While the reduction of 1, 25 (OH)$_2$D by increased FGF23 is likely to reduce intestinal phosphate absorption and contribute to maintaining serum phosphate level, it may induce or aggravate secondary hyperparathyroidism. However, the role of FGF23 in the development of secondary hyperparathyroidism is complex because FGF23 was shown to directly inhibit production and secretion of PTH [24]. With the progression of CKD, the expression of Klotho in the kidneys and parathyroid glands were shown to decrease that likely leads to impaired actions of FGF23 [25].

Elevated serum FGF23 levels and low vitamin D may further reduce Klotho expression in the kidney and parathyroid tissue in CKD patients, because FGF23 and vitamin D can downregulate and upregulate Klotho expression, respectively. Decline in Klotho expression exacerbates FGF23 resistance in the kidney and parathyroid gland, further increasing FGF23, decreasing vitamin D, and increasing PTH. This vicious cycle (Fig. 3) may contribute

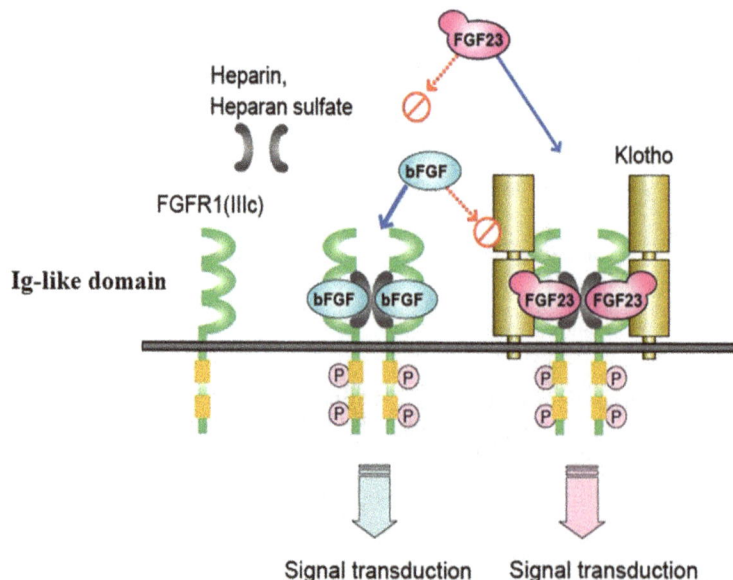

Fig. 2 Interaction between FGF23 and Klotho. Cited from [10]

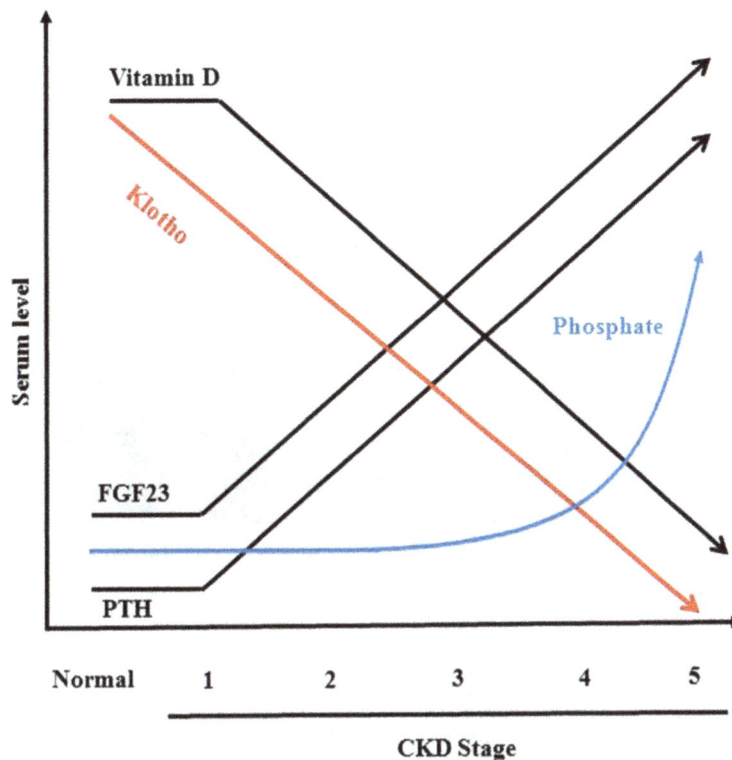

Fig. 3 Changes in phosphate-regulating factors during CKD progression. Cited from [26]

to the pathophysiology of deranged phosphate metabolism in CKD patients [26]. In the advanced stages of CKD, increased FGF23 can no longer compensate for dietary phosphate overload, resulting in overt hyperphosphatemia, vitamin D deficiency, and parathyroid hyperplasia. The fact that patients with advanced stage CKD have extremely high serum levels of biologically active FGF23 has raised the possibility that the elevated serum FGF23 levels may activate FGF signaling in tissues that do not innately express Klotho, which may then contribute to systemic complications in ESRD.

It has been reported that calcimimetics decrease plasma FGF23 concentration in hemodialysis patients, and the decrease in plasma FGF23 concentration seems to be related to the decrease in serum phosphate concentration [27]. Chertow et al. reported the results of the Evaluation of Cinacalcet Therapy to Lower Cardiovascular Events (EVOLVE) trial in 3883 patients receiving long-term hemodialysis treatment [28]. In an unadjusted intention-to-treat (ITT) analysis, cinacalcet had no significant benefit on the primary composite outcome (death or first non-fatal myocardial infarction, hospitalization for unstable angina, heart failure, or peripheral vascular events) but significantly reduced the incidence of heart failure. In an adjusted ITT analysis and lag-censoring analysis, the effect of cinacalcet on the primary outcome

was significant. ITT analyses adjusted for baseline characteristics suggest that treating secondary hyperparathyroidism with cinacalcet results in significant reduction in the risk of death or cardiovascular events.

Role of FGF23 in CV disease
Serum FGF23 levels were independently associated with left ventricular mass index and the risk of new-onset LVH in the Chronic Renal Insufficiency Cohort (CRIC) study [29]. Negishi et al. reported that FGF23 was significantly associated with LVH, and they suggested that FGF23 could be a novel biomarker of left ventricular overload, which is closely associated with an increased risk of death in hemodialysis patients [30]. We demonstrated that hemodialysis patients with LVH were more likely to have higher systolic blood pressure and LVH was significantly associated with female gender and higher serum phosphate levels in addition to serum FGF23 levels (Fig. 4) [31]. An experimental study by Faul et al. demonstrated that FGF23 induced rat cardiomyocyte hypertrophy through FGFR-dependent activation of the calcineurin-NFAT signaling pathway in a Klotho-independent manner [32]. FGFR-4 is now considered the specific FGFR directly involved in the Klotho-independent activity of FGF23 in the myocardium [33]. FGF23 activates only FGFR-4 in cardiomyocytes, thereafter stimulating PLC-γ-calineurin-

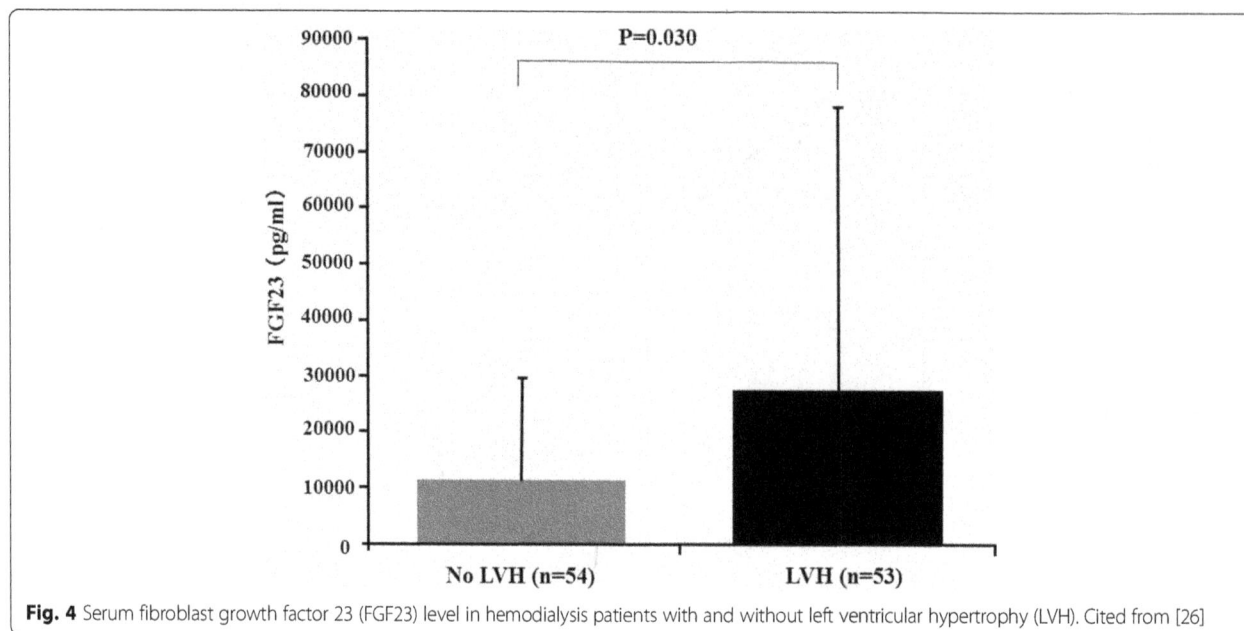

Fig. 4 Serum fibroblast growth factor 23 (FGF23) level in hemodialysis patients with and without left ventricular hypertrophy (LVH). Cited from [26]

NFAT cell signaling [34]. Knock-out mice lacking FGFR-4 did not develop LVH in response to high FGF23 levels, while gain-of-function transgenic mutants of FGFR-4 spontaneously led to LVH [35]. Leifhelt-Nestler et al. recently reported that FGF23/FGFR4-mediated LVH is reversible [36]. Moreover, data from 24 deceased patients with childhood-onset ESRD provides evidence that expression of FGFR-4 and activation of the PLC-γ-calcineurin-NFAT pathway were associated with cardiac expression of FGF23 in situ [36]. Reduced expression of Klotho in the same cardiac tissues supports the notion that high FGF23 levels concomitant with Klotho downregulation may favor activation of Klotho-independent pathways that lead to LVH. Thus, high serum FGF23 levels exert toxic effects via Klotho-independent pathways in myocardium. However, a potential effect of LVH on FGF23 remains unclear. Matsui et al. recently evaluated the effect of LVH on FGF23 using cardiomyocyte-specific calcineurin A transgenic mice and showed severe LVH with elevated serum FGF23 levels [37]. The FGF23 levels were elevated in cardio myocytes, but not osteocytes, suggesting that FGF23 and LVH might be linked in a vicious cycle, particularly in the setting kidney disease: LVH itself could increase FGF23, which, in turn, cause LVH progression.

FGF23 has been associated with abdominal aortic calcification in healthy older men [38]. In a study of 545 African Americans with diabetes, Freedman et al. found an independent association of FGF23 with coronary artery-calcified atherosclerotic plaque, but not with carotid and aortoiliac-calcified plaque [39]. Among 142 patients in CKD stages 2 through 5D, intact FGF23 was elevated and independently associated with aortic calcification

score, as assessed by multislice, spiral-computed tomography (CT) [40]. Morena et al. described a significant correlation between FGF23 expression and coronary artery calcification among 195 non-dialysis CKD patients [41]. Due to the considerable interaction between FGF23 and osteoprotegerin (OPG), these authors suggested that FGF23 expression represented a biomarker for severe vascular calcification, whereas OPG expression was associated with moderate coronary calcification [41]. More recently, Di Lullo et al. demonstrated an independent association between FGF23 expression and the extent of aortic valve calcification among 100 consecutive non-hospitalized CKD stage 3–4 patients [42].

Aortic calcification index, which is assessed on non-contrast CT, was independently associated with serum levels of intact FGF23 in 65 hemodialysis patients [43]. Although coronary artery and thoracic aortic calcium concentrations were not associated with serum FGF23 levels among 1501 patients from the CRIC study, secondary analysis revealed an association between serum FGF23 levels and thoracic aorta calcium concentrations among CKD patients with non-zero calcification scores [44]. This result was statistically significant, despite the significant association detected between serum phosphate levels and coronary calcium concentrations. The authors concluded that these types of studies are highly sensitive to the specific definition of vascular calcification, the site of interest, the sample size, and the proportion of subjects with a calcification score of zero [44].

FGF23 may even be associated with progression of vascular calcification, although there are discrepancies in these results. Khan et al. assessed coronary arterial calcification by electrocardiography-triggered multislice CT in 99 incident hemodialysis patients [45]. FGF23 was associated with progression of coronary calcification independently of serum phosphate levels and known risk factors [45]. Among 74 hemodialysis patients, progression of coronary artery calcification, assessed twice by scoring with a 1-year interval, was associated with serum levels of FGF23 and phosphate, as well as baseline coronary calcium scores [46]. Conversely, we reported higher FGF23 levels in hemodialysis patients with regression, rather than progression, of aortic arch calcification, at a 5-year follow-up, as assessed by simple chest radiographs [47].

Prognostic value of FGF23 in CKD patients

Previous studies suggest that elevated serum FGF23 level is strongly associated with increased mortality risk across the spectrum of CKD [48–50]. We have recently reported that serum FGF23 level was not associated with increased mortality risk in our cohort of prevalent hemodialysis patients [51], suggesting that the impact of FGF23 on mortality may be modified by gender and previous CV disease and is blunted by the grade of hyperphosphatemia in ESRD patients. However, the overall prognostic utility of FGF23 remains unclear. Previous observational studies have shown conflicting results. To resolve this uncertainty regarding FGF23 as a prognostic tool in patients with ESRD, Yang et al. conducted a systematic review to quantify the association between elevated FGF23 and long-term mortality among ESRD patients. They showed that elevated serum FGF23 levels were significantly associated with higher risk of all-cause mortality in ESRD patients, indicating FGF23 predicts poor prognosis in these patients [52]. The mechanism of the association between elevated serum FGF23 levels and mortality, however, remained unclear. Possible mechanisms may include that FGF23 suppresses vitamin D metabolism, stimulates the renin–angiotensin– aldosterone system, and increases production of inflammatory mediators. In addition, elevated circulating FGF23 concentration contributes directly to the high prevalence of LVH in CKD as mentioned above. These factors have shown a strong association with adverse outcomes in patients with CKD and ESRD.

FGF23 concentrations had been found to be associated with serum phosphate level, and FGF23 also leads to decreased synthesis of vitamin D as mentioned above. The effects of serum calcium, vitamin D, and PTH on serum FGF-23 concentration have not been studied. However, some medical administration including vitamin D supplementation, cinacalcet, and phosphate binders may influence serum calcium and phosphate level, further affect FGF23 concentration directly or indirectly [53]. Most of the included studies had adjusted for serum phosphate when calculating hazard ratios. However, four studies did not report medical treatment. Few studies adjusted medication. The medical treatment with phosphate binders and vitamin D may potentially be a confounding factor.

Conclusion

CV disease remains frequently complicated in CKD patients, representing the main cause of death in dialysis patients, because conventional therapies against atherosclerosis, vascular calcification, and CKD-MBD seem to provide no survival benefit to these patients. Thus, additional research is warranted to improve the understanding of vascular aging in CKD. Signaling through FGF23 and Klotho represents a critical element in the vascular consequences of CKD-MBD.

Results from clinical and experimental studies support a consistent, direct, protective effect of Klotho on LVH, atherosclerosis, and vascular calcification. However, additional research is needed to elucidate the precise localization of transmembrane Klotho expression within the heart and arterial walls, as well as the paracrine and endocrine effects of secreted Klotho on the vascular system. Concomitant reduction of Klotho and FGFR expression may be responsible for the onset and progression of (1) CKD-MBD via FGF23 resistance and (2) LVH, atherosclerosis, and vascular calcification resulting from impaired endogenous protection against vascular injury.

The classic Klotho-dependent activity of FGF23 on the kidney and parathyroid glands is accepted as a fundamental pathway for the maintenance of phosphate homeostasis and protection against the onset of CKD-MBD. However, many of the findings are conflicting. For example, experimental data and analysis of families with FGF23 deficiency confirm that defects in FGF23 signaling induce vascular damage with eventual critical impact. These data conflict with observational studies that report a direct association between high serum FGF23 levels and CV disease, suggesting a role for FGF23 as a biomarker of advanced CKD-MBD rather than a direct causative agent of vascular aging. As a second example, experimental data seem to suggest that LVH results from a direct Klotho-independent response to high serum FGF23 levels in cardiomyocytes. Although the direct activity exerted by FGF23 on the arteries is supported by several studies, data regarding whether this effect is protective or detrimental remain inconsistent.

Future perspectives

Future research in this field will shed light on several topics, such as Klotho-independent pathways activated by FGF23, and the precise and dynamic localization of Klotho-FGFR-FGF23 expression within the heart and arterial tissue. These studies should be designed to overcome several weaknesses in the literature, including (i) lack of information on gender, ethnicity, and genetic characteristics of human VSMC donors, which may interact with FGF23 on vascular calcification [54], (ii) frequent barriers encountered while dealing with translation from animal to human models and from in vitro to dynamic in vivo models, (iii) the specific characteristics and limitations of laboratory methods adopted for assessing Klotho and FGF23 levels, and (iv) the challenging reproduction and control of systemic conditions, such as inflammation, which may influence Klotho and FGF23 activity significantly in vivo.

Abbreviations
1, 25(OH)$_2$D: 1, 25 Dihydroxyvitamin D; CKD: Chronic kidney disease; CKD-MBD: Chronic kidney disease-mineral and bone disorder; CRIC: Chronic Renal Insufficiency Cohort; CV: Cardiovascular; ERK: Extracellular signal-regulated kinase; ESRD: End-stage renal disease; FGF23: Fibroblast growth factor 23; FGFR: Fibroblast growth factor receptor; LVH: Left ventricular hypertrophy; MAPK: Mitogen-activated protein kinase; NFAT: Calcineurin-nuclear factor of activated T cells; OPG: Osteoprotegerin; PiT: Sodium-dependent phosphate co-transporter; PLC: Phospholipase C; PTH: Parathyroid hormone; VSMC: Vascular smooth muscle cell

Acknowledgements
The authors acknowledge the medical staffs who contributed to this work in the Department of Medicines, Kidney Center, Tokyo Women's Medical University.

Author's contributions
KN searched the literature and prepared this article. The author read and approved the final manuscript.

Competing interests
The author declares no competing interests.

References
1. Masakane I, Taniguchi M, Nakai S, Tsuchida K, Goto S, Wada A, Ogata S, Hasegawa T, Hamano T, Hanafusa N, Hoshino J, Minakuchi J, Nakamoto H. Annual Dialysis data report 2015, JSDT renal data registry (JRDR). Ren Replace Ther. 2018;4:19.
2. Tanaka K, Watanabe T, Takeuchi A, Ohashi Y, Nitta K, Akizawa T, Matsuo S, Imai E, Makino H, Hishida A, CKD-JAC Investigators. Cardiovascular events and death in Japanese patients with chronic kidney disease. Kidney Int. 2017;91:227–34.
3. Collins AJ, Foley RN, Gilbertson DT, Chen SC. United States Renal Data System public health surveillance of chronic kidney disease and end-stage renal disease. Kidney Int Suppl. 2011;5:2–7.
4. Briet M, Burns KD. Chronic kidney disease and vascular remodelling: molecular mechanisms and clinical implications. Clin Sci. 2012;123:399–416.
5. Rhee CM, Kovesdy CP. Epidemiology: spotlight on CKD deaths increasing ortality worldwide. Nat Rev Nephrol. 2015;11:199–200.
6. Ketteler M, Elder GJ, Evenepoel P, Ix JH, Jamal SA, Lafage-Proust MH, Shroff R, Thadhani RI, Tonelli MA, Kasiske BL, Wheeler DC, Leonard MB. Revising KDIGO clinical practice guideline on chronic kidney disease-mineral and bone disorder: a commentary from a Kidney Disease: improving Global Outcomes controversies conference. Kidney Int. 2015;87:502–28.
7. Nitta K. Vascular calcification in patients with chronic kidney disease. Ther Apher Dial. 2011;15:513–21.
8. Hruska KA, Sugatani T, Agapova O, Fang Y. The chronic kidney disease – mineral bone disorder (CKD-MBD): advances in pathophysiology. Bone. 2017;100:80–6.
9. Bover J, Evenepoel P, Urena-Torres P, Vervloet MG, Brandenburg V, Mazzaferro S, Covic A, Goldsmith D, Massy ZA, Cozzolino M, CKD-MBD Working Group of ERA-EDTA. Pro: cardiovascular calcifications are clinically relevant. Nephrol Dial Transplant. 2015;30:345–51.
10. Nitta K, Nagano N, Tsuchiya K. Fibroblast growth factor 23/klotho axis in chronic kidney disease. Nephron Clin Pract. 2014;128:1–10.
11. Raggi P. Cardiovascular disease: coronary artery calcification predicts risk of CVD in patients with CKD. Nat Rev Nephrol. 2017;13:324–6.
12. Shroff R. Phosphate is a vascular toxin. Pediatr Nephrol. 2013;28:583–93.
13. Shanahan CM, Crouthamel MH, Kapustin A, Giachelli CM. Arterial calcification in chronic kidney disease: key roles for calcium and phosphate. Circ Res. 2011;109:697–711.
14. Reynolds JL, Joannides AJ, Skepper JN, McNair R, Schurgers LJ, Proudfoot D, Jahnen-Dechent W, Weissberg PL, Shanahan CM. Human vascular smooth muscle cells undergo vesicle-mediated calcification in response to changes in extracellular calcium and phosphate concentrations: a potential mechanism for accelerated vascular calcification in ESRD. J Am Soc Nephrol. 2004;15:2857–67.
15. Li X, Yang HY, Giachelli CM. Role of the sodium-dependent phosphate cotransporter, Pit-1, in vascular smooth muscle cell calcification. Circ Res. 2006;98:905–12.
16. Paloian NJ, Giachelli CM. A current understanding of vascular calcification in CKD. Am J Physiol Renal Physiol. 2014;307:F8915–F900.
17. Shimada T, Kakitani M, Yamazaki Y, Hasegawa H, Takeuchi Y, Fujita T, Fukumoto S, Tomizuka K, Yamashita T. Targeted ablation of Fgf23 demonstrates an essential physiological role of FGF23 in phosphate and vitamin D metabolism. J Clin Invest. 2004;113:561–8.
18. Martin A, David V, Quarles LD. Regulation and function of the FGF23/klotho endocrine pathways. Physiol Rev. 2012;92:131–55.
19. Mace ML, Gravesen E, Hofman-Bang J, Olgaard K, Lewin E. Key role of the kidney in the regulation of fibroblast growth factor 23. Kidney Int. 2015;88: 1304–13.
20. Kuro-o M, Matsumura Y, Aizawa H, Kawaguchi H, Suga T, Utsugi T, Ohyama Y, Kurabayashi M, Kaname T, Kume E, Iwasaki H, Iida A, Shiraki-Iida T, Nishikawa S, Nagai R, Nabeshima YI. Mutation of the mouse klotho gene leads to a syndrome resembling ageing. Nature. 1997;390:45–51.
21. Kurosu H, Ogawa Y, Miyoshi M, Yamamoto M, Nandi A, Rosenblatt KP, Raum MG, Schiavi S, Hu MC, Moe OW, Kuro-o M. Regulation of fibroblast growth factor-23 signaling by klotho. J Biol Chem. 2006;281:6120–3.
22. Gutierrez O, Isakova T, Rhee E, Shah A, Holmes J, Collerone G, Juppner H, Wolf M. Fibroblast growth factor-23 mitigates hyperphosphatemia but accentuates calcitriol deficiency in chronic kidney disease. J Am Soc Nephrol. 2005;16:2205–15.
23. Hasegawa H, Nagano N, Urakawa I, Yamazaki Y, Iijima K, Fujita T, Yamashita T, Fukumoto S, Shimada T. Direct evidence for a causative role of FGF23 in the abnormal renal phosphate handling and vitamin D metabolism in rats with early-stage chronic kidney disease. Kidney Int. 2010;78:975–80.
24. Ben-Dov IZ, Galitzer H, Lavi-Moshayoff V, Goetz R, Kuro-o M, Mohammadi M, Sirkis R, Naveh-Many T, Silver J. The parathyroid is a target organ for FGF23 in rats. J Clin Invest. 2007;117:4003–8.
25. Komaba H, Goto S, Fujii H, Hamada Y, Kobayashi A, Shibuya K, Tominaga Y, Otsuki N, Nibu K, Nakagawa K, Tsugawa N, Okano T, Kitazawa R, Fukagawa M, Kita T. Depressed expression of Klotho and FGF receptor 1 in hyperplastic parathyroid glands from uremic patients. Kidney Int. 2010;77:232–8.
26. John GB, Cheng CY, Kuro-o M. Role of Klotho in aging, phosphate metabolism, and CKD. Am J Kidney Dis. 2011;58:127–34.
27. Kuczera P, Adamczak M, Wiecek A. Cinacalcet treatment decreases plasma fibroblast growth factor 23 concentration in haemodialysis patients with chronic kidney disease and secondary hyperparathyroidism. Clin Endocrinol. 2014;80:607–12.
28. Chertow GM, Block GA, Correa-Rotter R, Drueke TB, Floege J, Goodman WG, Herzog CA, Kubo Y, London GM, Mahaffey KW, Mix TC, Moe SM, Trotman ML, Wheeler DC, Parfrey PS. Effect of cinacalcet on cardiovascular disease in patients undergoing dialysis. N Engl J Med. 2012;367:2482–94.
29. Scialla JJ, Xie H, Rahman M, Anderson AH, Isakova T, Ojo A, Zhang X, Nessel L, Hamano T, Grunwald JE, Raj DS, Yang W, He J, Lash JP, Go AS, Kusek JW, Feldman H, Wolf M, Chronic Renal Insufficiency Cohort (CRIC) Study

Investigators. Fibroblast growth factor-23 and cardiovascular events in CKD. J Am Soc Nephrol. 2014;25:349–60.

30. Negishi K, Kobayashi M, Ochiai I, Yamazaki Y, Hasegawa H, Yamashita T, Shimizu T, Kasama S, Kurabayashi M. Association between fibroblast growth factor 23 and left ventricular hypertrophy in maintenance hemodialysis patients. Comparison with B-type natriuretic peptide and cardiac troponin T. Circ J. 2010;74:2734–40.

31. Saito A, Onuki T, Echida Y, Otsubo S, Nitta K. Fibroblast growth factor 23 and left ventricular hypertrophy in hemodialysis patients. Int J Clin Med. 2014;5:1102–10.

32. Faul C, Amaral AP, Oskouei B, Hu MC, Sloan A, et al. FGF23 induces left ventricular hypertrophy. J Clin Invest. 2011;121(11):4393–408.

33. Juppner H, Wolf M. Klotho: FGF23 coreceptor and FGF23-regulating hormone. J Clin Invest. 2012;122:4336–9.

34. Grabner A, Amaral AP, Schramm K, Singh S, Sloan A, et al. Activation of cardiac fibroblast growth factor receptor 4 causes left ventricular hypertrophy. Cell Metab. 2015;22(6):1020–32.

35. Grabner A, Schramm K, Silswal N, Hendrix M, Yanucil C, Czaya B, Singh S, Wolf M, Hermann S, Stypmann J, Di Marco GS, Brand M, Wacker MJ, Faul C. FGF23/FGFR4-mediated left ventricular hypertrophy is reversible. Sci Rep. 2017;7:1993.

36. Leifheit-Nestler M, Grose Siemer R, Flasbart K, Richter B, Kirchhoff F, et al. Induction of cardiac FGF23/FGFR4 expression is associated with left ventricular hypertrophy in patients with chronic kidney disease. Nephrol Dial Transplant. 2016;31:1088–99.

37. Matsui I, Oka T, Kusunoki Y, Mori D, Hashimoto N, Matsumoto A, Shimada K, Yamaguchi S, Kubota K, Yonemoto S, Higo T, Sakaguchi Y, Takabatake Y, Hamano T, Isaka Y. Cardiac hypertrophy elevates serum levels of fibroblast growth factor 23. Kidney Int. 2018;94(1):60–71.

38. Schoppet M, Hofbauer LC, Brinskelle-Schmal N, Varennes A, Goudable J, Richard M, Hawa G, Chapurlat R, Szuic P. Serum level of the phosphaturic factor FGF23 is associated with abdominal aortic calcification in men: the STRAMBO study. J Clin Endocrinol Metab. 2012;97:575–983.

39. Freedman BI, Divers J, Russell GB, Palmer ND, Bowden DW, Carr JJ, Wagenknecht LE, Hightower RC, Xu J, Smith SC, Langefeld CD, Hruska KA, Register TC. Plasma FGF23 and calcified atherosclerotic plaque in African Americans with type 2 diabetes mellitus. Am J Nephrol. 2015;42:391–401.

40. Desjardins L, Liabeuf S, Renard C, Lenglet A, Lemke HD, Choukroun G, Drueke TB, Massy ZA, European Uremic Toxin (EUTox) Work Group. FGF23 is independently associated with vascular calcification but not bone mineral density in patients at various CKD stages. Osteoporos Int. 2012;23:2017–25.

41. Morena M, Jaussent I, Halkovich A, Dupuy AM, Bargnoux AS, Chenine L, Leray-Moragues H, Klouche K, Vernhet H, Canaud B, Cristol JP. Bone biomarkers help grading severity of coronary calcifications in non dialysis chronic kidney disease patients. PLoS One. 2012;7:e36175.

42. Di Lullo L, Gorini A, Bellasi A, Morrone LF, Rivera R, Russo L, Santoboni A, Russo D. Fibroblast growth factor 23 and parathyroid hormone predict extent of aortic valve calcifications in patients with mild to moderate chronic kidney disease. Clin Kidney J. 2015;8:732–6.

43. Nasrallah MM, El-Shehaby AR, Salem MM, Osman NA, El Sheikh E, Sharaf El Din UA. Fibroblast growth factor-23 (FGF-23) is independently correlated to aortic calcification in haemodialysis patients. Nephrol Dial Transplant. 2010; 25:2679–85.

44. Scialla JJ, Lau WL, Reilly MP, Isakova T, Yang HY, et al. Fibroblast growth factor 23 is not associated with and does not induce arterial calcification. Kidney Int. 2013;83:1159–68.

45. Khan AM, Chirinos JA, Litt H, Yang W, Rosas SE. FGF-23 and the progression of coronary arterial calcification in patients new to dialysis. Clin J Am Soc Nephrol. 2012;7(12):2017–22.

46. Ozkok A, Kekik C, Karahan GE, Sakaci T, Ozel A, Unsal A, Yildiz A. FGF-23 associated with the progression of coronary artery calcification in hemodialysis patients. BMC Nephrol. 2013;14:241.

47. Tamei N, Ogawa T, Ishida H, Ando Y, Nitta K. Serum fibroblast growth factor-23 levels and progression of aortic arch calcification in non-diabetic patients on chronic hemodialysis. J Atheroscler Thromb. 2011;18:217–23.

48. Gutiérrez OM, Mannstadt M, Isakova T, Rauh-Hain JA, Tamez H, Shah A, Smith K, Lee H, Thadhani R, Jüppner H, Wolf M. Fibroblast growth factor 23 and mortality among patients undergoing hemodialysis. N Engl J Med. 2008;359:584–92.

49. Isakova T, Xie H, Yang W, Xie D, Anderson AH, Scialla J, Wahl P, Gutiérrez OM, Steigerwalt S, He J, Schwartz S, Lo J, Ojo A, Sondheimer J, Hsu CY, Lash J, Leonard M, Kusek JW, Feldman HI, Wolf M, Chronic Renal Insufficiency Cohort (CRIC) Study Group. Fibroblast growth factor 23 and risks of mortality and end-stage renal disease in patients with chronic kidney disease. JAMA. 2011;305:2432–9.

50. Kendrick J, Cheung AK, Kaufman JS, Greene T, Roberts WL, Smits G, Chonchol M; HOST investigators: FGF-23 associates with death, cardiovascular events, and initiation of chronic dialysis. J Am Soc Nephrol 2011; 22: 1913–1922.

51. Sugimoto H, Ogawa T, Iwabuchi Y, Otsuka K, Nitta K. Relationship between serum fibroblast growth factor-23 level and mortality in chronic hemodialysis patients. Int Urol Nephrol. 2014;46:99–106.

52. Yang H, Luo H, Tang X, Zeng X, Yu Y, Ma L, Fu P. Prognostic value of FGF23 among patients with end-stage renal disease: a systematic review and meta-analysis. Biomarker Med. 2016;10:547–56.

53. Moe SM, Chertow GM, Parfrey PS, Kubo Y, Block GA, Correa-Rotter R, Drueke TB, Herzog CA, London GM, Mahaffey KW, Wheeler DC, Stolina M, Dehmel B, Goodman WG, Floege J. Cinacalcet, fibroblast growth factor-23, and cardiovascular disease in hemodialysis: the Evaluation of Cinacalcet HCl Therapy to Lower Cardiovascular Events (EVOLVE) trial. Circulation. 2015;132: 27–39.

54. Morita H, Takeda Y, Fujita S, Okamoto Y, Sakane K, Teramoto K, Ozeki M, Tasaki R, Kizawa S, Sohmiya K, Hoshiga M, Ishizaka N. Gender specific association between serum fibroblast growth factor 23/alpha-klotho and coronary artery and aortic valve calcification. J Atheroscler Thromb. 2015;22: 1338–46.

Permissions

List of Contributors

Norio Hanafusa and Ken Tsuchiya
Department of Blood Purification, Tokyo Women's Medical University, Tokyo, Japan

Takashi Shigematsu
Department of Nephrology, Wakayama Medical University, Wakayama 641-8509, Japan

Masayuki Okazaki, Mizuki Komatsu and Hiroshi Kawaguchi
Department of Nephrology, Jyoban Hospital, Fukushima, Japan

Shunji Shiohira
Department of Medicine, Kidney Center, Tokyo Women's Medical University, 8-1 Kawada-cho, Shinjuku-ku, Tokyo 162-8666, Japan
Department of Nephrology, Jyoban Hospital, Fukushima, Japan

Akihito Tanaka, Hibiki Shinjo, Minako Murata and Asami Takeda
Kidney Disease Center, Japanese Red Cross Nagoya Daini Hospital, 2-9, Myoken-cho, Showa-ku, Nagoya 466-8650, Japan

Daijo Inaguma
Kidney Disease Center, Japanese Red Cross Nagoya Daini Hospital, 2-9, Myoken-cho, Showa-ku, Nagoya 466-8650, Japan
Department ofNephrology, Fujita Health University School of Medicine, Toyoake, Aichi, Japan
Aichi Cohort Study of Prognosis in Patients Newly Initiated Into Dialysis (AICOPP), Aichi, Japan

Akihito Tanaka, Yu Watanabe, Eri Ito, Naoki Kamegai, Hiroya Shimogushi, Minako Murata, Hibiki Shinjo, Kiyomi Koike, Yasuhiro Otsuka and Asami Takeda
Kidney Disease Center, Japanese Red Cross Nagoya Daini Hospital, 2-9, Myoken-cho, Showa-ku, Nagoya 466-8650, Japan

Tomoaki Nakamura
Blood Purification Center, Japanese Red Cross Nagoya Daini Hospital, Nagoya, Japan

Daijo Inaguma
Kidney Disease Center, Japanese Red Cross Nagoya Daini Hospital, 2-9, Myoken-cho, Showa-ku, Nagoya 466-8650, Japan
Department of Nephrology, Fujita Health University School of Medicine, Toyoake, Aichi, Japan

Blood Purification Center, Japanese Red Cross Nagoya Daini Hospital, Nagoya, Japan

Yasuhiko Ito, Takayuki Katsuno, Yasuhiro Suzuki and Masashi Mizuno
Department of Nephrology and Renal Replacement Therapy, Nagoya University Graduate School of Medicine, 65 Tsurumai-cho, Showa-ku, Nagoya 466-8550, Japan

Hiroshi Kinashi
Department of Nephrology and Renal Replacement Therapy, Nagoya University Graduate School of Medicine, 65 Tsurumai-cho, Showa-ku, Nagoya 466-8550, Japan
Department of Pathology, University Medical Center Utrecht, Utrecht, The Netherlands

Yoichi Ohtake
Ebaraji-cho Nishi-ku Sakai, Osaka 593-8304, Japan

Yoko Yoshida, Hideki Kato and Masaomi Nangaku
Division of Nephrology and Endocrinology, The University of Tokyo Hospital, 7-3-1 Hongo, Bunkyo-ku 113-8655, Tokyo, Japan

Ryota Matsuzawa, Kentaro Kamiya and Kohei Nozaki
Department of Rehabilitation, Kitasato University Hospital, Sagamihara, Japan

Takashi Masuda
Department of Rehabilitation, School of Allied Health Sciences, Kitasato University, 1-15-1 Kitasato, Sagamihara, Kanagawa 252-0373, Japan
Department of Cardio-Angiology, Graduate School of Medical Sciences, Kitasato University, Sagamihara, Japan

Nobuaki Hamazaki
Department of Rehabilitation, Kitasato University Hospital, Sagamihara, Japan
Department of Cardio-Angiology, Graduate School of Medical Sciences, Kitasato University, Sagamihara, Japan

Shinya Tanaka
Department of Cardio-Angiology, Graduate School of Medical Sciences, Kitasato University, Sagamihara, Japan

Emi Maekawa
Department of Cardiovascular Medicine, Kitasato University School of Medicine, Sagamihara, Japan

Junya Ako
Department of Cardio-Angiology, Graduate School of Medical Sciences, Kitasato University, Sagamihara, Japan
Department of Cardiovascular Medicine, Kitasato University School of Medicine, Sagamihara, Japan

Hideyo Tsutsui
Research Center of Health, Physical Fitness, and Sports, Nagoya University, Furo-cho, Chikusa-ku, Nagoya 464-8601, Japan
Department of Hygiene and Public Health, Teikyo University School of Medicine, 2-11-1 Kaga, Itabashi-ku, Tokyo 173-8605, Japan
General Medical Education and Research Center, Teikyo University, 2-11-1 Kaga, Itabashi-ku, Tokyo 173-8605, Japan

Kyoko Nomura
Department of Hygiene and Public Health, Teikyo University School of Medicine, 2-11-1 Kaga, Itabashi-ku, Tokyo 173-8605, Japan

Aya Ishiguro
Department of Hygiene and Public Health, Teikyo University School of Medicine, 2-11-1 Kaga, Itabashi-ku, Tokyo 173-8605, Japan
Jean Hailes Research Unit, School of Public Health and Preventive Medicine, Monash University, Level 1, 549 St Kilda Rd, Melbourne, VIC 3004, Australia

Yoshinari Tsuruta
Meiyo Clinic, 64-3 Yatori-cho, Toyohashi 441-8023, Japan

Sawako Kato
Department ofNephrology, Nagoya University Graduate School of Medicine, 65 Tsurumai, Showa-ku, Nagoya 466-0064, Japan

Yoshinari Yasuda
Department of Chronic Kidney Disease Initiatives, Nagoya University Graduate School of Medicine, 65 Tsurumai, Showa-ku, Nagoya 466-0064, Japan

Shunya Uchida
Department of Internal Medicine, Teikyo University School of Medicine, 2-11-1 Kaga, Itabashi-ku, Tokyo 173-8605, Japan

Yoshiharu Oshida
Research Center of Health, Physical Fitness, and Sports, Nagoya University, Furo-cho, Chikusa-ku, Nagoya 464-8601, Japan

Norio Hanafusa and Ken Tsuchiya
Department of Blood Purification, Tokyo Women's Medical University, 8-1 Kawada-cho, Shinjuku-ku, Tokyo 162-8666, Japan

Kosaku Nitta
Department of Medicine, Kidney Center, Tokyo Women's Medical University, 8-1 Kawada-cho, Shinjuku-ku, Tokyo 162-8666, Japan

Takayasu Ohtake and Shuzo Kobayashi
Department of Nephrology, Immunology, and Vascular Medicine, Kidney Disease and Transplant Center, Shonan Kamakura General Hospital, 1370-1 Okamoto, Kamakura 247-8533, Japan

Daijo Inaguma, Shigehisa Koide, Kazuo Takahashi, Hiroki Hayashi, Midori Hasegawa and Yukio Yuzawa
Department of Nephrology, Fujita Health University, Toyoake, Aichi, Japan

Ikuto Masakane, Shiho Esashi, Asami Yoshida and Tetsuro Chida
Yabuki Hospital, Yamagata, Japan

Hiroaki Fujieda, Yoshiyuki Ueno and Hiroyuki Sugaya
Advanced Materials Research Labs, Toray Industries, Inc., 2-2 Sonoyama 3-chome, Otsu, Shiga, Japan

Bach Nguyen
Department of Nephrology and Dialysis, Thong Nhat Hospital, 01 Ly Thuong Kiet Street, Tan Binh Dist, Ho Chi Minh City, Vietnam

Fumiko Fukuuchi
Department of Nephrology and Dialysis, Hayama Heart Center, Hayama, Japan

Ai Katsuma, Takafumi Yamakawa, Yasuyuki Nakada, Izumi Yamamoto and Takashi Yokoo
Division of Nephrology and Hypertension, Department of Internal Medicine, The Jikei University School of Medicine, 3-25-8, Nishi-Shimbashi, Minato-ku, Tokyo 105-8461, Japan

Eiichi Sato
Division of Nephrology, Department of Medicine, Shinmatsudo Central General Hospital, 1-380 Shinmatsudo, Matsudo, Chiba 270-0034, Japan

Atsuko Kamijo-Ikemori
Department of Anatomy, St. Marianna University School of Medicine, Sugao, Miyamae-Ku, Kawasaki, Kanagawa 216-8511, Japan
Department of Nephrology and Hypertension, Department of Internal Medicine, St. Marianna University School of Medicine, Sugao, Miyamae-Ku, Kawasaki, Kanagawa 216-8511, Japan

Tsuyoshi Oikawa and Aya Okuda
CMIC HOLDINGS Co., Ltd., Hamamatsucho Bldg., 1-1-1 Shibaura, Minato-ku, Tokyo 105-0023, Japan

Takeshi Sugaya
CMIC HOLDINGS Co., Ltd., Hamamatsucho Bldg., 1-1-1 Shibaura, Minato-ku, Tokyo 105-0023, Japan
Department of Nephrology and Hypertension, Department of Internal Medicine, St. Marianna University School of Medicine, Sugao, Miyamae-Ku, Kawasaki, Kanagawa 216-8511, Japan

Kenjiro Kimura
Department of Internal Medicine, Japan Community Health Care Organization, Tokyo Takanawa Hospital, Tokyo, Japan

Tsukasa Nakamura
Division of Nephrology, Department of Medicine, Shinmatsudo Central General Hospital, 1-380 Shinmatsudo, Matsudo, Chiba 270-0034, Japan
Department of Nephrology and Hypertension, Department of Internal Medicine, St. Marianna University School of Medicine, Sugao, Miyamae-Ku, Kawasaki, Kanagawa 216-8511, Japan

Yugo Shibagaki
Department of Nephrology and Hypertension, Department of Internal Medicine, St. Marianna University School of Medicine, Sugao, Miyamae-Ku, Kawasaki, Kanagawa 216-8511, Japan

Hiroshi Nihei, Ken Sakai, Seiichiro Shishido and Atsushi Aikawa
Department of Nephrology, Faculty of Medicine, Toho University, 6-11-1 Omori-Nishi, Ota-ku, Tokyo 143-8541, Japan

Kazutoshi Sibuya
Department of Surgical Pathology, Faculty of Medicine, Toho University, Tokyo, Japan

Hideo Edamatsu
Department of Otolaryngology, Faculty of Medicine, Toho University, Tokyo, Japan

Kazuho Honda
Department of Anatomy, Showa University School of Medicine, 1-5-8 Hatanodai, Shinagawa-ku, Tokyo 142-8555, Japan

Chieko Hamada
Division of Nephrology, Juntendo Medical University Faculty of Medicine, 2-1-1 Hongo, Bunkyo-ku, Tokyo 113-8421, Japan

Kunio Kawanishi
Department of Surgical Pathology, Tokyo Women's Medical University, 8-1 Kawada-cho, Shinjuku-ku, Tokyo 162-8666, Japan

Masaaki Nakayama
Research Division of Chronic Kidney Disease and Dialysis Treatment, Tohoku University Hospital, 1-1 Seiryo-cho, Aoba-ku, Sendai-shi, Miyagi 980-0872, Japan

Masanobu Miyazaki
Miyazaki Clinic, 3-12 Shiratori-cho, Nagasaki-shi, Nagasaki 852-8042, Japan

Yasuhiko Ito
Department of Nephrology and Renal Replacement Therapy, Nagoya University Graduate School of Medicine, 65 Tsurumai-cho, Showa-ku, Nagoya 466-8550, Japan

Shigeru Nakai, Kazunori Kawaguchi, Kazuyoshi Sakai and Nobuya Kitaguchi
Faculty of Clinical Engineering Technology, Fujita Health University School of Health Sciences, Dengakugakubo 1-98, Kutsukake-cho, Toyoake, Aichi 470-1192, Japan

Kenji Wakai
Department of Preventive Medicine, Nagoya University Graduate School of Medicine, Tsurumai-cho 65, Showa-ku, Nagoya, Aichi 466-8550, Japan

Eiichiro Kanda
Department of Nephrology, Tokyo Kyosai Hospital, Nakameguro 2-3-8, Meguro-ku, Tokyo 153-8934, Japan

Kazuhiko Tsuruya
Department of Integrated Therapy for Chronic Kidney Disease, Graduate School of Medical Sciences, Kyushu University, 3-1-1 Maidashi, Higashi-ku, Fukuoka 812-8582, Japan
Department of Medicine and Clinical Science, Graduate School of Medical Sciences, Kyushu University, Fukuoka, Japan

Hisako Yoshida
Department of Integrated Therapy for Chronic Kidney Disease, Graduate School of Medical Sciences, Kyushu University, 3-1-1 Maidashi, Higashi-ku, Fukuoka 812-8582, Japan
Clinical Research Center, Saga University Hospital, Saga, Japan

Shunsuke Yamada, Kumiko Torisu, Shigeru Tanaka, Akihiro Tsuchimoto, Masahiro Eriguchi, Kiichiro Fujisaki, Kosuke Masutani and Takanari Kitazono
Department of Medicine and Clinical Science, Graduate School of Medical Sciences, Kyushu University, Fukuoka, Japan

Ryota Ikee
Department of Nephrology and Dialysis, H. N. Medic Kitahiroshima, 5-6-1 Kyoeicho, Kitahiroshima, Hokkaido 061-1113, Japan

Shinya Kawamoto, Yu Kaneko, Hideo Misawa, Katsuhiro Nagahori, Atsushi Kitazawa, Atsunori Yoshino and Tetsuro Takeda
Department of Nephrology, Dokkyo Medical University Saitama Medical Center, 2-1-50 Minami-Koshigaya, Koshigaya, Saitama 343-8555, Japan

Hirotoshi Kodama, Akihiro Fujinoki and Tatsuo Inoue
Division of Blood Purification Center, Kamifukuoka General Hospital, 931 Fukuoka, Fujimino, Saitama 356-0011, Japan

Akira Tsuji, Koujirou Ooshima and Kaori Ishizeki
Department of Blood Purification, National Defense Medical College Hospital, 3-2 Namiki, Tokorozawa, Saitama 359-8513, Japan

Manae Harada, Kei Yoneki and Atsuhiko Matsunaga
Department of Rehabilitation Sciences, Kitasato University Graduate School of Medical Sciences, 1-15-1 Kitasato, Minami-ku, Sagamihara, Kanagawa 252-0373, Japan

Ryota Matsuzawa
Department of Rehabilitation, Kitasato University Hospital, Sagamihara, Japan

Naoyoshi Aoyama
Department of General Medicine, Kitasato University School of Medicine, Sagamihara, Japan

Kaoru Uemura, Yoriko Horiguchi, Junko Yoneyama and Atsushi Yoshida
Sagami Junkanki Clinic, Sagamihara, Japan

Keika Hoshi
Department of Hygiene, Kitasato University School of Medicine, Sagamihara, Japan

Takaaki Watanabe and Takahiro Shimoda
Department of Rehabilitation Sciences, Kitasato University Graduate School of Medical Sciences, 1-15-1 Kitasato, Minami-ku, Sagamihara, Kanagawa 252-0373, Japan
Sagami Junkanki Clinic, Sagamihara, Japan

Yasuo Takeuchi and Shokichi Naito
Division of Nephrology, Department of Internal Medicine, Kitasato University School of Medicine, Sagamihara, Japan

E. K. Tannor
Department of Medicine and Renal Unit, Komfo Anokye Teaching Hospital, Kumasi, Ghana

Y. A. Awuku
Department of Medicine and Therapeutics, School of Medical Sciences, University of Cape Coast, Cape Coast, Ghana

V. Boima
Department of Medicine and Renal Unit, Korle-bu Teaching Hospital, Accra, Ghana

S. Antwi
Paediatric Nephrology Unit, Department of Child Health, Kwame Nkrumah University of Science and Technology/Komfo Anokye Teaching Hospital, Kumasi, Ghana

Kosaku Nitta
Department of Medicine, Kidney Center, Tokyo Women's Medical University, Tokyo, Japan

Satoko Sakurai, Masaomi Nangaku and Hideki Kato
Division of Nephrology and Endocrinology, The University of Tokyo Graduate School of Medicine, Tokyo, Japan

Norio Hanafusa
Department of Blood Purification, Kidney Center Tokyo Women's Medical University, 8-1 Kawada-cho, Shinjuku-ku, Tokyo 162-8666, Japan

Shinji Iizaka
School of Nutrition, College of Nursing and Nutrition, Shukutoku University, Chiba, Japan

Ryoko Murayama
Department of Advanced Nursing Technology, The University of Tokyo Graduate School of Medicine, Tokyo, Japan

Maki Hiratsuka, Katsushi Koyama, Kinya Sengo, Jun Yamamoto, Aiko Narita, Chiharu Ito, Satoshi Kominato, Arata Hibi, Keisuke Kamiya and Toshiyuki Miura
Department of Nephrology, Kariya-Toyota General Hospital, 5-15 Sumiyoshi-cho, Kariya-city, Aichi Prefecture 448-8505, Japan

Rumi Miyahara
Department of Pharmacy, Kariya-Toyota General Hospital, Kariya, Japan

Junichi Fujikawa
Department of Clinical Engineering Technology, Kariya-Toyota General Hospital, Kariya, Japan

Masayuki Tanemoto
Division of Nephrology, Department of Internal Medicine, 418-1 Kamihayami, Kuki, Saitama 346-8530, Japan
Dialysis Unit, Shin-Kuki General Hospital, 418-1 Kamihayami, Kuki, Saitama 346-8530, Japan

Yu Ishimoto, Yukio Kosako and Yukio Okazaki
Dialysis Unit, Shin-Kuki General Hospital, 418-1 Kamihayami, Kuki, Saitama 346-8530, Japan

Kojiro Nagai
Department of Nephrology, Institute of Biomedical Sciences, Tokushima University Graduate School, Tokushima, Japan
Tokushima University Graduate School, 3-18-15, Kuramoto-cho, Tokushima 770-8503, Japan

Sayo Ueda and Toshio Doi
Department of Nephrology, Institute of Biomedical Sciences, Tokushima University Graduate School, Tokushima, Japan

Kenji Tsuchida
Department of Dialysis Vascular Surgery, Tsuchida Dialysis Access Clinic, Osaka, Japan
Tsuchida Dialysis Access Clinic, 2-10-18, Fujiidera DH building 4F, Oka, Fujiidera City, Osaka 583-0027, Japan

Jun Minakuchi
Department of Kidney Disease (Dialysis and Transplantation), Kawashima Hospital, Tokushima, Japan

Muhammad A. Siddiqui
School of Health Sciences, Queen Margaret University, Edinburgh, UK

Professional Faculties, University of Calgary, Calgary, Canada

Suhel Ashraff
Diabetes and Endocrinology, James Cook University Hospital, Middlesbrough, UK

Derek Santos and Thomas Carline
School of Health Sciences, Queen Margaret University, Edinburgh, UK

Kosaku Nitta
Department of Medicine, Kidney Center, Tokyo Women's Medical University, 8-1 Kawada-cho, Shinjuku-ku, Tokyo 162-8666, Japan

Index

www.ingramcontent.com/pod-product-compliance
Lightning Source LLC
Chambersburg PA
CBHW080250230326
41458CB00097B/4243